The Regulation of Cerebral Blood Flow

The Regulation of Cerebral Blood Flow

Edited by

John Whitfield Phillis, Ph.D., D.Sc., D.V.Sc.
Chairman and Professor of Physiology
Department of Physiology
Wayne State University Medical School
Detroit, Michigan

CRC Press
Boca Raton Ann Arbor London Tokyo

Library of Congress Cataloging-in-Publication Data

The Regulation of cerebral blood flow / edited by John Whitfield
Phillis.
p. cm.
Includes bibliographical references and index.
ISBN 0-8493-5096-4
1. Cerebral circulation--Regulation. I. Phillis, J. W.
[DNLM: 1. Cerebrovascular Circulation--physiology. WL 302 R344]
QP108.5.C4R44 1993
612.8′24--dc 20
DNLM/DLC
for Library of Congress 92-48267
CIP

Direct all inquiries to CRC Press, Inc., 2000 Corporate Blvd., N.W., Boca Raton, Florida 33431.

International Standard Book Number 0-8493-5096-4

Library of Congress Card Number 92-48267

Printed in the United States of America 1 2 3 4 5 6 7 8 9 0

Printed on acid-free paper

PREFACE

Blood flow regulation, the process by which cellular requirements for the acquisition and disposal of metabolic substrates are satisfied, plays a crucial role in a variety of body systems. Neurons in the central nervous system, by virtue of their high energy demands, are particularly sensitive to any misalignment between their metabolic requirements and the local blood supply. *The Regulation of Cerebral Blood Flow* provides the reader with an authoritative account of the various mechanisms (intrinsic, neuronal, metabolic) by which the tone of the smooth muscle cells, which regulate cerebral vascular resistance, is controlled in health and disease. It is anticipated that this book, prepared with the assistance of a number of distinguished researchers in the field, will serve as a valuable reference for both researchers in the field and clinicians managing cerebrovascular disorders.

The subject matter has been organized to provide ready access to current research findings on the regulation of cerebral blood flow. Initial contributions include a discussion of the technicalities of measuring cerebral blood flow and describe the intrinsic properties of cerebral vascular smooth muscle and the ability of cerebral vessels to autoregulate blood flow. An extensive section is devoted to the neural regulation of cerebral blood flow. In addition to the conventional neurotransmitters, this section includes chapters on several new peptide neuroregulators of vascular smooth muscle and the novel neurotransmitters, nitric oxide and adenosine triphosphate. A comprehensive review of vascular responses to changes in oxygen and carbon dioxide levels in the blood leads into a major section on metabolic regulators of cerebral blood flow. The final section of the book is devoted to the influence of trophic factors on cerebral vascular responses e.g., age, injury, diabetes, trauma, hypertension, and migraine. In summary, the contents embrace virtually every aspect of this important field in a readily assimilable format.

THE EDITOR

Dr. John Whitfield Phillis, B.V.Sc., Ph.D., D.Sc., D.V.Sc. is Department Chairman and Professor of Physiology at the Wayne State University Medical School in Detroit, Michigan.

Dr. Phillis obtained his training at Sydney University, receiving the B.V.Sc. (Hon.) degree in 1958 and obtained his Ph.D. degree in 1961 at the Australian National University, Canberra. In 1970 he was awarded a D.Sc. degree by Monash University, Melbourne and in 1976 a D.V.Sc. degree by Sydney University. He served as Lecturer/Senior Lecturer at Monash University from 1963 to 1969; as Visiting Professor in Biophysics at Indiana University in 1969; as Professor of Physiology at the Medical School of the University of Manitoba, 1970 to 1973; as Professor and Chairman of the Department of Physiology at the University of Saskatchewan, 1973 to 1981; and in 1981, he assumed his present position.

Dr. Phillis is a member of the Pharmacological and Physiological Societies of Great Britain, the American Physiological Society, the Society for Neuroscience, and the International Brain Research Organization. He was formerly the President of the Canadian Physiological Society. Dr. Phillis has been on the Medical Research Council of Canada, a Visiting Professor at several universities, and was a Wellcome Visiting Professor at Tulane University. He is a past Editor of the *Canadian Journal of Physiology and Pharmacology,* is presently Co-Editor of *Progress in Neurobiology,* and serves on the Editorial Boards of *General Pharmacology* and *International Journal of Purine and Pyrimidine Research.* He has been the recipient of research grants from the Canadian Medical Research Foundation, the National Institutes of Health, the American Heart Association, and the American Diabetes Association (Michigan Affiliate).

Dr. Phillis is the author of over 300 papers and book chapters and one book; he has edited three books. His current research interests relate to the pharmacology of chemical transmission in the brain and treatment of stroke.

CONTRIBUTORS

M. Aldasoro, M.D.
Department of Physiology
University of Valencia
Valencia, Spain

William M. Armstead, Ph.D.
Department of Anesthesiology and Critical Care Medicine
Children's Hospital of Philadelphia
Philadelphia, Pennsylvania

Gilles Bonvento, Ph.D.
Laboratoire de Recherches Cérébrovasculoires Recherche
Centre National de la Recherche Scientifique, UA641
Paris, France

David W. Busija, Ph.D.
Department of Physiology & Pharmacology
Bowman Gray School of Medicine
Winston-Salem, North Carolina

Jan Fahrenkrug, M.D., D.M.Sc.
Department of Clinical Chemistry
Bispebjerg Hospital
University of Copenhagen
Copenhagen, Denmark

Frank M. Faraci, Ph.D.
Department of Internal Medicine
University of Iowa
Iowa City, Iowa

Masatoshi Fujishima, M.D.
Department of Internal Medicine
Kyushu University Medical School
Fukuoka, Japan

Harold Goldman, Ph.D.
Department of Pharmacology
Wayne State University
Detroit, Michigan

Mark J. Gorman, M.D.
Department of Neurology
Henry Ford Hospital
Detroit, Michigan

David R. Harder, Ph.D.
Department of Physiology
Medical College of Wisconsin
Milwaukee, Wisconsin

Sami I. Harik, M.D.
Departments of Neurology & Neuroscience
Case Western Reserve University
Cleveland, Ohio

Toru Itakura, M.D.
Department of Neurological Surgery
Wakayama Medical College
Wakayama, Japan

Hermes A. Kontos, M.D., Ph.D.
Department of Medicine
Medical College of Virginia
Richmond, Virginia

Wolfgang Kuschinsky, M.D.
Department of Physiology
University of Heidelberg
Heidelberg, Germany

Pierre Lacombe, Ph.D.
Laboratoire de Recherche Cérébrovasculoires Recherche
Centre National de la Recherche Scientifique, UA641
Paris, France

Charles W. Leffler, Ph.D.
Laboratory for Research in Neonatal Physiology
Department of Physiology and Biophysics
University of Tennessee
Memphis, Tennessee

S. Lluch, M.D.
Department of Physiology
University of Valencia
Valencia, Spain

M. C. Martinez, Ph.D.
Department of Physiology
University of Valencia
Valencia, Spain

William G. Mayhan, Ph.D.
Department of Physiology & Biophysics
University of Nebraska
Medical Center
Omaha, Nebraska

Tracy K. McIntosh, Ph.D.
Department of Neurosurgery
University of Pennsylvania
Philadelphia, Pennsylvania

Ikunobu Muramatsu, Ph.D.
Department of Pharmacology
Fukui Medical School
Fukui, Matsuoka, Japan

Tomio Okamura, M.D., Ph.D.
Department of Pharmacology
Shiga University of Medical Science
Ohtsu, Shiga, Japan

Koichi Okiyama, M.D.
Department of Neurosurgery
University of Pennsylvania
Philadelphia, Pennsylvania

Takashi Okuno, M.D.
Department of Neurological Surgery
Wakayama Medical College
Wakayama, Japan

William J. Pearce, Ph.D.
Department of Physiology
Division of Perinatal Biology
Loma Linda University
School of Medicine
Loma Linda, California

John W. Phillis, Ph.D., D.Sc., D.V.Sc.
Department of Physiology
Wayne State University
School of Medicine
Detroit, Michigan

Seizo Sadoshima, M.D.
Department of Internal Medicine
Kyushu University Medical School
Fukuoka, Japan

Lothar Schilling, M.D.
Department of Physiology
University of Munich
Munich, Germany

Oscar U. Scremin, M.D., Ph.D.
West Los Angeles DVA Medical Center
Department of Physiology
University of California
Los Angeles, California

Masaaki Shibata, Ph.D.
Laboratory for Research in Neonatal Physiology
Department of Physiology and Biophysics
University of Tennessee
Memphis, Tennessee

Yoshio Suzuki, M.D., Ph.D.
Department of Neurosurgery
Nagoya University School of Medicine
Nagoya, Japan

Noboru Toda, M.D., Ph.D.
Department of Pharmacology
Shiga University of Medical Science
Ohtsu, Shiga, Japan

Ursula Tuor, Ph.D.
Neonatology Research
The Hospital for Sick Children
Toronto, Ontario
Canada

J. M. Vila, Ph.D.
Department of Physiology
University of Valencia
Valencia, Spain

Michael Wahl, M.D.
Department of Physiology
University of Munich
Munich, Germany

Enoch P. Wei, Ph.D.
Department of Medicine
Medical College of Virginia
Richmond, Virginia

K. M. A. Welch, M.D.
Department of Neurology
Henry Ford Hospital
Detroit, Michigan

TABLE OF CONTENTS

I. INTRODUCTION

Chapter 1
Techniques for Measuring Cerebral Blood Flows 3
Harold Goldman

Chapter 2
Electrophysiological Mechanisms of Cerebral Arterial Muscle Activation: Influences of Environmental Stimuli 33
David R. Harder

Chapter 3
Cerebral Autoregulation 45
David W. Busija

II. NEURAL REGULATION OF CEREBRAL BLOOD FLOW

Chapter 4
The Role of Central Neural Pathways in the Regulation of Cerebral Blood Flow 65
David W. Busija

Chapter 5
Catecholaminergic Innervation of Cerebral Blood Vessels 79
Sami I. Harik

Chapter 6
Serotonin and the Cerebral Circulation 97
Gilles Bonvento and Pierre Lacombe

Chapter 7
Histaminergic Effects on Cerebral Hemodynamics 113
Lothar Schilling and Michael Wahl

Chapter 8
Cholinergic Control of Cerebral Blood Flow 129
Oscar U. Scremin

Chapter 9
Neuropeptide Y and the Cerebral Circulation 147
Ursula I. Tuor

Chapter 10
Neural Regulation of Cerebral Blood Flow: Vasoactive
Intestinal Peptide (VIP)....................165
Jan Fahrenkrug

Chapter 11
Calcitonin Gene-Related Peptide (CGRP)....................179
Yoshio Suzuki

Chapter 12
Tachykinins and Cerebral Blood Flow....................195
Toro Itakura and Takashi Okuno

Chapter 13
Vasopressin Receptors in Cerebral Arteries....................213
M. C. Martinez, J. M. Vila, M. Aldasoro, and S. Lluch

Chapter 14
Purinergic Transmission in Cerebral Arteries....................225
Ikunobu Muramatsu

Chapter 15
Role of Nitric Oxide in Cerebroarterial Relaxation....................233
Noboru Toda and Tomio Okamura

III. EXTERNAL FACTORS INFLUENCING CEREBRAL BLOOD FLOW

Chapter 16
Cerebral Vascular Responses to Hypoxia, Hyper- and Hypo-
Capnia and Hypotension....................249
John W. Phillis

IV. METABOLIC REGULATION OF CEREBRAL BLOOD FLOW

Chapter 17
Coupling of Blood Flow and Metabolism in the Brain....................269
Wolfgang Kuschinsky

Chapter 18
Cerebrovascular Flow Regulation by Adenosine....................281
Enoch P. Wei and Hermes A. Kontos

Chapter 19
Role of the Eicosanoids in Cerebral Hemodynamics....................297
Charles W. Leffler, William M. Armstead, and Masaaki Shibata

Chapter 20
Effects of Bradykinin in the Cerebral Microcirculation..................315
Michael Wahl and Lothar Schilling

V. TROPHIC INFLUENCES ON CEREBRAL BLOOD FLOW REGULATION

Chapter 21
Hypertension and the Autoregulation of Cerebral Blood Flow...........331
Seizo Sadoshima and Masatoshi Fujishima

Chapter 22
Cerebral Circulation During Aging......................................341
Frank M. Faraci

Chapter 23
Responses of Cerebral Blood Vessels During Diabetes Mellitus.........353
William G. Mayhan

Chapter 24
Effects of Traumatic Brain Injury on Cerebral Blood Flow..............367
Koichi Okiyama and Tracy K. McIntosh

Chapter 25
Cerebrovascular Regulation in the Fetus and Neonate...................381
William J. Pearce

Chapter 26
Cerebral Blood Flow and Migraine......................................399
Mark J. Gorman and K. M. A. Welch

INDEX...413

I. Introduction

Chapter 1

TECHNIQUES FOR THE MEASUREMENT OF CEREBRAL BLOOD FLOW

Harold Goldman

TABLE OF CONTENTS

I. Introduction 4
  A. Historical Background 5

II. Experimental Methods 5
  A. Tissue Indicator Uptake Methods 5
    1. Whole Brain Flow (Global) Measurements 7
    2. Tissue Equilibration Techniques 7
    3. Indicator Fractionation Techniques 10
      a. Permeable Radiolabeled Markers 10
      b. Radiolabeled Microspheres 12
  B. Hydrogen Clearance 14
  C. Doppler Flowmetry 15

III. Clinical Methods 17
  A. ^{133}Xenon Clearance 17
  B. Stable Xenon Enhanced Computed Tomography (Xe/CT) 19
  C. Single Photon Emission Computed Tomography (SPECT) 20
  D. Positron Emission Tomography (PET) 21

IV. Emerging Technology 23
  A. Ultrafast CT 23
  B. Very Fast NMR Imaging Technologies 24

References 26

0-8493-5096-0/93/$0.00 + $.50

I. INTRODUCTION

The central nervous system is a supersystem, a system of systems, that functions at a high metabolic rate most of the time. This supersystem is critically dependent on a unique, highly regulated vascular supply for rapid, on-demand, regional delivery of energy and structural substrates, the removal of toxic metabolic products, a tight control of its fluid, ionic, and temperature environment, and for transport of significant amounts of neuroendocrine information. Nowhere is the critical dependence of brain and spinal cord functions on blood flow more obvious than when the flow is interrupted for a few seconds.

A quantitative knowledge, therefore, of changes in regional perfusion (rCBF) of the central nervous system (CNS) has considerable investigational and clinical utility. As the dependent variable, regional perfusion provides an estimate of normal, altered, and pathophysiological functions and is useful in evaluating the regional effects of drugs. Given the usually tight coupling between regional blood flow, metabolism, and neuronal-behavioral functions, a measurement of local flow can contribute considerable insight into the operations of the CNS. The degree of uncoupling of these functions now can be determined by simultaneous measurements of flow and metabolism. Nervous tissue perfusion as the independent variable, e.g., a determinant of regional function, is often incorporated into studies of stroke and other cerebrovascular pathologies. From the author's point of view, it also provides a basis for the study of therapeutic interventions.

With the exception of direct blood sampling, virtually all blood flow methods are essentially indirect methods that depend on the measurement of movements of tracer solutes carried by the blood. Most employ metabolically inert substances, exogenously administered, and usually in tracer quantities. Exceptions include red-cell velocity measured by means of fiber optics and laser-Doppler flowmetry or bulk flow of blood ions in vessels detected by miniaturized electromagnetic flowmeters.

The key to improved techniques for the measurement of regional perfusion of the central nervous system has been mainly in the quantitative detection of tracer substances. It is the basis for the following review. The choice of a detection method depends on a balance between the need for regional specificity, the amount of acceptable intervention, the speed of measurement, and the cost.

Ideally, cerebral blood flow should be measured by a noninvasive technique, which does not require the use of anesthesia and has a high degree of spatial and temporal resolution so that mapping of regional functional states can be both highly detailed and dynamic. In reality, some of the current methods are capable of high spatial resolution, whereas others are able to provide good temporal resolution of dynamic changes in blood flow. No single blood flow technique has yet achieved good spatial and temporal resolution simultaneously, either in animal experimentation or in human studies. However, potentially useful but still expensive ways to resolve this problem may be presaged in recent technical advances in ultrafast versions of X-ray computed tomography and magnetic resonance imaging (MRI).

The types of methods discussed here, admittedly selective, have been grouped by the priority assigned by the author to high spatial resolution and minimal intervention. The first group is associated with experimental investigations mainly in animals, the latter with clinical assessments of flow. Table 1 summarizes important features of the various methods.

A. HISTORICAL BACKGROUND

The anatomy of the vasculature, especially in the brain, has been an area of interest and speculation for several thousand years.[1] However, the function of the vasculature was largely unrecognized or misunderstood until Harvey, in 1616, described the circulation of the blood and thereby transformed vascular anatomy into physiology.[2] This work was followed by Wepfer's studies of the role of the cerebral vasculature in apoplexy (1658)[3] and Willis's first functional description of the circle that bears his name (1664).[4] Quantitative measurements of cerebral blood flow were much slower to develop. More than 200 years later, von Schulten[5] cataloged three limited categories of cerebral blood flow measurement: (1) direct observations in the pia mater; (2) recordings of brain volume; and (3) measurement of the flow velocity in cerebral vessels.

Interest in cerebral circulation and its related technology grew more rapidly after 1860, e.g., Cybulski's photohematochometer (cited by Hill)[6] for flow measurements and a method for blood pressure measurement in the circle of Willis.[7] Progress continued with development of both global and local blood flow techniques: venous outflow from the lateral sinus in animals (1887);[8] small brain-insertable thermoelectric (heat clearance) flow probes (1929);[9,10] Kolin's clamp-on electromagnetic flow devices for blood vessels (1938);[11] and internal carotid bubble-flow meters (1943).[12] More recent blood flow methods have exploited unique properties of flow markers, e.g., radioactivity, radio-opacity, or nuclear magnetic resonance, to improve the spatial and temporal resolution of flow measurements and, at the same time, minimize the invasiveness of the measurement procedure. Moreover, derivative methods have been developed for measurements of local metabolic status which now permit the concurrent mapping of regional flow and function. Our ideas about the cerebral circulation and its functions have been dramatically shaped by the evolving technology.

II. EXPERIMENTAL METHODS

A. TISSUE INDICATOR UPTAKE METHODS

Most modern techniques for measurement of CNS blood flow, and for localized flow in particular, have grown out of the seminal work of Kety and

TABLE 1
Cerebrovascular Blood Flow Methodology

	Resolution	CNS tissue invasiveness	Total time/measure	Repeated measures	Continuous measures	Mapping usefulness
I. **Experimental Methods**						
Tissue uptake (Kety) global Fick: N_2O	Whole brain	No	Minutes	Yes	No	No
Regional						
Tissue equilibration	<1 mm^3	No	<1 min	No	No	Yes
Indicator fractionation						
Permeable radiolabeled markers	<1 mm^3	No	5–10 s	No	No	Yes
Radiolabeled microspheres	5–8 mm^3	No	5–10 s	Up to 5	No	Yes
H_2 Tissue washout (regional clearance)	3–5 mm^3	Yes	1–2 min	Yes	No	No
Laser-Doppler flowmetry	~1 mm^3	Yes	Instantaneous	Yes	Yes	No
II. **Clinical Measurements**						
^{133}Xe clearance	6–8 Cortical regions	No	15 min	Yes	No	Crude
Stable Xe enhanced computed tomography (Xe/CT)	10 mm^3 voxel[a]	No	6.5 min/3 slices	Yes	No	Yes
Single photon emission computed tomography (SPECT)	2–7 cm^3	No	4–20 min	Yes	No	Yes
Positron emission tomography (PET)	125–500 mm^3	No	<10 min	Yes	No	Yes
III. **Emerging Technology**						
Ultrafast CT	300 mm^3	No	<1 min	Yes	No	Yes
Echo-planar MRI	8–18 mm^3	No	64 msec/scan 20 s/40 planes	Yes	No	Yes

[a] System error limits accurate estimations of flow to 600 mm^3.

his associates,[13-17] which in turn was based on concepts first enunciated in 1870 by Adolph Fick.[18]

Fick's major physiologic synthesis was the idea that related the blood flow in an organ or tissue with respiratory gas transport; specifically, that the ratio of uptake of oxygen or carbon dioxide by a tissue to its arterio-venous difference was a measure of the blood perfusion of that tissue. This concept was later adapted and restated by Kety and Schmidt[13] to measure global cerebral blood flow in humans employing the inspiration of an exogenous, nonmetabolized substance, N_2O.

1. Whole Brain Flow (Global) Measurements

The original Kety contributions began with a theoretical and technical advancement in the measure of global whole brain blood flow by means of the nitrous oxide (N_2O) inhalational method. Kety's central idea was based on Fick's idea that the amount of an inhaled, highly diffusible inert gas taken up by a tissue per unit of time is equal to the quantity brought to the tissue by the arterial blood minus the quantity carried away in the venous blood. Thus, at a time when the N_2O contents of the brain and its effluent blood reached a virtual equilibrium (usually 10 min), i.e., when the brain neither gained nor lost indicator, brain content of N_2O and blood flow (CBF) could be estimated from the histories of the differential rates of change in the arterial and venous concentrations of N_2O prior to steady state conditions. A mean global cerebral blood flow of 54 ± 12 ml/100 g · min^{-1} was determined in this manner in 14 young, healthy males in the 1940s.[14] The same technique could then be applied to oxygen and glucose uptake so that from a knowledge of the CBF and the characteristic A-V differences of these substrates it was then possible to calculate oxygen and glucose utilization rates from the Fick principle.

Advantages: The method is simple, repeatable, and can be used in conscious animals and humans to provide estimates of whole brain perfusion. It is useful for purposes of clinical investigation but not for the assessment of pathology.

Disadvantages: Although application of this method is not invasive, in the nervous system it does require catheterization of the carotid artery and femoral vein for blood sampling. Brain weight has to be estimated. Estimates of regional circulation and regional mapping of blood flow are not possible.

Such techniques have been largely replaced by the less invasive, more convenient xenon-133 (^{133}Xe) clearance methods described below.

2. Tissue Equilibration Techniques

In spite of the usefulness of overall estimates of cerebral blood flow, the original Kety technique did not lend itself to detailed regional measurements in complex, heterogeneous structures such as the CNS because it was not possible to determine very local venous concentrations of indicator.

In an effort to circumvent the limitations of the global method, Kety devised a shorter term, *equilibration technique* which included autoradiographic detection of the regional brain contents of highly diffusible, radiolabeled tracers, e.g., ([^{131}I]triiodomethane, ^{14}C-antipyrine, later [^{131}I]-iodoantipyrine) and a mathematical expression of blood flow in terms of three measurable variables: regional content of tracer, the tracer's tissue-blood partition coefficient, and the integrated arterial tracer concentration curve from the time of initial intravenous administration to the death of the experimental animal.[15,17,19] The latest version of this method is fully described by Ginsberg.[20]

The equations originally developed by Kety[15] to describe the exchange of inert, diffusible indicators between the blood and tissues can be used to estimate blood flow. That is, if the time-course of the arterial concentration of the indicator after administration is known and if the partition coefficient of the indicator between blood and tissue is known, then the indicator content of the tissue at time T, i.e., at the end of the experiment, can be described as a function of tissue blood flow. Tissue content of indicator is determined by means of autoradiography in this high spatial resolution method.

Among the most widely used of indirect tracer methods, autoradiographic techniques allow simultaneous estimations of flow in many brain and spinal cord regions of experimental animals. Important supplementary techniques have been introduced which also permit analysis, sometimes simultaneously with rCBF, of flow-related variables such as glucose metabolism,[21-23] regional pH,[24] and protein synthesis.[25]

In this method, the indicator is assumed to be metabolically inert, rapidly exchangeable, and highly diffusible, i.e., completely extracted in a single capillary passage. Indicator passage between the blood and tissue is considered to be bidirectional, instantaneous, uniformly distributed, and is adequately described by a completely exchangeable two-compartment system. Additionally, the blood flow rate is assumed to be constant during measurement.

The differential equation for blood-tissue exchange in this situation is based on the Fick principle and is

$$dC_i/dt = F(C_a - C_i/\lambda) \tag{1}$$

The solution to this equation is

$$C_i(T) = F \int_0^T Ca(t)\, e^{[-(T-t)F/\lambda]} dt \tag{2}$$

Equation 2 is the operational equation of the "tissue equilibration" technique, where

t = the variable time, (min)
T = time at the end of the experimental period, (min)

$C_i(T)$ = indicator concentration per unit weight of tissue at time T, $(\mu C_i \cdot g^{-1})$
λ = estimated equilibrium tissue-blood partition coefficient of the indicator, $(ml \cdot g^{-1})$
F = blood flow rate per unit weight of tissue $(ml \cdot g^{-1} \cdot min^{-1})$
C_a = arterial concentration of the indicator $(\mu C_i \cdot ml^{-1})$

In practice, an anesthetized animal is catheterized and allowed to recover from anesthesia under the restraint of a ''loose-fitting'' body cast. This is followed by intravenous administration of an inert, highly diffusible radioactive tracer. Arterial blood is sampled over a 30 to 45 s time period, after which the animal is quickly killed. Terminal samples of brain (or spinal cord) are obtained, and quantitative measurements of the indicator in all blood and CNS samples are made. Equation 2 is used to calculate blood flow.

The autoradiographic technique for tissue sampling is usually applied to frozen coronal or parasagittal sections with alternate sections used for histological identification. Multiregional distribution of ^{14}C or ^{3}H radiolabeled tracers is analyzed by means of film microdensitometry. Properly applied to well frozen tissue, the autoradiographic technique allows very high spatial resolution measurements (<1 mm^3) in essentially permanent records of regional blood flow.

As efforts have increased to examine perfusion in adjacent microregions in varying functional states, more attention has focused on the rapid freezing of brains at the end of an experiment in order to minimize errors of intercompartmental diffusion of readily diffusible indicators such as iodoantipyrine.[26] This is especially appropriate with a short-term indicator fractionation method, which is described below.

Advantages: This method lends itself to the detailed mapping of rCBF. A derivative method permits similar mapping of regional glucose utilization rates and provides a powerful, relatively inexpensive companion investigative tool.[27]

Disadvantages: This technique usually employs some form of stressful animal restraint which may perturb flow measurements. The data is derived for a single time point and the animal must be killed. Regional values for λ, usually assumed, are averages derived from ''normal'' animals, which may not apply in some altered or pathological states. Most of the inert, diffusible tracers used in blood flow determinations are diffusion-limited at some flow rate. As a consequence rCBF can be progressively underestimated at higher flow rates. In the case of the most commonly used indicator, ^{14}C-iodoantipyrine, rCBF becomes significantly underestimated above flow rates of 1.8 $ml \cdot min^{-1} \cdot g^{-1}$, e.g., under conditions encountered in hypercapnia.[28-30] The use of more lipid soluble indicators,[31,32] including radiolabeled nicotine[33,34] or a benzodiazepine,[30,35,123] may circumvent this problem.

The Kety indicator equilibration technique has been incorporated into human studies by Lassen,[36] which utilize extracranial detection of gamma-emitting gaseous tracers,[85] krypton, or ^{133}xenon. Refinements, which include complex detector arrays and computed tomographic imaging,[37-39] are discussed later.

3. Indicator Fractionation Techniques

a. Permeable Radiolabeled Markers

The Fick Principle has given rise to two current types of high resolution, multiregional experimental methods: (1) the tissue saturation[40] or *equilibration* method established by Kety, Sokoloff, and co-workers[17,19,41] just described, and (2) the *indicator fractionation* technique, traceable to the initial studies of Stewart[42,43] and Hamilton,[44] which have been refined by Sapirstein,[45,46] Goldman and Sapirstein,[47] Van Uitert and Levy,[28,48] Gjedde,[27] Sage,[49] Jones,[50] and are described here. The theoretical bases, applications and limitations of the two types of methods have been elegantly reviewed by Patlak, Fenstermacher, and Blasberg.[51,52]

As originally formulated by Sapirstein,[45] the indicator fractionation technique was applied to blood flow measurement in virtually any tissue except the brain and spinal cord. This exception was due to the use of indicators, such as ^{42}K or ^{86}Rb, which do not freely traverse the blood-brain barrier. The method subsequently was adapted for estimation of rCBF by Goldman and Sapirstein.[47] Like the Kety indicator equilibration method, this approach is the basis of several of the experimental and clinical rCBF techniques discussed below. Technically, several of its features resemble those of the Kety-Sokoloff method. However, the methods differ in certain important respects.

The indicator fractionation method deals mainly with the early unidirectional delivery of an indicator in a tissue, i.e., measurement takes place at a time before significant backflux has occurred and tissue content of indicator is not yet in equilibrium with the venous effluent. Therefore, knowledge of the regional partition coefficient of the indicator is not important. The killing time consequently is shorter, and accurate timing of the experimental procedure becomes more critical. The indicator can be readily diffusible (e.g., iodoantipyrine), highly diffusible but sequestered in the tissue for some protracted time (e.g., benzodiazepine), or nondiffusible (e.g., microspheres).

Flow, F_i, is derived from a knowledge of three variables: U_i, the tissue content of indicator at the termination time T; J, the injected dose of indicator, i.e., in effect the body uptake of indicator at time T; and the cardiac output, CO.

The basic equation of the original Sapirstein method is

$$U_i/J \approx F_i/CO \qquad (3)$$

Equation 3 states in effect, that when a readily diffusible indicator, such as iodoantipyrine, is administered in a single, intravenous injection and the killing time is short, then the pattern of indicator distribution in the brain will be the same as the fractional distribution of the cardiac output. Flow measurement can be expressed in two ways: (1) the "flow fraction", as a percentage of the cardiac output per unit time or (2) in perfusion units, e.g., ml $\cdot$ $min^{-1} \cdot g^{-1}$, if the cardiac output is known.

The cardiac output can be determined simultaneously if the amount of the injected indicator is known, from the following equation:

$$CO = J/\int_0^T Ca'dt \approx J/\int_0^\infty Ca\,dt \qquad (4)$$

where Ca′ describes the arterial indicator dilution curve obtained by substituting extrapolated points after recirculation for the real ones according to Hamilton.[53]

The Kety and Sapirstein equations are equivalent if the killing time is sufficiently short to minimize indicator backflux. Under such conditions Equation 1 can be simplified to

$$dA/dt = F \cdot Ca \qquad (5)$$

and the solution to this equation is equivalent to the Sapirstein Equation 3:[47,51]

$$C_i(T) = F\int_0^T Ca(t)\,dt \qquad (6)$$

In current practice, integration of the arterial concentration-time curve is usually performed mechanically by the creation of an "artificial organ", i.e., by withdrawing a sample of blood into a syringe at a constant rate during the entire measurement period, and determining the radioactivity of the indicator. Tissue indicator is usually determined by the same autoradiographic technique described earlier or by microdissection from frozen sections. As noted earlier, the measurement time must be short for accurate estimates of very local flows, particularly when high flow rates are anticipated. Consequently, rapid freezing of tissue must be employed to prevent postmortem diffusion of iodoantipyrine. Alternatively, the use of highly diffusible but readily trapped radiolabeled indicators, such as nicotine[33,34] or benzodiazepines,[30,35,123] may prove useful. A version of the indicator fractionation method in which the radiolabeled indicator is carried by 15-μm microspheres achieves the same end, i.e., complete microvascular trapping of the indicator. In contrast to the conventional, single time-point "indicator equilibrium" or "indicator fractionation" techniques, multiple measures of flow (up to five) can be made by the microsphere technique to assess the effects of different experimental conditions. This version of the indicator fractionation technique is discussed below.

Advantages: The advantages of the indicator-fractionation are similar to those obtained with the tissue-equilibration method, including high spatial resolution. A knowledge of regional partition coefficients for the indicator is not required. The method can be performed in conscious, unrestrained animals as small as an adult rat and, with modifications, in smaller animals, e.g., the immature rat.[54-56] The method is faster than the tissue-equilibration method so that the constant blood flow requirement is easier to meet.

Disadvantages: As in the case of the tissue equilibration technique, the data is derived for a single time point and the animal must be killed. Additionally, in cases of elevated rCBF, even a highly diffusible radiotracer, e.g., iodoantipyrine, emerges more rapidly into the cerebral venous effluent (backflux) and very short (1 to 2 s) study intervals must be employed in order not to violate the assumptions of the method. Thus, the indicator fractionation technique may be impractical in circumstances where elevated rates of rCBF cannot be predicted. Patlak[51] showed that the relative error due to backflux is proportional to the product TF/λ and is dependent on the shape of the arterial input function. This combined error can be reduced by employing a close cardiac intravenous bolus administration, a short study duration, and restricting the use of the method to normal- or low-flow states. Alternatively, these problems may be circumvented by employing an indicator, such as nicotine[33,34] or diazepam,[30] which has a very rapid influx but a considerably retarded backflux, even under high flow conditions. The suitability of diazepam has been verified at high rCBF (>7 ml · min^{-1} · g^{-1}) by means of a variant of the indicator fractionation technique which employs radiolabeled microspheres.[30]

Our own work with the indicator fractionation technique (unpublished observations) has shown that ^{14}C-diazepam uptake in several high-flow nervous tissues, e.g., pineal gland and posterior pituitary gland (3 to 4 ml · min^{-1} · g^{-1}), provides estimates of blood flow equal to those determined by the original Sapirstein method[57,58] and much higher blood flow estimates than can be obtained with the use of iodoantipyrine. Regional contents of diazepam remain constant throughout the brain for at least 1 min after injection before significant backflux is detected. The retarded backflux of diazepam also noted by others[30] has been attributed, in part, to its significant binding in nervous tissue.[59]

b. Radiolabeled Microspheres

This blood flow method is based on the embolization of end-organ capillaries by radiolabeled microspheres. The microsphere uptake method is an extension of the indicator fractionation technique in which the major limitation of indicator backflux from tissue to blood is bypassed. As a consequence, the technique is often used as a benchmark for other blood flow methods, particularly for flow measurements in tissues with high perfusion rates. The application of the current version of this method is detailed by Warner.[60] Its theoretical basis is summarized by Equation 6.

The following special requirements for microspheres to act as accurate, single capillary pass markers of blood flow were described by Rudolph and Heymann.[63]

1. It is essential that the microspheres be well-mixed at the injection site. This continues to be a problem, especially with some types of microspheres which have a specific gravity approaching 1.5. Microsphere materials technology has evolved considerably since the introduction of glass spheres in 1947.[61] Efforts to improve their rheologic properties led to the use of albumin[62] in 1969 and, more recently, to lighter plastic formulations.[60]
2. The spheres must distribute in the blood stream in proportion to the actual flow.
3. They must be completely trapped on the first capillary transit in brain and spinal cord tissues in proportion to their perfusion rates. In the CNS, this is accomplished with 15-μm diameter spheres (>97%).[64,65]
4. They must not significantly perturb circulatory functions. Since this is not strictly true, particularly in the CNS and heart, a 1% capillary blockage is usually regarded as an upper limit.
5. The spheres must remain lodged and radioactive until counted. Leakage of the tracer from the microsphere must be minimal.

Measurement is accomplished by the use of carbonized or plastic microspheres with a mean diameter of 15 μm. Microspheres can be radiolabeled with a variety of gamma emitters[65,66] which can be discriminated by differential gamma spectrometry. Currently, microspheres are available with specific gravities of 1.23 to 1.40, which have a rheology closer to that of red blood cells (1.098). The experimental protocols are essentially the same as described for other indicator fractionation techniques, with certain important modifications. These include the vigorous agitation of microspheres just prior to each injection to minimize clumping, and require steady administration into the left auricle or ventricle of the heart, usually over a 10 to 20 s period.

Advantages: This technique averts problems with backflux, tissue-blood partitioning, and recirculation. It provides accurate measurements at high blood flow rates because it is not affected by problems of tracer diffusibility or efflux. Used carefully, flow determination can be repeated up to five times employing microspheres labeled with a different isotope each time in concert with differential gamma radiation spectroscopy. This permits regional flow estimations under multiple experimental conditions in the same animal. The number of repetitions is based on a balance between the minimum numbers of spheres required to permit good counting statistics and the local infarctions which are produced by these microemboli. The technique has been validated by means of the Kety equilibration method and the indicator (iodoantipyrine) fractionation method.

Disadvantages: The capillary obstruction caused by microspheres produces localized ischemia and microinjury. It is therefore invasive and irreversible. The amount of microspheres that is required for accurate counting in any tissue is limited by potential functional changes produced by ischemic damage; CNS and coronary perfusions are especially critical. Additionally, despite the utility of multiple determinations, instantaneous knowledge of flow changes is not available, thereby precluding judicious alteration of the course of an experiment on the basis of previous information.

B. HYDROGEN CLEARANCE

Blood flow determinations in highly localized brain regions can be determined repeatedly by means of hydrogen clearance polarography[67] (Farrar, 1987). The polarographic platinum black electrode was first used for blood flow measurements by Misrahy and Clark[68] and further developed for H_2 detection by Aukland et al.[69] H_2 is an ideal gas for clearance methods. It is metabolically inert, not usually found in body tissues; it has a high diffusion coefficient and, therefore reaches equilibrium with brain tissues quickly; and it has a very low water:gas partition coefficient (0.018), thereby minimizing recirculation problems.

Flow estimation is dependent on the detection of tissue desaturation of H_2, which like the previously discussed methods, is based on the Fick principle. It utilizes a simplified version of Equation 2, the operational equation of Kety's "tissue equilibration" technique, which is valid for saturation or desaturation studies depending on the boundary conditions that are set.

For H_2 clearance where $\lambda \approx 1$, when Ca is constant and zero during desaturation, Equation 2 reduces to

$$C_{brain}(t) = Ca(0)e^{-Ft} \tag{7}$$

where C(0) is the concentration at $t = 0$.

In practice, portions of the skull in anesthetized animals are carefully removed to expose the brain surface and very sharp platinum electrodes are implanted through the dura by means of a microdrive, which minimizes tissue injury due to lateral movements. Nevertheless, the penetration of the electrode into the brain creates a region of impaired cells and fluid accumulation at the electrode surface which acts as a diffusion barrier, preferably one that stabilizes at a thickness of less than 200 μm.

Electrodes are sealed in place with cold-curing dental acrylic over a Gelfoam layer. An electrode is polarized to a positive voltage with respect to a Ag/AgCl or stainless steel reference electrode. Usually, a period of 30 to 60 min is required for electrode and diffusion barrier stabilization. The animal is then allowed to breathe a mixture of air and hydrogen gas for a period of time to reach essentially complete brain tissue saturation. Optimum saturation time for the measurement of H_2 clearances from two brain compartments, i.e., gray and white matter, is about 5 min which allows a good signal-to-noise ratio in the CNS. The inspired air is quickly switched to room air and desaturation measurement begins. Repeated measurements can be made at 15 to 20 min intervals for up to 10 h.

Preparation of electrodes is well described by Farrar.[67] Polarization voltages are usually about +350 mV with respect to the Ag/AgCl reference electrodes; about +600 mV for stainless steel. This is sufficient to oxidize all of the local H_2, forming hydrogen ^+H ions and electrons which are accepted by the platinum electrode causing a H_2 gradient between the bulk tissue and oxidizing surface. The electrode current is related to the diffusion-limited amount of hydrogen reaching the electrode. Under properly controlled conditions, the current is a linear function of the hydrogen ion concentration provided that the thickness of the diffusion layer remains constant and the reaction at the electrode surface remains sufficiently vigorous.

Advantages: Like the microsphere method, the H_2 clearance technique permits multiple, but discontinuous measurements over a long period of time, up to 10 h. This can be accomplished in a relatively small amount of tissue (about 3 mm^3). The course of the experiment can be altered depending on previous flow measurements. The relatively uncomplicated polarographic method relies on simple, inexpensive system design and uncomplicated data analysis. With hydrogen gas, the partition coefficient (λ) is essentially equal to one and is stable even in damaged tissue (i.e., it is independent of the water content). Hydrogen electrodes can be used in concert with other polarographic electrodes to explore relationships between blood flow and other parameters such as tissue pH, oxygen tension, and various ionic concentrations in brain microregions. Flows in multiple regions can be sampled simultaneously by means of arrays of electrodes.[70]

Disadvantages: Although there is rough agreement between estimates of local blood flow derived by the hydrogen clearance method and other methods, such as venous outflow,[69] 133-xenon,[71] radioactive microspheres,[121] and ^{14}C-antipyrine,[72] there is considerable variation. This is due mainly to the likelihood that these methods did not sample the same volumes of tissue. Other limitations and potential sources of errors include the following: significant movement artifacts requiring the use of anesthesia; local hyperemia due to tissue injury by the needle electrode; reduced blood flows due to edema and tissue compression; loss of autoregulation; trauma-induced baseline shifts and distorted clearance curves; possible indicator recirculation between vascular compartments; and permanent electrode inactivation by substances other than ^+H.

C. DOPPLER FLOWMETRY

Acoustic (ultrasound) Doppler technology,[73] e.g., flow-induced frequency shift between transmitted and reflected beams of ultrasound, offers the capability to noninvasively record blood flow velocity from major basal intracranial arteries.[74,75] Currently, both acute and chronic volume flow measurements can be made in small and large vessels, from 1 to 30 mm in diameter. Although it has considerable clinical utility,[74,75] this methodology is not suited for flow measurements in microvascular beds.

Laser-Doppler flowmetry (LDF) is an adaptation of Doppler vascular technology which does allow direct, continuous evaluation of regional cerebral microcirculation either through tissue implantation or cranial windows. It has *both* experimental and clinical applications. LDF employs small fiber optics (0.84 mm) to illuminate and sample reflected low-power laser light in a small volume of tissue. It relies on detection of a Doppler Shift in radiation caused by red blood cell (RBC) movement in microvessels. Information about RBC velocity and density per unit volume in a local microvascular bed is derived with a microcomputer. The product of blood velocity and blood volume is proportional, but not identical, to the local perfusion rate. Although the proportionality factor usually remains constant after an initial fiber placement, it is neither constant nor predictable between regions or tissues.

LDF has been used to continuously estimate blood flow by measuring blood cell flux in a variety of tissues, including the CNS.[76-79] Like the H_2 clearance technique, LDF is used to estimate highly localized microcirculation, i.e., on the order of 1 mm^3. However, like H_2 measurements, correlation with microsphere-derived data is not always good, probably for the same reasons, i.e., the surveyed tissue volumes differ.

Although most recent cerebrovascular measurements in animals have employed anesthetics, the fiber optics conceivably can be fixed in place for long-term cortical recordings in conscious animals, e.g., at a pial site. However, current dimensions of the fiber optics may still be limiting if the implantation site is parenchymal. Nevertheless, clinical applications include measurement and monitoring of blood flow in premature infants.

Advantages: The main advantage of LDF is its ability to sample changes in microcirculatory flow continuously using a relatively atraumatic modality, i.e., low energy laser light. Unlike previously mentioned methods, it can be used clinically for monitoring perfusion of epidural, cortical, and subcortical regions.

Disadvantages: The current LDF technique for measurements in the CNS requires some tissue exposure for surface measurements and is invasive when used in a needle configuration. Additionally, the method is very motion sensitive and is affected by ambient light conditions. The method is unable to report flow directly in conventional units, i.e., $ml \cdot min^{-1} \cdot g^{-1}$, preventing direct comparisons with published results derived by other techniques. Although such measurements are proportional to perfusion, the proportionality factor varies between tissues.

III. CLINICAL METHODS

Clinical methods for determining CNS blood flow have been developed for investigational, as well as diagnostic and postsurgical or trauma monitoring. Recent efforts have stressed noninvasiveness, repeatability, and fast measurements. In addition, there has been a movement towards more detailed three-dimensional spatial and dynamic temporal resolution for accurate time-dependent mapping of regional blood flow in the brain and spinal cord. Some of these methods can be used in concert with simultaneous mapping of regional metabolism for accurate estimates of regional functional status of nervous tissues. The promise of these newer techniques for investigational purposes is obvious.

The conceptual bases for blood flow measurements by means of these mechanically and electronically sophisticated instruments remain those outlined by Kety. Aside from hardware and software, there have been substantial refinements in knowledge of diffusion equilibria, in multicompartmental analyses, and in the well-known "convolution integral" or arterial indicator input function developed by Kety for use in the autoradiographic method for local CNS blood flow measurements.

A. ^{133}XENON CLEARANCE

Clinical cerebral blood flow measurement employing xenon gas illustrates the role of technological development over the last 30 years.[39,80] In its radioactive form, xenon has replaced N_2O for the measurement of global CBF. Moreover, detection of the tracer by means of multiple, extracranial gamma radiation detectors placed over each cerebral hemisphere has simplified more localized routine clinical measurements for both investigative and diagnostic purposes. Commercially available systems consisting of arrays of up to 256 fixed detectors (NaI:photomultiplier) can sample comparatively detailed cortical blood flows in a variety of normal and disease conditions.[37] More recently, the use of radiodense, nonradioactive xenon to enhance fast X-ray computerized tomographic (CT) scans of human brain and spinal cord has permitted noninvasive, three-dimensional estimations of blood flows with improved spatial resolution.

The substitution of krypton-85 for nitrous oxide, followed soon after by the more energetic gamma emitter ^{133}Xe, and extracranial scintillation counting yielded a direct measure of a tracer within a tissue and, by employing modifications of the Kety Equation 2, estimates of blood flow in a broad variety of clinical applications. The ^{133}Xe technique has yielded insights into mechanisms of blood flow regulation in both health and disease and provided substantial information in a variety of neurological and psychiatric disturbances.[81]

In current practice, in the noninvasive version of this method, ^{133}Xe is usually administered by means of inhalation of a gas (or intravenous injection of the gas in a saline solvent). End-tidal tracer concentrations are monitored for about 1 min to obtain the ^{133}Xe input function, Ca, and brain clearance of the tracer is monitored by extracranial detectors for about 15 min. Radioactivity is usually captured bilaterally at the surface of the head by means of arrays of 4 to 256 collimated NaI crystals attached to photomultiplier detectors. Newer instruments rely on multiple, miniaturized cadmium telluride gamma detectors and small personal computers to markedly reduce their size and improve portability. Some of these devices are small enough for use in pediatric applications and animal studies if high spatial resolution is not essential.[82]

These methods of ^{133}Xe delivery have resulted in errors related to prolonged input times and appreciable recirculation of the indicator. This, in addition to the extracranial contamination of gray and white matter signals, stimulated the development of complex mathematical modeling of input and, especially, output clearance curves.[83,84] Normally, a two-compartment analysis of the ^{133}Xe clearance curves is performed using a correction for recirculation of the indicator. Under most circumstances, the determination of the arterial time-concentration integral is performed by using the less traumatic sampling of the end-tidal content of ^{133}Xe. Ordinarily, there is little difference between rCBF values based on delivery of the tracer by the inhalational or intravenous routes of administration. The choice usually depends on technical, economic, and psychological factors. However, the use of end-tidal air in subjects with pulmonary disease as an approximation of the arterial time-concentration curve will lead to underestimation of CBF.[85] Such errors can be circumvented by using the intravenous injection version of this method.

Advantages: This method is superior to the global N_2O method of Kety and Schmidt[13,14] because it provides somewhat more detail. The ^{133}Xe inhalation (or intravenous) technique is still useful because of its lack of invasiveness and low radiation dose. It has been used extensively to obtain normative data and in longitudinal studies.[80] The method is suited to monitoring therapeutic intervention, particularly in intensive care and operating room environments. Although the inhalational technique is not as accurate as the injection version, its ease of use for repeated measurements, portability, and relatively low cost has made it a popular choice for clinical investigations. It is regarded as the method of choice for problems that appear to involve more or less the whole brain such as dementia or head trauma.

Disadvantages: Spatial resolution with this method is limited by massive cross-talk between hemispheres and by Compton scattering. Even when arrays containing up to 32 detectors per hemisphere are employed the actual resolution is quite gross, perhaps limited to 6 to 8 brain areas. The ^{133}Xe inhalation (tissue equilibration) method is insensitive to smaller, high flow components that are better detected by bolus fractionation methods, and is insensitive to very low-flow components, i.e., infarctions that are better visualized tomographically.

B. STABLE XENON ENHANCED COMPUTED TOMOGRAPHY (Xe/CT)

The drawbacks of the classical ^{133}Xe clearance techniques have stimulated the introductions of new technologies for purposes of clinical diagnosis and management, as well as experimental studies of cerebral circulation. The theoretical bases for these methods nevertheless remain the Kety formulations and the operational Equation 2.

There are at least five tomographic methods for faster, higher resolution measurement of blood flow, each in varying stages of development. Most use computer-assisted image reconstructions based on a series of lateral projections of regional signals emanating from the head (and spinal cord). The first of the three methods is stable xenon computerized tomography and is described next. Others include single photon emission CT (SPECT), positron emission tomography (PET), Ultrafast CT, and very fast MRI, e.g., echo-planar MRI (EPI).

The Xe/CT method, introduced about 1978,[86,87] couples the use of the radioenhancement properties of *stable* xenon with updated applications of the Kety tissue equilibration formulation for inert gas clearance and the high resolution imaging technology of transmission X-ray computerized tomography. Since, along with estimates of blood flow, the newer versions of this method also provide information about the actual regional partition coefficients for xenon,[88] there no longer is a need to assume "normal" partition coefficients for xenon for the calculation of regional blood flow. This modification is particularly useful in cases of pathophysiology where regional λ may be abnormal. Additional improvements have increased the accuracy of measurements of xenon uptake and clearances, new ways to determine the input arterial concentration, better ways to postprocess the flow image, better head holders, and faster scanners with higher signal-to-noise characteristics.[89]

In practice, xenon is administered in high concentrations (up to 33%) by inhalation during X-ray irradiation of the head. The sensitivity of current instruments to movement requires head constraint for about 6 min during the acquisition of baseline and enhanced scans. X-ray exposure for each measurement is considerable, 8 to 28 cGy* for each plane or "slice" of brain examined. A delay period of 15 to 25 min between studies is usually required to permit reliable flow estimates in low-flow brain regions. The technique has been used in normal and head-injured patients[90] and has been validated with the radiolabeled microsphere technique in baboons.[91]

Advantages: This method provides CBF information about well-defined cortical and deep brain regions not readily obtained with more conventional ^{133}Xe CBF studies. This is particularly evident, for example, in difficult

* 1 Gy = 1 Gray = 100 RAD (Radiation absorbed dose).

studies of cerebrovascular responsivity to carbon dioxide.[92] The equipment for this method is relatively inexpensive for sophisticated imaging.

Disadvantages: The xenon indicator is expensive. The signal-to-noise ratio, i.e., the degree of image enhancement, is low with this method, even at high concentrations of xenon. The general anesthetic properties of xenon preclude the use of high levels (>33%). The vasoactivity of such concentrations of xenon can produce a variable degree of flow enhancement.

C. SINGLE PHOTON EMISSION COMPUTED TOMOGRAPHY (SPECT)

The second tomographic technique, single photon emission CT (SPECT), utilizes the indicator fractionation method for the estimation of rCBF.[124] It employs highly diffusible, relatively short-lived tracers, e.g., usually ^{123}I-labeled amines, which are trapped in brain tissue after an initial capillary pass and behave as "liquid microspheres".[93] Kuhl has demonstrated that the initial distribution of compounds such as *N*-isopropyl-^{123}I-*p*-iodoamphetamine (IMP) in the brain provides good estimates of rCBF over a wide range of flows.[94] These tracer substances freely pass the blood-brain barrier but are rapidly converted to highly bound metabolites which are retained for several minutes, sufficient for tomographic imaging. The consequences of variations in partition coefficients and backfluxes of the indicator and its polar metabolites are minimal during this time. The Kety equations are simplified considerably in such circumstances and regional blood flow can be estimated from the ratio of the regional content of indicator and its integrated arterial concentration (Equation 6).

In practice, the tracer is injected intravenously. At the same time, the arterial concentration-time curve is determined mechanically by withdrawing a sample of arterial blood into a syringe at a constant rate during the entire measurement period and determining the radioactivity of indicator.

Tissue radioactivity is detected either with arrays of fixed sensors surrounding the head or a gamma camera which rotates around the head. Fixed multidetector systems permit more rapid scanning (5 to 7.5 min) of a 2-cm slice in a region of interest with a useful spatial resolution of about 2 cm^3. The standard rotating gamma camera provides a lower resolution alternative, but it surveys larger volumes of tissue than multidetector systems and usually is more readily available. Improvements in both types of detector systems have significantly increased the resolution and speed of measurements.

Lassen has introduced a hybrid method in which the time course of ^{133}Xe through the brain is monitored by means of a very fast rotating SPECT-type gamma camera.[38] Such advanced devices consist of multiple gamma cameras, each containing arrays of detectors which rotate rapidly about a fixed head. Spatial resolution of about 6 cm^3 can be achieved in up to six 2-cm thick slices of brain. The tracer, unlike stable xenon or ^{123}I-labeled compounds, is commercially available at a reasonable cost and is readily detectable with a relatively high signal-to-noise ratio.

In practice, two groups of measurements are made over a total time of 5 min in a subject breathing tracer amounts of ^{133}Xe. During the time interval of 0 to 2.5 min, multiple tomographic images are constructed from a series of rapid scans of at least three slices of brain. The bolus fractionation principle is applied during this early phase to derive most of the blood flow information, i.e., when adjustments related to partition coefficients are not required. The tissue equilibrium principle is applied in the remaining time, 2.5 to 4.5 min, to correct for slight overestimations of regional perfusion in low-flow regions that are obtained during the first phase. In this late phase, a partition coefficient for xenon distribution between brain tissue and blood is assumed to be 0.85.[38]

In addition, a single nonmoving probe placed over the upper part of the right lung is used to record the shape of the lung tracer content, which normally represents the shape of the arterial input curve to the brain. Although there is good agreement between the end-tidal and arterial ^{133}Xe curves in healthy adults, the validity of such an estimate has been questioned recently in subjects with pulmonary disease, where end-tidal tracer concentrations no longer reflect arterial levels.[85] Such distortions consistently underestimate arterial concentration and, therefore, blood flow.

Advantages: These methods are simple, atraumatic, short-term (4 to 20 min), repeatable at intervals from a few hours to 2 days depending on the indicator, and relatively inexpensive. They have found application in a variety of clinical investigations of normal brain activity, including visual, motor, and language functions and have been used to characterize cerebral blood flow in pathologic states, such as migraine, stroke, Alzheimer's disease, and epilepsy.

Disadvantages: The higher costs, the relatively short half-life of ^{123}I-iodinated compounds, and the necessarily high radiation dose compared to ^{133}Xe are significant limitations. On the other hand, Compton scattering constitutes a major source of error with the ^{133}Xe indicator, reducing resolution and making the tomograph significantly nonlinear in low- or no-flow regions. Expensive gamma detecting counting devices are necessary to detect the low-photon fluxes from the target tissue. The use of compounds that lend themselves to indicator fractionation techniques, which are labeled with more energetic sources, e.g., technetium-99^{m}, may prove to be better alternatives to ^{123}I-labeled tracers, particularly if employed with more sensitive gamma cameras.[95]

D. POSITRON EMISSION TOMOGRAPHY (PET)

The third technique, positron emission tomography (PET), is based on coincidence counting of annihilation photons from a variety of positron emitting indicator compounds which are labeled with short-lived isotopes, e.g., ^{77}Kr, ^{15}O, ^{13}N, ^{18}F, ^{68}Ga, ^{75}Br. The method enables the simultaneous estimation of regional perfusion and metabolism.[96-100] The technique has been developed primarily for research studies of the pathophysiology of cerebrovascular and other CNS diseases. It is a relatively noninvasive method permitting repeated determinations of regional blood flow, separately and in combination with metabolism, with a fair degree of spatial resolution.[96] The method provides a way to approach a pathological state from different tracer pathways, e.g., acute stroke at a time when there may be substantial uncoupling between blood flow and oxygen utilization. PET applications also include studies of cerebral hemodynamics, blood-brain barrier transport functions, and neurotransmitter receptor distributions.

The problems which have been discussed earlier, concerning the external localization of a source of radiation within the brain, are generally overcome by using the unique properties of positron-emitting isotopes. Paired, opposing detectors utilizing coincidence circuitry are able to record the gamma photons produced by positron annihilation. In tomographic systems, corrections can be made for radiation absorption by tissue surrounding the photon source and the (Compton) scattering of photons that leads to false tissue localization. This is a significant limitation with all external counting methods. The coincidence circuitry permits accurate spatial discrimination of different photon generating sources. Modern scanners usually consist of rotating arrays of paired barium fluoride detectors (up to 4096) arranged in four or more rings which produce a seven-slice tomograph. Tomographic images have been improved by administration of relatively large amounts of radioactivity, 50 to 75 mCi, which improve signal-to-noise characteristics, and the development of multi-plane ("slice") technology, which allows a larger portion of the brain to be imaged following a single tracer injection.

In practice, the head and system attenuation of radiation is measured before the subject is examined by employing a rotating tracer source. The subject is fitted with a mask which delivers the tracer by inhalation or, alternatively, is catheterized to permit injection and measurement of the arterial concentration of the tracer. The head is immobilized and positioned in the PET scanner. The most widely used approach to the measurement of rCBF by PET is a modified Kety equilibrium technique using ^{15}O-labeled CO_2, delivered at a constant rate by inhalation. The catalytic action of carbonic anhydrase in the lung rapidly transfers the ^{15}O label to water, the indicator for flow measurements. Most indicators are administered by inhalation, and end-tidal radioactivity in the expired air is routinely used to determine the shape of the arterial input curve. A weighted partition coefficient based on prior experimental evidence is used for each indicator. The procedure is usually completed in 10 min or less. The repetition time of the method depends on the half-life of the tracer.

The most widely used tracer, ^{15}O-labeled water is a biologically inert, chemically stable, and naturally occurring body constituent with no untoward physiologic or pharmacologic side effects and it is easily synthesized in large millicurie quantities. It has a 2 min half-life and large amounts can be administered repeatedly with only limited radiation exposure. However, it should be noted that water is diffusion limited, so that its extraction is incomplete in high-flow regions, and flow consequently tends to be underestimated. This problem has been circumvented by the use of more lipid-soluble indicators, such as ^{18}F-fluoromethane.

Advantages: A principle advantage of PET is the capability to examine a variety of physiologic functions in addition to rCBF. Since most of a human brain can be repeatedly monitored and the time courses of regional radioactive contents followed, local metabolic processes as well as blood flows can be quantitatively monitored both spatially and temporally. The productivity of PET has been described by Jones[99] as a technology which appears to have "advanced further than the ability to interpret recorded data."

Disadvantages: The logistics of coordinating the multidisciplinary effort needed to effect an innovative PET program are very complex. The initial and operating costs of a PET program are very high. This is complicated by the difficulties related to high speed synthesis of compounds containing short-lived tracers. The molecular synthesis involving short-lived radionuclides is specialized and labor-intensive since it must be performed rapidly and yet yield substances which are sufficiently pure for human subjects. It also requires a close-by cyclotron and a system for rapid delivery of indicators to the measurement site. It is not surprising, therefore, that PET technology is limited to a few centers. However, some of these formidable difficulties may be circumvented by emerging technologies.

IV. EMERGING TECHNOLOGY

A. ULTRAFAST CT

It has been realized for some time that CT scans of the transit of a radiocontrast agent might be used to noninvasively measure rCBF with a high degree of spatial resolution,[101,102] provided that an accurate history of that transit could be captured in a series of CT "snapshots". Changes in concentration of the contrast agent in a region of interest (ROI) could be obtained from the CT images and rCBF could be derived from such changes by the application of indicator dilution theory. Older attempts to use this technique were handicapped by the long times required to generate sufficient numbers of scans to accurately characterize each indicator transit. Such limitations have been substantially reduced by the development of ultrafast scanners with short image acquisition times of 50 to 100 msec and an interscan delay of 600 msec.[102]

In experimental trials,[102] heads of mechanically ventilated anesthetized dogs were placed onto a plastic rest within the CT scanner, a bolus of iodinated contrast agent was mechanically injected intravenously, and a series of 20 CT scans (100 msec/scan) were made of a single brain slice, 6-mm thick. The method has been validated employing the radiolabeled microsphere method in both normal and abnormal brains of dogs.[102]

The dynamic CT method for estimating rCBF is based on the estimation of regional fractional vascular volume (V_b) and mean transit time (t_f) of blood containing a non-diffusible contrast agent. These are derived from a knowledge of the concentration-time integrals (AUC or areas under the curves) and mean transit times (t) of the indicator in the ROI and arterial blood

$$rCBF = n[(AUC_{ROI}/AUC_{PA})/(\langle t_{ROI}\rangle - \langle t_{PA}\rangle)] \quad (8)$$

where n is a correction factor for the difference in hematocrit between the ROI and a nearby artery, PA; AUC_{ROI} is the concentration-time integral in the ROI; AUC_{PA} is the concentration-time integral in that nearby artery; $\langle t_{ROI}\rangle - \langle t_{PA}\rangle$ represents the derivation of the mean transit time of the indicator, corrected for the difference in arrival time of the bolus in the ROI and the artery.[101]

Advantages: The ultrafast CT method has clinical potential for measurement of rCBF in both normal and pathological tissues. The method is relatively noninvasive, requiring only the introduction of a single venous catheter. The studies can be short. Trial studies indicate that rCBF can be measured in about 300 mm^3 of tissues in up to four different levels of brain. Multiple studies can be made with additional administrations of contrast agent at intervals of 10 to 15 min. Ultrafast CT has the potential for being useful in the diagnosis and management of cerebrovascular disorders and for experimental studies in large animals.

Disadvantages: Accurate determination of mean transit times is most critical in high-flow areas. Compared to studies employing microspheres, significant nonlinearities in flow measurements were observed at flow rates exceeding 1.2 $ml \cdot min^{-1} \cdot g^{-1}$, suggesting that the fastest acceptable mean transit time with current instrumentation is about 1 s.[102] Accurate values for tissue and peripheral blood hematocrits are essential since these vary considerably.[103,104] Hemodynamic alterations related to the arterial vasodilation induced by hyperosmotic contrast agents may limit the accuracy of subsequent measurements. The current radiation dose of 8 to 9 cGy/20 scans limits the number of measurements that can be made safely.

B. VERY FAST NMR IMAGING TECHNOLOGIES

The monitoring of cerebral circulation by imaging techniques based on nuclear magnetic resonance (NMR) is a major activity in nuclear medicine investigations of tissue perfusion. MRI[105] is a genuinely noninvasive imaging modality. MRI also has the potential for high quality anatomical mapping. In addition, recent introduction of fast (<1 s) and ultra-fast (50 to 100 msec) MRI techniques has facilitated the mapping of *time-dependent* changes in functional variables, e.g., regional metabolite concentrations, vascular flow,[106,107] diffusion,[108] blood volumes,[109] and tissue perfusion[110-114] in moving organs, under normal and pathological conditions.

All atomic nuclei that contain odd numbers of protons or neutrons or of both, i.e., which possess a mechanical spin and a magnetic moment, can serve as indicators in NMR-based imaging techniques. Example of stable isotopes which have medical applications include ^{1}H, ^{2}H, ^{7}Li, ^{13}C, ^{19}F, ^{23}Na, and ^{31}P. In NMR,[115,116,122] magnetic nuclear spins which are aligned by a large uniform magnetic field are resonantly excited by a radio-frequency (RF) field. The resonant frequency is proportional to the intensity of the magnetic field. In MRI, strong external magnetic field *gradients* are applied across the imaging region. As a consequence, different points in space can be identified with different resonant frequencies. Thus, it becomes possible to locate nuclear spins in space by the characteristic frequencies of their RF emissions. The signal amplitude at a given frequency is a measure of the spin concentration in that space. During the past two decades, a wide variety of techniques have been developed for manipulating combinations of magnetic field gradients to generate two- and three-dimensional images. The theoretical aspects of nuclear magnetic resonance imaging,[111] and perfusion studies with fast imaging, in particular are well-reviewed elsewhere.[117] A review of the latest stage in the evolution of high-speed MRI, Echo-Planar Imaging (EPI)[110] describes both its theoretical and considerable biomedical potential.

In practice, the subject is treated in much the same way as in a CT procedure, except for the use of different types of indicators, and imaging hardware. Recently, rapid EPI imaging of capillary transits of nondiffusible, paramagnetic tracers, such as chelates of gadolinium, have been used to estimate regional blood volumes.[109] If the arterial input function of that tracer is also determined, then, as in the case of ultrafast CT, regional perfusion can be obtained.[118]

In animal studies, slower MRI methods employing highly diffusible tracers, such as ^{19}F-freon and $^{2}H_2O$, have been used to determine blood flow with the Kety tissue equilibration technique in cat brains,[112,119] rat livers,[120] and mouse tumors.[114] Theoretically, complex cerebrovascular studies in small animals are feasible with EPI technique, particularly since the considerably faster speed of the method virtually eliminates motion artifacts, and thereby improves resolution.

Advantages: This method offers relatively fast, repeatable, high-resolution measurements of rCBF and other important CNS variables, sometimes concurrently. It provides the opportunity for the simultaneous examination of morphologic and functional relationships in real-time. The method is free from ionizing radiation and allows free choice of the image-plane orientation. The results obtained with EPI parallel those of PET, except that the signal-to-noise and spatial characteristics are much better. In EPI, images can be obtained thousands of times faster than with conventional spin-echo MRI. Also, since images can be obtained and displayed in much less than 1 s, fields of view can be selected in real-time, and tissue image contrasts can be optimized under visual control.

Disadvantages: The intense magnetic fields encountered in conventional MRI are normally safe for the subject. EPI differs from conventional MRI in that very large gradient fields are switched rapidly, resulting in peak rates of change of 50 to 100 Tesla/s, particularly when high-resolution at ultra-short image acquisition times is desired. Some neural stimulation has been observed with field changes that exceed 80 T/s. Although the upgrading of existing MRI installations is possible, EPI technology is still evolving rapidly and is not generally available for either experimental or investigational use.

REFERENCES

1. **Bell, B. A.,** Early study of cerebral circulation and measurement of cerebral blood flow, in *Cerebral Blood Flow: Physiologic and Clinical Aspects,* Wood, J. H., Ed., McGraw-Hill, New York, 1987, Chapt. 1.
2. **Harvey, W.,** *Exercitatio Anatomica de Motu Cordis et Sanguinis in Animalibus,* Fitzer, Frankfort, 1628, (Translated by Leake, C. D., Thomas, Springfield, IL, 1928).
3. **Wepfer, J. J.,** *Observations Anatomicae, Ex Cadaveribus Eorum, Quos Sustulit Apoplexia, cum Exercitatione de Eius Loc Affecto,* Suterus, J. C., Shaffhausen, 1658.
4. **Willis, T. and Wren, C.,** *Cerebri Anatome: Cui Accessit Nervorum Descriptio et Usus,* Flesher, J., London, 1664.
5. **Von Schulten, M. W.,** Untersuchungen uber den hirndruck, mit besonder rucksicht auf sine einwirkung auf die Circulation-verhaltnisse des Avges, *Arch. Klin. Chir.,* 32, 455, 733, and 947, 1885.
6. **Hill, L. E.,** *The Physiology and Pathology of the Cerebral Circulation,* Churchill, London, 1896.
7. **Hürthle, K.,** Beiträge zur Hämodynamik Dritte Abhandlung: Untersuchungen über die Innervation der Hirngefässe, *Pfluegers Arch. Ges. Physiol.,* 14, 561, 1889.
8. **Gärtner, G. and Wagner, J.,** Über den Hirnkreislauf, *Wein. Med. Wochenschr.,* 37, 601 and 640, 1887.
9. **Rein, H.,** Verber Besonderheiten der Blutzirculation in der Arteria carotis, *Z. Biol.,* 89, 307, 1929.
10. **Gibbs, F. A.,** A thermoelectric blood flow recorder in the form of a needle, *Proc. Soc. Exp. Biol. Med.,* 31, 141, 1933.
11. **Katz, L. N. and Kolin, A.,** The flow of blood in the carotid artery of the dog under various circumstances as determined with the electromagnetic flowmeter, *Am. J. Physiol.,* 122, 788, 1938.
12. **Dumke, P. R. and Schmidt, C. F.,** Quantitative measurements of cerebral blood flow in the macaque monkey, *Am. J. Physiol.,* 138, 421, 1943.
13. **Kety, S. S. and Schmidt, C. F.,** The determination of cerebral blood flow in man by the use of nitrous oxide in low concentrations, *Am. J. Physiol.,* 143, 53, 1945.
14. **Kety, S. S. and Schmidt, C. F.,** The nitrous oxide method for the quantitative determination of cerebral blood flow in man: theory, procedure and normal values, *J. Clin. Invest.,* 27, 476, 1948.
15. **Kety, S. S.,** The theory and applications of the exchange of inert gas at the lungs and tissues, *Pharmacol. Rev.,* 3, 1, 1951.
16. **Kety, S. S., Landau, W. M., Rowland, L. P., and Sokoloff, L.,** Estimation of regional circulation in the brain by the uptake of an inert gas, *Fed. Proc.,* 14, 85, 1955.

17. **Sakurada, O., Kennedy, C., Jehle, J., Brown, J. D., Carbin, G. L., and Sokoloff, L.,** Measurement of local cerebral blood flow with iodo [^{14}C] antipyrine, *Am. J. Physiol.,* 234, H59, 1978.
18. **Fick, A.,** Über die Messung des Blutquantums in den Herzventrikeln, *Sitz ber Physik-Med Ges Wurzburg,* 2, 16, 1870.
19. **Landau, W. M., Freygang, W. A., Jr., Rowland, L. P., Sokoloff, L., and Kety, S. S.,** The local circulation of the living brain: values in the unanesthetized and anesthetized cat, *Trans. Am. Neurol. Assoc.,* 80, 125, 1955.
20. **Ginsberg, M. D.,** Autoradiographic measurement of local cerebral blood flow, in *Cerebral Blood Flow: Physiologic and Clinical Aspects,* Wood, J. H., Ed., McGraw-Hill, New York, 1987, 299.
21. **Sokoloff, L., Reivich, M., Kennedy, C., DesRosiers, M. H., Patlak, C. S., Pettigrew, K. D., Sakurada, O., and Shinohara, M.,** The (14C)deoxyglucose method for the measurement of local glucose utilization: Theory, procedure, and normal values in the conscious and anesthetized albino rat, *J. Neurochem.,* 28, 897, 1977.
22. **Phelps, M. E., Mazziotta, J. C., and Huang, S. C.,** Study of cerebral function with position, *J. Cereb. Blood Flow Metab.,* 2, 113, 1982.
23. **Baron, J. C., Frackowiak, R. S. J., Herholz, K., Jones, T., Lammertsma, A. A., et al.,** Use of PET methods for the measurement of cerebral energy metabolism and hemodynamics in cerebrovascular disease, *J. Cereb. Blood Flow Metab.,* 9, 723, 1989.
24. **Kobatake, K., Sako, K., Izawa, M., Yamamoto, Y. L., and Hakim, A. M.,** Autoradiographic determination of brain pH following middle cerebral artery occlusion in the rat, *Stroke,* 15, 540, 1984.
25. **Dwyer, B. E., Donatoni, P., and Wasterlain, C. G.,** A quantitative autoradiographic method for the measurement of local rates of brain protein synthesis, *Neurochem. Res.,* 7, 563, 1982.
26. **Williams, J. L., Shea, M., Furlan, A. J., Little, J. R., and Jones, S. C.,** Importance of freezing time when iodoantipyrine is used for measurement of cerebral blood flow, *Am. J. Physiol.,* 261, H252, 1991.
27. **Gjedde, A., Hansen, A. J., and Siemkowicz, E.,** Rapid simultaneous determination of regional blood flow and blood-brain glucose transfer in brain of rat, *Acta Physiol. Scand.,* 108, 321, 1980.
28. **Van Uiert, R. L. and Levy, D. E.,** Regional brain blood flow in the conscious gerbil, *Stroke,* 9, 67, 1978.
29. **Tomita, M. and Gotoh, F.,** Local cerebral blood flow values as estimated with diffusible tracers: validity of assumptions in normal and ischemic tissue, *J. Cereb. Blood Flow Metab.,* 1, 403, 1981.
30. **Takasato, Y., Rapoport, S. I., and Smith, Q. R.,** An in situ perfusion technique to study cerebrovascular transport in the rat, *Am. J. Physiol.,* 247, H484, 1984.
31. **Leo, A., Hansch, C., and Elkins, D.,** Partition coefficients and their uses, *Chem. Rev.,* 71, 525, 1971.
32. **Rapoport, S. I., Ohno, K., and Pettigrew, K. D.,** Drug entry into the brain, *Brain Res.,* 172, 354, 1979.
33. **Oldendorf, W. H.,** Brain uptake of metabolites and drugs following carotid arterial injections, *Trans. Am. Neurol. Assoc.,* 96, 46, 1971.
34. **Bradbury, W. B., Patlak, C. S., and Oldendorf, W. H.,** Analysis of brain uptake and loss of radiotracers after carotid injection, *Am. J. Physiol.,* 229, 1110, 1975.
35. **Drewes, L. R., Mies, G., Hossmann, K.-A., and Stöcklin, G.,** Blood-brain transfer and regional distribution of bromo-benzodiazepine, *Brain Res.,* 401, 55, 1987.
36. **Lassen, N. A. and Perl, W.,** *Tracer Kinetic Methods in Medical Physiology,* Raven Press, New York, 1979.
37. **Lassen, N. A., Henriksen, L., and Paulson, O.,** Regional cerebral blood flow in stroke by ^{133}Xenon in halation and emission tomography, *Stroke,* 12, 284, 1981.

38. **Lassen, N. A.,** Cerebral blood flow tomography using Xenon-133 inhalation-methodological considerations, in *Cerebral Blood Flow and Metabolism Measurement,* Hartmann, A. and Hoyer, S., Eds., Springer-Verlag, Heidelberg, 1985, 224.
39. **Lassen, N. A.,** Basic principles of CBF measurement by Xenon-133 and external recording by multiple stationary detectors, in *Handbook of Regional Cerebral Blood Flow,* Knezevic, S., Maximilian, V. A., Mubrin, Z., Prohovnik, I. and Wade, I., Eds., Laurence Erlbaum, Assoc., Hillsdale, NJ, 1988, Chapt. 2.
40. **Lacombe, P., Meric, P., and Seylaz, J.,** Validity of cerebral blood flow measurements obtained with quantitative tracer techniques, *Brain Res. Rev.,* 2, 105, 1980.
41. **Freygang, W. H., Jr. and Sokoloff, L.,** Quantitative measurement of regional circulation in the central nervous system by the use of radioactive inert gas, *Adv. Biol. Med. Physics,* 6, 263, 1958.
42. **Stewart, G. N.,** Researches on the circulation time in organs and on the influences which affect it, *J. Physiol.,* 15, 1, 1894.
43. **Stewart, G. N.,** Researches on the circulation time and on the influences which affect it. IV. The output of the heart, *J. Physiol.,* 22, 159, 1897.
44. **Hamilton, W. F., Moore, J. W., Kinsman, J. M., and Spurling, R. G.,** Studies on the circulation. IV. Further analysis of the injection method and of changes in hemodynamics under physiological and pathological conditions and pathological conditions, *Am. J. Physiol.,* 99, 534, 1932.
45. **Sapirstein, L. A.,** Regional blood flow by fractional distribution of indicators, *Am. J. Physiol.,* 193, 161, 1958.
46. **Sapirstein, L. A. and Hanusek, G.,** Cerebral blood flow in the rat, *Am. J. Physiol.,* 193, 272, 1958.
47. **Goldman, H. and Sapirstein, L.,** Brain blood flow in the conscious and anesthetized rat, *Am. J. Physiol.,* 224, 122, 1973.
48. **Van Uitert, R. L., Sage, J. I., Levy, D. E., and Duffy, T. E.,** Comparison of radiolabelled butanol and iodoantipyrine as cerebral blood flow markers, *Brain Res.,* 222, 365, 1981.
49. **Sage, J. I., Van Uitert, R. L., and Duffy, T. E.,** Simultaneous measurement of cerebral blood flow and unidirectional movement of substances across the blood-brain barrier: theory, method, and application to leucine, *J. Neurochem.,* 36, 1731, 1981.
50. **Jones, S. C., Korfali, E., and Marshall, S. A.,** Cerebral blood flow with the indicator fractionation of [^{14}C] Iodoantipyrine: effect of P_aCO_2 on cerebral venous appearance time, *J. Cereb. Blood Flow Metab.,* 11, 236, 1991.
51. **Patlak, C. S., Blasberg, R. G., and Fenstermacher, J. D.,** An evaluation of errors in the determination of blood flow by the indicator fractionation and tissue equilibration (Kety) methods, *J. Cereb. Blood Flow Metab.,* 4, 47, 1984.
52. **Blasberg, R. G., Patlak, C. S., and Fenstermacher, J. D.,** Selection of experimental conditions for the accurate determination of blood-brain transfer constants from single-time experiments. A theoretical analysis, *J. Cereb. Blood Flow Metab.,* 3, 215, 1983.
53. **Hamilton, W. F.,** The physiology of cardiac output, *Circulation,* 8, 527, 1953.
54. **Lyons, D. T., Vasta, F., and Vannucci, R. C.,** Regional cerebral blood flow in the immature rat, *Pediatric Res.,* 21, 471, 1987.
55. **Bryan, R. M., Jr., Myers, C. L., and Page, R. B.,** Regional neurohypophysial and hypothalamic blood flow in rats during hypercapnia, *Am. J. Physiol.,* 255, R295, 1988.
56. **Ringle, M., Bryan, R. M., and Vannucci, R. C.,** Regional cerebral blood flow during hypoxia-ischemia in the immature rat: comparisons of iodoantipyrine and iodoamphetamine as radioactive tracers, *Dev. Brain Res.,* 59, 231, 1991.
57. **Goldman, H. and Wurtman, R.,** Flow of blood to the pineal body of the rat, *Nature,* 203, 87, 1964.
58. **Goldman, H.,** Vasopressin modulation of the distribution of the blood flow in the unanesthetized rat, *Neuroendocrinology,* 1, 23, 1965.

59. **Mohler, H. and Okada, T.,** Benzodiazepine receptor: demonstration in the central nervous system, *Science,* 198, 849, 1977.
60. **Warner, D. S., Kassell, N. F., and Boarini, D. J.,** Microsphere cerebral blood flow determination, in *Cerebral Blood Flow: Physiologic and Clinical Aspects,* Wood, J. H., Ed., McGraw-Hill, New York, 1987, Chapt. 17.
61. **Prinzmetal, M., Simkin, B., Bergman, H. C., and Kruger, H. E.,** Studies on the coronary circulation. II. The collateral circulation of the normal human heart by coronary perfusion with radioactive erythrocytes and glass spheres, *Am. Heart J.,* 33, 420, 1947.
62. **Rhodes, B. A., Zolle, I., Buchanan, J. W., and Wagner, H. N.,** Radioactive albumin microspheres for studies of the pulmonary circulation, *Radiology,* 92, 1453, 1969.
63. **Rudolph, A. M. and Heymann, M. A.,** The circulation of the fetus in utero: methods for studying distribution of blood flow, cardiac output, and organ blood flow, *Circ. Res.,* 21, 163, 1967.
64. **Alm, A.,** Radioactively labelled microspheres on regional blood flow determinations; a study on monkeys with 15 and 35 μm spheres, *Acta Physiol. Scand.,* 95, 60, 1975.
65. **Marcus, M. L., Heistad, D. D., Ehrhardt, J. C., Abboud, F. M.,** Total and regional cerebral blood flow measurement with 7-, 10-, 15-, 25-, and 50-μ microspheres, *J. Appl. Physiol.,* 40, 501, 1976.
66. **Heistad, D. D., Marcus, M. L., and Busija, D. W.,** Measurement of cerebral blood flow in experimental animals with microspheres: Applications of the method, in *Cerebral Metabolism and Neural Function,* Passonneau, J. V., Ed., Williams & Wilkins, Baltimore, 1980.
67. **Farrar, J. K.,** Hydrogen clearance technique, in *Cerebral Blood Flow: Physiologic and Clinical Aspects,* Wood, J. H., Ed., McGraw-Hill, New York, 1987, Chapt. 16.
68. **Misrahy, G. A. and Clark, L. C.,** Use of the platinum black cathode for local blood flow measurements in vivo, 20th Int. Physiol. Cong. (Aug), Brussels, Belgium 650, (Abstr.) 1956.
69. **Aukland, K., Bower, B. F., and Berliner, R. W.,** Measurement of local blood flow with H_2 gas, *Circ. Res.,* 14, 164, 1964.
70. **Young, W.,** H_2 clearance measurement of blood flow: a review of technique and polarographic principle, *Stroke,* 11, 552, 1980.
71. **Rowan, J. O., Reilly, P., Farrar, J. K., and Teasdale, G.,** The Xenon-133 and hydrogen clearance methods — A comparative analysis, in *Blood Flow and Metabolism in the Brain,* Harper, A. M., Jennet, W. B., Miller, J. D., and Rowan, J. O., Eds., Churchill Livingstone, Edinburgh, 1975, 7.9.
72. **Fieschi, C., Bozzao, L. Agnoli, A., Nardini, M., and Bartolini, A.,** The hydrogen method of measuring local blood flow in subcortical structures of the brain: including a comparative study with the ^{14}C-antipyrine method, *Exp. Brain Res.,* 7, 111, 1969.
73. **Kaneko, Z.,** First steps in the development of the Doppler flowmeter, *Ultrasound Med. Biol.,* 12, 1877, 1986.
74. **Aaslid, R., Markwalder, T.-M., and Nornes, H.,** Non-invasive transcranial Doppler ultrasound recording of flow-velocity in basal cerebral arteries, *J. Neurosurg.,* 57, 769, 1982.
75. **Newell, D. W. and Aaslid, R.,** Transcranial Doppler: Clinical and experimental uses, *Cerebrovasc. Brain Metab. Rev.,* 4, 122, 1992.
76. **Haberl, R. L., Heizer, M. L., Marmarou, A., and Ellis, E. F.,** Laser-Doppler assessment of brain microcirculation: effect of systemic alterations, *Am. J. Physiol.,* 256, H1247, 1989.
78. **Rosenblum, B. R., Bonner, R. F., and Oldfield, E. H.,** Intraoperative measurement of cortical blood flow adjacent to cerebral AVM using laser-Doppler velocimetry, *J. Neurosurg.,* 66, 396, 1987.
79. **Arbit, E., DiResta, G. R., Bedford, R. R., Shak, N. K., and Galicich, J. H.,** Intraoperative measurement of cerebral and tumor blood flow with laser-Doppler flowmetry, *Neurosurgery,* 24, 166, 1989.

80. **Obrist, W. D. and Wilkinson, W. E.,** Regional cerebral blood flow measurement in humans by Xenon-133 clearance, *Cerebrovasc. Metab. Rev.*, 2, 283, 1990.
81. **Jaggi, J. L. and Obrist, W. D.,** Regional cerebral blood flow determined by ^{133}Xenon clearance, in *Cerebral Blood Flow: Physiologic and Clinical Aspects,* Wood, J. H., Ed., McGraw-Hill, New York, 1987, Chapt. 11.
82. **Jaggi, J. L., Lipp, A. E., and Duc, G.,** Measurement of cerebral blood flow with a non-invasive Xenon-133 method in pre-term infants, in *Physiologic Foundations of Prenatal Care,* Stern, L., Orzalesi, M., and Friis-Hansen, B., Eds., Elsevier, New York, Vol. 3, 1989, Chapt. 25.
83. **Obrist, W. D., Thompson, H. K., Jr., King, C. H., and Wang, H. S.,** Determination of regional cerebral blood flow by inhalation of ^{133}Xenon, *Circ. Res.*, 20, 124, 1967.
84. **Mallett, B. L. and Veall, N.,** The measurement of regional cerebral clearance rates in man using Xenon-133 inhalation and extracranial recording, *Clin. Sci.*, 29, 179, 1965.
85. **Obrist, W. D., Wang, H. S., Wilkinson, W. E., and Harel, D.,** The non-invasive 133Xe method: Influence of the input function on computed rCBF values, in *Handbook of Regional Cerebral Blood Flow,* Knezevic, S., Maximilian, V. A., Mubrin, Z., Prohovnick, I., and Wade, I., Eds., Laurence Erlbaum, Assoc., Hillsdale, NJ, 1988.
86. **Drayer, B. P., Wolfson, S. K., Jr., Reinmuth, O. M., Dujovny, M., Boehake, M., and Cook, E. E.,** Xenon enhanced computed tomography for the analysis of cerebral integrity, perfusion, and blood flow, *Stroke,* 9, 123, 1978.
87. **Kelcz, F., Hilal, S. K., Hartwell, P., and Joseph, P. M.,** Computed tomographic measurement of xenon brain-blood partition coefficient and implication for regional cerebral blood flow: a preliminary report, *Radiology,* 127, 385, 1978.
88. **Gur, D., Wolfson, S. K., Jr., Yonas, H., Good, W. F., Shabason, L., Latchaw, R. E., Miller, D. M., and Cook, E. E.,** Progress in cerebrovascular disease: local cerebral blood flow by xenon enhanced CT, *Stroke,* 13, 750, 1982.
89. **Yonas, H. W., Gur, D., Latchaw, R. E., and Wolfson, S. K.,** Xenon computed tomographic blood flow mapping, in *Cerebral Blood Flow: Physiologic and Clinical Aspects,* Wood, J. H., Ed., McGrawHill, New York, 1987, Chapt. 13.
90. **Fatouros, P. P., Wist, A. O., Marmarou, A., DeWitt, D. S., Keenan, R. L., and Kishore, P. R. S.,** Development, validation, and use of stable xenon-enhanced computed tomography at the Medical College of Virginia, in *Cerebral Blood Flow Measurement with Stable Xenon-Enhanced Computed Tomography,* Yonas, H., Ed., Raven Press, New York, 1992, 22.
91. **DeWitt, D. S., Fatouros, P. P., Wist, A. O., et al.,** Stable xenon versus radiolabeled microsphere cerebral blood flow measurements in baboons, *Stroke,* 20, 1716, 1989.
92. **Marion, D. W. and Bouma, G. J.,** The use of stable Xenon-enhanced computed tomographic studies of cerebral blood flow to define changes in cerebral carbon dioxide vasoresponsivity caused by severe head injury, *Neurosurgery,* 29, 869, 1991.
93. **Winchell, H. S., Horst, W. D., Bravn, L., Oldendorf, W. H., Hattner, R., and Parker, H.,** N-isopropyl-[I-123] p-iodoamphetamine: single-pass brain uptake and washout; binding to brain synaptosomes and localization in dog and monkey brain, *J. Nucl. Med.*, 21, 947, 1980.
94. **Kuhl, D. E., Barrio, J. R., Huang, S. C., Selin, C., Ackermann, R. F., Lear, J. L., Wu, T. H., Lin, T. H., and Phelps, M. E.,** Quantifying local cerebral blood flow by N-isopropyl-p-(123-I) iodoamphetamine (imp) tomography, *J. Nucl. Med.*, 23, 196, 1982.
95. **Ell, P. J., Hocknell, J. M. L., Jarritt, P. H., Cullum, I., Lui, D., Campos-Costa, D., Nowotnik, D. P., Pickett, R. D., Canning, L. R., and Neirinckx, R. D.,** A Tc-99-labelled radiotracer for the investigation of cerebrovascular disease, *Nucl. Med. Commun.*, 6, 437, 1985.
96. **Powers, W. J. and Raichle, M. E.,** Positron emission tomography and its application to the study of cerebrovascular disease in man, *Stroke,* 16, 361, 1985.

97. **Phelps, M. E., Mazziotta, J. C., and Schelbert, H. R., Eds.,** *Positron Emission Tomography and Autoradiographic Principles and Applications for the Brain and Heart,* Raven Press, New York, 1986.
98. **Herscovitch, P. and Powers, W. J.,** Measurement of regional cerebral blood flow by positron emission tomography, in *Cerebral Blood Flow: Physiologic and Clinical Aspects,* Wood, J. H., Ed., McGraw-Hill, New York, 1987, Chapt. 15.
99. **Jones, T.,** Measurement of regional tissue physiology using positron emission tomography, *News in Physiological Science,* 3, 230, 1988.
100. **Berridge, M. S., Adler, L. P., Nelson, A. A., Cassidy, E. H., Muzic, R. F., Bednarczyk, E. M., and Miraldi, F.,** Measurement of human cerebral blood flow with [^{15}O] butanol and positron emission tomography, *J. Cereb. Blood Flow Metab.,* 11, 707, 1991.
101. **Axel, L.,** Cerebral blood flow determination by rapid-sequence computed tomography, *Radiology,* 137, 679, 1980.
102. **Gobbel, G. T., Cann, C. E., Iwamoto, H. S., and Fike, J. R.,** Measurement of regional cerebral blood flow using ultrafast computed tomography: theoretical aspects and experimental validation, *Stroke,* 22, 768, 1991.
103. **Gibson, J. G., Seligman, A. M., Peakock, W. C., Aub, J. C., Fine, J., and Evans, R. D.,** The distribution of red cells and plasma in large and minute vessels of the normal dog, determined by radioactive isotopes of iron and iodine, *J. Clin. Invest.,* 25, 848, 1946.
104. **Cremer, J. E. and Seville, M. P.,** Regional brain blood flow, blood volume and haematocrit values in the adult rat, *J. Cereb. Blood Flow Metab.,* 3, 254, 1983.
105. **Mansfield, P.,** Multiplanar image formation using NMR spin echoes, *J. Phys. C.,* 10, L55, 1977.
106. **Axel, L.,** Blood flow effects in magnetic-resonance imaging, *Am. J. Roentgenol.,* 143, 1157, 1984.
107. **Firmin, D. N., Klipstein, R. H., Hounsfield, G. L., Paley, M. P., and Longmore, D. B.,** Echo-planar high-resolution flow velocity mapping, *Magn. Reson. Med.,* 12, 316, 1987.
108. **Moseley, M. E., Kucharczyk, J., Mintorovitch, J. Cohen, Y., Kurhanew, J., Derugin, N., Asgari, H., and Norman, D.,** Diffusion-weighted MR imaging of acute stroke: Correlation with T2-weighted and magnetic susceptibility-enhanced MR imaging in cats, *Am. J. Neuroradiol.,* 11, 423, 1990.
109. **Belliveau, J. W., Kennedy, D. N., McKinstry, R. C., Buchbinder, B. R., Weisskoff, R. M., Cohen, M. S., Vevea, J. M., Brady, T. J., and Rosen, B. R.,** Functional mapping in the human visual cortex by magnetic resonance imaging, *Science,* 254, 716, 1991.
110. **Stehling, M. K., Turner, R., and Mansfield, P.,** Echo-planar imaging: magnetic resonance imaging in a fraction of a second, *Science,* 254, 43, 1991.
111. **Hall, L. D. and Williams, S. C. R.,** Nuclear magnetic resonance imaging, in *Cerebral Blood Flow: Mathematical Models, Instrumentation, and Imaging Techniques,* Rescigno, A. and Boicelli, A., Eds., Plenum Press, New York, 1986, 185.
112. **Detre, J. A., Subramanian, V. H., Mitchell, M. D., Smith, D. S., Kobayashi, A., Zaman, A., and Leigh, J. S., Jr.,** Measurement of regional cerebral blood flow in cat brain using intracarotid ^2H_2O and ^2H NMR imaging, *Magn. Reson. Med.,* 14, 389, 1990.
113. **Rosen, B. R., Belliveau, J. W., and Chien, D.,** Perfusion imaging by nuclear magnetic resonance, *Magn. Reson. Q.,* 5, 263, 1989.
114. **Evelhoch, J. L., Larcombe-McDouall, J. B., Mattiello, J., and Simpson, N. F.,** Measurement of relative regional tumor blood flow in mice by deuterium NMR imaging, *Magn. Reson. Med.,* 24, 42, 1992.
115. **Bloch, F., Hansen, W. W., and Packard, M.,** Nuclear induction, *Phys. Rev.,* 69, 127, 1946.

116. **Purcell, E. M., Torrey, H. C., and Pound, R. V.,** Resonance absorption by nuclear magnetic moments in a solid, *Phys. Rev.*, 69, 37, 1946.
117. **Turner, R.,** Perfusion studies and fast imaging, in *Cerebral Blood Flow: Mathematical Models, Instrumentation, and Imaging Techniques,* Rescigno, A. and Boicelli, A., Eds., Plenum Press, New York, 1986, 245.
118. **Rosen, B. R., Belliveau, J. W., Vevea, J. M., and Brady, T. J.,** Perfusion imaging with NMR contrast agents, *Magn. Reson. Med.*, 14, 249, 1990.
119. **Ewing, J. R., Branch, C. A., Helpern, J. A., Smith, M. B., Butt, S. M., and Welch, K. M. A.,** Cerebral blood flow measured by indicator dilution in cats, *Stroke,* 20, 259, 1989.
120. **Ackerman, J. H., Ewy, C. S., Becker, N. N., and Shalwitz, R. A.,** Deuterium nuclear magnetic resonance measurements of blood flow and tissue perfusion employing ^2H_2O as a freely diffusible tracer, *Proc. Natl. Acad. Sci.*, 34, 4099, 1987.
121. **Heiss, W.-D. and Traupe, H.,** Comparison between hydrogen clearance and microsphere technique for RCBF measurement, *Stroke,* 12, 161, 1981.
122. **Mansfield, P. and Grannell, P. K.,** NMR diffraction in solids, *J. Phys. C.*, 6, L422, 1973.
123. **Gjedde, A., Drewes, L. R., and Christensen, B.,** Brain uptake of a fluid microsphere: comparison of flunitrazepam, water, and iodoantipyrine transfer across the blood-brain barrier, *J. Cereb. Blood Flow Metab.*, 3, 8, 1983.
124. **Holman, L. and Hill, T. C.,** Perfusion imaging with single-photon emission computed tomography, in *Cerebral Blood Flow: Physiologic and Clinical Aspects,* Wood, J. H., Ed., McGraw-Hill, New York, 1987, Chapt. 14.

Chapter 2

ELECTROPHYSIOLOGICAL MECHANISMS OF CEREBRAL ARTERIAL MUSCLE ACTIVATION: INFLUENCES OF ENVIRONMENTAL STIMULI

David R. Harder

TABLE OF CONTENTS

I. Introduction 34

II. Membrane Potential and Regulation of Tone in Cerebral Arterial Muscle 34
- A. K^+ Currents in Cerebral Arterial Muscle 35
- B. Ca^{2+} Channels in Cerebral Arterial Muscle 37

III. Physical and Environmental Factors Affecting Membrane Electrical Events in Cerebral Arterial Muscle 37
- A. Transmural Pressure and Electromechanical Coupling in Cerebral Arterial Muscle 37
- B. Effect of P_{O_2} on Membrane Properties of Cerebral Arterial Muscle 40
- C. Effect of P_{CO_2} and pH on Electrophysiological Properties of Cerebral Arterial Muscle 41

References 42

0-8493-5096-0/93/$0.00 + $.50

I. INTRODUCTION

The Final Common Pathway for the regulation of cerebral arterial tone is activation of the vascular muscle cells. The determinates of this response and whether this response occurs in a normal or abnormal way depends upon cellular mechanisms responsible in bringing about that muscle cell activation. The degree of activation of cerebral arterial muscle is largely influenced by electrical events occurring at the plasma membrane. Recent findings have demonstrated that the electrophysiological properties of arterial muscle, in general, and specifically cerebral arterial muscle, can be directly and/or indirectly influenced by local environmental conditions, which have been demonstrated to modify and/or control cerebral vascular reactivity. Local metabolic influences include such things as pH, P_{CO_2}, oxygen, and the mechanical forces of pressure and flow. This chapter will separate these local influences from metabolic and neural-humoral control. The reason for such separation is that these environmental stimuli appear to set a basal level of vascular tone upon which the second-to-second and minute-to-minute regulation of nutritional flow occurs. This chapter will focus upon the influence of the gaseous and physical environmental factors upon the cellular and ionic mechanisms responsible for arterial muscle cell activation.

II. MEMBRANE POTENTIAL AND REGULATION OF TONE IN CEREBRAL ARTERIAL MUSCLE

Electrophysiological events occurring at the plasma membrane regulate many cellular functions within excitable cells. With respect to arterial muscle, one of the principal events regulated, to a large extent by changes in resting membrane potential in nondividing differentiated cells, is activation of contractile elements and cell shortening. The precise degree of membrane control involved in activation of arterial muscle varies, depending upon the nature of the stimulus initiating the event.

The resting membrane potential (E_m) of cerebral arterial muscle studied in an organ bath is between -60 and -70 mV.[1,2] This E_m is established and maintained largely by the muscle cell permeability to K^+. The slope of the relationship between E_m and extracellular K^+ approaches 60 mV per tenfold change (decade) between 10 and 100 m*M* $[K]_o$.[1] This is the value predicted by constant field theory for a K^+ selective membrane.[3] The contributions of other ion species, namely, Na^+ and Cl^-, are small.[4]

It is difficult to determine the contribution of active transport to the E_m in cerebral arterial muscle. Reduction of extracellular K^+ depolarizes cerebral arterial muscle;[1] however, it is difficult to determine if this is due to a primary inhibition of Na-K ATPase or reduction in K^+ conductance (g_K). Application of ouabain to cat basilar artery results in a 12 mV depolarization;[5] on face value one could conclude that most of this depolarization was due to inhibition

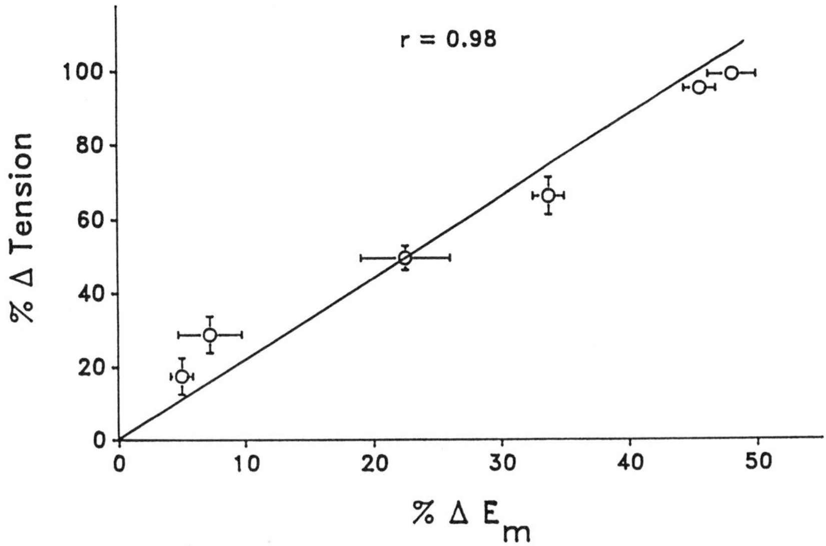

FIGURE 1. Relationship between change in membrane potential (ΔE_m) and development in tension (Δ tension) in isolated cat cerebral arteries. Activation was induced by increasing doses of serotonin beginning at 3×10^{-9} *M*. (From Harder, D. R. and Waters, A., *Intl. Rev. Cytol.*, 89, 1, 1984. With permission.)

of Na-K ATPase except for the finding that ouabain may also inhibit g_K in arteriolar smooth muscle.[6] Thus, one can conclude that the electrogenic transport of Na^+ and K^+ in cerebral arterial muscle contributes to the E_m; however, it is difficult to determine the exact extent.

There is very tight coupling between electrical and mechanical events in cerebral arterial muscle. The high degree of electromechanical coupling in cat cerebral arteries is depicted in Figure 1. As can be seen, a change of only a few mV will elicit a substantial increase in tension. In K^+ depolarized canine carotid arteries, a 3 mV depolarization results in a large contraction.[7]

Cerebral arterial muscle is capable of generating action potentials in response to membrane depolarization.[1,8] The primary ion species carrying the inward current is Ca^{2+}. Action potential amplitude is not affected by tetrodotoxin and is markedly reduced by verapamil and inorganic Ca^{2+} channel blockers.[8]

A. K^+ CURRENTS IN CEREBRAL ARTERIAL MUSCLE

A number of K^+ channels have been identified in arterial muscle. These channels are voltage activated and have been characterized based upon their sensitivity to known blockers of g_K, namely, 4-aminopyridine (4-AP) and tetraethylammonium (TEA).[4] Thus far, three physiologically relevant types of K^+ channels which probably play a role in the regulation of vascular

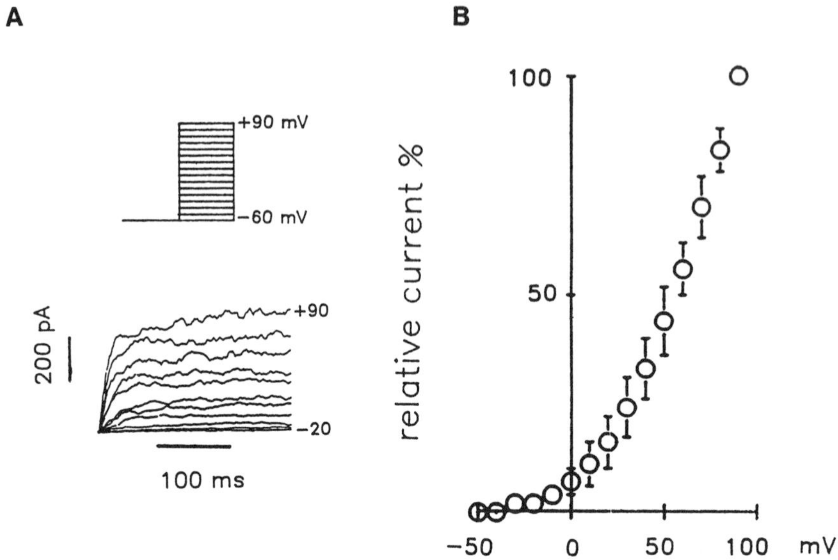

FIGURE 2. Data obtained from voltage-clamped cat cerebral arterial smooth muscle cells. (A) Actual recordings of outward current in a patch-clamped cell (bottom trace), and the command step protocol (top panel) used to produce the current traces. Holding potential (HP) was −60mV. (B) Normalized (% relative current) current/voltage (I/V) relationships obtained from 12 voltage-clamped cells. The vertical bars are standard deviations of the mean values. (From Bonnet, P. et al., *Pfluegers Arch.*, 418, 292, 1991. With permission.)

muscle activation have been identified; these are a delayed rectifier K^+ channel,[9] a Ca^{2+} regulated outward current,[10-13] and an ATP-sensitive K^+ channel.[14] The Ca^{2+}-sensitive K^+ channel is activated as intracellular Ca^{2+} increases, but may be sensitive to extracellular Ca^{2+} as well. The ATP-sensitive K^+ channel is turned off as intracellular ATP increases beyond some critical value and is sensitive to sulfonylurea blockers. The ATP-sensitive channel may not be sensitive only to ATP but may also be regulated by a variety of intracellular mediators including pH.[15,16]

A delayed rectifier K^+ current has been described in cerebral arterial muscle studied in the whole cell voltage clamp mode, which is sensitive to 4-AP and is activated at depolarizing voltages beyond −30 mV (Figure 2).[17]

Single channel recording from cellattached cat cerebral arterial muscle cells demonstrates up to three channel types (unpublished observations). The largest of these three channel types exhibits a unitary conductance around 200 pS and expresses a marked increase in open time probability (NP_o) upon elevation of intracellular Ca^{2+} in excised inside-out membrane patches. This Ca^{2+}-sensitive K^+ channel (K^+_{Ca}) will be discussed in more detail later.

B. Ca^{2+} CHANNELS IN CEREBRAL ARTERIAL MUSCLE

Two primary types of Ca^{2+} channels have been described in arterial muscle based upon the voltage ranges at which activation occurs and their sensitivity to dihydropyridines. An L-type Ca^{2+} channel is sensitive to dihydropyridines and is maintained in a conductive state during prolonged depolarization.[18] The second type of Ca^{2+} current in arterial muscle is referred to as a "T-type" current. It is transient in nature, has a lower threshold for activation, and is insensitive to dihydropyridines.[19]

Voltage-dependent Ca^{2+} channels have been identified in cerebral arterial muscle. Two types of Ca^{2+} channel have been identified in cell-attached patches of rabbit cerebral arteries with unitary conductances of 9 and 5 pS using barium as the charge carrier.[20] In rat cerebral arteries, a voltage-dependent Ca^{2+} channel with a conductance of 30 pS (80 m*M* Ba^{2+} as the charge carrier) has also been identified.[21] In a recent review Nelson et al.[22] have identified a voltage-dependent Ca^{2+} channel from rabbit cerebral arteries recorded in solutions containing 10 m*M* Ca^{2+} in which the probability of opening was significantly reduced as the membrane was hyperpolarized beyond -40 mV and in which serotonin markedly increased the frequency of opening and mean open time. In guinea pig basilar artery, an L-type Ca^{2+} current has been identified using 10 m*M* Ba^{2+} as the charge carrier with a peak current in the whole cell mode of 292 pA at $+15$ mV.[23] From these studies it is clear that voltage-operated Ca^{2+} channels probably play an important role in the activation of cerebral arterial muscle and that neurohumoral agents such as serotonin can activate this particular conductance system.

III. PHYSICAL AND ENVIRONMENTAL FACTORS AFFECTING MEMBRANE ELECTRICAL EVENTS IN CEREBRAL ARTERIAL MUSCLE

Agents which depolarize or hyperpolarize cerebral arterial muscle will activate or inhibit activation, respectively. A recent review by Hirst and Edwards[4] has covered the electrophysiological responses to many of the relevant neurotransmitters and humoral agents affecting arterial muscle that are also relevant to cerebral vascular muscle. This discussion will focus on the effects of transmural pressure, P_{O_2}, P_{CO_2}, and pH on electrophysiological properties of cerebral arterial muscle.

A. TRANSMURAL PRESSURE AND ELECTROMECHANICAL COUPLING IN CEREBRAL ARTERIAL MUSCLE

Increasing transmural pressure in isolated cerebral arterial segments depolarizes muscle cells, induces spontaneous action potential generation, and reduces internal diameter.[24] Increasing transmural pressure in cat middle cerebral arteries from 20 to 160 mmHg decreased E_m from -68 to around -36 mV. The slope relating the change in E_m to the change in pressure increased as Ca^{2+} was elevated in the perfusion media and decreased upon reduction of Ca^{2+} below control levels.[24] The frequency of spontaneous electrical spike activity in these isolated pressurized cerebral arteries increased as transmural pressure was increased from 100 to 140 mmHg. These findings suggest that either pressure or the subsequent mechanical deformation of the vascular muscle wall activates arterial muscle by depolarizing the membrane and increasing Ca^{2+} permeability.

The ''sensor'' translating the mechanical stimulus into the observed biophysical processes in arterial muscle is not yet well defined. Similar phenomenon have been documented in a variety of vascular beds.[25,26] Over the past 5 years a number of laboratories have examined the role of the vascular endothelium in this regard; however, there is currently a good bit of controversy centered around the best way to remove the endothelium and in which vascular beds the endothelium may play a role.[27,28] Endothelial contractile factors have been identified in the aorta. Endothelin is a potent vasoactive peptide which has been shown to open Ca^{2+} channels and, therefore, is a prime candidate for a pressure-released endothelial contractile factor.[29] However, endothelin has not been shown to be released from pressurized cerebral arteries and generally does not fit the profile necessary to act as a mediator in this regard.[29]

An obvious possibility for a ''pressure-sensor'' in arterial muscle is a ''stretch-activated'' ion channel either in the vascular muscle, endothelial cell, or both. Such mechanosensitive ion channels have been described in a wide variety of cell types including smooth muscle and aortic endothelial cells.[30] The majority of mechanosensitive ion channels are nonspecific and exhibit conductance for multiple ion species with the greatest level of selectivity being either for cations or anions.[30] These mechanosensitive channels are generally studied under patch clamp conditions and usually conduct current with a sufficiently large magnitude to have a large effect on E_m, and, therefore, must be considered as a plausible mediator for the muscle cell depolarization and action potential generation observed in cerebral arteries upon elevations in transmural pressure.

Several reports have demonstrated that inhibition of protein kinase C(PKC) can inhibit pressure-induced activation of arteries and that phorbol esters augment myogenic tone.[31,32] PKC is activated by 1,2-diacylglycerol (1,2-DAG) formed via metabolism of phosphoinositide lipids.[33] Activation of phospholipase C(PLC) through a membrane receptor G protein complex, or possibly mechanical deformation, cleaves phosphatidylinositol 4,5-biphosphate (Ptd-Ins 4,5 P_2) into the hydrophobic 1,2-DAG and water-soluble inositol 1,4,5-triphosphate (IP_3). IP_3 elevates intracellular Ca^{2+} by its action on intracellular stores. 1,2-DAG serves as a second messenger to activate PKC, which has many cellular functions including phosphorylation of membrane ion channels.[34,35] At present, it is not known how pressure activates PKC; however, we have preliminary data demonstrating that IP_3 is elevated in dog renal arteries as transmural pressure is increased, suggesting that pressure stimulates PLC activity in the arterial wall.[36]

Recent studies from our laboratory have demonstrated that inhibition of cytochrome P-450 enzymes markedly attentuates pressure-induced myogenic tone and that increasing substrate availability by supplying exogenous arachidonic acid enhances the myogenic response. We have also identified a cytochrome P-450 arachidonic acid (AA) metabolite from renal artery microsomal fractions which coelutes with 20-hydroxyeicosatetraenoic acid (20-HETE) upon reverse-phase HPLC.

There are two primary sources for the release of AA in arterial muscle, namely, from phosphatidylcholine by the action of phospholipase A_2 and from 1,2-DAG through the action of DAG lipase.[37] Given our findings, and those of others, that PLC activity is enhanced upon pressure-induced activation of arteries, it seems likely that the source of AA for production of 20-HETE is from 1,2-DAG.

When 20-HETE is applied to isolated dog renal arterial muscle cells loaded with the fluorescent Ca^{2+} probe FURA-2, we typically observe a large increase in signal indicating a large rise in $[Ca]_i$. In addition, we have a good deal of data demonstrating that isolated 20-HETE contracts and depolarizes renal arterial muscle by an action which is to inhibit K^+ channel activity. These effects of 20-HETE are most likely not due to nonspecific actions of fatty acids in that the effect of AA on isolated renal arterial membrane patches is to markedly increase K^+ channel activity.

Thus, 20-HETE fulfills the requirements as a potential mediator of pressure-induced myogenic tone, i.e., (1) inhibition of its formation blocks the myogenic response to pressure; (2) increasing the concentration of the substrate (AA) for 20-HETE enhances the response to pressure; and (3) the product itself has an action on isolated vessels mimicking the response to pressure. An overall scenario encompassing these ideas is depicted in Figure 3.

The E_m at a transmural pressure of 100 to 120 mmHg is between -40 and -45 mV.[24] Taken at face value, this would mean that at a normal level of arterial pressure the E_m is always at or near a mechanical threshold of around -50 mV *in vivo*. This level of E_m also brings the plasma membrane closer to the operational voltages for K^+ and Ca^{2+} channels than we had previously thought, derived from the studies done in nonpressurized arterial preparations or single cells.[4] The operational voltage range for K^+ channels begins at around -30 mV and for Ca^{2+} channels at around -40 mV.[4,22] Thus, the higher the pressure and the greater the degree of depolarization, the more reactive the arterial muscle to influences which operate via ionic- or voltage-dependent mechanisms. Indeed, in cat cerebral arteries, as transmural pressure is elevated, the sensitivity to serotonin increases by an entire order of magnitude between 60 and 140 mmHg.[38]

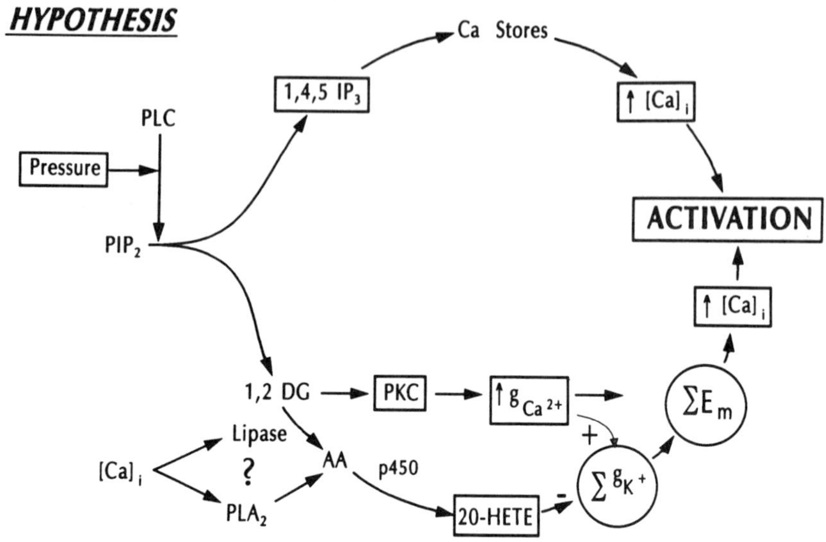

FIGURE 3. Proposed mechanism for pressure-induced activation of arterial muscle.

B. EFFECT OF P_{O_2} ON MEMBRANE PROPERTIES OF CEREBRAL ARTERIAL MUSCLE

The direct effects of O_2 on cerebral arterial muscle are difficult to determine. Siegel and Grote[39] have shown that reducing P_{O_2} from 160 to 40 torr hyperpolarizes and relaxes muscle cells within canine carotid arteries. However, there are several reports that hypoxia enhances EDRF release, and EDRF hyperpolarizes cerebral arterial muscle.[40] Thus, it is difficult to ascertain the direct effect of reducing O_2 on cerebral arterial muscle from the indirect effects of EDRF.

Recently, however, Pearce et al.[41] have demonstrated that hypoxia relaxes rabbit common carotid arteries, demonstrating a direct effect of hypoxia on arterial muscle. Hypoxia also inhibits Ca^{2+} dependent action potential generation in cat cerebral arteries.[42] In other vascular muscle preparations, hypoxia is thought to reduce tone by increasing the activity of an ATP sensitive K^+ channel.[43] As discussed previously, when the level of intracellular ATP drops, there is an increase in single K^+ channel activity. It is, therefore, a seemingly logical mechanism that hypoxia will reduce intracellular ATP, increase outward current, hyperpolarize, and then relax arterial muscle. However, the predominant K^+ channel type found in cerebral arterial muscle cells is the K^+_{Ca}. The K^+_{Ca} is a large conductance channel, around 200 pS in excised membrane patches or when studied in cell attached membrane patches in symmetrical K^+. We have shown that reduction of O_2 from 20 to $<3\%$ significantly increases the probability of opening (NP_o) and mean open time in both cell-attached or excised membrane patches. Given the large con-

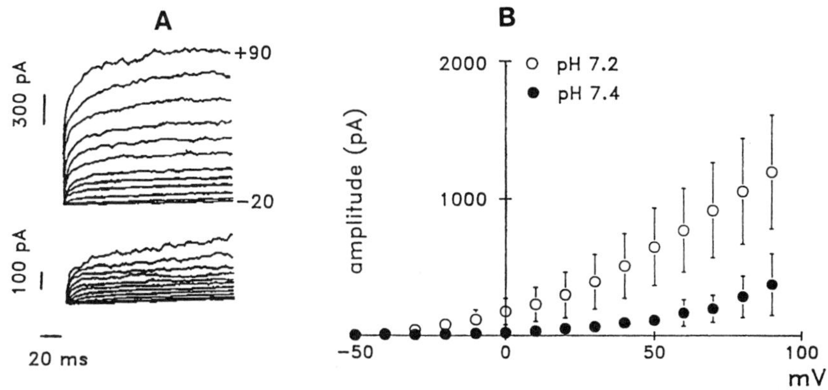

FIGURE 4. Figure depicting the effect of reduction of extracellular pH on outward K^+ currents in isolated, patch-clamped cat cerebral arterial muscle cells. Note: the large increase in peak outward current as pH is lowered from 7.43 to 7.2. (From Bonnet, P. et al., *Pfluegers Arch.*, 418, 292, 1991. With permission.)

ductance of the K^+_{Ca} and its predominance in cerebral arterial muscle, it is not difficult to imagine that even a small increase in activity can hyperpolarize cerebral arterial muscle and mediate relaxation. It is interesting to note that in pulmonary arteries where hypoxia contracts, reduction of PO_2 reduces the activity of the K^+_{Ca}, which would be expected to depolarize and contract.[44]

C. EFFECT OF P_{CO_2} AND pH ON ELECTROPHYSIOLOGICAL PROPERTIES OF CEREBRAL ARTERIAL MUSCLE

Reduction of extracellular pH either by increases in P_{CO_2} or H^+ dilates cerebral arteries. This dilation is mediated by membrane hyperpolarization in isolated cat cerebral arteries.[45] Reduction of P_{CO_2} or elevation of pH while maintaining P_{CO_2} constant depolarizes and contracts cat cerebral arteries.[46] Both of these effects are apparently mediated at least in part by changes in g_K, i.e., reduction of pH or elevation of P_{CO_2} increases the slope of the curve relating changes in E_m to changes in $[K]_o$ consistent with an increase in g_K, while increasing pH or reducing P_{CO_2} reduces the slope of this curve indicating a decrease in g_K according to constant field theory.[3]

Recently we have been able to assess directly the effect of pH on K^+ currents in isolated cerebral arterial muscle cells. In patch-clamped cat cerebral arterial muscle, reduction of pH from 7.4 to 7.20 greatly increases the peak outward current by 35% in 60% of the cells studied in this regard.[17] Figure 4 summarizes the effect of reducing pH on outward K^+ currents in cerebral arterial muscle. It is possible that H^+ may have a direct effect on K^+ channels in that the data in Figure 4 was recorded in the whole cell mode in which the cell cytoplasm is dialyzed and contiguous with the pipette solutions containing 10 m*M* HEPES, which would be expected to buffer any significant changes in intracellular pH. It is also possible that changing pH on either side of the plasma membrane affects channel conductances by altering the "field potential" and, thus, the conformational state of the channel proteins. Given that pH can affect many cellular processes, it is difficult to determine which effect may act directly on ion channels or which may be secondary. A recent report suggests that pH does not affect outward currents in the guinea pig basilar artery.[47]

REFERENCES

1. **Harder, D. R.,** Comparison of electrical properties of middle cerebral and mesenteric artery in cat, *Am. J. Physiol.,* 239, C23, 1980.
2. **Harder, D. R. and Madden, J. A.,** in *Neural Regulation of Brain Circulation,* Elsevier, Amsterdam, 1986, 81.
3. **Sperelakis, N.,** Origin of the cardiac resting potential, in *Handbook of Physiology — The Cardiovascular System,* Vol. 1, Berne, R. M., Ed., American Physiology Society, Bethesda, MD, 1979, 187.
4. **Hirst, G. D. S. and Edwards, F. R.,** Sympathetic neuroeffector transmission in arteries and arterioles, *Physiol. Rev.,* 69, 546, 1989.
5. **Waters, A. and Harder, D. R.,** Altered membrane properties of cerebral vascular smooth muscle following subarachnoid hemorrhage: an electrophysiological study, *Stroke,* 16, 990, 1985.
6. **Hirst, G. D. S. and Van Helden, D. F.,** Ionic basis of the resting potential of submucosal arterioles in the ileum of the guinea-pig, *J. Physiol. (London),* 333, 53, 1982.
7. **Siegel, A., Wiesert, G., Ehehalt, R., and Bertusche, O.,** Membrane basis of vascular regulation, in *Ionic Actions on Vascular Smooth Muscle,* Betz, E., Ed., Springer-Verlag, New York, 1976, 48.
8. **Hirst, G. D. S., Silverberg, G. D., and Van Helden, D. F.,** The action potential and underlying ionic currents in proximal rat middle cerebral arterioles, *J. Physiol.,* 371, 289, 1986.
9. **Okabe, K., Kitamura, K., and Kuriyama, H.,** Features of 4-aminopyridine sensitive outward current observed in single smooth muscle cells from rabbit pulmonary artery, *Pfluegers Arch.,* 409, 561, 1987.
10. **Wilde, D. W. and Lee, K. S.,** Outward potassium currents in freshly isolated smooth muscle cells of dog coronary arteries, *Circ. Res.,* 65, 1718, 1989.
11. **Benham, C. D., Bolton, T. B., Lang, R. J., and Takewaki, T.,** Calcium activated potassium channels in single smooth muscle cells of rabbit jejunum and guinea-pig mesenteric artery, *J. Physiol.,* 371, 45, 1986.
12. **Inoue, R., Kitamura, K., and Kuriyama, H.,** Two Ca-dependent K-channels classified by the application of tetraethylammonium distribute to smooth muscles membranes of the rabbit portal vein, *Pfluegers Arch.,* 405, 173, 1985.
13. **Ohya, Y., Kitamara, K., and Kuriyama, H.,** Cellular calcium regulates outward currents in rabbit intestinal smooth muscle, *Am. J. Physiol.,* 252, C401, 1987.
14. **Standen, N. B., Quayle, J. M., Davies, N. W., Brayden, J. E., Huang, Y., and Nelson, M. T.,** Hyperpolarizing vasodilators activate ATP-sensitive K^+ channels in arterial smooth muscle, *Science,* 245, 309, 1989.
15. **Ashcroft, F. M.,** Adenosine 5′-triphosphate-sensitive potassium channels, *Annu. Rev. Neurosci.,* 11, 97, 1988.

16. **Davies, N. W.,** ATP-sensitive K^+ channels in skeletal muscle are modulated by intracellular protons, *Nature,* 343, 375, 1990.
17. **Bonnet, P., Rusch, N. J., and Harder, D. R.,** Characterization of an outward K^+ in freshly dispersed cerebral arterial muscle cells, *Pfluegers Arch.,* 418, 292, 1991.
18. **Benham, C. D., Hess, P., and Tsien, R. W.,** Two types of calcium channels in single smooth muscle cells from rabbit ear artery studied with whole-cell and single channel recordings, *Circ. Res.,* 61(Suppl. 1), 110, 1987.
19. **Bean, B. P., Sturek, M., Puga, A., and Hermsmeyer, K.,** Calcium channels in muscle cells isolated from rat mesenteric arteries: modulation by dihydropyridine drugs, *Circ. Res.,* 59, 229, 1986.
20. **Quayle, J. M. and Nelson, M. T.,** Calcium currents through single calcium channels in smooth muscle cells from cerebral arteries, *Biophys. J.* (Abstr.), 57, 301a, 1990.
21. **Quayle, J. M., McCarron, J., Halpern, W., and Nelson, M. T.,** Calcium channels and tone in normotensive and hypertensive rat resistance sized arteries, *Biophys. J.* (Abstr.), 57, 301a, 1990.
22. **Nelson, M. T., Patlak, J. B., Worley, J. F., and Standen, N. B.,** Calcium channels, potassium channels, and voltage dependence of arterial smooth muscle tone, *Am. Physiol. Soc.* (Brief Review), C3, 1990.
23. **Simard, M. J.,** Calcium channel currents in isolated smooth muscle cells of the guinea pig, *Pfluegers Arch.,* in press.
24. **Harder, D. R.,** Pressure-dependent membrane depolarization in cat middle cerebral artery, *Circ. Res.,* 55, 197, 1984.
25. **Smeda, J. S. and Daniel, E. E.,** Elevations in arterial pressure induce the formation of spontaneous action potentials and alter neurotransmission in canine ileum arteries, *Circ. Res.,* 62, 1104, 1988.
26. **Osol, G. and Halpern, W.,** Myogenic properties of cerebral blood vessels from normotensive and hypertensive rats, *Am. J. Physiol.,* 249 (*Heart Circ. Physiol.,* 18), H914, 1985.
27. **McCarron, J. G., Osol, G., and Halpern, W.,** Myogenic responses are independent of the endothelium in rat pressurized posterior cerebral arteries, *Blood Vessels,* 26, 315, 1989.
28. **Osol, G., Cipolla, M. and Knutson, S.,** A new method for mechanically denuding the endothelium of small (50–150 μm) arteries with a human hair, *Blood Vessels,* 26, 320, 1989.
29. **Yanagisawa, M., Kurihara, H., Kimura, S., Tomobe, Y., Kobayashi, M., Mitsui, Y., Yazaki, Y., Goto, K., and Masaki, T.,** A novel potent vasoconstrictor peptide produced by vascular endothelial cells, *Nature,* 332, 411, 1988.
30. **Morris, C. E.,** Mechanosensitive ion channels, *J. Membrane Biol.,* 113, 93, 1990.
31. **Hill, M. A., Falcone, J. C., and Meininger, G. A.,** Evidence for protein kinase C involvement in arteriolar myogenic reactivity, *Am. J. Physiol.,* 259, H1586, 1990.
32. **Laher, I. and Bevan, J. A.,** Staurosporine, A protein kinase C inhibitor attenuates Ca^{2+}-dependent stretch-induced vascular tone, *Biochem. Biophys. Res. Commun.,* 158, 58, 1989.
33. **Berridge, M. J.,** Inositol triphosphate and diacylglycerol: two interacting second messengers, *Annu. Rev. Biochem.,* 56, 159, 1987.
34. **DeRiemer, S. A., Strong, J. A., Alpert, K. A., Greengard, D., and Kaczmarek, L. K.,** Enhancement of calcium current in "Aplysia" neurones by phorbol ester and protein kinase C, *Nature,* 313, 313, 1985.
35. **Heagerty, A. M. and Ollerenshaw, J. D.,** The phosphoinositide signalling system and hypertension, *J. Hypertension,* 5, 515, 1987.
36. **Harder, D. R., Narayanan, J., Ma, Y. H., and Roman, R. J.,** Activation of phospholipase C and induction of 2nd messengers in pressurized renal arteries, *FASEB J.,* 6, A1733, 1992.

37. **Ohanian, J., Ollerenshaw, J., Collins, P., and Heagerty, A.,** Agonist-induced production of 1,2-diacylglycerol and phosphatidic acid in intact resistance arteries, *J. Biol. Chem.*, 265, 8921, 1990.
38. **Harder, D. R.,** Increased sensitivity of cat cerebral arteries to serotonin upon elevation of transmural pressure, *Pfluegers Arch.*, 411, 698, 1988.
39. **Siegel, G. and Grote, J.,** P_{O_2} induced changes of membrane potential and tension in vascular smooth musculature, in *Oxygen Sensing in Tissues,* Acker, H., Ed., Springer-Verlag, Berlin, 1988, 131.
40. **Broyden, J. E. and Wellman, G. C.,** Endotheliumdependent dilation of feline cerebral arteries: role of membrane potential and cyclic nucleotides, *J. Cerebral Blood Flow Metab.*, 9, 256, 1989.
41. **Pearce, W. J., Ashwal, S., and Cuevas, J.,** Direct effects of graded hypoxia on intact and denuded rabbit cranial arteries, *Am. J. Physiol.*, 257, H824, 1989.
42. **Lombard, J. H., Smeda, J., Madden, J. A., and Harder, D. R.,** Effect of reduced oxygen availability upon myogenic depolarization and contraction of cat middle cerebral artery, *Circ. Res.*, 58, 565, 1986.
43. **Daut, J., Maior-Rudolph, W., Von Beckerath, N., Mehrke, G., Ganther, K., and Goedel-Meinen, L.,** Hypoxic dilation of coronary arteries is medicated by ATP sensitive potassium channels, *Science,* 24, 1341, 1990.
44. **Post, J. M., Hume, J. R., Archer, S. L., and Weir, E. K.,** Direct role of potassium channel inhibition in hypoxic pulmonary vasoconstriction, *Am. J. Physiol.*, 262, C882, 1992.
45. **Harder, D. R.,** Effect of H^+ and elevated P_{CO_2} on membrane electrical properties of cat cerebral arteries, *Pfluegers Arch.*, 349, 182, 1982.
46. **Harder, D. R. and Madden, J. A.,** Cellular mechanism of force development in cat middle cerebral artery by reduced P_{CO_2}, *Pfluegers Arch.*, 403, 402, 1985.
47. **West, G. A., Leppla, D. C., and Simond, J. M.,** Effects of external pH on ionic currents in smooth muscle cells from the basilar artery of the guinea pig, *Circ. Res.*, 71, 201, 1992.
48. **Harder, D. R. and Waters, A.,** Electrical activation of arterial muscle, *Intl. Rev. Cytol.*, 89, 1, 1984.

Chapter 3

CEREBRAL AUTOREGULATION

David W. Busija

TABLE OF CONTENTS

I. Introduction 46

II. Perfusion Pressure/Blood Flow Relationship 46

III. Mechanisms of Autoregulation 48

IV. Factors Affecting Autoregulation 51
- A. Resting Tone 51
- B. Neural Influences 51
- C. Brain Injury 53

V. Concluding Remarks 54

References 54

0-8493-5096-0/93/$0.00 + $.50

I. INTRODUCTION

A characteristic feature of the cerebral circulation is its ability to maintain total and regional blood flows relatively constant over a wide range of arterial blood pressures.[1] The independence of cerebral blood flow (CBF) from arterial blood pressure typically is called *cerebral autoregulation*. To maintain relatively constant blood flow in the face of increasing or decreasing arterial blood pressure, the cerebral resistance vessels must constrict or dilate, respectively. The importance of autoregulation is that it allows blood flow to match metabolic needs in spite of fluctuations in arterial blood pressure by maintaining capillary perfusion pressure at levels to ensure adequate capillary exchange. At higher arterial blood pressures, autoregulatory responses of larger resistance vessels result in attenuation of microvascular pressure and protection of downstream vessels from damage.[2]

Cerebral autoregulation is a topic that has received considerable attention for the last three decades. While it is clear that cerebral autoregulation occurs, and that a number of factors are able to modulate vascular responses, the underlying mechanisms driving cerebrovascular adjustments to changes in arterial blood pressure are controversial. The purpose of this contribution is to discuss the characteristics and mechanisms of autoregulation in the cerebral circulation.

II. PERFUSION PRESSURE/BLOOD FLOW RELATIONSHIP

Although autoregulation is typically discussed in terms of arterial blood pressure vs. blood flow, usually for convenience and simplicity, it is more precise to use the term *perfusion pressure* instead of arterial blood pressure. In the cerebral circulation, perfusion pressure is defined as the difference between arterial blood pressure and cerebral venous pressure or cerebrospinal fluid (CSF) pressure, depending on which of the latter values is higher. Under most physiological conditions, cerebral venous and CSF pressures are relatively low[3,4] and are often assumed to be negligible. However, during a variety of conditions, such as increased airway pressure, postural movements, reventilation following asphyxia, reperfusion following cerebral ischemia, brain injury, and during hydrocephalus, cerebral venous and CSF pressures can be quite large relative to arterial blood pressure[3-12] and need to be considered in resistance calculations.

Under steady state conditions in awake and anesthetized animals, and in man, CBF is maintained relatively constant over mean arterial blood pressures ranging from 50 to 130 mmHg.[13-17] Whether CBF in the *autoregulatory range* actually stays constant or varies somewhat (perhaps increasing or decreasing by 2 to 7%/10 mmHg when arterial blood pressure is elevated or decreased, respectively) is controversial.[18] However, during hemorrhagic hypotension, brainstem blood flow often increases, probably due to increased metabolic rate.[13,19] Nonetheless, even allowing for minor changes in blood flow, it is clear that there is a relatively flat part to the arterial pressure/CBF relationship. Cerebral blood flow also is maintained relatively constant when perfusion pressure is decreased somewhat by increasing cerebral venous or CSF pressures.[20,21] However, at mean arterial blood pressures below 60 mmHg, CBF begins to fall because the driving pressure of blood is insufficient to allow adequate perfusion. There is some degree of regionality in these responses. In general, during low arterial blood pressure conditions and during increased CSF pressure, blood flow is better maintained in brainstem compared to more rostral areas of the brain.[17,21] On the other hand, when arterial blood pressure increases to beyond approximately 130 mmHg, CBF increases as the ability of the resistance vessels to compensate is exceeded. This ***vascular failure*** is represented by an inability of the vessels to constrict enough to match the increase in intravascular pressure and by mechanical failure of vascular smooth muscle to maintain constriction.[22-25] In the latter situation, cerebral resistance vessels become dilated and passively respond to changes in arterial blood pressure. As during arterial hypotension, during increases in arterial blood pressure, blood flow in the brainstem is better maintained than in rostral areas of the brain.[26,27] Also, blood-brain barrier integrity during arterial hypertension is better maintained in brainstem than in cerebrum and cerebellum.[26]

Autoregulation to perfusion pressure changes is a general feature of most regional circulations. Thus, in the absence of neural influences and changes in circulating constrictor agents, blood flow in skeletal muscle, heart, and kidney, as well as in other organs, is maintained relatively constant over a wide range of arterial blood pressure values.[12]

Depending upon the normal resting mean arterial blood pressure, the cerebral autoregulatory curve could be shifted either to the left or right. In the fetus or neonate, where arterial blood pressures are lower than in adults, there is a maintenance of CBF to arterial pressures as low as 35 mmHg,[27-33] and CBF can be maintained for at least 60 min at these low arterial blood pressure levels.[19] However, the upper limit of cerebral autoregulation is shifted to lower arterial blood values.[34] On the other hand, just the opposite situation exists for chronically hypertensive individuals, where the cerebral autoregulatory curve is shifted to the right.[35-41] Chronic arterial hypertension is associated with cerebrovascular changes such as hypertrophy of elastic tissue and smooth muscle.[42-47] In previously hypertensive people and animals, pharmacological reduction in resting arterial blood pressure restores the autoregulatory range towards normal.[35,48,49]

Cerebral autoregulation is a relatively robust response and occurs even following development of atherosclerosis. Although intracranial arteries usually are spared by atherosclerosis, large extracranial arteries often have extensive intima proliferation and restricted lumens.[50] However, the distal resistance vessels are able to compensate and maintain CBF at normal levels during arterial hypotension,[50-52] whereas increases in CBF in response to arterial hypercapnia are attenuated.[50,53]

The normally presented cerebral autoregulatory curve is based on steady state conditions. Thus, perfusion pressure is changed and maintained at a new level for several minutes and then CBF is determined. Only a few studies have looked at the time course of cerebral autoregulation, and they have found that compensatory adjustments to changes in arterial blood pressure occur very quickly; arterial/arteriolar diameter and CBF begin to change within 10 s and vascular responses are largely completed by 60 s.[54-60] Increases in blood flow at the onset of rapid increases in arterial blood pressure are greatest in cerebral cortex, and lowest in white matter in cats, but roughly equivalent in dogs.[57] Arteries and arterioles *in vitro* also show rapid responses to increases in intraluminal pressure.[61-63]

In apparent contrast to many other regional circulations, in the cerebral circulation relatively large arteries, such as the internal carotid artery, circle of Willis, basilar artery, and proximal branches coming off the latter two structures, are important resistance vessels[2,64,65] and play an important role in autoregulatory responses. The relative importance of *large* and *small* resistance vessels during cerebral autoregulation is dependent upon prevailing conditions, such as level of arterial blood pressure, arterial blood gases, degree of neural influences, and vessels' wall status.

Thus, autoregulation is an important mechanism in the cerebral circulation. Characteristics of cerebral autoregulation include rapidity of responses and plasticity to changing conditions such as normal arterial blood pressure and atherosclerosis.

III. MECHANISMS OF AUTOREGULATION

Considerable controversy exists concerning mechanisms underlying autoregulatory responses in the cerebral circulation. Possible mechanisms include neurogenic, myogenic, and metabolic factors.

Early studies indicated that reflexes, involving the arterial baroreceptors, play an important role in cerebral autoregulation. Thus, it was reported that activation of arterial baroreceptors to simulate arterial hypertension leads to cerebral vasoconstriction via relax pathways.[66,67] However, more recent studies in dogs and monkeys have suggested that arterial baroreceptors are not involved in this response.[68,69] In addition, the section of sympathetic nerves supplying cerebral vessels does not alter steady state cerebrovascular responses to alterations in arterial pressure within the autoregulatory range.[4,17,57,70] Thus, it seems unlikely that nerves are necessary for autoregulatory responses of cerebral vessels. An interesting but not yet replicated finding is that lesions of the nucleus tractus solitarii abolishes cerebrovascular autoregulatory responses to increases in arterial blood pressure.[71] In contrast, lesions of the anteroventral portion of the third cerebral ventricle, which is critical for cardiovascular regulation, do not prevent maintenance of CBF in the rat during hemorrhagic hypotension.[72] However, it seems unlikely that nerves are necessary for autoregulation to occur. In organs and tissues with intact circulations that can be studied *in vitro,* where neural influences are abolished, such as the kidney and cardiac and skeletal muscle, autoregulation is excellent.[12] Nonetheless, as described in the next section, sympathetic and trigeminal nerves can modify the pressure-flow relationship during severe hypertension, and sympathetic/parasympathetic nerves may affect CBF during arterial hypotension in some species.

Metabolic factors also have been proposed as important mediators of autoregulation. Changes in perfusion pressure may alter local concentrations of vasoactive substances which will in turn affect vascular tone. Thus, increased perfusion pressures will result in the increased washout of dilator metabolites while the opposite effects occur at reduced perfusion pressures. Metabolic factors currently thought to play an important role in cerebral autoregulation include extracellular fluid (ECF) concentrations of H^+, K^+, adenosine, and prostaglandins. All four of these substances are potent cerebrovascular dilator agents.[1] The best evidence that arterial/arteriolar dilator responses during arterial hypotension are due to metabolic factors comes from a study by Kontos et al.,[73] in which they showed that pial arteriolar dilation during hypotension was abolished by superfusion with a fluorocarbon equilibrated with 100% oxygen. Similarly, increased cerebral venous pressure also caused dilation of pial arterioles, and this dilation was reversed to mild constriction during hyperoxia.[6] Thus, relative tissue hypoxia might be a stimulus for dilation during hypotension. However, the connection between tissue hypoxia and dilation is unclear. Wahl and Kuschinsky[74] measured perivascular $[H^+]$ and $[K^+]$ near pial arterioles when arterial blood pressure was varied over the range of 60 to 200 mmHg and found that levels of these substances did not change even though arterioles responded to changes in arterial blood pressure. This study supports an earlier report concerning K^+.[75] On the other hand, a number of investigators have found that tissue or interstitial fluid adenosine concentration doubles when arterial blood pressure is decreased in rats or piglets.[76-78] Interstitial fluid levels of adenosine are more important to consider since much of whole tissue adenosine is sequestered within cells and thereby unavailable to directly affect vascular tone.[79] Increases in interstitial adenosine levels during arterial hypotension were abolished by artificial CSF with a PaO_2 of 152 mmHg.[77] Further, blockade of adenosine receptors with 8-phenyltheophylline impaired cerebrovascular dilator responses to arterial hypotension.[78] Brain ECF levels of prostaglandins also appear to be important in autoregulatory responses to arterial hypotension in piglets. During arterial hypotension, CSF levels of two dilator prostaglandins, namely PGE_2 and prostacylin, increase severalfold,[80] as does prostacyclin in cerebral venous blood.[19,81] In addition, administration of indomethacin, an inhibitor of prostaglandin production, abolishes maintenance of CBF to arterial hypotension in both anesthetized and awake piglets.[19,81] Several other studies support the concept that prostanoids contribute to cerebrovascular dilation during hypotension in neonates[82] and adults[83] although other investigators have not shown this effect.[84] Thus, it appears that adenosine and prostaglandins might be important determinants of CBF during decreases in arterial blood pressure. On the other hand, evidence is scant concerning the role of these substances during arterial hypertension, and thus their role is unclear.

Another approach to support the metabolic concept comes from studies in which perfusion pressure is changed by increasing either cerebral venous blood or CSF pressure. This approach should result in increased extracellular fluid concentrations of metabolites, but with arterial inflow pressure remaining the same. Wei and Kontos[6] found that increased cerebral venous pressure resulted in pial arteriolar dilation; a response consistent with a fall in overall cerebrovascular resistance. Similarly, Wagner and Traystman[20] found that when cerebral venous pressure was elevated in dogs, CBF was maintained. In studies in piglets, we found that increased airway pressure caused a fall in cerebral perfusion pressure, but pial arterioles dilated and CBF was maintained.[3,5] Autoregulatory responses were associated with increased CSF levels of both PGE_2 and prostacyclin and increased cerebral venous concentrations of prostacyclin.[5,85]

It has been suggested that myogenic factors also are involved in autoregulatory responses. Thus, changes in intravascular pressure rather than ECF metabolite levels constitute the stimulus for contraction or relaxation of cerebral resistance vessels. Myogenic mechanisms would represent events intrinsic to the vessel wall. Numerous investigators have shown that cerebral arterioles *in vitro* develop tone[61,62,86-88] and that this tone can be augmented by increasing intraluminal pressure[61-63,86-91] via a calcium-dependent mechanism.[63,90] Associated with maintained tone or increased tone during increased intraluminal pressures is progressive mooth muscle depolarization.[90] It is unclear whether intrinsic vascular responses to pressure are endothelium-dependent. Harder et al.[89] have shown that endothelium removal abolishes maintenance or constriction of tone during increased intraluminal pressure and that an *endothelium-derived factor* is transferable to intact vessel segments. However, the nature of this agent is not known. In contrast, McCarron et al.[91] have shown that myogenic responses are present even when endothelium is removed. The reason for this discrepancy in findings concerning the role of endothelium is unclear and may involve species differences (cat vs. rat, respectively) or other methodological differences.

Although cerebral autoregulation is a well studied phenomenon, the mechanisms involved in maintenance of CBF are unclear. It appears that metabolic factors might be more important during decreases in arterial blood pressure, while myogenic factors might be more important during arterial hypertension.

Likely metabolic stimuli include prostaglandins and adenosine. Myogenic constriction might be an intrinsic property of vascular smooth muscle or could require prior activation of endothelium and subsequent release of a constrictor factor. Resting tone, although present even *in vitro,* might be due to a combination of myogenic and metabolic influences. In addition, it seems likely that neural influences might be able to modify or facilitate autoregulatory responses.

IV. FACTORS AFFECTING AUTOREGULATION

A number of factors can affect the normal arterial blood pressure/blood flow relationship in the cerebral circulation. These include resting tone, neural influences, and brain injury.

A. RESTING TONE

Arterial hypercapnia and hypoxia dilate cerebral resistance vessels and increase CBF. If the cerebrovascular dilation is severe enough, then cerebral autoregulation is inhibited or abolished and CBF passively follows changes in arterial blood pressure.[13,92-96] During decreases in arterial blood pressure, additional capacity for the resistance vessels is limited because of the prior dilation.[97] However, since basal CBF is already elevated by arterial hypercapnia and hypoxia, oxygen delivery to brain tissues is still sufficient to meet the needs of the brain despite a fall in blood flow, except when arterial blood pressure approaches 50 mmHg during hypoxia.[13,96] During increases in arterial blood pressure, the ability of the arteries and arterioles to constrict is limited probably by acidosis and the presence of other metabolic factors both inside and outside smooth muscle cells. If indeed cerebral resistance vessels constrict during arterial hypertension by a mechanism involving protein kinase C activation, then it would not be surprising that acidosis or a metabolite would interfere with vascular constriction. We have shown that pial arteriolar constriction due to protein kinase C activation by phorbol esters is reversed to dilation by arterial hypercapnia or application of artificial CSF high in K^+.[98] On the other hand, prior vasoconstriction might augment autoregulatory responses. For example, electrical stimulation of sympathetic nerves, which constricts large cerebral arteries, and is usually begun just prior to increasing arterial blood pressure, limits increases in CBF during moderate and severe hypotension.

B. NEURAL INFLUENCES

Cerebral blood vessels are supplied extensively by several different types of innervation, including sympathetic, parasympathetic, and sensory fibers.[1] In addition, it has been suggested that central pathways, existing exclusively within the brain itself, supply innervation to cerebral resistance vessels (see Chapter 4). Thus, the potential exists for nerves to play a role in cerebral autoregulation. While it is clear that cerebral autoregulation occurs despite removal of various neural influences, it is clear that nerves can modulate various features such as speed of vascular responses and the range over which autoregulation occurs.

Sympathetic nerves clearly are able to modify the cerebrovascular response to changes in arterial blood pressure. When arterial blood pressure is raised abruptly but is still within the autoregulatory range in anesthetized cats, there is a transient rise in CBF before autoregulatory adjustments are able to restore CBF back to control.[57] Under these conditions, electrical stimulation of sympathetic nerves is able to dramatically attenuate this cerebral hyperemia.[57] Since minor fluctuations in arterial blood pressure occur in everyday life, as a consequence of postural, emotional, and activity changes,[12,99] it seems likely that sympathetic activation could limit hyperperfusion of the brain. When mean arterial blood pressure is increased to values greater than the upper limit of autoregulation, CBF increases. During these conditions, electrical stimulation of sympathetic nerves severely blunts increases in CBF.[100,101] In addition, disruption of the bloodbrain barrier caused by severe arterial hypertension is reduced by stimulation of sympathetic nerves.[100,101] The reason that sympathetic nerves appear to have more pronounced effects during elevations in arterial blood pressure than during normotension is unclear. However, there are several possible explanations. First, the initial vascular stretch that occurs with the beginning of arterial hypertension might increase responsiveness to constrictor stimuli.[102] Second, constriction of large arteries and arterioles, which receive more extensive sympathetic innervation than small arterioles, during sympathetic stimulation might protect downstream vessels from forced dilation during sudden increases in arterial blood pressure. Since large sustained increases in arterial blood pressure can occur during stressful conditions such as weight lifting,[99] it is easy to see why a protective role of sympathetic nerves can be so important to prevent inappropriate cerebral hyperemia and damage to the blood brain barrier. It is possible to demonstrate the importance of sympathetic influences on restricting increases in CBF and blood-brain barrier disruption during arterial hypertension in several animal models. During sino-aortic deafferentation, which results in intense sympathetic discharge and doubling of arterial blood pressure, CBF increases severalfold.[103] However, intact sympathetic fibers supplying cerebral blood vessels attenuate increases in CBF and barrier disruption. Similarly, stimulation of carotid chemoreceptors in awake, but paralyzed and ventilated dogs caused an abrupt increase in arterial blood pressure and a 40% increase in CBF when sympathetic nerves were sectioned.[104] However, in dogs with intact sympathetic nerves, CBF did not increase despite arterial hypertension. Finally, under bicuculline-induced seizure conditions, where CBF increases several times above normal due to both elevated cerebral metabolic rate and arterial hypertension, intact sympathetic nerves limit increases in CBF.[105] Other types of nerves might affect cerebral autoregulatory responses under these conditions. Moskowitz et al.[106] have found that trigeminal fibers oppose pial arteriolar constriction during arterial hypertension and promote disruption of the blood-brain barrier.

Sympathetic nerves might also have important effects on cerebrovascular responses during arterial hypotension, but the results are conflicting. In anesthetized cats and dogs, or in awake cats, piglets, or rabbits, sympathetic nerves have no detectable effect on CBF.[13,17,107-109] However, in awake monkeys, and dogs at arterial pressures between 40 to 60 mmHg,[110,111] sympathetic nerves modestly reduce CBF. Reasons for differences in responses are unclear. Nonetheless, the potential exists for sympathetic nerves to have detrimental effects on CBF under these conditions. Parasympathetic nerves also appear to have a modest effect in promoting dilation during hemorrhagic hypotension in rats. The chronic section of parasympathetic nerves that innervate cerebral blood vessels results in impaired autoregulation.[112] However, sectioning of trigeminal fibers does not affect autoregulation.[112]

Sympathetic nerves could also contribute to cerebral autoregulatory adjustments in an indirect fashion. It has been shown that sympathetic nerves contribute to development of vascular hypertrophy during development of arterial hypertension.[42-44] Vascular hypertrophy allows the cerebral circulation to withstand the higher blood pressure and extends the autoregulatory curve to the right. By enhancing vessel mass and wall thickness, sympathetic nerves can contribute to protection against cerebral hemorrhages and infarcts.[43,44]

Thus, neural influences are able to modify basic autoregulatory responses. In some cases neural effects clearly are beneficial, such as with sympathetic effects during arterial hypertension. However, in other cases, such as trigeminal effects during arterial hypertension, neural influences appear to be detrimental.

C. BRAIN INJURY

A number of pathological conditions result in loss or diminution of cerebral autoregulation. These include cerebral ischemia/reperfusion, asphyxia/reventilation, subarachnoid hemorrhage, and trauma. Depending upon type and severity of insult, alterations in cerebrovascular autoregulatory ability may occur quickly or take time to develop and may or may not be reversible.

Global or local cerebral ischemia followed by reperfusion results in complex changes in CBF, and in most models results in loss of vascular responses to changes in arterial blood pressure as well as to many other stimuli. For example, we have found in newborn pigs following 20 min of global ischemia, normal dilatory response to arterial hypotension is reversed to constriction at 2 to 3 h and 24 h.[113] Impairment of cerebral autoregulation also has been reported in human patients following cerebral ischemia.[114-116] Similar to ischemia/reperfusion, prolonged arterial hypoxia followed by a return to normoxia is able to inhibit cerebrovascular dilation to arterial hypotension in lambs and babies.[117-120] The impairment of cerebrovascular responses under these conditions seems to involve mechanisms involving free oxygen radicals.[119-122]

Trauma to cerebral arteries and arterioles may reduce normal responsiveness to alterations in arterial blood pressure. For example, excessive surgical manipulation of cerebral vessels eliminates autoregulatory responses.[123] Another type of trauma, namely concussive brain injury, leads to impairment of cerebral autoregulatory responses in man and animals.[124,125] The mechanism for this altered responsiveness appears to involve the severe arterial hypertension that accompanies head trauma[125] and the resultant production of free radicals.[126,127]

Yet another stimulus which is able to attenuate cerebrovascular dilatory responses to arterial hypotension is chronic presence of blood on the cortical surface.[128] Rupture of cerebral arteries results in subarachnoid hemorrhage. In contrast to this response, dilator responses to topical isoproterenol were intact. The effects of blood on cerebrovascular responsiveness to arterial hypotension were not present immediately, but developed over 1 to 4 days. Although it is not clear what mechanisms are involved in this change in cerebrovascular responsiveness, it has been shown that blood has the capability of generating free radicals.[129]

It is clear that as a consequence of different types of brain injury, the ability of the cerebral circulation to make appropriate adjustments to changes in arterial blood pressure is compromised. This impaired autoregulatory ability could lead to further vascular damage. A common mechanism for cerebrovascular damage following several types of brain injury appears to involve free radicals.

V. CONCLUSIONS

The cerebral circulation has the ability to maintain CBF relatively constant over a wide range of arterial blood pressures. Although autoregulatory responses under a variety of conditions have been studied extensively, the mechanisms involved in regulating responses are still elusive, but may involve primarily a metabolic mechanism for decreases in arterial blood pressure and primarily a myogenic mechanism for increases in arterial blood pressure. Neural influences can modify this basic response. In addition, brain injury can lead to events which severely limit the ability of the cerebral circulation to respond appropriately to changes in arterial blood pressure.

REFERENCES

1. **Busija, D. W. and Heistad, D. D.,** Factors involved in physiological regulation of cerebral blood flow, *Rev. Physiol. Biochem. Pharmacol.*, 101, 161, 1984.
2. **Faraci, F. M. and Heistad, D. D.,** Regulation of large cerebral arteries and cerebral microvascular pressure, *Circ. Res.*, 66, 8, 1990.

3. **Mirro, R., Leffler, C. W., Armstead, W., Beasley, D. G., and Busija, D. W.,** Indomethacin restricts cerebral blood flow during pressure ventilation of newborn pigs, *Ped. Res.*, 24, 59, 1988.
4. **Sadoshima, S., Thames, M., and Heistad, D.,** Cerebral blood flow during elevation of intracranial pressure: role of sympathetic nerves, *Am. J. Physiol.*, 241, H78, 1981.
5. **Mirro, R., Armstead, W., Busija, D. W., Green, R., and Leffler, C.,** Increasing ventilation pressure increases cortical subarachnoid cerebrospinal fluid prostanoids in newborn pigs, *Ped. Res.*, 22, 647, 1987.
6. **Wei, E. P. and Kontos, H. A.,** Increased venous pressure causes myogenic constriction of cerebral arterioles during local hyperoxia, *Circ. Res.*, 55, 249, 1984.
7. **Fried, A. and Shapiro, K.,** Subtle deterioration in shunted childhood hydrocephalus, *J. Neurosurg.*, 65, 211, 1986.
8. **Luce, J. M., Huseby, J. S., Kirk, W., and Butler, J.,** Mechanism by which positive end-expiratory pressure increases cerebrospinal fluid pressure in dogs, *J. Appl. Physiol.*, 52, 231, 1982.
9. **Lupton, B. A., Hill, A., Roland, E. H., Whitfield, M. F., and Flodmark, O.,** Brain swelling in the asphyxiated term newborn: pathogenesis and outcome, *Pediatrics,* 82, 139, 1988.
10. **McPhee, A. J., Kotagal, U. R., and Kleinman, L. I.,** Cerebrovascular hemodynamics during and after recovery from acute asphyxia in the newborn dog, *Ped. Res.*, 19, 645, 1985.
11. **Fanconi, S. and Duc, G.,** Intratracheal suctioning in sick preterm infants: prevention of intracranial hypertension and cerebral hypoperfusion by muscle paralysis, *Pediatrics,* 79, 538, 1987.
12. **Berne, R. M. and Levy, M. N.,** *Cardiovascular Physiology,* C. V. Mosby, St. Louis, 1981.
13. **Busija, D. W.,** Sympathetic nerves reduce cerebral blood flow during hypoxia in awake rabbits, *Am. J. Physiol.*, 247, H446, 1984.
14. **Harper, S. T., Bohlen, H. G., and Rubin, M. J.,** Arterial and microvascular contributions to cerebral cortical autoregulation in rats, *Am. J. Physiol.*, 246, H17, 1984.
15. **Rapela, C. E. and Green, H. D.,** Autoregulation of canine cerebral blood flow, *Circ. Res.*, 14(Suppl. 1), 205, 1964.
16. **Harper, A. M.,** Autoregulation of cerebral blood flow: influence of the arterial blood pressure on the blood flow through the cerebral cortex, *J. Neurol. Neurosurg. Psychiatry,* 29, 398, 1966.
17. **Mueller, S. M., Heistad, D. D., and Marcus, M. L.,** Total and regional cerebral blood flow during hypotension, hypertension, hypocapnia. Effect of sympathetic denervation in dogs, *Circ. Res.*, 41, 350, 1977.
18. **Heistad, D. D. and Kontos, K. A.,** Cerebral Circulation, in *Handbook of Physiology,* American Physiological Society, Bethesda, MD, 137, 1983.
19. **Leffler, C. W., Busija, D. W., Beasley, D. G., and Fletcher, A. M.,** Maintenance of cerebral circulation during hemorrhagic hypotension in newborn pigs: role of prostanoids, *Circ. Res.*, 59, 562, 1986.
20. **Wagner, E. M. and Traystman, R. J.,** Cerebral venous outflow and arterial microsphere flow with elevated venous pressure, *Am. J. Physiol.*, 244, H505, 1983.
21. **Sadoshima, S., Thames, M., and Heistad, D.,** Cerebral blood flow during elevation of intracranial pressure: role of sympathetic nerves, *Am. J. Physiol.*, 241, H78, 1981.
22. **Auer, L. M.,** The pathogenesis of hypertensive encephalopathy, *Acta Neurochir. Suppl.*, 29, 1, 1978.
23. **Kontos, H. A., Wei, E. P., Dietrich, W. D., Navari, R. M., Povlishock, J. T., Ghatak, N. R., Ellis, E. F., and Patterson, J. L., Jr.,** Mechanism of cerebral arteriolar abnormalities after acture hypertension, *Am. J. Physiol.*, 240, H511, 1981.

24. **Kontos, H. A., Wei, E. P., Navari, R. M., Levasseur, J. E., Rosenblum, W. I., and Patterson, J. L.**, Responses of cerebral arteries and arterioles to acute hypotension and hypertension, *Am. J. Physiol.*, 234, H371, 1978.
25. **MacKenzie, E. T., Standgaard, S., Graham, D. I., Jones, J. V., Harper, A. M., and Farrar, J. K.**, Effects of acutely induced hypertension in cats on pial arteriolar caliber, local cerebral blood flow, and the blood-brain barrier, *Circ. Res.*, 39, 33, 1976.
26. **Baumbach, G. L. and Heistad, D. D.**, Heterogeneity of brain blood flow and permeability during acute hypertension, *Am. J. Physiol.*, 249, H629, 1985.
27. **Burke, A. M., Greenberg, J. H., Sladky, J., and Reivich, M.**, Regional variation in cerebral perfusion during acute hypertension, *Neurology,* 37, 94, 1987.
28. **Hernandez, M. J., Brennan, R. W., and Bowman, G. S.**, Autoregulation of cerebral blood flow in the newborn dog, *Brain Res.*, 184, 199, 1980.
29. **Purves, M. J. and James, I. M.**, Observations on the control of cerebral blood flow in the sheep fetus and newborn lamb, *Circ. Res.*, 25, 651, 1969.
30. **Pasternak, J. F. and Groothuis, D. R.**, Autoregulation of cerebral blood flow in the newborn Beagle puppy, *Bio. Neonate,* 48, 100, 1985.
31. **Ashwal, S., Dale, P. S., and Longo, L. D.**, Regional cerebral blood flow: studies in the fetal lamb during hypoxia, hypercapnia, acidosis, and hypotension, *Ped. Res.*, 18, 1309, 1984.
32. **Laptook, A. R., Stonestreet, B. S., and Oh, W.**, Brain blood flow and O_2 delivery during hemorrhagic hypotension in the piglet, *Ped. Res.*, 17, 77, 1983.
33. **Laptook, A., Stonestreet, B. S., and Oh, W.**, Autoregulation of brain blood flow in the newborn piglet: regional differences in flow reduction during hypotension, *Early Human Dev.*, 6, 99, 1982.
34. **Fletcher, A. M., Leffler, C. W., and Busija, D. W.**, Effects of hypertension and sympathetic denervation on cerebral blood flow in newborn pigs, *Am. J. Vet. Res.*, 50, 754, 1989.
35. **Barry, D. I., Vorstrup, S., Jarden, J. O., Graham, D. I., Svendsen, U. G., Brandstrup, O., and Strandgaard, S.**, Chronic antihypertensive treatment normalizes autoregulation of cerebral blood flow in hypertension, *J. Cereb. Blood Flow Metab.*, 3, S656, 1983.
36. **Jones, J. V., Fitch, W., MacKenzie, E. T., Standgaard, S., and Harper, A. M.**, Lower limit of cerebral blood flow autoregulation in experimental renovascular hypertension in the baboon, *Circ. Res.*, 39, 555, 1976.
37. **Overbeck, H. W., Berne, R. M., Chien, S., Cowley, A. W., Haddy, F. J., Heistad, D. D., Honig, C. R., Kirkendall, W., Rapela, C. E., Wells, R., Abboud, F. M., Lindheimer, M. D., and Yipintsoi, T.**, Report of the hypertension task force of the National Heart, Lung, and Blood Institute, *Hypertension,* 2, 342, 1980.
38. **Strandgaard, S., Jones, J. V., MacKenzie, E. T., and Harper, A. M.**, Upper limit of cerebral blood flow autoregulation in experimental renovascular hypertension in the baboon, *Circ. Res.*, 37, 164, 1975.
39. **Strandgaard, S., MacKenzie, E. T., Sengupta, D., Rowam, J. O., Lassen, N. A., and Harper, A. M.**, Upper limit of autoregulation of cerebral blood flow in the baboon, *Circ. Res.*, 34, 435, 1974.
40. **Strandgaard, S., Olesen, J., Skinhøj, M., and Lassen, N. A.**, Autoregulation of brain circulation in severe arterial hypertension, *Br. Med. J.*, 1, 507, 1973.
41. **Sadoshima, S., Yoshida, F., Ibayashi, S., Shiokawa, O., and Fujishima, M.**, Upper limit of cerebral autoregulation during development of hypertension in spontaneously hypertensive rats — effect of sympathetic denervation, *Stroke,* 16, 477, 1985.
42. **Hart, M., Heistad, D. D., and Brody, M. J.**, Effect of chronic hypertension and sympathetic denervation on wall/lumen ratio of cerebral arteries, *Hypertension,* 2, 419, 1980.

43. **Sadoshima, S., Busija, D., Brody, M., and Heistad, D.,** Sympathetic nerves protect against stroke in stroke-prone hypertensive rats, *Hypertension,* 3, I124, 1981.
44. **Sadoshima, S., Busija, D. W., and Heistad, D. D.,** Mechanisms of protection against stroke in stroke-prone spontaneously hypertensive rats, *Am. J. Physiol.,* 244, H406, 1983.
45. **Nordborg, C., Fredriksson, K., and Johansson, B. B.,** The morphometry of consecutive segments in cerebral arteries of normotensive and spontaneously hypertensive rats, *Stroke,* 16, 313, 1985.
46. **Harper, S. L. and Bohlen, H. G.,** Microvascular adaptation in the cerebral cortex of adult spontaneously hypertensive rats, *Hypertension,* 6, 408, 1984.
47. **Johansson, B. B.,** Cerebral vascular bed in hypertension and consequences for the brain, *Hypertension,* 6, III81, 1984.
48. **Strandgaard, S.,** Autoregulation of cerebral blood flow in hypertensive patients. The modifying influence of prolonged antihypertensive treatment on the tolerance to acute, drug-induced hypotension, *Circulation,* 53, 720, 1976.
49. **Hoffman, W. E., Miletich, D. J., and Albrecht, R. F.,** Cerebrovascular response to hypotension in hypertensive rats. Effect of antihypertensive therapy, *Anesthesiology,* 58, 326, 1983.
50. **Heistad, D. D., Marcus, M. L., Piegors, D. J., and Armstrong, M. L.,** Regulation of cerebral blood flow in atherosclerotic monkeys, *Am. J. Physiol.,* 239, H539, 1980.
51. **Agnoli, A., Fieschi, C., Bozzao, L., Battistini, N., and Prencipe, M.,** Autoregulation of cerebral blood flow. Studies during drug induced hypertension in normal subjects and in patients with cerebral vascular diseases, *Circulation,* 38, 800, 1968.
52. **Simard, D., Olesen, J., Paulson, O. B., Lassen, N. A., and Skinhøj, M.,** Regional cerebral blood flow and its regulation in demintia, *Brain,* 94, 273, 1971.
53. **Novack, P., Shenkin, H. A., Bortin, L., Goluboff, B., and Soffe, A. M.,** The effects of carbon dioxide inhalation upon the cerebral blood flow and cerebral oxygen consumption in vascular disease, *J. Clin. Invest.,* 32, 696, 1953.
54. **Nornes, H., Knutgen, H. B., and Wikeby, P.,** Cerebral arterial blood flow and aneurysm surgery, *J. Neurosurg.,* 47, 819, 1977.
55. **Symon, L., Held, K., and Doroch, N. W. C.,** A study of regional autoregulation in the cerebral circulation to increased perfusion pressure in normocapnia and hypercapnia, *Stroke,* 4, 139, 1973.
56. **Kontos, H. A., Wei, E. P., Navari, R. M., Levasseur, J. E., Rosenblum, W. I., and Patterson, J. L., Jr.,** Responses of cerebral arteries and arterioles to acute hypotension and hypertension, *Am. J. Physiol.,* 234, H371, 1978.
57. **Busija, D. W., Heistad, D. D., and Marcus, M. L.,** Effects of sympathetic nerves on cerebral vessels during acute, moderate increases in arterial pressure in dogs and cats, *Circ. Res.,* 46, 696, 1980.
58. **Busija, D. W., Heistad, D. D., and Marcus, M. L.,** Continuous measurement of cerebral blood flow in anesthetized cats and dogs, *Am. J. Physiol.,* 241, H228, 1981.
59. **Aaslid, R., Lindegaard, K. F., Sorteberg, W., and Nornes, H.,** Cerebral autoregulation dynamics in humans, *Stroke,* 20, 45, 1989.
60. **Florence, G. and Seylaz, J.,** Rapid autoregulation of cerebral blood flow: a laser-Doppler flowmetry study, *J. Cereb. Blood Metabol.,* 12, 674, 1992.
61. **Osol, G., Laher, I., and Cipolla, M.,** Protein kinase C modulates basal myogenic tone in resistance arteries from the cerebral circulation, *Circ. Res.,* 68, 359, 1991.
62. **Osol, G. and Halpern, W.,** Myogenic properties of cerebral vessels from normotensive and hypertensive rats, *Am. J. Physiol.,* 249, H914, 1985.
63. **Vinall, P. E. and Simeone, F. A.,** Cerebral autoregulation: an *in vitro* study, *Stroke,* 12, 640, 1981.
64. **Kontos, H. A., Wei, E. P., Navari, R. M., Levasseur, Rosenblum, W. I., and Patterson, J. L., Jr.,** Responses of cerebral arteries and arterioles to acute hypotension and hypertension, *Am. J. Physiol.,* 234, H371, 1978.

65. **Heistad, D. D., Marcus, M. L., and Abboud, F. M.,** Role of large arteries in regulation of cerebral blood flow in dogs, *J. Clin. Invest.*, 62, 761, 1978.
66. **Ponte, J. and Purves, M. J.,** The role of the carotid body chemoreceptors and carotid sinus baroreceptors in the control of cerebral blood vessels, *J. Physiol. (London)*, 237, 315, 1974.
67. **James, I. M. and MacDonell, L.,** The role of baroreceptors and chemoreceptors in the regulation of the cerebral circulation, *Clin. Sci.*, 49, 465, 1975.
68. **Heistad, D. D. and Marcus, M. L.,** Total and regional cerebral blood flow during stimulation of carotid baroreceptors, *Stroke*, 7, 239, 1976.
69. **Rapela, C. E., Green, H. D., and Denison, A. B., Jr.,** Baroreceptor reflexes and autoregulation of cerebral blood flow in the dog, *Circ. Res.*, 21, 559, 1967.
70. **Busija, D. W.,** Unilateral and bilateral sympathetic effects on cerebral blood flow during normocapnia, *Am. J. Physiol.*, 19, H498, 1986.
71. **Ishitsuka, T., Iadecola, C., Underwook, M. D., and Reis, D. J.,** Lesions of nucleus tractus solitarii globally impair cerebrovascular autoregulation, *Am. J. Physiol.*, 251, H269, 1986.
72. **Bealer, S. L. and Busija, D. W.,** Redistribution of cardiac output after hyothalamic lesions and hemorrhage, *Exp. Brain Res.*, 69, 107, 1987.
73. **Kontos, H. A., Wei, E. P., Raper, A. J., Rosenblum, W. I., Navari, M., and Patterson, J. L., Jr.,** Role of tissue hypoxia in local regulation of cerebral microcirculation, *Am. J. Physiol.*, 234, H582, 1978.
74. **Wahl, M. and Kuschinsky, W.,** Unimportance of perivascular H^+ and K^+ activities for the adjustment of pial arterial diameter during changes of arterial blood pressure in cats, *Pfluegers Arch.*, 382, 203, 1979.
75. **Perez-Hernandez, M. J. and Anderson, D. K.,** Autoregulation of cerebral blood flow and its relation to cerebrospinal fluid pH, *Am. J. Physiol.*, 231, 929, 1976.
76. **Winn, H. R., Welsh, J. E., Rubio, R., and Berne, R. M.,** Brain adenosine production in rat during sustained alteration in systemic blood pressure, *Am. J. Physiol.*, 239, H636, 1980.
77. **Park, T. S., Van Wylen, D. G. L., Rubio, R., and Berne, R. M.,** Brain interstitial adenosine and sagittal sinus blood flow during systemic hypotension in piglet, *J. Cereb. Blood Flow Metabol.*, 8, 822, 1988.
78. **Laudignon, N., Beharry, K., Farri, E., and Aranda, J. V.,** The role of adenosine in the vascular adaptation of neonatal cerebral blood flow during hypotension, *J. Cereb. Blood Flow Metabol.*, 11, 424, 1991.
79. **Ueland, P. M. and Saebø, J. C.,** Sequestration of adenosine in crude extract from mouse liver and other tissues, *Biochim. Biophys. Acta*, 581, 341, 1979.
80. **Leffler, C. W. and Busija, D. W.,** Prostanoids and pial arteriolar diameter in hypotensive newborn pigs, *Am. J. Physiol.*, 252, H687, 1987.
81. **Leffler, C. W., Busija, D. W., and Beasley, D. G.,** Effect of therapeutic dose of indomethacin on the cerebral circulation of newborn pigs, *Ped. Res.*, 21, 188, 1987.
82. **Ment, L. R., Stewart, W. B., Duncan, C. C., Cole, J., and Pitt, B. R.,** Beagle puppy model of perinatal cerebral infarction. Acute changes in regional cerebral prostaglandins during hemorrhagic hypotension, *J. Neurosurg.*, 63, 899, 1985.
83. **Shohami, E. and Sidi, A.,** Accumulation of prostacyclin in rat brain during hemorrhagic hypotension — possible role of PGI_2 in autoregulation, *J. Cereb. Blood Flow Metabol.*, 4, 107, 1984.
84. **Pickard, J. D. and MacKenzie, E. T.,** Inhibition of prostaglandin synthesis and the response of baboon cerebral circulation to carbon dioxide, *Nature New Biol.*, 245, 187, 1973.
85. **Mirro, R., Leffler, C. W., Armstead, W. M., and Busija, D. W.,** Pressure ventilation increases brain vascular prostacyclin production in newborn pigs, *Ped. Res.*, 28, 609, 1990.

86. **Harder, D. R.,** Pressure-induced myogenic activation of cat cerebral arteries is dependent on intact endothelium, *Circ. Res.,* 60, 102, 1987.
87. **Nakayama, D.,** Calciumdependent contractile activation of cerebral artery produced by quick stretch, *Am. J. Physiol.,* 242, H760, 1982.
88. **Dacey, R. G. and Duling, B. R.,** A study of rat intracerebral arterioles: methods, morphology and reactivity, *Am. J. Physiol.,* 243, H598, 1982.
89. **Harder, D. R., Sanchez-Ferrer, C., Kauser, K., Stekiel, W. J., and Rubanyi, G. M.,** Pressure releases a transferable endothelial contractile factor in cat cerebral arteries, *Circ. Res.,* 65, 193, 1989.
90. **Harder, D. R.,** Pressure-dependent membrane depolarization in cat middle cerebral artery, *Circ. Res.,* 55, 197, 1984.
91. **McCarron, J., Osol, G., and Halpern, W.,** Myogenic responses are independent of endothelium in rat posterior cerebral arteries, *Blood Vessels,* 26, 315, 1990.
92. **Tweed, W. A., Cote, J., Pash, M., and Lou, H.,** Arterial oxygenation determines autoregulation of cerebral blood flow in the fetal lamb, *Ped. Res.,* 17, 246, 1983.
93. **Häggendal, E. and Johansson, B.,** Effects of arterial carbon dioxide tension and oxygen saturation on cerebral blood flow autoregulation in dogs, *Acta Physiol. Scand.,* 66(Suppl. 2–8), 27, 1965.
94. **Iwabuchi, T., Kutsuzawa, T., Keda, K. I., and Nakamura, T.,** Effects of blood gases on the pressure-flow relationships in canine cerebral circulation, *Stroke,* 4, 65, 1973.
95. **Kogure, K., Scheinberg, P., Reinmuth, O. M., and Fujishima, M.,** Effects of hypoxia on cerebral autoregulation, *J. Appl. Physiol.,* 29, 223, 1970.
96. **Hohimer, A. R., Chao, C. R., and Bissonnette, J. M.,** The effect of combined hyoxemia and cephalic hypotension on fetal cerebral blood flow and metabolism, *J. Cereb. Blood Flow Metabol.,* 11, 99, 1991.
97. **Tuor, U. I. and Farrar, J. K.,** Pial vessel caliber and cerebral blood flow during hemorrhage and hypercapnia in the rabbit, *Am. J. Physiol.,* 247, H40, 1984.
98. **Busija, D. W. and Chen, J.,** Reversal by increased CSF [H^+] and [K^+] of phorbol ester-induced arteriolar constriction in piglets, *Am. J. Physiol.,* 263, 1455, 1992.
99. **Seals, D. R., Washburn, R. A., Hanson, P. G., Painter, P. L., and Nagle, F. J.,** Increased cardiovascular response to static contraction of larger muscle groups, *J. Appl. Physiol.,* 54, 434, 1983.
100. **Bill, A. and Linder, J.,** Sympathetic control of cerebral blood flow in conscious rabbits — a microsphere study, *Acta Physiol. Scand.,* 96, 114, 1976.
101. **Heistad, D. D. and Marcus, M. L.,** Effect of sympathetic stimulation on permeability of the blood-brain barrier to albumin during acute hypertension in cats, *Circ. Res.* 38, 20, 1979
102. **Toda, N., Hatano, Y., and Hayaski, S.,** Modifications by stretch of the mechanical response of isolated cerebral and extracerebral arteries to vasoactive agents, *Pfluegers Arch.,* 374, 73, 1978.
103. **Gross, P. M., Heistad, D. D., Strait, M. R., Marcus, M. L., and Brody, M. J.,** Cerebral vascular responses to physiological stimulation of sympathetic pathways in cats, *Circ. Res.,* 44, 288, 1979.
104. **Vatner, S. F., Priano, L. L., Rutherford, J. D., and Manders, W. T.,** Sympathetic regulation of the cerebral circulation by the carotid chemoreceptor reflex, *Am. J. Physiol.,* 238, H594, 1980.
105. **Mueller, S. M., Heistad, D. D., and Marcus, M. L.,** Effect of sympathetic nerves on cerebral vessels during seizures, *Am. J. Physiol.,* 237, H178, 1979.
106. **Moskowitz, M. A., Kuo, C., Leemar, S. E., Jesser, M. E., and Kontos, H. A.,** Trigeminalectomy moifies pial arteriolar responses to hypertension and noradrenaline, *Am. J. Physiol.,* 24, H1, 1988.
107. **Heistad, D. D., Marcus, M. L., and Gross, P. M.,** Effects of sympathetic nerves on cerebral vessels in dog, cat and monkey, *Am. J. Physiol.,* 235, H544, 1978.

108. **Armstead, W. M., Leffler, C. W., Busija, D. W., Beasley, D. G., and Mirro, R.,** Adrenergic and prostanoid mechanisms in control of cerebral blood flow in hypotensive newborn pigs, *Am. J. Physiol.,* 254, H671, 1988.
109. **Heistad, D. D., Gross, P. M., Busija, D. W., and Marcus, M. L.,** Cerebral vascular response to loading and unloading of arterial baroreceptors, in *Arterial Baroreceptors and Hypertension,* Sleight, P., Ed., Oxford Univ. Press, Oxford, 1980, 210.
110. **Marcus, M. L. and Heistad, D. D.,** Effects of sympathetic nerves on cerebral blood flow in awake dogs, *Am. J. Physiol.,* 5, H549, 1979.
111. **Fitch, W., MacKenzie, E. T., and Harper, A. M.,** Effects of decreasing arterial blood pressure in cerebral blood flow in the baboon, *Circ. Res.,* 37, 550, 1975.
112. **Koketsu, N., Moskowitz, M. A., Kontos, H. A., Yokota, M., and Shimizu, T.,** Chronic parasympathetic sectioning decreases regional cerebral blood flow during hemorrhagic hypotension and increases infarct size after middle cerebral artery occlusion in spontaneously hypertensive rats, *J. Cereb. Blood Flow Metabol.,* 12, 613, 1992.
113. **Leffler, C. W., Busija, D. W., Beasley, D. G., Armstead, W. M., and Mirro, R.,** Postischemic cerebral microvascular responses to norepinephrine and hypotension in newborn pigs, *Stroke,* 20, 541, 1989.
114. **Fieschi, C., Agnioli, A., Battistini, N., Bozzao, L., and Prencipe, M.,** Derangement of regional cerebral blood flow and of its regulatory mechanisms in acute cerebrovascular lesions, *Neurology,* 18, 1166, 1968.
115. **Meyer, J. S., Shimazu, K., Fukuuchi, Y., Ohuchi, T., Okamoto, S., Koto, A., and Ericsson, A. D.,** Impaired neurogenic cerebrovascular control and dysautoregulation after stroke, *Stroke,* 4, 169, 1973.
116. **Meyer, J. S., Shimazu, K., Okamoto, S., Koto, A., Ohuchi, T., Sari, A., and Ericsson, A. D.,** Effects of alpha adrenergic blockade on autoregulation and chemical vasomotor control of CBF in stroke, *Stroke,* 4, 187, 1973.
117. **Tweed, A., Cote, J., Lou, H., Gregory, G., and Wade, J.,** Impairment of cerebral blood flow autoregulation in the newborn lamb by hypoxia, *Ped. Res.,* 20, 516, 1986.
118. **Lou, H. C., Lassen, N. A., and Friis-Hansen, B.,** Impaired autoregulation of cerebral blood flow in the distressed newborn infant, *J. Ped.,* 94, 118, 1979.
119. **Rosenberg, A. A.,** Cerebral blood flow and O_2 metabolism after asphyxia in neonatal lambs, *Ped. Res.,* 20, 778, 1986.
120. **Rosenberg, A. A., Murdaugh, E., and White, C. W.,** The role of oxygen free radicals in postasphyxia cerebral hypoperfusion in newborn lambs, *Ped. Res.,* 26, 215, 1989.
121. **Armstead, W. M., Mirro, R., Busija, D. W., and Leffler, C. W.,** Postischemic generation of superoxide anion by newborn pig brain, *Am. J. Physiol.,* 24, H401, 1988.
122. **Pourcyrous, M., Leffler, C. W., and Busija, D. W.,** Brain superoxide anion generation during asphyxia and reventilation in newborn pigs, *Ped. Res.,* 28, 618, 1990.
123. **Sagawa, K. and Guyton, A. C.,** Pressure-flow relationships in isolated canine cerebral circulation, *Am. J. Physiol.,* 200, 711, 1961.
124. **Langfitt, T. W., Weinstein, J. D., and Kassell, N. F.,** Vascular factors in head trauma, in *Head Injury,* Caveness, W. F. and Walker, A. E., Eds., Lippincott, Philadelphia, 1966, 172.
125. **Wei, E. P., Dietrich, W. D., Povlishock, J. T., Navari, R. M., and Kontos, H. A.,** Functional, morphological, and metabolic abnormalities of the cerebral microcirculation after concussive brain injury in cats, *Circ. Res.,* 46, 37, 1980.
126. **Wei, E. P., Kontos, H. A., Dietrich, W. D., Povishock, J. T., and Ellis, E. F.,** Inhibition by free radical scavengers and by cyclooxygenase inhibitors of pial arteriolar abnormalities from concussive brain injury in cats, *Circ. Res.,* 48, 95, 1981.
127. **Kontos, H. A. and Wei, E. P.,** Superoxide production in experimental brain injury, *J. Neurosurg.,* 64, 803, 1986.

128. **Busija, D. W. and Leffler, C. W.,** Selective attenuation by perivascular blood of prostanoid-dependent cerebrovascular dilation in piglets, *Stroke,* 22, 484, 1991.
129. **Mirro, R., Armstead, W. M., Busija, D. W., and Leffler, C. W.,** Blood-induced superoxide anion generation by newborn pig cerebral cortex, *Am. J. Physiol.*, 257, H1560, 1989.

II. Neural Regulation of Cerebral Blood Flow

Chapter 4

THE ROLE OF CENTRAL NEURAL PATHWAYS IN THE REGULATION OF CEREBRAL BLOOD FLOW

David W. Busija

TABLE OF CONTENTS

I. Overview 66

II. Locus Ceruleus 66

III. Raphé Nucleus 68

IV. Fastigial Nucleus 69

V. Other Areas 71

VI. Conclusions 71

References 72

0-8493-5096-0/93/$0.00 + $.50

I. OVERVIEW

Direct activation of perivascular nerves is a means by which alterations in cerebrovascular tone can be made quickly to anticipate or match changing hemodynamic or metabolic conditions. Although it is well established that cerebral blood vessels receive extensive and diverse innervation from the periphery, and that activation of peripheral nerves can influence cerebrovascular tone, considerable controversy exists concerning whether cerebral blood vessels are functionally innervated from fibers whose pathways are only through the brain.[1-4] A requirement of central innervation is that these fibers should influence cerebral blood flow (CBF) independently of changes in metabolic rate. Although there is suggestive anatomical evidence that central innervation exists, these pathways supply cerebral blood vessels in a nontraditional manner. Nerve endings from central pathways always are separated from small arteries and arterioles by an intervening basement membrane as well as by the presence of perivascular glia, and apparently do not reach the adventio-medial border.[5,6] Thus, diffusion distances for neurotransmitters are relatively greater than in conventional neuromuscular mechanisms. In contrast, peripheral fibers enter the cranium with the cerebral blood vessels, travel with the vessels during considerable distances, and then end in the adventio-medial border.[7-11] Capillaries do not appear to be innervated by peripheral fibers.[7] In addition, denervation experiments have documented the decrease in levels of neurotransmitters associated with sympathetic, parasympathetic, and sensory innervations of cerebral vessels. At present, no such documentation is available for central pathways innervating cerebral resistance vessels. However, there is evidence that capillaries in some well defined areas are innervated by central pathways.[5,12-14] In addition, an unexplored possibility is that the primary targets of central innervation are glia and not neurons or blood vessels, and that vascular effects are dependent upon activation of glia and release of glia-derived vasoactive substances.[6] Nonetheless, in spite of the dearth of anatomical evidence for direct, central innervation of cerebral blood vessels, something which is difficult to document conclusively, there are several provocative physiological studies that indicate that these pathways do exist and can influence cerebral blood flow or capillary permeability. Putative origins of these pathways are the locus ceruleus, raphé nucleus, fastigial nucleus, and several other brain areas. The purpose of this contribution is to discuss the possibility that cerebral blood vessels could be innervated by neurons whose pathways exist solely in the brain.

II. LOCUS CERULEUS

The first brain area to receive extensive attention as a possible source of central innervation was the locus ceruleus. The locus ceruleus is a nucleus located in the pons and has a widespread distribution of noradrenergic fibers to virtually the entire brain, including cerebral cortex, hippocampus, cerebellum, hypothalamus, medulla, and pons.[15] Some fibers appear to end in the vicinity of brain capillaries in discrete brain areas but there is little evidence that resistance vessels are supplied by the locus ceruleus.[5,13,16-18] However, even the issue of central innervation of capillaries has been questioned.[16,19] Because the locus ceruleus receives afferent input concerning vascular status of the body (i.e., arterial blood pressure and volume, arterial blood pCO_2),[20-22] it is conceivable that vascular innervation from this nucleus could constitute the efferent part of a reflex arc involving control of cerebrovascular tone or capillary permeability.

Results from studies of effects of chronic surgical (electrolytic lesions) or chemical denervation (6-hydroxydopamine) of the locus ceruleus on resting CBF are conflicting. Chronic denervation has been reported to increase resting CBF[23,24] while others have not found changes in CBF.[25-27] Chronic denervation also does not change the cerebral metabolic rate.[27] Further, results from studies of effects of locus ceruleus denervation on cerebrovascular responsiveness to arterial hypercapnia have also been controversial. Several groups showed an attenuation of increases in CBF,[23,25,28] while others did not see such an effect or saw an increased responsiveness to arterial hypercapnia.[24,27,29] Reasons for differences are unclear, but could be due to species studied, methods used to characterize cerebral blood flow, mode of denervation (surgical vs. chemical), or other aspects of the study. However, it is unlikely that cerebrovascular dilation caused by arterial hypercapnia is due to activation of neural pathways. For example, cerebral arteries relax to hypercapnia or acidosis *in vitro,*[30,31] dilate *in vivo* when extracellular pH falls,[32,33] and also dilate in spite of administration of various receptor blockers or denervation of putative peripheral dilator pathways.[34,35] Also, locus ceruleus lesions do not attenuate the dilation to arterial hypoxia.[27] Lastly, lesions of the locus ceruleus do not alter cerebral blood flow or metabolic responses to bicuculline-induced seizures.[36]

In contrast to the results from the chronic denervation studies, in which the results have been inconsistent, it is clear that electrical stimulation of the locus ceruleus results in widespread decreases in CBF[3741] in rats, cats, and monkeys. Pharmacological blockade of $\alpha_2$adrenoceptors blocked the decrease in CBF with stimulation.[42] However, it seems unlikely that this change in CBF is due to a direct effect of nerves on cerebral resistance vessels. For example, locus ceruleus stimulation decreases the firing rate of distant neurons[41,43,44] and reduces the cerebral metabolic rate in proportion to decreases in blood flow.[39,45] In contrast to the above studies, Mraovitch et al.[46] reported that locus ceruleus stimulation did not change CBF and suggested that previous studies had inadvertently activated the nearby parabrachial nucleus, which they have shown to decrease CBF and metabolic rate. Thus, it is unlikely that the locus ceruleus provides significant, direct innervation to cerebral resistance vessels.

Hartman and colleagues have reported that electrical stimulation of the locus ceruleus increases blood-brain barrier permeability to water by about 50% with[18] or without[37,47] decreasing CBF. These studies are in some ways similar to those of Iadecola et al.,[48] who showed a possible modification in blood-brain barrier permeability, in this case to plasma catecholamine, during stimulation of the dorsal medullary reticular formation. On the other hand, chronic lesions of the locus ceruleus failed to show a change in blood-brain barrier permeability.[26] Thus, I believe that the issue of whether the locus ceruleus normally plays an important role in regulation of blood-brain barrier permeability is still open.

III. RAPHÉ NUCLEUS

Early evidence[49] provided the basis for suggesting that serotoninergic fibers, possibly from the raphé nucleus, supply cerebral blood vessels. Almost all of the serotonin-containing neurons within the brain arise from the raphé nucleus of the midbrain, where they project to many rostral areas of the brain.[50-54] Biochemical and immunohistological approaches have documented the presence of serotonin in the adventia or walls of the cerebral resistance vessels of various sizes (circle of Willis, pial arterioles, parenchymal arterioles) in a wide range of species including man.[54-62] Destruction of the raphé nucleus greatly attenuates or abolishes the presence of serotonin associated with cerebral blood vessels.[54,59,60] In addition, electrical stimulation of the raphé nucleus reduced perivascular serotonin concentration, while the levels of the metabolite 5-hydroxyindoleacetic acid were increased.[60] The connection between cerebral arteries and the raphé nucleus is further documented by retrograde tracing experiments.[63] Although effects of exogenous serotonin have been examined extensively both *in vitro* and *in vivo,*[64-66] only one study has been done on effects of raphé nucleus stimulation on CBF. Evidence of functional innervation is provided by studies that show reduced CBF[67] without corresponding changes in metabolic rate[68] with electrical stimulation of the raphé nucleus; changes in regional CBF with stimulation did not correspond on a regional basis with density or distribution of serotonergic projections.

Recent studies, however, have questioned the concept of direct serotoninergic innervation to cerebral blood vessels. Thus, a number of investigators have found that removal of the superior cervical ganglia, which supply sympathetic innervation to cerebral blood vessels, virtually eliminates the presence of serotonin in these vessels.[66,69-71] Although peripheral blood vessels have been reported to take up and store serotonin in smooth muscle and endothelial cells, this process has not been documented in cerebral blood vessels. Further, careful flushing of vessels to remove blood prior to dissection and preparation prevents significant accumulation of serotonin in cerebral blood vessels.[72] As it turns out sympathetic nerve endings have a high affinity uptake system for serotonin, and once loaded with serotonin, co-release serotonin with norepinephrine during depolarization.[66,70] Potential pools for serotonin include mast cells, blood, and neuronal release.[73,74] Some investigators still maintain that while serotonin in large cerebral arteries is due to uptake by sympathetic nerve endings, pial arterioles are innervated directly via the raphé nucleus.[75,76] Thus, the evidence is strongly against direct serotoninergic innervation of cerebral blood vessels. However, it seems likely that serotonin can be taken up normally by sympathetic nerves and is coreleased upon neural activation.

IV. FASTIGIAL NUCLEUS

Perhaps the most extensively studied intracerebral pathway is that of the fastigial nucleus. The fastigial nucleus is located in the cerebellum and appears to be involved in arousal, and predatory, eating, and drinking behaviors.[77] The pathway to cerebral cortex is complex, but may be multisynaptic. Neurons originating or passing through the fastigial nucleus of the cerebellum might have synapses on basal forebrain nuclei which supply cortex with cholinergic innervation or simply pass throughout this area. Fibers from the fastigial nucleus also supply closer anatomical structures in the brainstem and the spinal cord. Electrical activation of the fastigial nucleus increases arterial blood pressure and heart rate,[78,79] increases release of renin,[80] adrenal catecholamines,[81] and vasopressin,[82] and has been reported to increase cephalic[83] and brain blood flows.[83-89] In addition, fastigial nucleus stimulation also increases myocardial blood flow and reduces renal and duodenum blood flows.[90] The overall cardiovascular effect is termed the fastigial pressor response.[78] It has been reported that separate loci mediate the pressor response and the CBF response,[88,91] although there is evidence for close association of pathways in some areas. The blood flow response occurs in virtually every area of the brain, with the largest increases approximately (100%) in cerebral cortex and the smallest increase (about 50%) occurring in the brainstem. Blood flow also increases in the spinal cord.[91] Increases are not immediate, but rather appear after a delay of about 20 to 25 s.[89,92] Increases in CBF occur even in the absence of arterial hypertension. Increases in blood flow are independent of changes in metabolic rate within cerebral cortex as in many other brain regions, but in other areas, especially brainstem, increases in blood flow are parallel to increases in the metabolic rate.[87] In contrast to the fastigial nucleus, stimulation of another caudal area of the brain, namely the dorsal medullary reticular formation, has been reported to similarly increase both blood flow and metabolic rate in many brain areas.[93] Directly stimulating the magnocellular nucleus of the basal forebrain/substantia innominate, which may be activated by fastigial nucleus stimulation, increases cortical blood flow.[94,95] Increases in cortical blood flow are abolished by lesions of the basal forebrain[96] or by systemic administration of atropine,[89,97] or substantially reduced by topical application of atropine,[98] thereby establishing the cholinergic nature of the response. Involvement of local neurons is suggested by experiments employing cortical application of ibotenic acid, which destroys local neurons but not cholinergic innervation, and abolishes increases in cortical blood flow with stimulation.[99] Electrical stimulation of the fastigial nucleus also reduces ischemic infarction size caused by middle cerebral artery occlusion in rats by 40 to 70%.[100]

However, there is evidence to the contrary that suggests caution in accepting the importance of the fastigial nucleus as a site of control of CBF. First, chronic lesions of the basal forebrain have been reported to decrease metabolic rate in the cerebral cortex,[101] providing evidence that this area supplies both neurons and possibly blood vessels. However, it is possible that separate pools of fibers from this area independently supply neurons or vessels, or that basal forebrain nuclei are unrelated to fastigial nucleus projections. Second, as mentioned earlier, there still is no documentation that central cholinergic nerves actually innervate resistance vessels. However, it is possible that neurons and/or glia are the ultimate terminations of innervation,[6] and that these cells in turn release vasodilator stimuli. Indeed, Iadecola[102] has reported that inhibition of nitric oxide synthase abolishes the cerebrovascular dilation due to fastigial nucleus stimulation. Third, the actual origin of the dilator pathway is unclear. While electrical stimulation of the fastigial nucleus results in increases in CBF, chemical stimulation of cell bodies of neurons in this area results in reduced CBF.[103] Thus, it is possible that electrical stimulation activates axons travelling through the fastigial nucleus, rather than activating only locally-originating neurons. Fourth, several studies from one institution have presented data which indicate that fastigial nucleus stimulation does not alter CBF. These authors found that fastigial nucleus stimulation does not increase cortical blood flow substantially in chloralose anesthetized cats or rats.[90,92,104] However, blood flow to caudate nucleus, pons, and medulla did increase in cats by 20 to 25% during stimulation.[90] In response to those studies, Iadecola et al.[91] have shown that larger doses of chloralose than they used in earlier studies blunted or eliminated dilation due to fastigial nucleus stimulation. Indeed, the CBF response appears to be particularly susceptible to anesthetic effects, being eliminated by barbituate[89] or halothane anesthesia.[91] The fastigial pressor response is blunted by additional barbituate[89] but not chloralose.[91,92] Why large doses of chloralose should almost completely block cerebrovascular dilation associated with fastigial nucleus stimulation is unclear. In chloralose anesthetized cats, cerebral resistance vessels still dilate to arterial hypercapnia and hypoxia, during seizures, and in response to topical application of many different substances.[34,35] Although there is considerable evidence indicating that the fastigial nucleus could play a role in regulation of the cerebral circulation via central pathways, I believe that the importance of dilator pathways to the cerebral blood vessels has not yet been proved.

V. OTHER AREAS

There is evidence that other brain areas might be involved in regulation of the cerebral circulation via central pathways. However, results concerning other specific brain areas have usually only been reported by a few papers from one laboratory. Therefore, independent confirmation of results often is lacking. Nonetheless, these studies provide interesting new information. One area, the centromedian-parafascicular complex of the thalamus, when electrically stimulated, has been reported to increase CBF in the absence of changes in metabolic rate.[105,106] Thus, in this respect, the centromedian-parafascicular complex is similar to the fastigial nucleus. Another area, the dorsal medullary reticular formation, has been reported to increase both CBF and metabolic rate when electrically stimulated.[48,107-109] An interesting aspect of these studies is that adrenally derived catecholamines, possibly acting through a modified blood-brain barrier or another yet, undefined mechanism, are responsible for a considerable part of the increased CBF. A third area, namely the parabrachial nucleus of the pons, is able to cause decreases in CBF and metabolic rate, when stimulated, in virtually every brain area studied except medulla and hypothalamus.[46] Thus, CBF and metabolic rate changes during stimulation of this area are similar to responses to stimulation of the nearby locus ceruleus. A fourth area, the nucleus tractus solitarii, appears to interact with the cerebral circulation in an unusual fashion. Lesions of this area caused loss of cerebral autoregulation to increases in arterial blood pressure to most areas of the brain, while cerebrovascular responsiveness to arterial hypercapnia or hypoxia was intact.[110]

VI. CONCLUSIONS

Considerable interest has focused on the possibility that cerebral blood vessels are innervated by pathways that exist entirely within the brain, and that activation of these pathways can alter CBF independently of changes in metabolic rate and can alter characteristics of the blood-brain barrier. At present, anatomical evidence establishing such connections is not well documented. However, it could be that other types of cells, such as glia, are innervated by central pathways, and that these cells release vasoactive substances when activated. On the other hand, functional studies have provided evidence that central innervation may play a role in control of cerebral blood flow. Further studies, however, are needed to conclusively establish the importance of central innervation in regulation of cerebral hemodynamics.

REFERENCES

1. **Busija, D. W. and Heistad, D. D.,** Factors involved in physiological regulation of cerebral blood flow, *Rev. Physiol. Biochem. Pharmacol.,* 101, 161, 1984.
2. **Busija, D. W., Sadoshima, S., Marcus, M. L., and Heistad, D. D.,** Functional significance of sympathetic innervation of cerebral vessels. Can the issue now be resolved?, in *Trends in Autonomic Pharmacology,* S., Kalsner, Ed., Urban and Schwarzenber, Baltimore, 1982, 187.
3. **Busija, D. W.,** Nervous control of the cerebral circulation, in *Nervous Control of Blood Vessels,* Gardiner, S. M. and Bennett, T., Eds., Harwood, London, in press.
4. **Heistad, D. D. and Kontos, H. A.,** Cerebral circulation, in *Handbook of Physiology, Section 2; The Cardiovascular Center, Vol. 3, Peripheral Circulation and Organ Blood Flow,* Shepherd, J. D. and Abboud, F. M., Eds., Academic Press, New York, 1983, 137.
5. **Rennels, M. L., Forbes, M. S., Anders, J. J., and Nelson, E.,** Innervation of the microcirculation in the central nervous system and other tissues, in *Neurogenic Control of the Brain Circulation,* Owman, C. and Edvinsson, L., Eds., Pergamon Press Oxford, 1977, 91.
6. **Stone, E. A. and Ariano, M. A.,** Are glia cells targets of the central noradrenergic system? A review of the evidence, *Brain Res. Rev.,* 14, 297, 1989.
7. **Nielsen, K. C. and Owman, C.,** Adrenergic innervation of pial arteries related to the circle of Willis in the cat, *Brain Res.,* 6, 773, 1967.
8. **Edvinsson, L., Owman, C., Rosengrent, E., and West, K. A.,** Concentration of noradrenaline in pial vessels, choroid plexus, and iris during 2 weeks after sympathetic ganglionectomy or decentralization, *Acta Physiol. Scand.* 85, 201, 1972.
9. **Edvinsson, L., Fahrenkrug, J., Hanko, J., Owman, C., Sundler, F., and Uddman, R.,** VIP (vasoactive intestinal polypeptide)-containing nerves of intracranial arteries in mammals, *Cell Tissue Res.,* 208, 135, 1980.
10. **Norregaard, T. and Moskowitz, M. A.,** Substance P and the sensory innervation of intracranial and extracranial feline cephalic arteries, *Brain,* 108, 517, 1985.
11. **Suzuki, N., Hardebo, J. E., and Owman, C.,** Origins and pathways of choline acetyltransferase — positive parasympathetic nerve fibers to cerebral vessels in rats, *J. Cereb. Blood Flow Metab.,* 8, 697, 1988.
12. **McDonald, D. M. and Rasmussen, G. L.,** An ultrastructural analysis of neurites in the basal lamina of capillaries in the chinchilla cochlear nucleus, *J. Comp. Neurol.,* 173, 475, 1977.
13. **Swanson, L. W., Connelly, M. A., and Hartman, B. K.,** Ultrastructural evidence for central monoaminergic innervation of blood vessels in the paraventricular nucleus of the hypothalamus, *Brain Res.,* 136, 166, 1977.
14. **Rennels, M. L. and Nelson, E.,** Capillary innervation in the mammalian central nervous system: an electron microscopic demonstration, *Am. J. Anat.,* 144, 233, 1975.
15. **Amaral, D. G. and Sinnamon, H. M.,** The locus ceruleus: neurobiology of a central noradrenergic nucleus, *Prog. Neurobiol.* 9, 147, 1977.
16. **Edvinsson, L., Lindvall, M., Nielsen, K. C., and Owman, C.,** Are brain vessels innervated also by central (non-sympathetic) adrenergic neurones?, *Brain Res.,* 63, 496, 1973.
17. **Hartman, B. K., Zide, D., and Udenfriend, D.,** The use of dopamine beta hydroxylase as a marker for the central noradrenergic nervous system in rat brain, *Proc. Natl. Acad. Sci. U.S.A.,* 69, 2722, 1972.
18. **Hartman, B. K., Swanson, L. W., Raichle, M. E., Preskorn, S. H., and Clark, H. B.,** Central adrenergic regulation of cerebral microvascular permeability and blood flow; anatomic and physiologic evidence, *Adv. Exp. Med. Biol.,* 131, 113, 1980.

19. **Jones, B. E.,** Relationship between catecholamine neurons and cerebral blood vessels studied by their simultaneous fluorescent revelation in the rat brainstem, *Brain Res. Bull.*, 9, 33, 1982.
20. **Carlsson, A., Holmin, T., Lindquist, M., and Siesjö, B.,** Effect of hypercapnia and hypocapnia on tryptophan and tyrosine hydroxylation in rat brain, *Acta Physiol. Scand.*, 99, 503, 1977.
21. **Elam, M., Svensson, T. H., and Thoren, P.,** Differentiated cardiovascular afferent regulation of locus ceruleus neurons and sympathetic nerves, *Brain Res.*, 358, 77, 1985.
22. **Svensson, T. H. and Thoren, P.,** Brain noradrenergic neurons in the locus ceruleus: inhibition by blood volume load through vagal afferents, *Brain Res.*, 172, 174, 1979.
23. **Bates, D., Weinshilboum, R. M., Campbell, R. J., and Sundt, T., Jr.** The effect of lesions in the locus ceruleus on the physiological responses of the cerebral blood vessels in cats, *Brain Res.*, 136, 431, 1977.
24. **Yokote, H., Itakura, T., Nakai, K., Kamei, I., Imai, H., and Komai, N.** The role of the central catecholamine neuron in cerebral circulation, *J. Neurosurg.*, 65, 370, 1986.
25. **Reddy, S. V. R., Yaksh, T. L., Anderson, R. E., and Sundt, T. M., Jr.** Effect in cat of locus ceruleus lesions on the response of cerebral blood flow and cardiac output to altered p_aCO_2, *Brain Res.*, 365, 278, 1986.
26. **McCulloch, J., Savaki, H. E., and Angerson, W.,** Regional water permeability in the CNS of conscious rats: effects of hypercapnia and locus ceruleus lesions, in *Cerebral Blood Flow: Effects of Nerves and Neurotransmitters*, Heistad, D. D. and Marcus, M. L., Eds., Elsevier North Holland, New York, 1982, 509.
27. **Dahlgren, N., Lindvall, O., Sakabe, T., Stenevi, U., and Siesjö,** Cerebral blood flow and oxygen consumption in the rat brain after lesions of the noradrenergic locus ceruleus system, *Brain Res.*, 209, 11, 1981.
28. **Mendelow, A. D., McCalden, T. A., Hattingh, J., et al.,** The effect of chemical sympathectomy on cerebrovascular reactivity and cerebral metabolism, in *International Symposium on Neurogenic Control of the Brain Circulation*, Owman, C. and Edvinsson, L., Eds., Pergamon Press, Oxford, 1977, 429.
29. **Edvinsson, L., Hardebo, J. E., and MacKenzie, E. T.,** Effects of intraventricular 6-hydroxydopamine on cerebrovascular CO_2 reactivity in anesthetized rats, *Acta Physiol. Scand.*, 101, 122, 1977.
30. **Harder, D. R. and Madden, J. A.,** Cellular mechanism of force development in cat middle cerebral artery by reduced CO_2, *Pfluegers Arch.*, 403, 402, 1985.
31. **Toda, N., Hatano, Y., and Mori, K.,** Mechanisms underlying response to hypercapnia and bicarbonate of isolated dog cerebral arteries, *Am. J. Physiol.*, 257, H141, 1989.
32. **Kontos, H. A., Raper, A. J., and Patterson, J. L.,** Analysis of vasoactivity of local pH, PCO_2, and bicarbonate on pial vessels, *Stroke*, 8, 358, 1977.
33. **Wagerle, L. C. and Mishra, O. P.,** Mechanism of CO_2 response in cerebral arteries of the newborn pig: role of phospholipase, cyclooxygenase, and lipoxygenase pathways, *Circ. Res.*, 62, 1019, 1988.
34. **Busija, D. W. and Heistad, D. D.,** Effects of cholinergic nerves on cerebral blood flow in cats, *Circ. Res.*, 48, 62, 1980.
35. **Busija, D. W. and Heistad, D. D.,** Atropine does not attenuate cerebral vasodilation during hypercapnia, *Am. J. Physiol.*, 242, H683, 1982.
36. **Ingvar, M., Lindvall, O., Folbergrová, J., .and Siesjö, B. K.,** Influence of lesions of the noradrenergic locus ceruleus system on the cerebral metabolic response to bicuculline-induced seizures, *Brain Res.*, 264, 225, 1983.
37. **Raichle, M. E., Hartman, B. K., Eichling, J. O., and Sharpe, L. G.,** Central noradrenergic regulation of cerebral blood flow and vascular permeability, *Proc. Natl. Acad. Sci. U.S.A.*, 72, 3726, 1975.
38. **Goadsby, P. J., Lambert, G. A., and Lance, J. W.,** Differential effects on the internal and external carotid circulation of the monkey evoked by locus ceruleus stimulation, *Brain Res.*, 249, 247, 1982.

39. **Buckweitz, E., Edelman, N. H., and Weiss, H. R.,** Effect of locus ceruleus stimulation on regional cerebral oxygen consumption in the cat, *Brain Res.*, 325, 107, 1985.
40. **De La Torre, J. C.,** Local cerebral blood flow following stimulation of locus ceruleus in monkeys and rats, in *Neurogenic Control of the Brain Circulation,* Owman, C. and Edvinsson, L., Eds., Pergamon Press, Oxford, 1977, 433.
41. **Katayama, Y., Aeno, Y., Tsukiyama, T., and Tsubakawa, T.,** Long lasting suppression of firing of cortical neurons and decrease in cortical blood flow following training pulse stimulation of the locus ceruleus in the cat, *Brain Res.*, 216, 173, 1981.
42. **Goadsby, P. G., Lambert, G. A., and Lance, J. W.,** The mechanism of cerebrovascular vasoconstriction in response to locus ceruleus stimulation, *Brain Res.*, 326, 213, 1985.
43. **Hoffer, B. J., Siggins, G. R., Oliver, A. P., and Bloom, F. E.,** Activation of the pathway from locus ceruleus to rat cerebellar Purkinje neurons: pharmacological evidence of noradrenergic central inhibition, *J. Pharmacol. Exp. Therap.*, 181, 553, 1973.
44. **Segal, M. and Bloom, F. E.,** The action of norepinephrine in the rat hippocampus. IV. The effects of locus ceruleus stimulation on evoked hippocampal unit activity, *Brain Res.*, 107, 513, 1976.
45. **Abraham, W. C., Delanay, R. L., Dunn, A. J., and Zornetzer, S. F.,** Locus ceruleus stimulation decreases deoxyglucose uptake in ipsilateral mouse cerebral cortex, *Brain Res.*, 172, 387, 1979.
46. **Mravoitch, S., Iadecola, C., Ruggiero, D. A., and Reis, D. J.,** Widespread reductions in cerebral blood flow and metabolism elicited by electrical stimulation of the parabrachial nucleus in rat, *Brain Res.*, 341, 283, 1985.
47. **Raichle, M. E., Grubb, R. L., Jr., and Eichling, J. O.,** Neural and hormonal regulation of brain water permeability, in *Neurogenic Control of the Brain Circulation,* Owman C. and Edvinsson, L., Eds., Pergamon Press, Oxford, 1977, 465.
48. **Iadecola, C.,** Adrenal catecholamines participate in the cerebrovascular vasodilation elicited by electrical stimulation of the dorsal medullary reticular formation in rat, *Acta Physiol. Scand.*, (Suppl.) 552, 74, 1986.
49. **Chan-Palay, V.,** Serotonin axons in the supra- and sub-ependymal plexuses and in the leptomeninges; their roles in local alterations of cerebrospinal and vasomotor activity, *Brain Res.*, 102, 103, 1976.
50. **Dahlström, A. and Fuxe, K.,** Evidence for the existence of monoamine-containing neurons in the central nervous system, *Acta Physiol. Scand.*, 62, 1, 1965.
51. **Azmitia, E. C. and Segal, M.,** An autoradiographic analysis of the differential ascending projections of the dorsal and median raphé nuclei in the rat, *J. Comp. Neurol.*, 179, 641, 1978.
52. **Parent, A., Descarries, L., and Baudet, A.,** Organization of ascending serotonin systems in the adult rat brain. A radioautographic study after intraventricular administration of [$^{+}$H]5-hydroxytryptamine, *Neuroscience,* 6, 115, 1981.
53. **Steinbusch, H. W. M.,** Distribution of serotonin immunoreactivity in the central nervous system of the rat-cell bodies and terminals, *Neuroscience,* 6, 557, 1981.
54. **Edvinsson, L., Degueurce, A., Duverger, D., MacKenzie, E. R., and Scatton, B.,** Central serotonergic nerves project to the pial vessels of the brain, *Nature (London),* 306, 55, 1983.
55. **Edvinsson, L., Birath, E., Uddman, R., Lee, T. J.-F., Duverger, D., MacKenzie, E. T., and Scatton, B.,** Indoleaminergic mechanisms in brain vessels: localization, concentration, uptake and *in vitro* response of 5-hydroxytryptamine, *Acta Physiol. Scand.*, 121, 291, 1984.
56. **Griffith, S. G. and Burnstock, G.,** Immunohistochemical demonstration of serotonin in nerves supplying human cerebral and mesenteric blood vessels, *Lancet,* 1, 561, 1983.
57. **Griffith, S. G., Lincoln, J., and Burnstock, G.,** Serotonin as a neurotransmitter in cerebral arteries, *Brain Res.*, 247, 388, 1982.

58. **Moskowitz, M. A., Liebmann, J. E., Reinhard, J. F., and Schlosberg, A.,** Raphé origin of serotonin-containing neurons within choroid plexus of the rat, *Brain Res.*, 169, 590, 1979.
59. **Reinhard, J. F., Liebmann, J. E., Schlosberg, A. J., and Moskowitz, M. A.,** Serotonin neurons project to small blood vessels in the brain, *Science,* 206, 85, 1979.
60. **Scatton, B., Duverger, D., L'Heureux, R., Serrano, A., Fage, D., Nowicki, J.-P., and MacKenzie, E. T.,** Neurochemical studies on the existence, origin and characteristics of the serotonergic innervation of small pial vessels, *Brain Res.*, 345, 219, 1985.
61. **Di Carlo, V.,** Histochemical evidence for a serotonergic innervation of the microcirculation in the brain stem, in *Neurogenic Control of the Brain Circulation,* Owman, C. and Edvinsson, L., Eds., Pergamon Press, Oxford, 1977, 55.
62. **Di Carlo, V.,** Perivascular serotoninergic neurons: somatodendritic contacts and axonic innervation of blood vessels, *Neurosci. Lett.*, 51, 295, 1984.
63. **Tsai, S. H., Lin, S. Z., Wang, S. D., Liu, J. C., and Shih, C. J.,** Retrograde localization of the innervation of the middle cerebral artery with horseradish peroxidase in cats, *Neurosurgery,* 16, 463, 1985.
64. **Chang, J.-Y. and Owman, C.,** Serotonin potentiates noradrenalin-induced vasoconstriction through 5-HT_1-type receptors in guinea pig basilar artery, *J. Cereb. Blood Flow Metab.*, 9, 713, 1989.
65. **Harper, A. M. and MacKenzie, E. T.,** Effects of 5-hydroxytryptamine on pial arteriolar calibre in anesthetized cats, *J. Physiol.*, 271, 721, 1977.
66. **Saito, A. and Lee, T. J.-F.,** Serotonin as an alternative transmitter in sympathetic nerves of large cerebral arteries of the rabbit, *Circ. Res.*, 60, 220, 1987.
67. **Bonvento, G., Lacombe, P., and Seylaz, J.,** Effects of electrical stimulation of the dorsal raphé nucleus on local cerebral blood flow in the rat, *J. Cereb. Blood Flow Metab.*, 9, 251, 1989.
68. **Cudennec, A., Duverger, D., Serrano, A., Scatton, B., and MacKenzie, E. T.,** Influence of ascending serotonergic pathways on glucose use in the conscious rat brain. II. Effects of electrical stimulation of the rostral raphé nuclei, *Brain Res.*, 444, 227, 1988.
69. **Chang, J.-Y. and Owman, C.,** Immunohistochemical and pharmacological studies on 5-HT nerves and receptors in brain vessels, *Acta Physiol. Scand.*, 127, 49, 1986.
70. **Chang, J.-Y., Ekblad, E., Kannisto, P., and Owman, C.,** Serotonin uptake into cerebrovascular nerve fibers of rat, visualization by immunohistochemistry, disappearance following sympathectomy, and release during electrical stimulation, *Brain Res.*, 492, 79, 1989.
71. **Alafaci, C., Cowen, T., Crockard, H. A., and Burnstock, G.,** Cerebral perivascular serotonergic fibers have a peripheral origin in the gerbil, *Brain Res. Bull.*, 16, 303, 1986.
72. **Yu, J.-G. and Lee, T. J.-F.,** 5-hydroxytryptamine-containing fibers in cerebral arteries of the cat, rat and guinea pig, *Blood Vessels,* 26, 33, 1989.
73. **Jackowski, A., Crockard, A., Burnstock, G., and Lincoln, J.,** Alterations in serotonin and neuropeptide Y content of cerebrovascular sympathetic nerves following experimental subarachnoid hemorrhage, *J. Cereb. Blood Flow Metab.*, 9, 271, 1989.
74. **Edvinsson, L., Cervós-Navarro, J., Larsson, L.-I., Owman, C., and Rönnberg, A.-L.,** Regional distribution of mast cells containing histamine, dopamine, or 5-hydroxytryptamine in mammalian brain, *Neurology,* 27, 878, 1977.
75. **Bonvento, G., Lacombe, P., MacKenzie, E. T., Fage, D., Benavides, J., Rouquier, L., and Scatton, B.,** Evidence for differing origins of the serotonergic innervation of major cerebral arteries and small pial vessels in the rat, *J. Neurochem.*, 56, 681, 1991.
76. **Bonvento, G., Lacombe, P., MacKenzie, E. T., Rouquier, L., Scatton, B., and Seylaz, J.,** Differential effects of electrical stimulation of the dorsal raphé nucleus and of cervical sympathectomy on serotonin and noradrenaline concentrations in major cerebral arteries and pial vessels in the rat, *J. Cereb. Blood Flow Metab.*, 10, 123, 1990.

77. **Reis, D. J., Doba, N., and Nathan, M. A.,** Predatory attack, grooming, and consummatory behaviors evoked by electrical stimulation of cat cerebellar nuclei, *Science Wash. DC,* 182, 845, 1973.
78. **Miura, M. and Reis, D. J.,** A blood pressure response from fastigial nucleus and its relay pathways in the brainstem, *Am. J. Physiol.,* 219, 1330, 1970.
79. **Dormer, K. J. and Stone, H. L.,** Cerebellar pressor response in the dog, *Am. J. Physiol.,* 41, 574, 1976.
80. **Koyama, S., Ammons, W. S., and Manning, J. W.,** Altered renal vascular tone and plasma renin activity due to fastigial and baroreceptor activation, *Am. J. Physiol.,* 239L, H232, 1980.
81. **Del Bo, A., Ross, C., Pardal, J. F., Saavedra, J. M., and Reis, D. J.,** Fastigial stimulation in rats releases adrenomedullary catecholamines, *Am. J. Physiol.,* 244, R801, 1983.
82. **Del Bo, A., Sved, A. F., and Reis, D. J.,** Fastigial stimulation releases vasopressin in amounts which elevate arterial pressure, *Am. J. Physiol.,* 244, H687, 1983.
83. **Goadsby, P. J. and Lambert, G. A.,** Electrical stimulation of the fastigial nucleus increases total cerebral blood flow in monkey, *Neurosci. Lett.,* 107, 141, 1989.
84. **Doba, N. and Reis, D. J.,** Changes in regional blood flow and cardiodynamics evoked by electrical stimulation of the fastigial nucleus in cat and their similarity to orthostatic reflexes, *J. Physiol. (London),* 222, 729, 1972.
85. **McKee, J. C., Denn, M. J., and Stone, H. L.,** Neurogenic cerebral vasodilation from electrical stimulation of the cerebellum in the monkey, *Stroke,* 7, 179, 1976.
86. **Nakai, M., Iadecola, C., and Reis, D. J.,** Global cerebral vasodilation by stimulation of rat fastigial cerebellar nucleus, *Am. J. Physiol.,* 243, H226, 1972.
87. **Nakai, M., Iadecola, C., Ruggiero, D. A., Tucker, L. W., and Reis, D. J.,** Electrical stimulation of cerebellar fastigial nucleus increases cerebrocortical blood flow without change in local metabolism: evidence for an intrinsic system in brain for primary vasodilation, *Brain Res.,* 260, 35, 1983.
88. **Mraovitch, S., Pinard, E., and Seylaz, J.,** Two neural mechanisms in rat fastigial nucleus regulating systemic and cerebral circulation, *Am. J. Physiol.,* 251, H153, 1986.
89. **Iadecola, C. and Reis, D. J.,** Continuous monitoring of cerebrocortical blood flow during stimulation of the cerebellar fastigial nucleus: a study by laser-doppler flowmetry, *J. Cereb. Blood Flow Metab.,* 10, 608, 1990.
90. **Williams, J. L., Heistad, D. D., Siems, J. L., and Talman, W. T.,** Effects of stimulation of fastigial nucleus on cerebral blood flow in cats, *Am. J. Physiol.,* 257, H297, 1989.
91. **Iadecola, C., Springston, M. E., and Reis, D. J.,** Dissociation by chloralose of the cardiovascular and cerebrovascular responses evoked from the cerebellar fastigial nucleus, *J. Cereb. Blood Flow Metab.,* 10, 375, 1990.
92. **Talman, W. T., Dragon, D. M. N., Heistad, D. D., and Ohta, H.,** Cerebrovascular effects produced by electrical stimulation of fastigial nucleus, *Am. J. Physiol.,* 261, H707, 1991.
93. **Iadecola, C., Nakai, M., Mraovitch, Ruggiero, D. A., Tucker, L. W., and Reis, D. J.,** Global increase in cerebral metabolism and blood flow produced by focal electrical stimulation of dorsal medullary reticular formation in rat, *Brain Res.,* 272, 101, 1983.
94. **Lacombe, P., Sercombe, R., Verrecchia, C., Philipson, V., MacKenzie, E. T., and Seylaz, J.,** Cortical blood flow increases induced by stimulation of the substantia innominata of the unanesthetized rat, *Brain Res.,* 491, 1, 1989.
95. **Kurosawa, M., Sato, A., and Sato, Y.,** Well-maintained responses of acetylcholine release and blood flow in the cerebral cortex to focal electrical stimulation of the nucleus basalis of Meynert in aged rats, *Neurosci. Lett.,* 100, 198, 1989.
96. **Iadecola, C., Mraovitch, S., Meeley, M. P., and Reis, D. J.,** Lesions of the basal forebrain in rat selectively impair the cortical vasodilation elicited from cerebellar fastigial nucleus, *Brain Res.,* 279, 41, 1983.

97. **Iadecola, C., Underwood, M. D., and Reis, D. J.,** Muscarinic cholinergic receptors mediate the cerebrovasodilation elicited by stimulation of the cerebellar fastigial nucleus in rat, *Brain Res.,* 368, 375, 1986.
98. **Arneric, S. P., Iadecola, C., Underwood, M. D., and Reis, D. J.,** Local cholinergic mechanisms participate in the increase in cortical cerebral blood flow elicited by electrical stimulation of the fastigial nucleus in rat, *Brain Res.,* 411, 212, 1987.
99. **Iadecola, C. Arneric, S. P., Baker, H. D., Tucker, L. W., and Reis D. J.,** Role of local neurons in cerebrocortical vasodilation elicited from cerebellum, *Am. J. Physiol.,* 252, R1082, 1987.
100. **Reis, D. J., Berger, S. B., Underwood, M. D., and Khayata, M.,** Electrical stimulation of cerebellar fastigial nucleus reduces ischemic infarction elicited by middle cerebral artery occlusion in rat, *J. Cereb. Blood Flow Metab.,* 11, 810, 1991.
101. **Orzi, F., Diana, G., Casamenti, F., Palombo, E., and Fieschi, C.,** Local cerebral glucose utilization following unilateral and bilateral lesions of the nucleus basalis magnocellularis in the rat, *Brain Res.,* 462, 99, 1988.
102. **Iadecola, C.,** Nitric oxide participates in the cerebral vasodilation elicited from cerebellar fastigial nucleus, *Am. J. Physiol.: Reg. Int. Physiol.,* 263, R1156, 1992.
103. **Chida, K., Iadecola, C., and Reis, D. J.,** Global reduction in cerebral blood flow and metabolism elicited from intrinsic neurons of fastigial nucleus, *Brain Res.,* 500, 177, 1989.
104. **Williams, J. L., Murray, M. A., Schalk, K. A., and Heistad, D. D.,** Cerebral blood flow during fastigial pressor response in cats, *Am. J. Physiol.,* 258, H729, 1990.
105. **Mraovitch, S. and Seylaz, J.,** Metabolism-independent cerebral vasodilation elicited by electrical stimulation of the centromedian-parafascicular complex in rat, *Neurosci. Lett.,* 83, 269, 1987.
106. **Mraovitch, S., Lasbennes, F., Calando, Y., and Seylaz, J.,** Cerebrovascular changes elicited by electrical stimulation of the centromedian-parafascicular complex in the rat, *Brain Res.,* 380, 42, 1986.
107. **Iadecola, C., Lacombe, P. M., Underwood, M. D., Ishitsuka, T., and Reis, D. J.,** Role of adrenal catecholamines in cerebrovasodilation evoked from brain stem, *Am. J. Physiol.,* 252, H1183, 1987.
108. **Iadecola, C., Nakai, M., Arbit, E., and Reis, D. J.,** Global cerebral vasodilation elicited by focal electrical stimulation of the dorsal medullary reticular formation in anesthetized rat, *J. Cereb. Blood Flow Metab.,* 3, 270, 1983.
109. **Lacombe, P. M., Iadecola, C., Underwood, M. D., Sved, A. F., and Reis, D. J.,** Plasma epinephrine modulates the cerebrovasodilation evoked by electrical stimulation of dorsal medulla, *Brain Res.,* 506, 93, 1990.
110. **Ishitsuka, T., Iadecola, C., Underwood, M. D., and Reis, D. J.,** Lesions of nucleus tractus solitarii globally impair cerebrovascular autoregulation, *Am. J. Physiol.,* 251, H269, 1986.

Chapter 5

CATECHOLAMINERGIC INNERVATION OF CEREBRAL BLOOD VESSELS

Sami I. Harik

TABLE OF CONTENTS

I. Introduction 80

II. Cervical Sympathetic Innervation of the Brain's Macrovessels 80
- A. The Anatomical Evidence 80
- B. The Physiological Evidence (*In Vivo* Studies) 81
- C. The Pathophysiological Evidence 82
- D. The Pharmacological Evidence 83
  - 1. *In Vitro* Studies 83
  - 2. *In Vivo* Studies 84

III. Central Noradrenergic Innervation of the Brain's Microvessels 84
- A. The Anatomical Evidence 84
- B. The Physiological Evidence 85
- C. The Pathophysiological Evidence 86
- D. The Biochemical and Pharmacological Evidence 87

IV. Concluding Remarks 89

References 90

0-8493-5096-0/93/$0.00 + $.50

I. INTRODUCTION

The brain is a complicated and fastidious organ that requires a large and uninterrupted blood flow, about one fifth of the cardiac output at rest, for the delivery of oxygen and metabolic substrates (largely glucose) and for the removal of waste products. Because the brain accepts only brief or no debt, regional cerebral blood flow (CBF) must match regional brain metabolism. The mechanisms that control CBF and ensure this coupling have been the subject of much controversy, particularly the neural control of the brain circulation. Claude Bernard showed the profound effects of autonomic nerves on the peripheral circulation, especially the splanchnic circulation.[1] However, despite the extensive anatomical evidence that date back to Willis[2] demonstrating nerve fibers in the walls of cerebral blood vessels, the physiological significance of such innervation is still shrouded in ambiguity. Until recently, texts of physiology (e.g., Reference 3) did not consider the cerebrovascular innervation important in controlling the brain circulation which was traditionally attributed to products of brain metabolism such as carbon dioxide. The demonstration by Roy and Sherrington[4] in 1890 of the powerful effect of carbon dioxide on CBF has withstood the test of time.

The lack of evidence of vigorous neural effects on the brain's circulation prompted a plethora of reports that exceed those pertaining to other circulatory beds and unleashed an extensive debate that resulted in several symposia[5,6] and reviews.[7-10] The purpose of this chapter is to examine the anatomical, biochemical, physiological, and pharmacological evidence that pertains to the catecholaminergic innervation of the brain vasculature. Because there is little evidence supporting a dopaminergic or adrenergic innervation, the discussion will be restricted to the noradrenergic innervation. In the first part, I will discuss the larger blood vessels from the base of the brain to the pial surface, which are believed to receive their noradrenergic innervation from the cervical sympathetic ganglia. Then, I shall discuss the intraparenchymal blood vessels down to capillaries, which are thought to receive their noradrenergic innervation principally from the nucleus locus ceruleus (LC).

II. CERVICAL SYMPATHETIC INNERVATION OF THE BRAIN'S MACROVESSELS

A. THE ANATOMICAL EVIDENCE

Nerve fibers are known to exist in the walls of brain arteries and arterioles in man and other experimental animals. Although they were suspected to be of sympathetic origin, their noradrenergic nature was not established until specific histochemical fluorescence methods for catecholamines were used.[11-16] Ultrastructural studies confirmed the presence of these nerves and allowed assessment of their density and the distance between nerve endings and smooth muscles.[13,17-21] These noradrenergic fibers are known to originate from the cervical sympathetic ganglia because they degenerate after ablation of the ganglia.[13,14,16,22,23] The sympathetic noradrenergic innervation is evident in the large arteries at the base of the brain and in the major fissures, and extends to pial arteries and veins. The density of this innervation is said to decrease with the decreasing size of the vessels, and arteries are more densely innervated than veins. Also, arterial branches of the posterior circulation are less densely innervated than those of the carotid system.[16]

To summarize, the anatomy of the sympathetic noradrenergic innervation of the brain macrovasculature does not appear to be much different from that of other systemic vascular beds. Yet, the functional significance of this innervation was questioned, leading some writers to label it as ''vestigial''.

B. THE PHYSIOLOGICAL EVIDENCE (*IN VIVO* STUDIES)

There is a large number of reports on the effects of stimulation or ablation of cervical sympathetic nerves on the cerebral circulation, with markedly different conclusions. Perhaps the larger number of publications on the sympathetic innervation of the brain circulation than on other circulatory beds emphasizes the controversial role of this innervation. In most studies, the cervical sympathetic nerves were stimulated or ablated and CBF was measured, or changes in the diameter of pial vessels were determined. Even in those latter studies, which involved relatively straightforward acute animal experiments, the results were often conflicting, even studies performed in the same laboratory.[24,25] However, most investigators since Forbes and Wolff[26] consistently noted some constriction of pial vessels with cervical sympathetic stimulation.[27,28] It should be noted that the effect of these relatively minor decrements in the pial arterial diameter on CBF is not known.

The physiological studies of the influence of sympathetic nerves on the cerebral circulation concentrated mostly on changes in CBF. The popularity of CBF studies was, and continues to be, rooted in the dogma of the tight coupling between CBF and cerebral metabolism, so that alterations in brain neurophysiology are thought to be always associated with appropriate CBF changes. Another reason for the popularity of CBF studies is the ready availability of several methods that allow CBF measurements. Although many of these studies revealed minor or no effects of stimulation or ablation of the cervical sympathetic nerves on CBF, a few studies showed major changes, e.g., D'Alecy and Feigl measured a 70% drop in CBF during cervical sympathetic stimulation in the dog.[29] This particular study used the venous outflow method which was later found to suffer from methodological problems.[30] The majority of the reports on the effects of cervical sympathetic stimulation or ablation on CBF are summarized in the tables of Reference 8. The results are conflicting, but in general, when an effect was seen, it was modest and appeared more prominent when arterial carbon dioxide tension was altered.[27,31-33] These studies are consistent with the general idea that cervical sympathetic nerve activation causes constriction of cerebral resistance vessels, which becomes more evident when this vascular bed is dilated by hypercapnia.

There are few studies that assessed an end point other than CBF after cervical sympathetic stimulation or ablation. One of those described a transient increase in the brain vascular permeability to water.[34] Two other reports described marked constriction of cerebral veins after cervical sympathetic stimulation.[35,36] Also, studies from the same group reported a drop in intracranial pressure under normal and increased intracranial pressure conditions.[37,38] Cerebral veins are well endowed with noradrenergic nerve fibers,[39] which is unusual for rostral venous systems. This innervation may have a role in the control of intracranial pressure.

Several cogent points can be extracted from these studies. First, changes in pial vessel diameter or in CBF were mostly weak. This supported the contention that the sympathetic innervation of the brain macrovessels is either an anatomical redundancy or that noradrenergic receptors in the resistance vessels are "unusual" or absent. Second, studies that reported a vigorous effect of cervical sympathetic stimulation or ablation utilized methods of measuring CBF that were of questionable validity, while studies that used microspheres for CBF measurements did not report significant changes. Third, there may be prominent differences among species. The dog appears to be least likely to show effects of cervical sympathetic stimulation while primates are more sensitive.

C. THE PATHOPHYSIOLOGICAL EVIDENCE

Because of the lack of vigorous effects of cervical sympathetic stimulation or ablation on CBF in most studies that were performed under basal conditions, the effects of the sympathetic innervation were studied under pathophysiological conditions such as acute and chronic hypertension. The cerebral circulation is considered to be autoregulated, meaning that brain perfusion remains constant over a large range of arterial perfusion pressure. Acute cervical sympathectomy was shown to lower the limits of autoregulation[33] while cervical sympathetic stimulation increases the upper limits of autoregulation.[40,41] In addition, activation of the cervical sympathetics decreases or attenuates the increased CBF that is often associated with increased arterial pressure.[42-45] However, other studies have shown that these issues are complicated and do not obey any known unifying mechanism.[46,47]

Perhaps more important is the role of the sympathetic innervation in chronic hypertension. It is generally accepted that hypertrophy of arteries and arterioles occurs in chronic hypertension, and the brain vasculature is no exception. Sympathetic denervation decreases the wall thickness of the central ear artery[48] and of cerebral arteries[49] of rabbits, and pial arterioles of rats.[50] In stroke-prone spontaneously hypertensive rats that had a unilateral cervical sympathectomy at 3 weeks of age, Hart et al. found 1 year later that the wall-to-lumen ratio was significantly reduced on the denervated side.[51] This and other findings,[52,53] prompted some investigators to champion the "trophic" role of sympathetic nerves which promotes hypertrophy of arterial and arteriolar walls to enable these vessels to respond better to constrictor stimuli, to improve autoregulation, and to protect the blood-brain barrier from the perils of chronic hypertension.[54] On the other hand, these protective effects were questioned by Johansson and her associates who did not find significant differences in the radii or media areas of the internal carotid, middle cerebral, posterior communicating, and pial arteries between sympathectomized and nonsympathectomized spontaneously hypertensive rats.[55] Also, unlike the results of an earlier study,[52] the cerebrovascular lesions in stroke-prone spontaneously hypertensive rats did not differ between sympathectomized and control sides.[55] Thus, the ''trophic'' role of the sympathetic innervation on the cerebral macrovasculature in chronic hypertension, like other roles ascribed to this innervation, remains controversial.

D. THE PHARMACOLOGICAL EVIDENCE

1. *In Vitro* Studies

The contractility of segments of the major arteries at the base of the brain and of pial arteries from a variety of mammals, in response to the application of catecholamines and their agonists and antagonists, and to electrical field stimulation of their intramural nerves, was examined in numerous studies (see Reference 56 for review). In general, norepinephrine (NE) and other α-noradrenergic agonists cause only a modest contraction of cerebral arterial strips amounting to less than 20% of their capacity to contract. The more disturbing fact is that the concentrations of NE that are needed to obtain threshold or EC_{50} effects are 2 or more orders of magnitude higher than those needed to obtain these results in similar preparations from other arteries from the same animal species. These studies were extended to human cerebral arteries that were either obtained at surgery or at autopsy soon after death, with similar results. These findings are compatible with the controversial results of physiological studies. Bevan and Van Riper[56] list several possible explanations: first, greater distances exist between the noradrenergic varicosities and the smooth muscle layer of cerebral blood vessels. This may explain the poor results obtained from electrical field stimulation studies but is unlikely to be relevant in experiments in which excess NE is added to the physiological medium of arterial strips. Second, the density of α-noradrenergic receptors in cerebral blood vessels may be low. This idea is based on *in vitro* studies of arterial strip contraction (circular logic) but is not confirmed by modern methods for measuring receptor density and affinity. Also, brain vascular α-noradrenergic receptors may be abnormal with a lower affinity of binding. However, the affinity of prazosin for cerebral arterial α-noradrenergic receptors is comparable to that of other arteries, which prompted speculation that the peculiarity of these receptors is that they are restricted to the agonist recognition site.[57] Third, there may be inefficient coupling of α-noradrenergic receptors to the contractile elements of cerebral blood vessels. Fourth, the effects of noradrenergic mechanisms in cerebral vessels could be multifactorial, with many of these factors canceling each other.

2. *In Vivo* Studies

Two types of *in vivo* pharmacological studies of the effects of noradrenergic agents on the cerebral circulation were performed. In one, NE or its agonists and antagonists were injected systemically or into the brain's arteries, simulating the physiological release of catecholamines into the blood stream. The results of these experiments are complicated because these agents have major systemic effects (e.g., changes in blood pressure and cardiac output) which may cause autoregulatory changes that are independent of their actions on the cerebral vasculature. Also, these agents could affect brain metabolism and physiology in a manner that alters CBF. In any case, the intravenous administration of NE decreased CBF in the dog (this effect was blocked by phentolamine, an α_1-noradrenergic receptor antagonist)[58] and in the caudate nucleus, but not in the lateral geniculate body in rats.[16] In another study, NE infusion in dogs increased CBF and, curiously, this effect was blocked by propranolol, a β-noradrenergic receptor antagonist.[59] Confusing results were also obtained when noradrenergic agents were injected into the cerebral arterial circulation. CBF decreased in isolated brain preparations[60-63] and in intact animals.[59,64] On the other hand, CBF did not decrease during intracarotid infusion of NE in the baboon[65] and in man.[66] To add to the confusion, intravenous or intraarterial injections of isoproterenol induced different responses in CBF in intact animals and in the perfused brain preparation. In man, no change in regional CBF was detected when isoproterenol or propranolol were injected into the carotid artery.[67]

The extravascular application of catecholamines would mimic the effects of these neurotransmitters when they are released from nerve endings in the vessel wall. This could be achieved by superfusing the brain surface or by the microinjection of catecholamines in the walls of the vessels and noting the response by direct visual inspection. Most studies that used these techniques showed constriction of cerebral blood vessels.[28,68] The effects of superfusion of the cerebral cortex with NE also resulted in vessel constriction in some studies[25,69,70] but not in others.[24,71] The effects of NE were blocked by phentolamine,[28,70] indicating that this effect is mediated by α-noradrenergic receptors. Consistent with this conclusion, the application of isoproterenol to brain vessels caused only mild effects indicating the absence of a functionally significant population of β-adrenergic receptors.[24,70,72]

III. CENTRAL NORADRENERGIC INNERVATION OF THE BRAIN'S MICROVESSELS

A. THE ANATOMICAL EVIDENCE

Hartman et al. were the first to suggest the possibility of central noradrenergic innervation of cerebral microvessels in their study of dopamine beta-hydroxylase immunoreactivity in the rat brain.[73] Their suggestion, which was based on the close proximity of dopamine beta-hydroxylase immunoreactive nerve fibers emanating primarily from the nucleus LC to brain arterioles and capillaries, was later strengthened by the findings of Edvinsson et al.,[74] de la Torre,[75] and Swanson et al.[76] These nerve fibers had delicate varicosities which were distinctly different from those of the cervical sympathetic nerve fibers.[74] The ultrastructural evidence suggesting the innervation of pericytes and endothelial cells of brain microvessels constituted supporting evidence.[77] However, as discussed previously in the case of the cervical sympathetics, this anatomical evidence does not prove innervation, since these nerves may be coursing through and not necessarily innervating brain microvessels.

B. THE PHYSIOLOGICAL EVIDENCE

Following the publication of the aforementioned structural results, the logical physiological and pharmacological studies were performed. LC stimulation caused a transient increase in the blood-brain barrier permeability to water.[78] Also, noradrenergic agonists, such as the tricyclic antidepressants, induced similar responses.[79] The physiological significance of the altered permeability of brain endothelium to water remains unknown. The lipid bilayer of cell membranes is quite permeable to water, and the cerebral endothelium is not an exception. The first pass extraction of radiolabeled water by the brain exceeds 80%. Nevertheless, the latter two studies focused attention on important functions of brain capillaries: permeability and transport. Until then, studies of the innervation of the brain circulation concentrated on CBF for reasons that were discussed earlier. Two studies of the effect of LC stimulation on CBF were reported with conflicting results. The studies of de la Torre et al. showed decreased CBF in the rat,[80] while Goadsby et al. showed increased CBF and decreased carotid vascular resistance in the cat, which was more prominent ipsilaterally and which was curiously blocked by bilateral interruption of the facial nerve.[81] These studies should be interpreted with caution because of varying methodologies of CBF determinations and because of problems inherent in the specificity of the neural structures of the brain stem that were stimulated.

There are several reports on the effects of LC ablation on cerebral vascular function. Many investigators took advantage of the predominantly ipsilateral nature of the ceruleo-cortical pathways and performed unilateral LC lesions so that the contralateral cortex, with its normal complement of NE, could be used as an internal control,[82] thereby minimizing the confounding systemic factors. The first study on the cerebral vascular effects of LC lesion demonstrated that bilateral electrolytic lesions increased resting CBF and abolished the hypercapnia-induced increase in CBF, without interfering with autoregulation in anesthetized cats.[83] Unfortunately, electrolytic lesions are likely to produce destruction of brain stem structures other than LC neurons, and the bilaterality of the lesion did not allow side-to-side comparisons. On the other hand, Dahlgren et al. found no effect of dorsal noradrenergic tract ablations on CBF in anesthetized rats,[84] and McCulloch et al. also could not find an effect of LC ablation on CBF or on the permeability × surface area (PS) product of water in conscious rats.[85]

We also were unable to document a significant effect of unilateral LC lesion on CBF in awake and anesthetized rats (unpublished observations). However, because noradrenergic receptors on cerebral microvessels are predominantly of the β_2 subtype (see below), we suspected that the central noradrenergic innervation of brain microvessels is more likely to subserve vasodilation and increased CBF. For this reason, we studied the effect of unilateral LC lesion on CBF and brain capillary water permeability in rats when the cerebral circulation was maximally dilated, such as during brief status epilepticus induced by the intravenous administration of bicuculline.[86,87] These studies showed that unilateral LC lesions failed to alter CBF or the regional PS product for water during normotensive status epilepticus, despite the fact that regional CBF increased by two- to threefold.[86,87] In another study designed to determine whether LC lesion reduces the hypercapnia-induced increased CBF in conscious rats, we found that LC lesion had no such effect.[88] On the other hand, the administration of intracisternal 6-hydroxydopamine attenuated the cerebrovascular reactivity to hypercapnia in baboons.[89] To confuse matters further, Edvinsson et al. reported increased cerebrovascular reactivity to hypercapnia in rats injected with 6-hydroxydopamine into their cerebral ventricles.[90] In the latter two studies the lesions were not restricted to the central noradrenergic systems because 6-hydroxydopamine, given by intracisternal or intraventricular routes, destroys several brain monoaminergic systems. Thus, the existing evidence for a role of the putative central noradrenergic innervation of cerebral microvessels in the control of CBF is hopelessly controversial.

LC lesions markedly decreased or abolished the increased cerebral blood volume that is consistently induced by brief trains of electrical impulses applied directly to the cerebral cortex.[91,92] It is not clear whether this effect is a consequence of NE depletion on cerebral metabolism or whether it is mediated via the central noradrenergic innervation of brain microvessels.

C. THE PATHOPHYSIOLOGICAL EVIDENCE

Probably the most solid evidence for central noradrenergic innervation of the brain microvasculature is based on studies of cerebrovascular permeability to macromolecules such as albumin and horseradish peroxidase in experimental animals subjected to acute hypertensive insults. Harik and McGunigal demonstrated that hypertension induced by catecholamine infusions or seizures caused significantly more albumin leakage into forebrain structures ipsilateral to LC lesion.[93] However, hypertension of the same magnitude induced by angiotensin did not cause increased albumin leakage in the NE-depleted cortex. This protective effect of the putative central noradrenergic innervation of the brain microvasculature is consistent with prior reports that neonatal 6-hydroxydopamine treatment[94] and intracisternal 6-hydroxydopamine injections[95] (to ablate central monoaminergic neurons) increased the vulnerability of the blood-brain barrier to acute hypertension in rats. To determine the mechanism by which the increased leakage of macromolecules occurs in the NE-depleted cerebral cortex after LC lesion, ultrastructural studies were performed using horseradish peroxidase as a tracer. Leakage occurred during catecholamine-induced hypertension, and it was more prominent ipsilateral to LC lesion.[96] The increased permeability affected mainly the arterioles which showed enhanced pinocytosis as the principal mechanism of tracer extravasation.[96] The results of all of these studies imply that the central noradrenergic innervation plays an important role in maintaining the integrity of the blood-brain barrier during acute hypertension, particularly when induced by agents that stimulate noradrenergic receptors.

D. THE BIOCHEMICAL AND PHARMACOLOGICAL EVIDENCE

If brain microvessels are truly innervated by noradrenergic nerves, then they should possess surface membrane molecules that recognize NE, i.e., noradrenergic receptors. There are several methods for studying such receptors. Prior to the advent of cellular and molecular pharmacology, receptors were studied by assessing one of their functions after the administration of the natural agonists. In cerebral macrovessels for example, NE would be added to the medium bathing vessel strips, and the contraction that ensued was measured. This assumes that NE causes cerebral arteries to contract. Because the exact function of NE, if any, in the cerebral microvasculature is not known, this line of research could not be pursued. The development of methods for isolating highly enriched and metabolically active brain microvessels allowed studies of their receptors using standard receptor binding methods. The presence of noradrenergic receptors in isolated brain microvessels was first reported in 1980 by Harik et al.[97] and Peroutka et al.[98] and was subsequently confirmed by several groups using a variety of ligands in a number of mammalian species including man.[99-105] The dominant noradrenergic receptor in cerebral microvessels is the β-noradrenergic receptor. Based on the differential affinity of binding to specific agonists and antagonists, the vast majority of the β-noradrenergic receptors are believed to be of the β_2 subtype.[99,104] Because β-noradrenergic receptors usually mediate their actions via cyclic AMP as the second messenger, the existence of these receptors in cerebral microvessel preparations was biologically anchored by showing that β-noradrenergic receptor agonists stimulate the formation of cyclic AMP in isolated cerebral microvessels and that this stimulation is blocked by specific β-antagonists.[106-108]

α_2-noradrenergic receptors were also identified in brain microvessels by ligand binding.[98,99,103,104] The second messenger by which these α_2 receptors mediate their function in brain microvessels remains unknown. On the other hand, the existence of a substantial density of α_1-noradrenergic receptors in brain microvessels is controversial. Harik et al. initially found no detectable

WB-4101 binding to α_1 receptors in rat brain microvessels and only minimal binding in pig brain microvessels,[99] while Peroutka et al. found a respectable amount of α_1 receptors using the same ligand in bovine brain microvessels.[98] More recent studies using better α_1 ligands (prazosin and HEAT) demonstrated the presence of α_1-noradrenergic receptors in human brain microvessels, but their density is low.[103,104] The effects of α_1-noradrenergic receptor stimulation in brain microvessels may be mediated by an altered phosphatidylinositol metabolism.[109]

The presence of noradrenergic receptors in brain microvessels indicates that these vessels can react to NE, but does not prove innervation by the central noradrenergic system, since these receptors, for example, may be there to respond to circulating NE. It is now generally accepted that ablation of the noradrenergic innervation to many organs, including the brain, results in an increased density of β-noradrenergic receptors in these organs, which probably underlies the phenomenon of "denervation supersensitivity".[110] This strategy was recently applied to microvessels isolated from the cerebral cortex ipsilateral to LC lesion. LC lesion induced a robust increase in the density of β_2-noradrenergic receptors in microvessels isolated from the NE-depleted cerebral hemisphere.[104] This denervation supersensitivity of cerebral microvessel β-noradrenergic receptors after LC lesion was as robust as that obtained after chronic reserpine treatment.[104] Because reserpine depletes central and peripheral NE stores, these results suggest that β-noradrenergic receptors of rat cerebral microvessels respond predominantly to NE from LC terminals. If the β-noradrenergic receptors of brain microvessels respond to NE from central noradrenergic systems, then these receptors are probably located on the abluminal side of capillaries. However, proof of the exact anatomical location of any of the noradrenergic receptors of cerebral blood vessels must await future ultrastructural investigations.

Because of the known degeneration of the central noradrenergic neurons, especially those of the LC, in Alzheimer disease, Kalaria and Harik assessed noradrenergic receptors of microvessels isolated from the cerebral cortex, obtained at autopsy from patients with Alzheimer disease. They found a significantly higher density of α_2- and β_2-noradrenergic receptors in cerebral microvessels from Alzheimer disease patients than in age-matched controls.[105] These findings may have consequences concerning the cerebral microvascular functions in this disease.

Further support for the notion that central noradrenergic innervation of cerebral microvessels from the LC influences the permeability of the blood-brain barrier was provided by the finding that LC lesion causes a marked loss in specific [^{3}H]ouabain binding sites in isolated cerebral microvessels.[111] Because ouabain binds to the catalytic unit of Na^+/K^+-ATPase, this finding implies decreased Na^+/K^+-ATPase activity. Na^+/K^+-ATPase has a polar distribution in cerebral microvessels, which constitute the blood-brain barrier, and is credited with controlling brain Na^+ and K^+ concentrations.

IV. CONCLUDING REMARKS

There is little question that brain macrovessels, from the larger ones at the base of the brain and until they penetrate into the brain tissue, have sympathetic noradrenergic nerve fibers in their adventitia to a degree that is comparable to that of the blood vessels of other organs. These nerves originate in the cervical sympathetic ganglia. Similar but less robust anatomical evidence also suggests noradrenergic innervation of intraparenchymal cerebral microvessels from the LC. However, anatomical evidence by itself does not prove innervation, and the functional role of this putative innervation was questioned. It is clear that alterations in CBF in response to stimulation or ablation of the sympathetic nerves or the LC, or to the application of NE *in vivo* and *in vitro,* are much less robust than similar experiments in other circulatory beds. Most of these experiments assumed that the effect of NE on the cerebral circulation is to cause constriction of the smooth muscles of resistance vessels thereby decreasing their diameters and CBF. Modern biochemical and pharmacological investigations of isolated cerebral microvessels now clearly show that α_2- and β_2-noradrenergic receptors exist, and a low density of α_1-noradrenergic receptors may also be present. The fact that cerebral microvessels possess noradrenergic receptors means that they can react to NE, but that again does not prove innervation, since it is possible for these receptors to interact with blood-borne NE. On the other hand, the fact that β-noradrenergic receptors upregulate when the LC is destroyed strongly suggests that these receptors receive their NE from LC neurons. Because these small vessels do not have much muscle elements and may be beyond the majority of the resistance part of the cerebral circulation, it is probable that this innervation is concerned mostly with alterations in capillary permeability and control of blood-brain barrier functions. While this conclusion cannot be extended to the cerebral macrovasculature for lack of appropriate data, the possibility that the noradrenergic innervation of the cerebral macrovasculature may not be related to changes in resistance and CBF should also be entertained.

Unlike the arterial system, the venous system has not received its fair share of studies regarding the influence of its noradrenergic innervation. From the structural viewpoint, cerebral veins are innervated, and stimulation of the cervical sympathetics was shown to cause their contraction. The functional significance of these observations needs further examination, particularly the relationship to changes in vascular permeability and intracranial pressure.

Perhaps the most compelling evidence for a functional role of the noradrenergic innervation of the brain vasculature derives from pathophysiological studies. For the cervical sympathetic innervation, most of that work was performed in acute and chronic hypertensive animals and the results pointed to a prominent effect of this innervation in maintaining autoregulation and protection of the blood-brain barrier functions. However, in chronic hypertension, the ''trophic'' effects of the neural innervation remain controversial.

For the intrinsic innervation of cerebral microvessels, there is considerable evidence for the importance of this innervation in protecting the blood-brain barrier from the leakage of macromolecules. An important avenue for future research concerns the effect of this innervation on permeability and transport of water-soluble nutrients and ions across the blood-brain barrier. The report that Na^+/K^+-ATPase may be decreased in brain microvessels after LC lesion supports this contention.

The final message of this chapter is that the noradrenergic innervation of the brain circulation is functional, and that rumors to the effect that it is vestigial, unusual, or otherwise impotent were greatly exaggerated and perhaps resulted from ignorance of the real functions of this innervation.

REFERENCES

1. **Bernard, C.,** *Lecons sur la Physiologie et la Pathologie du Systeme Nerveux,* Vol. 1, J. B. Bailliere et fils, Paris, 1858, 376.
2. **Willis, T.,** *Cerebri Anatome,* Martin and Allestry, London, 1664.
3. **Schmidt, C. F.,** *Handbook of Physiology,* American Physiological Society, Washington, D.C., 1960, 70.
4. **Roy, C. S. and Sherrington, C. S.** The regulation of the blood supply of the brain, *J. Physiol. (London),* 11, 85, 1890.
5. **Owman, C. and Edvinsson, L.,** *Neurogenic Control of the Brain Circulation,* Pergamon Press, Oxford, 1977.
6. **Heistad, D. D. and Marcus, M. L.,** *Cerebral Blood Flow: Effects of Nerves and Neurotransmitters,* Elsevier, New York, 1982.
7. **Edvinsson, L. and MacKenzie, E. T.,** Amine mechanisms in the cerebral circulation, *Pharmacol. Rev.,* 28, 275, 1977.
8. **Heistad, D. D. and Marcus, M. L.,** Evidence that neural mechanisms do not have important effects on cerebral blood flow, *Circ. Res.,* 42, 295, 1978.
9. **Purves, M. J.,** Do vasomotor nerves significantly regulate cerebral blood flow?, *Circ. Res.,* 43, 485, 1978.
10. **Kuschinsky, W. and Wahl, M.,** Local chemical and neurogenic regulation of cerebrovascular resistance, *Physiol. Rev.,* 58, 656, 1978.
11. **Falck, B., Mchedlishivili, G. I., and Owman, C. H.,** Histochemical demonstration of adrenergic nerves in cortex-pia of rabbit, *Acta Pharmacol. Toxicol.* 23, 133, 1965.
12. **Nielsen, K. C. and Owman, C.,** Adrenergic innervation of pial arteries related to the circle of Willis in the cat, *Brain Res.,* 6, 773, 1967.
13. **Iwayama, T., Furness, J. B., and Burnstock, G.,** Dual adrenergic and cholinergic innervation of the cerebral arteries of the rat, *Circ. Res.,* 26, 635, 1970.
14. **HernandezPerez, M. J. and Stone, H. L.,** Sympathetic innervation of the circle of Willis in the Macaque monkey, *Brain Res.,* 80, 507, 1974.
15. **Edvinsson, L.,** Neurogenic mechanisms in the cerebrovascular bed, *Acta Physiol. Scand.,* 427(Suppl.), 5, 1975.
16. **Sercombe, R., Aubineau, P., Edvinsson, L., Mamo, H., Owman, C., Pinard, E., and Seylaz, J.,** Neurogenic influence on local cerebral blood flow. Effect of catecholamines on sympathetic stimulation as correlated with the sympathetic innervation, *Neurology,* 25, 954, 1975.

17. **Nelson, E. and Rennels, M.,** Innervation of intracranial arteries, *Brain,* 93, 475, 1970.
18. **Nielsen, K. C., Owman, C., and Sporrong, B.,** Ultrastructure of the autonomic innervation apparatus in the main pial arteries of rats and cats, *Brain Res.,* 27, 25, 1971.
19. **Nelson, E., Takayanagi, T., Rennels, M. L., and Kawamura, J.,** The innervation of human intracranial arteries: a study by scanning and transmission electron microscopy, *J. Neuropathol. Exp. Neurol.,* 31, 526, 1972.
20. **Dahl, E.,** The innervation of the cerebral arteries, *J. Anat.,* 115, 53, 1973.
21. **Cervos-Navarro, J. and Matakas, F.,** Electron microscopic evidence for innervation of intracerebral arterioles in the cat, *Neurology,* 24, 282, 1974.
22. **Edvinsson, L., Owman, C. H., Rosengren, E., and West, K. A.,** Concentration of noradrenaline in pial vessels, choroid plexus, and iris during two weeks after sympathetic ganglionectomy or decentralization, *Acta Physiol. Scand.,* 85, 201, 1972.
23. **Itakura, T., Yamamoto, K., Tohyama, M., and Shimizu, N.,** Central dual innervation of arterioles and capillaries in the brain, *Stroke,* 8, 360, 1977.
24. **Raper, A. J., Kontos, H. A., Wei, E. P., and Patterson, J. L.,** Unresponsiveness of precapillary vessels to catecholamines and sympathetic nerve stimulation, *Circ. Res.,* 31, 257, 1972.
25. **Wei, E. P., Raper, A. J., Kontos, H. A., and Patterson, J. L.,** Permanence of response of pial arteries to norepinephrine and sympathetic nerve stimulation, *Stroke,* 6, 654, 1975.
26. **Forbes, H. S. and Wolff, H. G.,** Cerebral circulation. III. The vasomotor control of cerebral vessels, *Arch. Neurol. Psychiatry,* 18, 1057, 1928.
27. **Kobayashi, S., Waltz, A. J., and Rhoton, A. L.,** Effects of stimulation of cervical sympathetic nerves on cortical blood flow and vascular reactivity, *Neurology,* 21, 297, 1971.
28. **Kuschinsky, W. and Wahl, M.,** Alpha-receptor stimulation by endogenous and exogenous norepinephrine and blockade by phentolamine in pial arteries of cats, *Circ. Res.,* 37, 168, 1975.
29. **D'Alecy, L. G. and Feigl, E. O.,** Sympathetic control of cerebral blood flow in dogs, *Circ. Res.,* 31, 267, 1972.
30. **Traystman, R. J. and Rapela, C. E.,** Effect of sympathetic nerve stimulation on cerebral and cephalic blood flow in dogs, *Circ. Res.,* 36, 620, 1975.
31. **James, I. M., Millar, R. A., and Purves, M. J.,** Observations on the extrinsic neural control of cerebral blood flow in the baboon, *Circ. Res.,* 25, 77, 1969.
32. **Harper, A. M., Deshmukh, V. D., Rowan, J. O., and Jennett, W. B.,** The influence of sympathetic nervous activity on cerebral blood flow, *Arch. Neurol.,* 27, 1, 1972.
33. **Fitch, W., MacKenzie, E. T., and Harper, A. M.,** Effects of decreasing arterial pressure on cerebral blood flow in the baboon: influence of sympathetic nervous system, *Circ. Res.,* 37, 550, 1975.
34. **Grubb, R. L., Jr., Raichle, M. E., and Eichling, J. O.,** Peripheral sympathetic regulation of brain water permeability, *Brain Res.,* 144, 204, 1978.
35. **Auer, L. M. and Johansson, B. B.,** Pial venous constriction during cervical sympathetic stimulation in the cat, *Acta Physiol. Scand.,* 110, 203, 1980.
36. **Auer, L. M., Lund, S., and Johansson, B. B.,** Reaction of pial arteries and veins to sympathetic stimulation in the cat, *Stroke,* 12, 528, 1981.
37. **Auer, L. M. and Johansson, B. B.,** Cervical sympathetic nerve stimulation decreases intracranial pressure in the cat, *Acta Physiol. Scand.,* 113, 565, 1981.
38. **Auer, L. M., Sayama, I., Johansson, B. B., and Leber K.,** Sympathoadrenergic modulation of cerebral blood volume during increased ICP, in *Intracranial Pressure,* Ishii, S., Nagai, H., and Brock, M., Eds., Springer-Verlag, Berlin, 1983, 342.
39. **Owman, C., Edvinsson, L., and Nielsen, K. C.,** Autonomic neuroreceptor mechanisms in brain vessels, *Blood Vessels,* 11, 2, 1974.
40. **Bill, A. and Linder, J.,** Sympathetic control of cerebral blood flow in acute arterial hypertension, *Acta Physiol. Scand.,* 96, 114, 1976.

41. **Edvinsson, L., Owman, C. H., and Seisjo, B. K.,** Physiological role of cerebral vascular sympathetic nerves in the autoregulation of cerebral blood flow, *Brain Res.,* 117, 519, 1976.
42. **Peerless, S. J. and Yasargil, M. G.,** Adrenergic innervation of the cerebral blood vessels in the rabbit, *J. Neurosurg.,* 35, 148, 1971.
43. **Gross, P. M., Heistad, D. D., Strait, M. R., Marcus, M. L., and Brody, M. J.,** Cerebral vascular responses to physiological stimulation of sympathetic pathways in cats, *Circ. Res.,* 44, 288, 1979.
44. **Busija, D. W., Heistad, D. D., and Marcus, M. L.,** Effect of sympathetic nerves on cerebral vessels during acute, moderate increases in arterial pressure in dogs and cats, *Circ. Res.,* 46, 696, 1980.
45. **Vanter, S. F., Priano, L. L., Rutherford, J. D., and Manders, W. T.,** Sympathetic regulation of the cerebral circulation by the carotid chemoreceptor reflex, *Am. J. Physiol.,* 238, H594, 1980.
46. **Aubineau, P., Reynier-Rebuffel, A. M., Bouchaud, C., Jousseaume, O., and Seylaz, J.,** Long-term effects of superior cervical ganglionectomy on cortical blood flow of nonanesthetized rabbits in resting and hypertensive conditions, *Brain Res.,* 338, 13, 1985.
47. **Lacombe, P., Miller, M.-C., and Seylaz, J.,** Sympathetic regulation of cerebral blood flow during reflex hypertension, *Am. J. Physiol.,* 249, H672, 1985.
48. **Bevan, R. D. and Tsuru, H.,** Functional and structural changes in the rabbit ear artery after sympathetic denervation, *Circ. Res.,* 49, 478, 1981.
49. **Bevan, R. D., Tsuru, H., and Bevan, J. A.,** Cerebral artery mass in the rabbit is reduced by chronic sympathetic denervation, *Stroke,* 14, 393, 1983.
50. **Baumbach, G. L., Heistad, D. D., and Siems, J. E.,** Effects of sympathetic nerves on composition and distensibility of cerebral arterioles in rats, *J. Physiol. (London),* 416, 123, 1989.
51. **Hart, M. N, Heistad, D. D., and Brody, M. J.,** Effect of chronic hypertension and sympathetic denervation on wall/lumen ratio of cerebral vessels, *Hypertension,* 2, 419, 1980.
52. **Sadoshima, S., Busija, D. W., and Heistad, D. D.,** Mechanisms of protection against stroke in stroke-prone spontaneously hypertensive rats, *Am. J. Physiol.,* H406, 1983.
53. **Sadoshima, S., Fuji, K., Yao, H., Ibayashi, S., and Fujishima, M.,** Effect of chronic sympathetic denervation on cerebrovascular hypertrophy during the development of hypertension in rat, *Brain Res.,* 379, 205, 1986.
54. **Baumbach, G. L. and Heistad, D. D.,** Trophic role of sympathetic nerves during hypertension, in *Neurotransmission and Cerebrovascular Function,* Vol. 2, Seylaz, J. and Sercombe, R., Eds., Elsevier, Amsterdam, 1989, 279.
55. **Johansson, B. B. and Nordborg, C.,** Denervation related morphological alterations in cerebral vessels during hypertension, in *Neurotransmission and Cerebrovascular Function,* Vol. 2, Seylaz, J. and Sercombe, R., Eds., Elsevier, Amsterdam, 1989, 267.
56. **Bevan, J. A. and Van Riper, D.,** Sympathetic influences on cerebrovascular tone, in *Neurotransmission and Cerebrovascular Function,* Vol. 2, Seylaz, J. and Sercombe, R., Eds., Elsevier, Amsterdam, 1989, 65.
57. **Bevan, J. A., Bevan, R. D., and Shreeve, S. M.,** Variable receptor affinity hypothesis, *FASEB J.,* 3, 1696, 1989.
58. **Ekstrom-Jodal, B., Von Essen, C., and Haggendal, E.,** Effects of noradrenaline in the cerebral blood flow in the dog, *Acta Neurol. Scand.,* 50, 11, 1974.
59. **James, I. M. and MacDonnell, L.,** Factors effecting the cerebrovascular response to noradrenaline in the dog, *Br. J. Pharmacol.,* 54, 129, 1975.
60. **Lowe, R. F. and Gilboe, D. D.,** Demonstration of alpha and beta adrenergic receptors in canine cerebral vasculature, *Stroke,* 2, 193, 1971.
61. **Oberdorster, G., Lang, R., and Zimmer, R.,** Direct effects of α- and β-sympathomimetic amines on the cerebral circulation of the dog, *Pfluegers Arch.,* 340, 145, 1973.

62. **Zimmer, R., Lang, R., and Oberdorster, G.,** Effects of catecholamine infusions on cerebral blood flow and oxygen consumption of the isolated perfused dog brain, *Stroke,* 5, 397, 1974.
63. **Muravchick, S. and Bergofsky, E. H.,** Adrenergic receptors and vascular resistance in cerebral circulation of the cat, *J. Appl. Physiol.,* 40, 79, 1976.
64. **Lluch, S., Reimann, C., and Glick, G.,** Evidence for the direct effect of adrenergic drugs on the cerebrovascular bed of the unanesthetized goat, *Stroke,* 4, 50, 1973.
65. **MacKenzie, E. T., McCulloch, J., O'Keane, M., Pickard, J. D., and Harper, A. M.,** Cerebral circulation and norepinephrine: Relevance of the blood-brain barrier, *Am. J. Physiol.,* 231, 483, 1976.
66. **Olesen, J.,** The effect of intracarotid epinephrine, norepinephrine, and angiotensin on the regional cerebral blood flow in man, *Neurology,* 22, 978, 1972.
67. **Olesen, J.,** Effect of intracarotid isoprenaline, propranolol, and prostaglandin E_1 on regional cerebral blood flow in man, in *Blood Flow and Metabolism in the Brain,* Harper, A. M., Jennett, W. B., Miller, J. D., and Rowan, J. O., Eds., Churchill Livingstone, Edinburgh, 1975, 4.10.
68. **Wahl, M., Kuschinksy, W., Bosse, O., Olesen, J., Lassen, N. A., Ingvar, D. H., Michaelis, J., and Thoureau, K.,** Effect of *l*norepinephrine on the diameter of pial arterioles and arteries in the cat, *Circ. Res.,* 31, 248, 1972.
69. **Rosenblum, W. I.,** Contractile response of pial arterioles to norepinephrine. Effects in the mouse, *Arch, Neurol.,* 31, 197, 1974.
70. **Rosenblum, W. I.,** Pial arteriolar responses in mouse brain revisited, *Stroke,* 7, 283, 1976.
71. **Rosenblum, W. I. and Zweifach, B. W.,** Cerebral microcirculation in the mouse brain. Spontaneous and drug-induced changes in flow and vascular diameter, *Arch. Neurol.,* 9, 414, 1963.
72. **Wahl, M., Kuschinsky, W., Bosse, O., and Neiss, A.,** Micropuncture evaluation of β-receptors in pial arteries of cats, *Pfluegers Arch.,* 348, 293, 1974.
73. **Hartman, B. K., Zide, D., and Udenfriend, S.,** The use of dopamine beta-hydroxylase as a marker for the central noradrenergic nervous system in rat brain, *Proc. Natl. Acad. Sci. U.S.A.,* 69, 2722, 1972.
74. **Edvinsson, L., Lindvall, M., Nielsen, K. C., and Owman, C. H.,** Are brain vessels innervated also by central (non-sympathetic) adrenergic neurons?, *Brain Res.,* 63, 496, 1973.
75. **de la Torre, J. C.,** Evidence for central innervation of intracerebral blood vessels: local cerebral blood flow measurements and histofluorescence analysis by the sucrose-phosphate-glyoxylic acid (SPG) method, *Neuroscience,* 1, 455, 1967.
76. **Swanson, L. W., Connelly, M. A., and Hartman, B. K.,** Ultrastructural evidence for central monoaminergic innervation of blood vessels in the periventricular nucleus of the hypothalamus, *Brain Res.,* 136, 166, 1977.
77. **Rennels, M. L. and Nelson, E.,** Capillary innervation in the mammalian central nervous system: an electron microscopic demonstration, *Am. J. Anat.,* 144, 233, 1975.
78. **Raichle, M. E., Hartman, B. K., Eichling, J. O., and Sharpe, L. G.,** Central noradrenergic regulation of cerebral blood flow and vascular permeability, *Proc. Natl. Acad. Sci. U.S.A.,* 72, 3726, 1975.
79. **Preskorn, S. H., Hartman, B. K., Raichle, M. E., and Clark, H. B.,** The effect of dibenzazepines (tricyclic antidepressants) on cerebral capillary permeability in the rat *in vivo, J. Pharmacol. Exp. Ther.,* 213, 313, 1980.
80. **de la Torre, J. C., Surgeon, J. W., and Walker, R. H.,** Effect of locus coeruleus stimulation on cerebral blood flow in selected brain regions, *Acta Neurol. Scand.,* 64(Suppl.), 104, 1977.
81. **Goadsby, P. J., Lambert, G. A., and Lance, J. W.,** Effects of locus ceruleus stimulation on carotid vascular resistance in the cat, *Brain Res.,* 278, 175, 1983.

82. **Harik, S. I., Duckrow, R. B., LaManna, J. C., Rosenthal, M., Sharma, V. K., and Banerjee, S. P.,** Cerebral compensation for chronic noradrenergic denervation induced by locus ceruleus lesion: recovery of receptor binding, isoproterenol-induced adenylate cyclase activity, and oxidative metabolism, *J. Neurosci.,* 1, 64, 1981.
83. **Bates, D., Weinshilboum, R. M., Campbell, R. J., and Sundt, T. H., Jr.,** The effects of lesions in the locus ceruleus on the physiological responses of the cerebral blood vessels in cats, *Brain Res.,* 136, 431, 1977.
84. **Dahlgren, N., Lindvall, O., Sakabe, T., Stenevi, U., and Seisjo, B. K.,** Cerebral blood flow and oxygen consumption in the rat brain after lesions of the noradrenergic locus ceruleus system, *Brain Res.,* 209, 11, 1981.
85. **McCulloch, J., Savaki, H. E., and Angerson, W.,** Regional water permeability in the CNS of conscious rats: effects of hypercapnia and locus ceruleus lesions, in *Cerebral Flow: Effects of Nerves and Neurotransmitters,* Heistad, D. D. and Marcus, M. L., Eds., Elsevier, New York, 1982, 509.
86. **Busto, R., Ginsberg, M. D., Harik, S. I., and Smith, D. W.,** Regional cerebral blood flow during bicuculline-induced status epilepticus: insensitivity to hemispheral norepinephrine depletion, in *Cerebral Blood Flow, Metabolism and Epilepsy,* Baldy-Moulinier, M., Ingvar, D. H., and Meldrum, B. S., Eds., John Libbey, London, 1984, 336.
87. **Ginsberg, M. D., Busto, R., and Harik, S. I.,** Regional bloodbrain barrier permeability to water and cerebral flow during status epilepticus: Insensitivity to norepinephrine depletion, *Brain Res.,* 337, 59, 1985.
88. **Harik, S. I., Prado, R., Busto, R., and Ginsberg, M. D.,** Increased cerebral blood flow during hypercapnia is not affected by lesion of the nucleus locus ceruleus, *Stroke,* 17, 1235, 1986.
89. **Mendelow, A. D., McCalden, T. A., Hattingh, J., Kramer, B., Rosendorff, C., and Eidelman, B. H.,** The effect of chemical sympathectomy on cerebral vascular reactivity and cerebral metabolism, in *Neurogenic Control of the Brain Circulation,* Owman, C. and Edvinsson, L., Pergamon Press, Oxford, England, 1977, 429.
90. **Edvinsson, L., Hardebo, J. E., and MacKenzie, E. T.,** Effects of intraventricular 6-hydroxydopamine on cerebrovascular CO_2 reactivity in anesthetized rats, *Acta Physiol. Scand.,* 101, 122, 1977.
91. **Harik, S. I., LaManna, J. C., Light, A. L., and Rosenthal, M.,** Cerebral norepinephrine: influence on cortical oxidative metabolism *in situ, Science,* 206, 69, 1979.
92. **LaManna, J. C., Harik, S. I., Light, A. L., and Rosenthal, M.,** Norepinephrine depletion alters cerebral oxidative metabolism in active state, *Brain Res.,* 204, 87, 1981.
93. **Harik, S. I. and McGunigal, T., Jr.,** The protective influence of the locus ceruleus on the blood-brain barrier, *Ann. Neurol.,* 15, 568, 1984.
94. **Johansson, B. B.,** Neonatal 6-hydroxydopamine treatment increases the vulnerability of the bloodbrain barrier to acute hypertension in conscious rats, *Acta Neurol. Scand.,* 60, 198, 1979.
95. **Ben-Menachem, E., Johansson, B. B., and Svensson, T. H.,** Increased vulnerability of the blood-brain barrier to acute hypertension following depletion of brain noradrenaline, *J. Neural. Transm.,* 53, 159, 1982.
96. **Nag, S. and Harik, S. I.,** Cerebrovascular permeability to horseradish peroxidase in hypertensive rats: effects of unilateral locus ceruleus lesion, *Acta Neuropathol. (Berlin),* 73, 247, 1987.
97. **Harik, S. I., Sharma, V. K., Wetherbee, J. R., Warren, R. H., and Banerjee, S. P.,** Adrenergic receptors of cerebral microvessels, *Eur. J. Pharmacol.,* 61, 207, 1980.
98. **Peroutka, S. J., Moskowitz, M. A., Reinhard, J. F., Jr., and Snyder, S. H.,** Neurotransmitter receptor binding in bovine cerebral microvessels, *Science,* 208, 610, 1980.
99. **Harik, S. I., Sharma, V. K., Wetherbee, J. R., Warren, R. H., and Banerjee, S. P.,** Adrenergic and cholinergic receptors of cerebral microvessels, *J. Cereb. Blood Flow Metab.,* 1, 329, 1981.

100. **Culvenor, A. J. and Jarrott, B.,** Comparison of β-adrenoceptors in bovine intracerebral microvessels and cerebral gray matter by [^{3}H]dihydroallopurinol binding, *Neuroscience,* 6, 1643, 1981.
101. **Kobayashi, H., Memo, M., Spano, P. F., and Trabucchi, M.,** Identification of beta-adrenergic receptor binding sites in rat brain microvessels using [^{125}H]iodohydroxybenzylpindolol, *J. Neurochem.,* 36, 1382, 1981.
102. **Kobayashi, H., Frattola, L., Ferrarese, C., Spano, P., and Trabucchi, M.,** Characterization of beta-adrenergic receptors on human cerebral microvessels, *Neurology,* 32, 1384, 1982.
103. **Ferrari-DiLeo, G. and Potter, L. T.,** Adrenoreceptors and muscarine receptors in human pial arteries and microvessels: a receptor binding, *J. Cereb. Blood Flow Metab.,* 5, 458, 1985.
104. **Kalaria, R. N., Stockmeier, C., and Harik, S. I.,** Brain microvessels are innervated by locus ceruleus noradrenergic neurons, *Neurosci. Lett.,* 97, 203, 1989.
105. **Kalaria, R. N. and Harik, S. I.,** α_2 and β_2-adrenergic receptors in cerebral microvessels in Alzheimer disease, *Neurosci. Lett.,* 106, 233, 1989.
106. **Baca, G. M. and Palmer, G. C.,** Presence of hormonally-sensitive adenylate cyclase receptors in capillary-enriched fractions from rat cerebral cortex, *Blood Vessels,* 15, 286, 1978.
107. **Herbst, T. J., Raichle, M. E., and Ferrendelli, J. A.,** β-adrenergic regulation of adenosine 3′,5′monophosphate concentration in brain microvessels, *Science,* 204, 330, 1979.
108. **Nathanson, J. A. and Glaser, G. H.,** Identification of β-adrenergic-sensitive adenylate cyclase in intracranial blood vessels, *Nature,* 278, 567, 1979.
109. **Zeleznikar, R. J., Quist, E. E., and Drewes, L. R.,** An alpha-adrenergic receptor-mediated phosphatidylinositol effect in canine cerebral microvessels, *Mol. Pharmacol.,* 24, 163, 1983.
110. **Sharma, V. K., Harik, S. I., Busto, R., and Banerjee, S. P.,** Effects of noradrenaline depletion on adrenergic and muscarinic cholinergic receptors in the cerebral cortex, hippocampus, and cerebellum, *Exp. Neurol.,* 72, 179, 1981.
111. **Harik, S. I.,** Blood-brain barrier Na^+/K^+pump: modulation by central noradrenergic innervation, *Proc. Natl. Acad. Sci. U.S.A.,* 83, 4067, 1986.

Chapter 6

SEROTONIN AND THE CEREBRAL CIRCULATION

Gilles Bonvento and Pierre Lacombe

TABLE OF CONTENTS

I. Introduction 98

II. Serotonergic Innervation of the Cerebral Vasculature 98

III. Cerebrovascular Effects of Exogenous 5-HT 99
- A. 5-HT Reactivity *In Vitro* 99
- B. 5-HT Reactivity *In Situ* 100
- C. Effects of Systemic Administration on CBF 100
- D. Effects on Energy Metabolism 100

IV. Cerebrovascular Effects of Pharmacological Manipulations of the Serotonergic System 101
- A. Effects on CBF 101
- B. Effects on Energy Metabolism 101

V. Cerebrovascular Effects of Endogenous 5HT 101
- A. Effects on CBF 101
- B. Effects on Energy Metabolism 102

VI. Cerebral Blood Flow — Metabolism Coupling 102

VII. Current Anatomical and Functional View of the Serotonergic Innervation of the Cerebral Vasculature 106

VIII. The Cerebrovascular Serotonergic System: Relevance to the Neurovascular Theory of Migraine 107

IX. Conclusion 108

References 108

0-8493-5096-0/93/$0.00 + $.50

I. INTRODUCTION

Serotonin or 5-hydroxytryptamine (5-HT) is located in several tissues including circulating platelets, central neurons, and cerebral mast cells. Release of 5-HT from any of these sites can affect the vascular smooth musculature. Most functional studies on the vascular effects of serotonin have shown that this amine is a powerful constrictor agent, but that it also induces vasodilatation in small pial arteries.[1] It has long been suspected to intervene in the pathogenesis of cerebral vasospasm following subarachnoid hemorrhage and more recently in a number of cerebrovascular diseases such as stroke, trauma, and migraine.[2]

Electrophysiological and behavioral studies showed that the spontaneous activity of serotonergic central neurons is considerably increased when the animals pass from sleep to the wake-arousal state, or during tonic expression of particular stereotyped behaviors, while their activity is suppressed during the execution of phasic behaviors, such as those associated with attention and orientation.[3] Thus, 5-HT appears to be a neuromodulator that can both depress and activate certain physiological functions.

The serotonergic innervation of cerebral blood vessels was first postulated in 1976,[4] and neurochemical results supported this assumption.[5-7] However, subsequent histochemical studies have not provided consistent results, and it was suggested that the serotonergic innervation was in fact the noradrenergic sympathetic innervation, due to an uptake mechanism of 5-HT (see below.)[8] More recent studies involving activation of the central serotonergic pathway, and immunohistochemical labeling of the tryptophan-hydroxylase (TPOH), the rate-limiting enzyme catalyzing 5-HT synthesis,[9] favor the earlier hypothesis of a serotonergic control of the cerebral circulation.[10]

Additional features of the serotonergic system are (1) its numerous receptor subtypes, (2) the dual, ''extrinsic-intrinsic'' system of putative cerebrovascular innervation (see below), (3) the species-dependency of this organization,[1] and (4) the correlation between the cerebrovascular effects of 5-HT and the preexisting vascular tone.[11] Moreover, this monoamine may intervene in the cerebrovascular bed at the capillary level by altering the permeability of the blood-brain barrier.[12] Such a complex system cannot be expected to have a ''single'' function, but rather various modulatory, adaptative and physiological roles that may include a link between brain function and blood flow.

II. THE SEROTONERGIC INNERVATION OF THE CEREBRAL VASCULATURE

Serotonergic innervation of cerebral vessels was first suggested by Chan-Palay[4] and Di Carlo[13] based on studies of tritiated 5-HT uptake and autoradiography. This suggestion has been investigated by several approaches (anatomical, histochemical, and neurochemical) that are summarized below (see Reference 14, for more complete review). Despite the numerous manipulations undertaken in a number of animal species, one major issue remained unresolved until recently: is cerebrovascular 5-HT present in authentic serotonergic nerve fibers or is it taken up by sympathetic terminals?

Early reports were based on immunohistochemical studies using an antibody directed against 5-HT and on neurochemical determination of 5-HT and its principal metabolite (5-HIAA) in the cerebral vessels. These studies indicated the existence of a serotonergic innervation of the cerebral vasculature.[6,7] 5-HT was then found to be taken up by noradrenergic sympathetic fibers. This contention was supported by the observation that the 5-HT positive nerve terminals on the major cerebral arteries disappeared after a superior cervical ganglionectomy.[8,15,16] The literature also contained controversial reports on the origin of such innervation. The rostral raphé nuclei were the first candidates on the basis of stimulation and lesion experiments. In the mid 1980s, Marco et al.[17] showed that the superior cervical ganglion could also be the origin of the cerebrovascular serotonergic nerves fibers.

Very recently, these conflicting results have been reconciled. There seems to be an authentic serotonergic network that invests the cerebrovascular bed. This innervation has been substantiated by visualization of numerous nerve fibers that are immunoreactive for TPOH.[9] The distribution of these nerve fibers has been compared with that of noradrenergic fibers (revealed by an antibody directed against dopamine-β-hydroxylase, DBH). In major cerebral arteries and small pial vessels, it appears that the two networks are distinct.[18] These anatomical results are corroborated by the neurochemical determination of a *de novo* synthesis of 5-HT in the cerebral vasculature.[19] With respect to the putative origin of these TPOH-immunoreactive (TPOH-I) nerve fibers, the superior cervical ganglion remains the main candidate since its ablation results in a near complete disappearance of the nerve terminals present in the large and small pial arteries.[18]

III. CEREBROVASCULAR EFFECTS OF EXOGENOUS 5-HT

A. 5-HT REACTIVITY *IN VITRO*

The *in vitro* pharmacological characterization of the serotonergic receptors of the cerebral vasculature has been well documented in a number of species. A comparative pharmacological study of 5-HT in isolated cerebral arteries was recently published.[20] Two major features can be drawn from these studies. First, the great majority of isolated cerebral arteries contract in response to 5-HT. The vasoconstriction is very potent, as it ranges from 40 to 100% of the maximum contraction elicited by 124 m*M* potassium used as reference.[21] But 5-HT can also induce vasorelaxation, provided that the arteries are precontracted with $PGF_{2\alpha}$ and pretreated with phenoxybenzamine.[22] This suggests that several components intervene in the response.

Second, the 5-HT receptor subtypes are not identical in all species examined, or even within the same species. The majority of cerebral arteries express a 5-HT_1 contractile response, although a mixed 5-HT_1/5-HT_2 characteristic is often observed. This diversity in the nature of the vascular serotonergic receptor subtypes is an important feature which must be kept in mind in studies related to the cerebrovascular influence of 5-HT.

B. 5-HT REACTIVITY *IN SITU*

When 5-HT is applied topically to the perivascular space of cerebral arteries, it induces dilatation or constriction, depending on the site of investigation and on the method employed. When applied via a cranial window, 5-HT vasodilates small pial arterioles (diameter less than 70 μm), whereas it constricts large arteries (diameter larger than 200 μm).[23] In contrast, 5-HT constricts both small and large arteries when it is superfused over the cortical surface.[24] The receptor subtype that mediates the relaxant response is not well characterized, but a recent communication suggests activation of 5-HT_{1C}/5-HT_2 receptors.[25] With respect to the contractile effect, the 5-HT_1 agonist, sumatriptan (used as antimigraine drug) constricts rat pial arterioles, when it is applied topically.[25] Finally, the endothelium-derived relaxing factor (EDRF or nitric oxide, NO) has recently been shown to inhibit the constrictor response of large cerebral arteries to serotonin.[26]

C. EFFECTS OF SYSTEMIC ADMINISTRATION ON CBF

As 5-HT does not cross the blood-brain barrier (BBB), its influence on the cerebral circulation cannot be directly assessed. The effects of systemically administered 5-HT on global measurements of cerebral blood flow (CBF) have been well characterized in baboons.[27] 5-HT does not affect CBF in control conditions, whereas it significantly decreases CBF after BBB disruption. Using the autoradiographic technique in the rat, intracarotid 5-HT injection 10 min after opening of the BBB produced a decrease in CBF in a number of brain regions supplied by the internal carotid artery, while increases were noted in other regions.[28]

A direct effect of 5-HT on the BBB permeability cannot be ruled out although it is not really consistent with the above results. Such an effect has recently been reported.[12] Increasing the plasma 5-HT concentration in anesthetized rat induced an increase in BBB permeability and a simultaneous decrease in blood flow. Pretreatment with a 5-HT_2 receptor antagonist prevented both effects. The authors suggested that 5-HT acts on the vesicular transport of endothelial cells.

D. EFFECTS ON ENERGY METABOLISM

Following BBB disruption, 5-HT administration in the baboon induced a global metabolic depression as evidenced by a decrease in oxygen consumption and in EEG activity.[27] Similarly in the rat, 5-HT significantly decreased glucose consumption in cortical areas and in the caudate nucleus, but only if the MAO (monoamine oxidase, the major catabolic enzyme for 5-HT) has been previously inhibited.[29] Thus, circulating 5-HT can induce a direct action on the cerebral circulation and metabolism provided, according to some investigators, that the structural or enzymatic properties of the BBB are impaired so that the monoamine can readily reach the cerebral parenchyma.

IV. CEREBROVASCULAR EFFECTS OF PHARMACOLOGICAL MANIPULATIONS OF THE SEROTONERGIC SYSTEM

A. EFFECTS ON CBF

To our knowledge, there has only been one pharmacological manipulation of the serotonergic system correlated with CBF. Ketanserine, a 5-HT_2 antagonist, was found to induce increases in CBF in the neocortex.[30] The result is in accordance with the vasodilatory action of ketanserine on the small pial arteries.[31] Thus, there is a consensus that the vasoconstrictor properties of serotonin are mediated via 5-HT_2 receptors of the cerebral vasculature.

B. EFFECTS ON ENERGY METABOLISM

Over the last few years, there have been several studies correlating the effects of serotonergic agonists or antagonists with local cerebral glucose utilization (lCGU).[32-37] Both agonists and antagonists induced decreases and increases in lCGU, depending on the cerebral regions studied and the concentrations used, so that no decisive conclusion can be drawn from these results. One major drawback of the systemic administration of these pharmacological agents is that they induce marked behavioral changes.[34,35] Most of the agents used also lack pharmacological specificity.[32,34]

Further experimental studies, including the local injection of specific serotonergic compounds directly in the raphé nuclei where the serotonergic receptors are well characterized, could provide a clearer picture of the functional nature of the serotonergic system.

V. CEREBROVASCULAR EFFECTS OF ENDOGENOUS 5-HT

A. EFFECTS ON CBF

Let us now consider the circulatory consequences of activating the ascending serotonergic system. The first studies conducted by Goadsby et al. on cats[38] and monkeys[39] reported a vasodilatation (decreased common carotid resistance) in response to electrical stimulation of the dorsal raphé nucleus (DRN).

More direct approaches to the cerebral perfusion in the rat have used autoradiography to measure CBF. In the α-chloralose anesthetized animal,

DRN electrical stimulation produced a widespread CBF decrease ranging from −13 to −26%.[40] The most pronounced decreases were observed in limbic system relays, such as the accumbens, amygdaloid, interpeduncular, and median raphé nuclei. By contrast, in the conscious rat, stimulation heterogeneously increased CBF in 9 structures, and there were no significant changes in 54 other structures examined.[41] An example of this apparent discrepancy is shown in Figure 1. It provides further functional evidence of the multiple actions of the serotonergic system on the cerebral circulation, differentiating the stable conditions of the immobilized animal from the conscious, behaving animal.[42] The situation seems to be more complicated since Underwood et al.[43] showed that increases or decreases in CBF can occur in the α-chloralose anesthetized rat, depending on the precise location of the stimulation sites within the DRN. Hence, there is spatial heterogeneity in the function of the serotonergic neurons.

B. EFFECTS ON ENERGY METABOLISM

Like the CBF studies, the metabolic effects of electrical stimulation of the raphé nuclei have been described in two experimental paradigms (anesthetized and conscious rats). In the gently restrained rat, raphé nuclei activation increased lCGU in a number of brain regions including the whole extrapyramidal system, the somatosensory cortex, and the thalamic nuclei.[44] These effects are probably serotonergic in nature, since prior pharmacologic serotonergic lesioning (using 5,7-DHT) totally abolished the metabolic responses to the stimulation. In the α-chloralose anesthetized rat, electrical activation of the DRN caused significant increases in lCGU (13 to 52%) in 8 brain structures out of 33 investigated. Increases were restricted to extrapyramidal (red nucleus, substantia nigra) and limbic nonspecific areas (dorsal tegmental area, habenular nuclei).[45] In contrast, electrolytic[46] or neurotoxic[47] lesioning of the serotonergic system had minimal effects on the integrated functional cerebral activity.

These results therefore indicate that the ascending serotonergic system could exert a phasic rather than a tonic influence on the cerebral circulation and metabolism, which is consistent with its multivalent influence.

VI. CEREBRAL BLOOD FLOW — METABOLISM COUPLING

Analysis of the relationships between cerebral blood flow and glucose utilization still remains a unique tool for distinguishing a "primary" vascular phenomenon from a "secondary" metabolic activation. Such an analysis is usually carried out using the statistical approach developed by McCulloch et al.[48] The logged mean lCBF values for each brain region in both conditions are plotted against the mean lCGU values. Subsequent comparisons can identify both a global resetting of the flow-metabolism relationship and the individual structures in which the lCBF/lCGU ratio is modified.

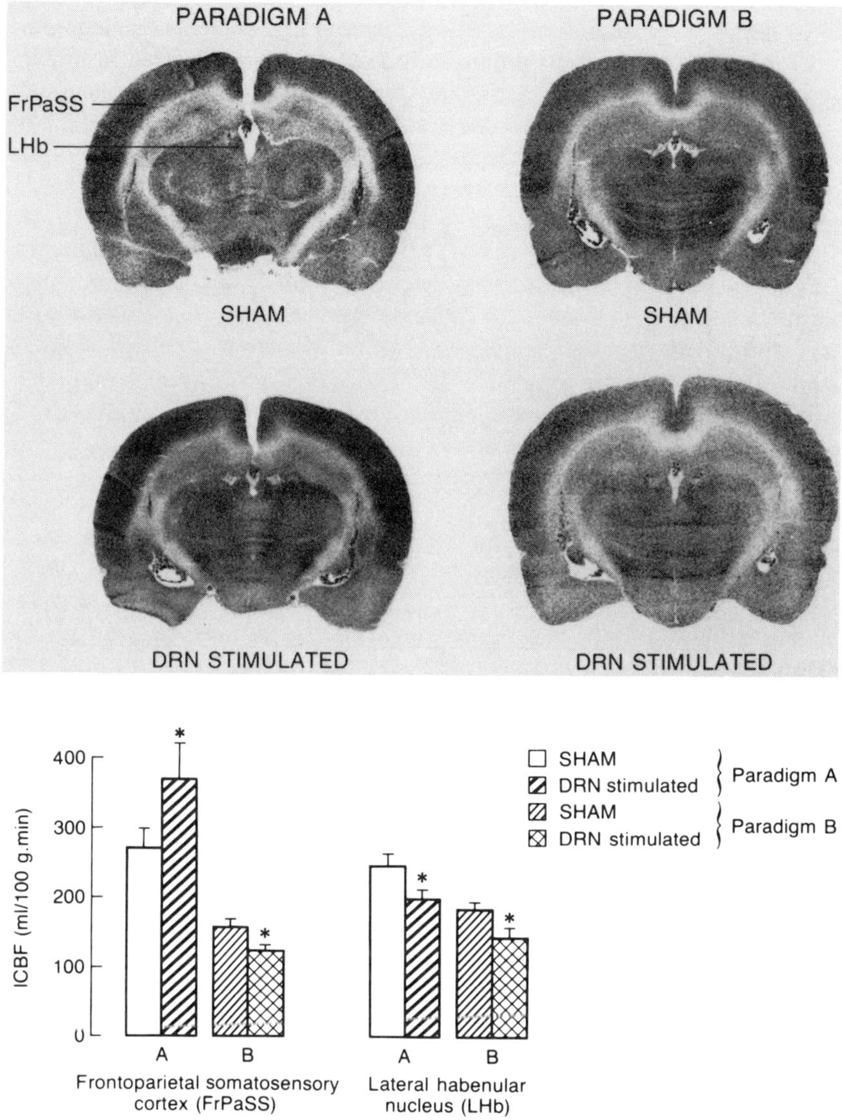

FIGURE 1. Cerebral blood flow (CBF) autoradiograms of sham and dorsal raphé nucleus (DRN) stimulated conscious (paradigm A) and anesthetized (paradigm B) rats. The quantitative CBF values (ml/100 g·min) measured in the frontoparietal somatosensory cortex (FrPass) and in the lateral habenular nucleus (LHb) are shown to demonstrate different results obtained with the two experimental paradigms.

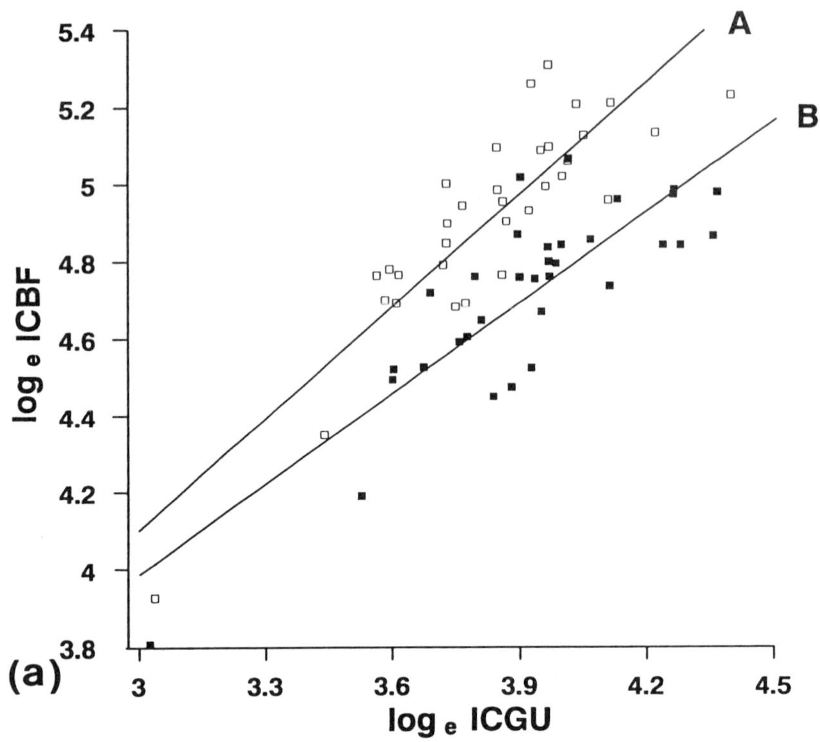

FIGURE 2a. Comparison of the relationship between local cerebral blood flow (lCBF) and local cerebral glucose utilization (lCGU) for anesthetized control (open squares) and dorsal raphé stimulated rats (filled squares). The regression lines and coefficients of correlation (r) derived from linear regression analysis are $y = 1.19 + 0.92\,x$; $r = 0.87$ for control (A), and $y = 1.62 + 0.79\,x$; $r = 0.84$ for raphé stimulated animals (B). Statistical analysis of the lCBF/lCGU ratio reveals that these two variables are uncoupled in 15 regions.

This statistical approach was used to analyze data obtained during DRN electrical stimulation both in anesthetized (Figure 2a)[45] and conscious rats (Figure 2b),[41] following chronic interruption of the ascending serotonergic system[49] and also during injection of a specific 5-HT_{1A} agonist.[50] Although these results must be interpreted cautiously because of statistical limitations,[51] the flow changes do not seem to be superimposable on the metabolic changes in any of the experimental conditions considered. Thus, it can be reasonably assumed that a primary vasoactive effect of 5-HT is, at least partly, responsible for the observed circulatory changes.

Such a lack of coupling between blood flow and oxidative metabolism was also reported after studies using positron emission tomography in man during physiological neural activation.[52] This dissociation could be due to a part of glucose being consumed anerobically, leading to lactate accumulation.

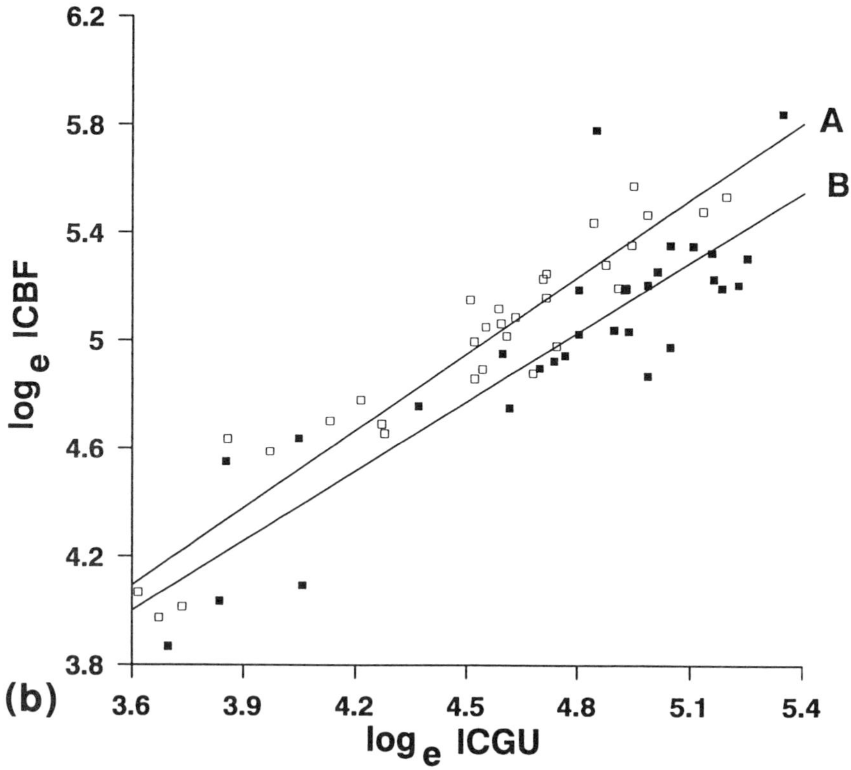

FIGURE 2b. Comparison of the relationship between local cerebral blood flow (lCBF) and local cerebral glucose utilization (lCGU) for conscious control (open squares) and dorsal raphé stimulated rats (filled squares). The regression lines and coefficients of correlation (r) derived from linear regression analysis are $y = 0.67 + 0.95\,x$; $r = 0.95$ for control (A) and $y = 0.91 + 0.86\,x$; $r = 0.87$ for raphé stimulated animals (B). Separately considering the regions reveals uncoupling in 18 regions to be statistically significant ($p < 0.05$) using uncorrected t test.

Enhancement of glycolysis has also been reported during photic stimulation[53] and electrical stimulation of the forepaw.[54] These data require further experimental support, through the measurement of lactate concentrations during serotonergic activation. This could be done using the autoradiographic method[55] or by microdialysis.[56]

To summarize, it appears that the 5-HT, possibly released in the vicinity of brain blood vessels from nerve terminals that arise from the mesencephalic raphé, could induce changes in the cerebral circulation via a neurovascular and/or a neurohumoral mechanism. As pointed out by Woods,[57] neurogenic coupling between brain activity and blood flow presents a metabolic advantage. By altering CO_2 washout and the extracellular pH, a circulatory control may orientate the glucose catabolism toward either the aerobic or anerobic pathways.

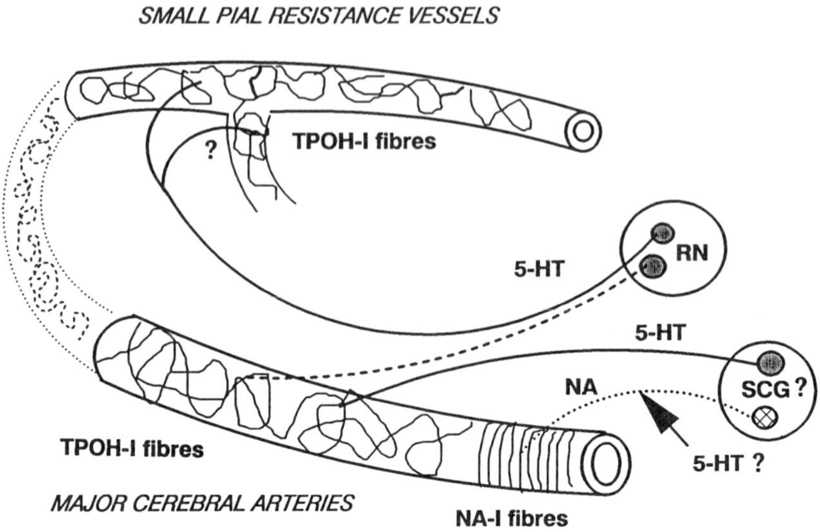

FIGURE 3. Schematic drawing of the current hypotheses for the origins of the cerebrovascular TPOH-immunoreactive (TPOH-I) fibers that may account for the effects of the rostral raphé nuclei (RN) stimulation (see text). An intracerebral source, the RN, sends projections to pial vessels via free TPOH-I fibers in the pia arachnoid membranes and probably the intraparenchymal arterioles (those which control the cerebral circulation). An anatomical link between the RN to the major cerebral arteries has not been demonstrated.

With respect to the extracerebral origin(s), the superior cervical ganglion (SCG) is the most likely candidate, since 5-HT-I but not TPOH-I cell bodies have been visualized in the ganglion. Nevertheless, the possibility exists that the TPOH-I fibers may pass through the SCG, and another autonomic ganglion (nodose) may contribute to this innervation. It is also unknown whether 5-HT and noradrenaline (NA) are at least partly colocalized in the same nerve fibers. Finally, 5-HT has been shown to be taken up and stored in sympathetic fibers that originate from the SCG, but the significance of this phenomenon has yet to be analyzed. The (?) indicate the points that do not yet have any anatomical support. (From Bonvento, G., et al., *Brain Res. Rev.*, 16, 257, 1991. With permission.)

VII. CURRENT ANATOMICAL AND FUNCTIONAL VIEW OF THE SEROTONERGIC INNERVATION OF THE CEREBRAL VASCULATURE

Two points have not been clarified in the data presented above: (1) the anatomical link between serotonergic neurons of the raphé nuclei and the pial arteries, either small or major, and (2) the cell bodies at the origin of the TPOH-I network that mostly supply the major cerebral arteries. This issue is illustrated in Figure 3.

The evidence of a link between the dorsal raphé nucleus and cortical circulation provided by functional studies[41,45] can be ascribed to the free TPOH-I fibers seen in the pia-arachnoid membrane.[18] These fibers may release

5-HT into the CSF and extracellular space when the DRN is activated, and thus influence the surrounding tissues including resistance vessels. Other effects of 5-HT on the cerebral parenchyma, especially interactions with the other neuronal systems, have also been described.[58,59]

Finally, another physiological consequence of raphé activation could involve the circumventricular organs, which have been shown to receive serotonergic fibers.[60-62] Such connections might indirectly influence the BBB permeability as already suggested for plasma catecholamines,[63] by selectively and specifically sensitizing these particular areas devoid of BBB to circulating agents.

The "extrinsic serotonergic" (TPOH-labeled) nerve fibers were discovered too recently for their function to be fully investigated. Since these fibers are closely associated with the sympathetic system, their function is probably related to the noradrenergic sympathetic innervation. The vasoconstriction in response to DRN stimulation is similar in magnitude to that which occurs in response to sympathetic stimulation.[64] This might indicate a common vascular mediator. Further cerebrovascular studies using pharmacologically specific approaches (neurotoxic treatments specific for either the adrenergic or serotonergic elements) may shed light on such things as the "escape phenomenon" of the sympathetic vasoconstriction.[65] This system may also intervene in pathological situations (see below), possibly in association with the sympathetic system.[66]

VIII. THE CEREBROVASCULAR SEROTONERGIC SYSTEM: RELEVANCE TO THE NEUROVASCULAR THEORY OF MIGRAINE

Although it has been suggested that serotonin is implicated in several brain pathologies such as injury or trauma (see Reference 67 for review), subarachnoid hemorrhage (see Reference 68 for review), and infarction,[69] there is no definite evidence on the origin of the 5-HT involved. The recent findings of 5-HT synthesizing nerve fibers on major cerebral vessels and pia-arachnoid membrane could probably substantiate several pathogenetic theories.

Migraine is one of the main examples of a condition involving a serotonergic dysfunction. The fact that 5-HT is a key neurotransmitter implicated in the pathophysiology of migraine relies on a number of pharmacological and biochemical findings accumulated over the last 30 years. Migraine was previously described as a purely vascular pathology; so, the platelets were logically considered as the major elements responsible for the alteration of the serotonergic metabolism that occur during a migraine attack. Further clinical and pharmacological observations revealed that such a hypothesis is no longer tenable (see Reference 70 for review). The "neurogenic" theory mainly developed by Lauritzen[71] likens migraine to the well-described cortical spreading depression of Leão. This phenomenon occurs in all neural tissues of all species; it induces pronounced, transient ionic and electrical changes accompanied by long lasting cerebrovascular changes.[71,72] But both the neurogenic and vascular hypotheses can account for only part of the numerous and complex symptoms of migraine.

Recently, a "neurovascular" theory that involves the central serotonergic system has gained ground.[73] This new hypothesis is based on the fact that most of the antimigraine compounds modify the electric activity of the central serotonergic neurons situated in the raphé nuclei. Since these neurons are sensitive to stressful stimuli known to participate in the initiation of the migraine crisis, it is tempting to believe that the ascending serotonergic system can act as an anatomical relay between the sensory stimulus and the nociceptive effector. In this context, the results suggesting that the ascending serotonergic system is functionally related to the vascular effector are highly relevant.

A more precise study of the relationships between the central serotonergic somata and the vascular bed (in particular toward the intraparenchymal vessels), together with a better characterization of the mechanisms responsible for the changes in CBF that occur during a migraine attack, could certainly provide fruitful information on the basic aspects of migraine.

IX. CONCLUSION

Serotonin probably occupies a pivotal place in the regulation of the cerebral circulation as a modulator: it is present throughout the brain and has a range of actions correlated with many subtypes of serotonergic receptors having specific tissue distributions. Its postulated role in the coupling between CBF and CGU is compatible with this view. Although the precise origin of the recently demonstrated TPOH-labeled nervous network endowing the large pial arteries is as yet unclear, it is probably closely related to the adrenergic sympathetic system originating in the SCG. Its physiological or pathological role must be investigated in conjunction to the sympathetic one. The role of serotonin in pathophysiological situations such as migraine, vasospasm, and ischemia remains to be further elucidated.

REFERENCES

1. **Young, A. R., Hamel, E., MacKenzie, E. T., Seylaz, J., and Verrecchia, C.,** The multiple actions of 5-hydroxytryptamine on cerebrovascular smooth muscle, in *Neuronal Messengers in Vascular Function,* Nobin, A., Owman, C., and Arneklo-Nobin, B., Eds., Elsevier, Amsterdam, 1987, 57.
2. **MacKenzie, E. T. and Scatton, B.,** Cerebral circulatory and metabolic effects of perivascular neurotransmitters, *CRC Crit. Rev. Clinical Neurobiol.,* 2, 357, 1987.

3. **Jacobs, B. L. and Fornal, C. A.,** Activity of brain serotonergic neurons in the behaving animal, *Pharmacol. Rev.,* 43(4), 563, 1991.
4. **Chan-Palay, V.,** Serotonin axons in the supra- and subependymal plexuses and in the leptomeninges; their roles in local alterations of cerebrospinal fluid and vasomotor activity, *Brain Res.,* 102, 103, 1976.
5. **Reinhard, J. F., Liebmann, J. E., Scholsberg, A. J., and Moskowitz, M. A.,** Serotonin neurons project to small blood vessels in the brain, *Science,* 206, 85, 1979.
6. **Edvinsson, L., Degueurce, A., Duverger, D., MacKenzie, E. T., and Scatton, B.,** Central serotonergic nerves project to the pial vessels of the brain, *Nature,* 306, 55, 1983.
7. **Scatton, B., Duverger, D., L'Heureux, R., Serrano, A., Fage, D., Nowicki, J. P., and MacKenzie, E. T.,** Neurochemical studies on the existence, origin and characteristics of the serotonergic innervation of small pial vessels, *Brain Res.,* 345, 219, 1985.
8. **Saito, A. and Lee, T. J. F.,** Serotonin as an alternative transmitter in sympathetic nerves of large arteries of the rabbit, *Circ. Res.,* 60, 220, 1987.
9. **Chedotal, A. and Hamel, E.,** Serotonin-synthesizing nerve fibers in rat and cat cerebral arteries and arterioles: immunohistochemistry of tryptophan-5-hydroxylase, *Neurosci. Lett.,* 116, 269, 1990.
10. **Edvinsson, L., Degueurce, A., Duverger, D., MacKenzie, E. T., Scatton, B., and Uddman, R.,** Coupling between cerebral blood flow and metabolism: a role for serotonin? in *Neurotransmitters the Cerebral Circulation (L.E.R.S. Monograph, Vol. 2),* MacKenzie, E. T. et al., Eds., Raven Press, New York, 1984, 121.
11. **Edvinsson, L., Birath, E., Uddman, R., Lee, T. J. F., Duverger, D., MacKenzie, E. T., and Scatton, B.,** Indoleaminergic mechanisms in brain vessels; localization, concentration, uptake and in vitro responses of 5-hydroxytryptamine, *Acta Physiol. Scand.,* 121, 291, 1984.
12. **Sharma, H. S., Olsson, Y., and Dey, P. K.,** Changes in blood-brain barrier and cerebral blood flow following elevation of circulating serotonin level in anesthetized rats, *Brain Res.,* 517, 215, 1990.
13. **Di Carlo, V.,** Histochemical evidence for a serotonergic innervation of the microcirculation in the brain stem, in *Neurogenic Control of the Brain Circulation,* Owman, C. and Edvinsson, L., Eds., Pergamon Press, Oxford, 1977, 55.
14. **Bonvento, G., MacKenzie, E. T., and Edvinsson, L.,** Serotonergic innervation of the cerebral vasculature: relevance to migraine and ischaemia, *Brain Res. Rev.,* 16, 257, 1991.
15. **Jackowski, A., Crockard, A., and Burnstock, G.,** 5-hydroxytryptamine demonstrated immunohistochemically in rat cerebrovascular nerves largely represents 5-hydroxytryptamine uptake into sympathetic nerve fibres, *Neuroscience,* 29, 453, 1989.
16. **Chang, J. Y., Ekblad, E., Kannisto, P., and Owman, C.,** Serotonin uptake into cerebrovascular nerve fibers of rat, visualization by immunochemistry, disappearance following sympathectomy, and release during electrical stimulation, *Brain Res.,* 492, 79, 1989.
17. **Marco, E. J., Balfagon, G., Salaices, M., Sanchez-Ferrer, C. F., and Marin, J.,** Serotonergic innervation of cat cerebral arteries, *Brain Res.,* 338, 137, 1985.
18. **Cohen, Z., Bonvento, G., Lacombe, P., Seylaz, J., MacKenzie, E. T., and Hamel, E.,** Cerebrovascular nerve fibers immunoreactive for tryptophan-5-hydroxylase in the rat: distribution, putative origin and comparison with sympathetic noradrenergic nerves, *Brain Res.,* 598, 203, 1992.
19. **Bonvento, G., Lacombe, P., MacKenzie, E. T., Fage, D., Benavides, J., Rouquier, L., and Scatton, B.,** Evidence for differing origins of the serotonergic innervation of major cerebral arteries and small pial vessels in the rat, *J. Neurochem.,* 56, 681, 1991.
20. **Parsons, A. A.,** 5-HT receptors in human and animal cerebrovasculature, *Trends Pharmacol. Sci.,* 12, 310, 1991.

21. **Young, A. R., Hamel, E., and MacKenzie, E. T.,** Recent studies on the serotonergic innervation of the cerebral circulation: a review, in *Neural Regulation of Brain Circulation,* Owman, C. and Hardebo, J. E., Eds., Elsevier, Amsterdam, 1986, 195.
22. **Edvinsson, L., Hardebo, J. E., and Owman, C.,** Pharmacological analysis of 5-hydroxytryptamine receptors in isolated intracranial and extracranial vessels of cat and man, *Circ. Res.,* 42, 143, 1978.
23. **Harper, A. M. and MacKenzie, E. T.,** Effects of 5-hydroxytryptamine on pial arteriolar calibre in anesthetized cats, *J. Physiol.,* 271, 735, 1977.
24. **Thompson, J. A., Wei, E. P., and Kontos, H. A.,** Inhibition by ketanserin of serotonin induced cerebral arteriolar constriction, *Stroke,* 15, 1021, 1984.
25. **Pryke, J. G.,** The effect of 5-HT on rat pial arterioles in vivo, *Br. J. Pharmacol.,* 98, 685P, 1989.
26. **Faraci, F. M. and Heistad, D. D.,** Endothelium-derived relaxing factor inhibits constrictor responses of large cerebral arteries to serotonin, *J. Cereb. Blood Flow Metab.,* 12, 500, 1992.
27. **Harper, A. M. and MacKenzie, E. T.,** Cerebral circulatory and metabolic effects of 5-hydroxytryptamine in anesthetized baboons, *J. Physiol.,* 271, 721, 1977.
28. **Grome, J. J. and Harper, A. M.,** The effects of serotonin on local cerebral blood flow, *J. Cereb. Blood Flow Metab.,* 3, 71, 1983.
29. **Grome, J. J. and Harper, A. M.,** Serotonin depression of local cerebral glucose utilization after monoamine oxidase inhibition, *J. Cereb. Blood Flow Metab.,* 5, 473, 1983.
30. **Dietrich, W. D., Busto, R., and Ginsberg, M. D.,** Effect of the serotonin antagonist ketanserin on the hemodynamic and morphological consequences of thrombotic infarction, *J. Cereb. Blood Flow Metab.,* 9, 812, 1989.
31. **Auer, L. M., Leber, K., and Sayama, I.,** Effect of serotonin and its antagonist ketanserin on pial vessels, *J. Cereb. Blood Flow Metab.,* 5, 517, 1985.
32. **Grome, J. J. and Harper, A. M.,** Local cerebral glucose utilization following indoleamine- and piperazine-containing 5-hydroxytryptamine agonists, *J. Neurochem.,* 46, 117, 1986.
33. **Wree, A., Zilles, K., Schleicher, A., Horvath, E., and Traber, J.,** Effects of the 5-HT_{1a} receptor agonist ipsapirone on the local cerebral glucose utilization of the rat hippocampus, *Brain Res.,* 436, 283, 1987.
34. **Ricchieri, G. L., Soncrant, T. T., Holloway, H. W., and Rapoport, S. I.,** Methiotepin reduces glucose utilization in forebrain regions of awake rats, *Psychopharmacology,* 93, 449, 1987.
35. **Kelly, P. A. T., Davis, C. J., and Goodwin, G. M.,** Differential patterns of local cerebral glucose utilization in response to 5-$hydroxytryptamine_1$ agonists, *Neuroscience,* 25, 907, 1988.
36. **Mitchell, E. A. and Pratt, J. A.,** Neuroanatomical structures involved in the action of the 5-HT_3 antagonist ondansetron: a 2-deoxyglucose autoradiographic study in the rat, *Brain Res.,* 538, 289, 1991.
37. **Freo, U., Soncrant, T. T., Holloway, H. W., and Rapoport, S. I.,** Dose- and time-dependent effects of 1-(2,5-dimetoxy-4-iodophenyl)-2-aminopropane (DOI), a serotonergic 5-HT_2 receptor agonist, on local cerebral glucose metabolism in awake rats, *Brain Res.,* 541, 63, 1991.
38. **Goadsby, P. J., Piper, R. D., Lambert, G. A., and Lance, J. W.,** Effects of stimulation of nucleus raphe dorsalis on carotid blood flow. II. The cat, *Am. J. Physiol.,* 48, R263, 1985.
39. **Goadsby, P. J., Piper, R. D., Lambert, G. A., and Lance, J. W.,** Effects of stimulation of nucleus raphe dorsalis on carotid blood flow. I. The monkey, *Am. J. Physiol.,* 248, R257, 1985.
40. **Bonvento, G., Lacombe, P., and Seylaz, J.,** Effects of electrical stimulation of the dorsal raphe nucleus on local cerebral blood flow in the rat, *J. Cereb. Blood Flow Metab.,* 9, 251, 1989.

41. **Cudennec, A., Duverger, D., and MacKenzie, E. T.,** Nature of the regional increases in cerebral blood flow induced by raphe stimulation in the conscious rat, *J. Cereb. Blood Flow Metab.*, 9(Suppl. 1), S375, 1989.
42. **Bonvento, G., Cudennec, A., Duverger, D., Lacombe, P., MacKenzie, E. T., and Seylaz, J.,** Experimental paradigms determine the cerebrovascular responses to dorsal raphe stimulation, in *Neurotransmission and Cerebrovascular Function I,* Seylaz, J. and MacKenzie, E. T., Eds., Elsevier, Amsterdam, 1989, 249.
43. **Underwood, M. D., Bakalian, M. J., Arango, V., Smith, R. W., and Mann, J. J.,** Regulation of cortical blood flow by the dorsal raphe nucleus: topographic organization of cerebrovascular regulatory regions, *J. Cereb. Blood Flow Metab.*, 12, 664, 1992.
44. **Cudennec, A., Duverger, D., Serrano, A., Scatton, B., and MacKenzie, E. T.,** Influence of ascending serotonergic pathways on glucose use in the conscious rat brain. II. Effects of electrical stimulation of the rostral raphé nuclei, *Brain Res.*, 244, 227, 1988.
45. **Bonvento, G., Lacombe, P., MacKenzie, E. T., and Seylaz, J.,** Effects of dorsal raphe stimulation on cerebral glucose utilization in the anesthetized rat, *Brain Res.*, 567, 325, 1991.
46. **Cudennec, A., Duverger, D., Nishikawa, T., McRae-Degueurce, A., MacKenzie, E. T., and Scatton, B.,** Influence of ascending serotonergic pathways on glucose use in the conscious rat brain. I. Effects of electrolytic or neurotoxic lesions of the dorsal and/or median raphé nucleus, *Brain Res.*, 244, 214, 1988.
47. **McBean, D. E., Sharkey, J., Ritchie, I. M., and Kelly, P. A. T.,** Chronic effects of the selective serotonergic neurotoxin, methylenedioxyamphetamine, upon cerebral function, *Neuroscience,* 38, 271, 1990.
48. **McCulloch, J., Kelly, P. A. T., and Ford, I.,** Effect of apomorphine on the relationship between local cerebral blood glucose utilization and local cerebral blood flow (with an appendix on its statistical analysis), *J. Cereb. Blood Flow Metab.*, 2, 487, 1982.
49. **McBean, D. E., Sharkey, J., Ritchie, I. M., and Kelly, P. A. T.,** Evidence for a possible role for serotonergic systems in the control of cerebral blood flow, *Brain Res.*, 537, 307, 1990.
50. **McBean, D. E., Sharkey, J., Ritchie, I. M., and Kelly, P. A. T.,** Cerebrovascular and functional consequences of 5-HT_{1A} receptor activation, *Brain Res.*, 555, 159, 1991.
51. **Ford, I., McColl, J. H., McCormack, A. G., and McCrory, S. J.,** Statistical issues in the analysis of neuroimages, *J. Cereb. Blood Flow Metab.*, 11, A89, 1991.
52. **Fox, P. T., Raichle, M. E., Mintun, M. A., and Dence, C.,** Nonoxidative glucose consumption during focal physiologic neural activity, *Science,* 241, 462, 1988.
53. **Prichard, J. W., Rothman, D. L., Novotny, E., Petroff, O. A. C., Kuwubara, T., Avison, M., Howseman, A., Hanstock, C. C., and Shulman, R. G.,** Lactate rise detected by ^{1}H NMR in human visual cortex during physiologic stimulation, *Proc. Natl. Acad. Sci. U.S.A.*, 88, 5829, 1991.
54. **Ueki, M., Linn, F., and Hossmann, K. A.,** Functional activation of cerebral blood flow and metabolism before and after global ischemia of rat brain, *J. Cereb. Blood Flow Metab.*, 8, 486, 1988.
55. **Paschen, W.,** Regional quantitative determination of lactate in brain sections. A bioluminescent approach, *J. Cereb. Blood Flow Metab.*, 5, 609, 1985.
56. **Kuhr, W. G. and Korf, J.,** Extracellular lactic acid as an indicator of brain metabolism: continuous on-line measurement in conscious, freely moving rats with intrastriatal dialysis, *J. Cereb. Blood Flow Metab.*, 8, 130, 1988.
57. **Woods, B. T.,** Metabolic advantage of neuronal coupling of regional brain activity and blood flow, *Ann. Neurol.*, 23, 629, 1988.
58. **Decker, M. W. and McGaugh, J. L.,** The role of interactions between the cholinergic system and other neuromodulatory systems in learning and memory, *Synapse,* 7, 151, 1991.

59. **Maura, G., Andrioli, G. C., Cavazzani, P., and Raiteri, M.,** 5-hydroxytryptamine$_3$ receptors sited on cholinergic axon terminals of human cerebral cortex mediate inhibition of acetylcholine release, *J. Neurochem.*, 58, 2334, 1992.
60. **Tramu, G., Pillez, A., and Leonardelli, J.,** Serotonin axons of the ependyma and circumventricular organs in the forebrain of the guinea pig: an immunohistochemical study, *Cell Tissue Res.*, 228, 297, 1983.
61. **Armstrong, D. M., Miller, R. J., Beaudet, A., and Pickel, V. M.,** Enkephalin-like immunoreactivity in rat area postrema: ultructural localization and coexistence with serotonin, *Brain Res.*, 310, 269, 1984.
62. **Lind, R. W.,** Bidirectional, chemically specified neural connections between the subfornical organ and the midbrain raphe system, *Brain Res.*, 384, 250, 1986.
63. **Lacombe, P. M., Iadecola, C., Underwood, M. D., Sved, A. F., and Reis, D. J.,** Plasma epinephrine modulates the cerebrovasodilation evoked by electrical stimulation of dorsal medulla, *Brain Res.*, 506, 93, 1990.
64. **Lacombe, P., Reynier-Rebuffel, A. M., Mamo, H., and Seylaz, J.,** Quantitative multiregional blood flow measurements during cervical sympathetic stimulation, *Brain Res.*, 129, 129, 1977.
65. **Sercombe, R., Lacombe, P., Aubineau, P., Mamo, H., Pinard, E., Reynier-Rebuffel, A. M., and Seylaz, J.,** Is there an active mechanism limiting the influence of the sympathetic system on the cerebral vascular bed? Evidence for vasomotor escape from sympathetic stimulation in the rabbit, *Brain Res.*, 164, 81, 1979.
66. **Dunn, A. J. and Welch, J.,** Stress- and endotoxin-induced increases in brain tryptophan and serotonin metabolism depend on sympathetic nervous system activity, *J. Neurochem.*, 57, 1615, 1991.
67. **Pappius, H. M.,** Brain injury: new insights into neurotransmitter and receptor mechanisms, *Neurochem. Res.*, 16,s36941, 1991.
68. **White, R. P.,** Pharmacodynamic features of delayed cerebral vasospasm, in *Cerebral Vasospasm,* Wilkins, R. H., Ed., Raven Press, New York, 1988, 373.
69. **Osterholm, J. L. and Bell, J.,** Experimental effects of free serotonin on the brain and its relation to brain injury, *J. Neurosurg.*, 31, 408, 1969.
70. **Fozard, J. R.,** 5-Hydroxytryptamine in the pathophysiology of migraine, in *Vascular Neuroeffector Mechanisms,* Bevan, J. A., et al., Eds., Elsevier, Amsterdam, 1985, 321.
71. **Lauritzen, M.,** Cortical spreading depression as a putative migraine mechanism, *Trends Neurosci.*, 10, 8, 1987.
72. **Lacombe, P., Sercombe, R., Correze, J. L., Springhetti, V., and Seylaz, J.,** Spreading depression induces prolonged reduction of cortical blood flow reactivity in the rat, *Exp. Neurol.*, 117, 278, 1992.
73. **Glover, M. and Sandler, V.,** Can the vascular and neurogenic theories of migraine finally be reconciled?, *Trends Pharmacol. Sci.*, 10, 1, 1989.

Chapter 7

HISTAMINERGIC EFFECTS ON CEREBRAL HEMODYNAMICS

L. Schilling and M. Wahl

TABLE OF CONTENTS

I. Introduction 114

II. Sources of Histamine in the Central Nervous System 114

III. Vasomotor Effects of Histamine 115
  A. Vasomotor Effects of Histamine *In Vivo* 115
  B. Vasomotor Effects of Histamine *In Vitro* 117
    1. Contractile Action of Histamine 117
    2. Relaxant Action of Histamine 118

IV. Effects of Histamine on Blood-Brain Barrier Permeability 119

V. Pathophysiological Importance of Histamine 121

References 122

0-8493-5096-0/93/$0.00 + $.50

I. INTRODUCTION

Histamine (HA) (β-imidazolyl ethylamine), derived from the amino acid precursor L-histidine, is involved in a variety of physiological functions.[1,2] Moreover, HA is also an important mediator of inflammation under various pathological conditions. The inflammatory response exerts profound influences on the cardiovascular system, including vasodilation and increase of vascular permeability. Since these reactions to HA have also been identified in the cerebral circulation, it has been hypothesized that HA may act as a mediator of secondary brain damage after cerebral insults.[3]

II. SOURCES OF HISTAMINE IN THE CENTRAL NERVOUS SYSTEM

Both neuronal and non-neuronal sources of HA have been identified in the brain. First evidence for a neurotransmitter function of HA was provided by neurochemical studies and lesion experiments.[4] Immunohistochemical studies using antibodies raised against HA[5,6] or the specific HA-synthesizing enzyme histidine-decarboxylase[7,8] revealed a high density of histaminergic perikarya in posterior hypothalamic nuclei from whence widespread projection pathways to almost all regions of the brain originate. The close contact between occasional varicose fibers exhibiting HA-like immunoreactivity and blood vessels in the hypothalamus[9] and in the cerebrum[10] of the rat also suggests a regional histaminergic cerebrovascular innervation.

The most important non-neuronal source of HA is probably mast cells. These have been found in the brain of many species, including man. According to Ibrahim[11] two types of mast cells may be distinguished. Type I mast cells are devoid of autofluorescence, but exhibit pronounced metachromasia to toluidine blue (typical for so-called connective tissue type mast cells). Although there is considerable intra- and interspecific variation, type I mast cells appear to be most abundant in the thalamus, but they have also been found in the cerebral cortex, hypothalamus, the leptomeninges, choroid plexus, and even in the hindbrain.[11-20] Such mast cells may be associated with intra- and extraparenchymal blood vessels, and they have also been detected in close proximity to nerves.[19] Thalamic mast cells may contribute up to 50% of whole brain HA content in rats,[21] and similar values have been inferred from studies on a mast cell-deficient (W/W^v) mouse strain.[22,23]

Type II mast cells termed "neurolipomastocytes"[11] exhibit a strong autofluorescence due to a high lipid content but barely stain metachromatically with toluidine blue. They may not contain heparin or vasoactive substances like histamine and are therefore not generally viewed as real mast cells.[17,18]

A further source of HA in the brain may be the blood vessel wall itself.[24-26] However, it is not clear which cell type(s) actually contain HA. It may stem from mast cells associated with the vessel wall,[24,25] but may also come from

TABLE 1
Compounds Used as Histaminergic Agonists and Antagonists in Cerebrovascular Research Defining HA Receptor Subtypes and Main Targets

Receptor Subtype	Agonist	Antagonist
	2-Pyridylethylamine	Mepyramine
H_1	2-Thiazolylethylamine	Chlorpheniramine
	2-Methylhistamine	
	Impromidine[a]	Burimamide[b]
	Dimaprit	Metiamide
H_2	4-Methylhistamine	Cimetidine
		Ranitidine
		Zolantidine
H_3	R(α)-methylhistamine	Thioperamide

Note: Most of the compounds are mentioned in the text.

[a] Also acts a H_3 receptor antagonist.
[b] Originally developed as H_2 receptor antagonist, but with a higher affinity towards H_3 receptor.

smooth muscle and endothelial cells[26] (similar to aortic smooth muscle and endothelium which have been shown to possess HA-forming capacity[27]).

III. VASOMOTOR EFFECTS OF HISTAMINE

Compounds acting as more-or-less specific activators or blockers of HA receptors have been used to identify receptor subtypes underlying histaminergic actions in cerebral blood vessels *in vitro* and *in vivo*. The compounds most often used are listed in Table 1 to enable the reader to associate compounds and receptors when mentioned in the text.

A. VASOMOTOR EFFECTS OF HISTAMINE *IN VIVO*

Intravascularly applied HA may not affect cerebral blood flow (CBF) as long as blood pressure is kept within the autoregulatory range since circulating HA does not readily cross the blood-brain barrier (BBB).[28] In those studies in which intravascular application of HA induced either a flow increase or a decrease of perfusion pressure,[29-34] disturbance of BBB permeability appears likely. In rats, intracarotid or intravenous application of HA increases CBF after transient opening of the BBB by a hyperosmotic bolus but has no effect under normal conditions.[35,36] Correspondingly, CBF may not change[37-39] or occasionally increase[37] after intravenous or intracarotid infusion of HA in man. In monkeys, systemic application of HA induces a transient increase of CBF[40] consistent with dilation of the anterior cerebral artery measured angiographically.[41] It is difficult to reconcile the contradictory results, but differences in histaminergic receptor population, sensitivity, or arrangement on smooth muscle cells and endothelium (see below) may be involved.

In a number of studies in which HA increased CBF, a blockade of H_2 receptors exerted a greater inhibitory effect than a blockade of H_1 receptors,[33-35] and these effects appeared to be additive.[33,34] Furthermore, impromidine and 2-pyridylethylamine both increased CBF in rats.[35] These results indicate involvement of H_1 and H_2 receptors in CBF response to HA; the latter may dominate.

When HA is applied extravascularly, an increase of cortical blood flow during superfusion[42] and of caudate nucleus flow during ventriculo-cisternal perfusion[43] is found. These results are consistent with the vasodilatory effect of topically applied HA in pial arteries first described by Forbes et al. more than 60 years ago.[44] Recently, these observations have been confirmed[42,45-49] and extended using specific agonists and antagonists. In cats perivascular microinjection of HA induces a concentration-related dilation of pial arterioles[45-47] but not of pial veins.[46] Lack of direct venomotor activity of HA therefore indicates that dilation of pial veins observed during cortical superfusion with HA[42,48] is an indirect effect and probably due to dilation of pial arteries. Wahl and Kuschinsky[45] were the first to demonstrate that pial arteriolar dilation was mainly due to H_2 receptor activation since the response was antagonized by cimetidine but barely influenced by mepyramine.[45] These results were substantiated by demonstrating that microapplication of impromidine induced a bigger dilation than 2-pyridylethylamine.[46,47] Activation of H_1 and H_2 receptors therefore appears to be involved in the dilatory action of extravascularly applied HA. This is in agreement with results obtained in CBF studies (see above).

Part of the vasomotor effects of HA may be due to interaction with different regulatory systems. In the cat, constriction of pial arterioles induced by sympathetic stimulation or exogenously applied noradrenaline is converted into dilation by simultaneous application of HA.[50] Inhibition of stimulation-induced constriction may partly be due to inhibition of noradrenaline release by prejunctional HA receptors.[51] However, a postsynaptic action must also be involved to account for the inhibitory effect of HA on noradrenaline-induced constriction of pial arteries.

In the piglet, cortical superfusion with HA elicits pial arteriolar dilation accompanied by an increase of prostanoid concentration, especially prostaglandin (PG) E_2, in the superfusion fluid.[49] This lead to the suggestion that prostanoids mediate HA-induced dilatation.

While extravascularly applied HA induces pial arterial dilation in most species studied, constriction occurs during cortical superfusion with HA in rabbits.[52] These findings agree with observations in rabbit-isolated cerebral arteries (see below) and are thought to be due to predomination of H_1 receptors in cerebral arteries of this species. Pial arterial constriction was also seen in mice during cortical superfusion with 200 μM HA while dilatation was observed at 100 μM.[53,54]

B. VASOMOTOR EFFECTS OF HISTAMINE *IN VITRO*

Isolated cerebral arteries kept under resting tension respond to HA with contraction. Since HA mostly induces concentration-dependent relaxation in precontracted arteries, both contractile and relaxant histaminergic receptors must be present in the cerebroarterial vessel wall, and activation of receptor subtypes may be influenced by vessel tone.

1. Contractile Action of Histamine

Contractile action of HA is found in cerebral arteries of various species.[47,55-68] Studies in dogs[61] and humans[56,63,66] suggest that big arteries, like the middle cerebral artery, appear to be more sensitive to the contractile action of HA than their distal branches. Contraction can be blocked by H_1 receptor antagonists[55,59,61,62,64,68] and is mimicked by 2-pyridylethylamine.[47,62,63,68] The H_2 receptors elicit no contractile activity, since neither impromidine and dimaprit elicit contraction,[47,68] nor does cimetidine affect histaminergic contraction.[47,64]

Location of the histaminergic receptors mediating contraction appears to vary between species. Results from studies in which the contractile effect of HA in cerebral arteries is compared with and without a functional endothelium favor a smooth muscle location in rabbits,[62,67] goats,[68] and distal portions of human middle cerebral artery,[66] but an endothelial location in canine basilar[65] and human proximal middle cerebral artery.[66] In the isolated dog basilar artery activation of endothelial H_1 receptors induces release of thromboxane A_2 as the contractile signal.[65] At present, it is not known whether the same coupling mechanism occurs in the human middle cerebral artery.

Histamine may exert its direct contractile activity via a number of mechanisms. Stimulation of inositol phospholipid hydrolysis, demonstrated in many cell types,[1] may be involved. Inositol phospholipid hydrolysis results in synthesis of inositol-1,4,5,trisphosphate which then releases Ca^{2+} from intracellular stores[69] to activate the contractile apparatus. Release of intracellular Ca^{2+} by HA has been demonstrated in smooth muscle cells of swine carotid artery.[70]

Activation of a cation channel (unselective) may also be involved in the contractile action of HA.[71-73] The resulting depolarization allows influx of Ca^{2+} through voltage-gated channels thus increasing cytosolic Ca^{2+} concentration. This may then induce or maintain activation of contractile proteins.[74] In feline isolated middle cerebral artery[71] and guinea pig basilar artery,[72,73] HA (above 1 μM) induced a concentration-related depolarization of smooth muscle cell membrane which was blocked by simultaneous application of mepyramine, the latter indicating mediation by H_1 receptors.[71]

In many tissues H_1 receptors are coupled to activation of guanylate cyclase.[1] However this does not appear to hold for vascular smooth muscle since in this tissue an increase in cytosolic cyclic guanosine monophosphate (cGMP) concentration induces relaxation rather than contraction.[75]

In contrast to its effect on pial arteries *in vivo*[50] (see above) HA has been shown to enhance release of noradrenaline from nerve terminals of isolated cerebral arteries of cats,[59,60,76,77] goats,[68] and humans.[78] Accordingly, contraction induced by field stimulation was potentiated by HA.[57,67,68] This apparent discrepancy may be due to the experimental conditions, especially the type and degree of vessel tone which determine the type of receptor activated by HA and thus its vasomotor action.

2. Relaxant Action of Histamine

The relaxant action of HA and the underlying mechanisms have been studied in precontracted vessels. In isolated human pial veins, HA induced a small relaxation in only two out of seven specimens.[79] This is consistent with a lack of venomotor effects of HA in micropuncture studies in cats *in situ*.[46]

When the relaxant effect of HA is compared with its contractile action (in noncontracted arteries) in the same study, relaxation usually occurs in a lower concentration range than contraction.[47,55,61] Relaxation is often related to H_2 receptor activation, since H_2 receptor antagonists diminish or even abolish HA-induced relaxation[16,47,55,61-64,66,80-82] and application of H_2 receptor agonists mimics histaminergic relaxation.[47,63,80,82] After damaging the endothelium, HA still elicits an H_2 receptor-mediated relaxation.[62,64,66,82] These results suggest that the H_2 receptor is located on the smooth muscle cells. The endothelium of cerebral arteries also carries relaxant histaminergic receptors which are apparently of the H_1 subtype in rat,[64,82] monkey, and man.[66] The relative contribution of endothelial H_1 receptors to the overall response appears to increase with decreasing vessel size since relaxation of small pial arteries in monkeys and man was blocked by H_2 receptor antagonists to a lesser degree than by H_1 receptor antagonists.[63,66]

In the rabbit isolated middle cerebral artery relaxant receptors of the H_1 and H_3 subtype may be located on the endothelium.[80,83,84] H_3-receptor mediation of relaxation was identified through antagonism by thioperamide and mimicry by R(α)-methyl-histamine.[84] The H_3 receptor was first identified on neurons and is also found on perivascular nerve terminals of peripheral arteries.[85] Whether H_3 receptors are also present on vascular nerve terminals of cerebral arteries has not yet been established.

The H_2 receptor is coupled to adenylate cyclase in a variety of tissues[1] including vascular smooth muscle.[86] The resulting increase in intracellular concentration of cyclic adenosine monophosphate (cAMP) induces relaxation by decreasing cytosolic Ca^{2+} concentration and diminishing the Ca^{2+} sensitivity of the contractile apparatus.[75] In addition to adenylate cyclase stimulation, H_2 receptor activation may elicit relaxation by inducing membrane hyperpolarization, which has been shown in isolated feline middle cerebral artery.[71] Although the mechanism underlying histaminergic hyperpolarization has not yet been elucidated, it is obviously not due to activation of ATP-modulated K^+ channels since glibenclamide, which acts as a blocker of this type of K^+ channel in cerebral arteries,[87,88] does not affect HA-induced relaxation of rat isolated basilar artery.[89]

The endothelial component of histaminergic relaxation is mediated by release of vasoactive factors from the endothelium. One of these factors appears to be nitric oxide or a nitric oxide containing moiety. Nitric oxide elicits relaxation by stimulating smooth muscle soluble guanylate cyclase.[90] In the presence of methylene blue, which inhibits soluble guanylate cyclase, HA-induced relaxation is shifted to higher concentrations in the isolated rat middle cerebral artery[82] and is slowed in monkey cerebral arteries.[66] In the isolated rabbit middle cerebral artery relaxation due to activation of H_3 receptor is partly blocked by an inhibitor of nitric oxide synthesis.[84] However, full blockade is only achieved by simultaneous application of inhibitors of nitric oxide and prostanoid synthesis,[84] indicating that release of both nitric oxide and relaxant prostanoid(s) is involved in mediating endothelium-dependent histaminergic relaxation. Comparable findings have been obtained in studies of acetylcholine-induced, endothelium-dependent relaxation in the rabbit isolated basilar artery.[91]

The mechanisms involved in vasomotor actions of HA in isolated cerebral arteries are summarized schematically in Figure 1.

IV. EFFECTS OF HISTAMINE ON BLOOD-BRAIN BARRIER PERMEABILITY

Although HA clearly increases BBB permeability, a number of investigators have failed to find tracer extravasation after intracarotid or intravenous application of HA[92-96] or during cortical superfusion.[42,97,98] The reasons for this are unclear, but may be related to techniques and methods, or even species differences. An increase of BBB permeability due to systematically applied HA has been unequivocally demonstrated using tracers with both low[99-104] and high molecular weight.[102,105] Furthermore, cortical superfusion with HA also increased BBB permeability as demonstrated by intravital fluorescence microscopy[48,106,107] and measurement of transmural electrical resistance of pial vessels.[108] These results imply that the histaminergic receptor mediating increase of cerebrovascular permeability is located on both the luminal and abluminal sides of the endothelial cells.

Intravital fluorescence microscopy as described by Wahl et al.[109] has been used to quantify tracer extravasation during cortical superfusion with HA, which is thought to mimic massive release from the parenchyma. Intravenously applied tracers were Na^+-fluorescein (mol wt 376) and fluorescein

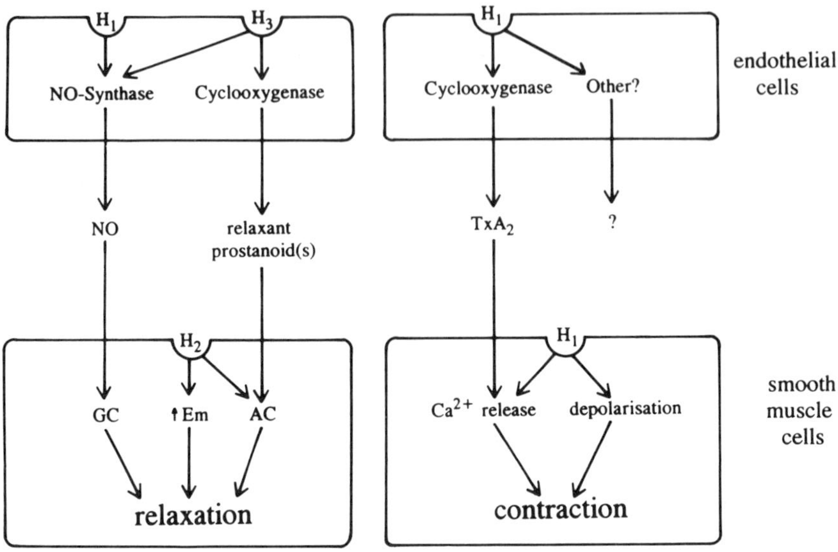

FIGURE 1. Scheme of pathways which may be involved in the vasomotor actions of HA in cerebral arteries. The contribution of each pathway to the overall effect of HA depends upon the vessel type, species, and experimental condition. AC, adenylate cyclase; GC, guanylate cyclase; TxA_2, thromboxane A_2; Em, membrane potential; NO, nitric oxide. While NO directly stimulates GC, the prostanoid effects (including those of TxA_2) are mediated by activation of smooth muscle membrane receptors.

isothiocyanate (FITC) labeled dextrans (mol wt 62,000 and 150,000). These tracers were restricted to the intravascular space during control superfusion with artificial cerebrospinal fluid but all three extravasated during superfusion with HA. The threshold concentration of HA required to induce extravasation was lowest for Na^+-fluorescein and increased with the size of the tracer used.[48] These results imply that HA opens functional "pores" with a diameter of at least 35 nm to allow leakage of FITC-dextran 150,000. Histamine thus induces an unspecific opening of the BBB in contrast to bradykinin, which elicits extravasation of Na^+-fluorescein only.[109,110]

In cerebral microvessel preparations from ox[111] and man,[112] H_1 binding sites have been identified, but H_2 receptors are also present. In fact, experimental evidence suggests H_2 receptors are even more important in modulating BBB function than H_1 receptors. Increase of BBB permeability by HA is diminished or even abolished by application of H_2 but not of H_1 receptor antagonists,[101,102,104,105,108,113] and it is mimicked in dogs by systemic application of 4-methylhistamine but not of 2-methylhistamine.[104] Moreover, cortical superfusion in cats with impromidine induces extravasation of Na^+-fluorescein at considerably lower concentrations than HA.[114]

The mechanism underlying histaminergic alteration of BBB permeability appears to involve activation of adenylate cyclase via H_2 receptors as suggested by studies performed in rat and guinea pig.[25,115,116] Furthermore, HA has been shown to stimulate synthesis of prostanoids, especially PGE_2[117] in brain microvessels. This may augment HA-induced activation of adenylate cyclase in an autocrine manner. The proposition of a mediator function for cAMP in HA-induced extravasation is strengthened by the observation that intravenous administration of dibutyryl-cAMP (a membrane permeable analogue of cAMP) or direct activation of adenylate cyclase by forskolin resulted in increased BBB permeability, similar to HA.[104,115]

The route of extravasation induced by HA is not yet clear. Stimulation of vesicular transport has been claimed to be a mechanism, since an increased number of vesicles is frequently found in cerebral capillaries after intravascular or intraventricular application of HA or dibutyryl-cAMP.[102,105,113,115,118] However, the very fast onset[108] of the increase of transendothelial ionic conductance induced by HA is obviously not compatible with vesicular transport but rather with opening of inter- or transendothelial gaps. Widening of interendothelial clefts by HA due to endothelial contraction has been suggested by Majno et al.[119] and intercellular gaps have been demonstrated in peripheral blood vessels after application of HA.[120] However, there is no evidence for the widening of tight junctions in cerebral blood vessels[102] or ultrastructural alterations as judged from freeze fracture studies.[105]

V. PATHOPHYSIOLOGICAL IMPORTANCE OF HISTAMINE

Due to its potent enhancement of permeability and dilatory effects on cerebral blood vessels, an increase of HA concentration in the brain interstitial fluid may increase CBF and induce brain edema. Under experimental conditions an increase in brain tissue content, or interstitial fluid concentration, of HA was found after such brain traumas as cold lesion,[121] stab wound,[122] or regional ischemia,[123,124] implying a pathophysiological role for HA under these conditions.

Further evidence for a mediator function of HA has been gained from experimental studies using HA receptor antagonists under different pathological conditions. Thus, increase in CBF during acute normocapnic hypoxia was attenuated by H_2 receptor blockade in dogs, while the hyperemic response during normoxic hypercapnia was not affected.[125] Furthermore, brain edema induced by severe hypoxemia due to experimental pneumothorax in piglets could be diminished by pretreatment with mepyramine and ranitidine.[126]

Radiation-induced brain edema may also involve release of HA. Metiamide was shown to decrease the degree of Evans blue extravasation induced by local brain radiation in different species.[127,128]

Histamine released from neurones may also be involved in the development of brain edema following seizures. This is concluded from a study in which ranitidine, given before and during seizure induction with kainate, decreased Evans blue extravasation in the thalamus.[129]

Contradictory results have been obtained in experimental models of brain trauma. Brain edema due to stab wound could be attenuated by pre- and posttreatment with high doses of cimetidine, but not mepyramine.[122] In contrast, brain edema induced in monkeys by cold lesion was not diminished by combined treatment with dexamethasone and chlorpheniramine.[130] Similarly, cold lesion-induced edema in rats was not blocked by pre- and posttreatment with either zolantidine or mepyramine.[131]

In summary, HA profoundly affects vasomotor and permeability function of cerebral blood vessels. Its involvement in the regulation of CBF or BBB permeability under physiological conditions is as yet unclear. However, it may be involved in various disease states affecting cerebral circulation. Whether HA acts as a mediator of vasogenic brain edema[3] is still unclear because convincing therapeutic results with HA receptor antagonists are still lacking.

REFERENCES

1. **Hill, S. J.,** Distribution, properties, and functional characteristics of three classes of histamine receptor, *Pharmacol. Rev.*, 42, 45, 1990.
2. **Schwartz, J.-C., Arrang, J.-M., Garbarg, M., Pollard, H., and Ruat, M.,** Histaminergic transmission in the mammalian brain, *Physiol. Rev.*, 71, 1, 1991.
3. **Wahl, M., Unterberg, A., Baethmann, A., and Schilling, L.,** Mediators of blood-brain barrier dysfunction and formation of vasogenic brain edema, *J. Cereb. Blood Flow Metab.*, 8, 621, 1988.
4. **Garbarg, M., Barbin, G., Feger, J., and Schwartz, J.-C.,** Histaminergic pathway in rat brain evidenced by lesions of the medial forebrain bundle, *Science*, 186, 833, 1974.
5. **Steinbusch, H. W. M. and Mulder, A. H.,** Immunohistochemical localization of histamine in neurons and mast cells in the rat brain, in *Handbook of Chemical Neuronanatomy*, Vol. 3, *Classical Transmitters and Transmitter Receptors in the CNS*, Part II, Björklund, A., Hökfelt, T., and Kuhar, M. J., Eds., Elsevier, Amsterdam, 1984, 126.
6. **Airaksinen, M. S. and Panula, P.,** The histaminergic system in guinea pig central nervous system: an immunocytochemical mapping study using an antiserum against histamine, *J. Comp. Neurol.*, 273, 163, 1988.
7. **Watanabe, T., Taguchi, Y., Hayaschi, H., Tanaka, J., Shiosaka, S., Tohyama, M., Kubota, H., Terano, Y., and Wada, H.,** Evidence for the presence of a histaminergic neuron system in the rat brain: an immunohistochemical analysis, *Neurosci. Lett.*, 39, 249, 1983.
8. **Smits, R. P. J. M., Steinbusch, H. W. M., and Mulder, A. H.,** The localization of histidine decarboxylase-immunoreactive cell bodies in the guinea-pig brain, *J. Chem. Neuroanat.*, 3, 85, 1990.
9. **Steinbusch, H. W. M. and Verhofstad, A. A. J.,** Immunocytochemical demonstration of noradrenaline, serotonin and histamine and some observations on the innervation of the intracerebral blood vessels, in *Neural Regulation of Brain Circulation*, Owman, C. and Hardebo, J. E., Eds., Elsevier, Amsterdam, 1986, 181.
10. **Takagi, H., Morishima, Y., Matsuyama, T., Hayashi, H., Watanabe, T., and Wada, H.,** Histaminergic axons in the neostriatum and cerebral cortex of the rat: a correlated light and electron microscopic immunocytochemical study using histidine decarboxylase as a marker, *Brain Res.*, 364, 114, 1986.

11. **Ibrahim, M. Z. M.,** The mast cells of the mammalian central nervous system. Part I. Morphology, distribution and histochemistry, *J. Neurol. Sci.,* 21, 431, 1974.
12. **Kelsall, M. A. and Lewis, P.,** Mast cells in the brain, *Fed. Proc.,* 23, 1107, 1964.
13. **Campbell, D. J. and Kiernan, J. A.,** Mast cells in the central nervous system, *Nature,* 210, 756, 1966.
14. **Flood, P. R. and Krüger, P. G.,** Fine structure of mast cells in the central nervous system of the hedgehog, *Acta Anat.,* 75, 443, 1970.
15. **Dropp, J. J.,** Mast cells in mammalian brain, *Acta Anat.,* 94, 1, 1976.
16. **Edvinsson, L., Owman, C., and Sjöberg, N.-O.,** Autonomic nerves, mast cells, and amine receptors in human brain vessels. A histochemical and pharmacological study, *Brain Res.,* 115, 377, 1976.
17. **Kiernan, J. A.,** A comparative survey of the mast cells of the mammalian brain, *J. Anat.,* 121, 303, 1976.
18. **Edvinsson, L., Cervos-Navarro, J., Larsson, L.-I., Owman, C., and Rönnberg, A.-L.,** Regional distribution of mast cells containing histamine, dopamine, or 5-hydroxytryptamine in the mammalian brain, *Neurology,* 27, 878, 1977.
19. **Marinkovic, S., Bogdanovic, D., Nestorovic, D., and Teofilovski, G.,** Mast cells in the middle cerebral artery wall, *Acta Med. Iugosl.* 33, 381, 1979.
20. **Dimitriadou, V., Lambracht-Hall, M., Reichler, J., and Theoharides, T. C.,** Histochemical and ultrastructural characteristics of rat brain perivascular mast cells stimulated with compound 48/80 and carbachol, *Neuroscience,* 39, 209, 1990.
21. **Goldschmidt, R. C., Hough, L. B., and Glick, S. D.,** Rat brain mast cells: contribution to brain histamine levels, *J. Neurochem.,* 44, 1943, 1985.
22. **Grzanna, R. and Shultz, L. D.,** The contribution of mast cells to the histamine content of the central nervous system: a regional analysis, *Life Sci.,* 30, 1959, 1982.
23. **Yamatodani, A., Maeyama, K., Watanabe, T., Wada, H., and Kitamura, Y.,** Tissue distribution of histamine in a mutant mouse deficient in mast cells. Clear evidence for the presence of non-mast cell histamine, *Biochem. Pharmacol.,* 31, 305, 1982.
24. **Jarrott, B., Hjelle, J. T., and Spector, S.,** Association of histamine with cerebral microvessels in regions of bovine brain, *Brain Res.,* 168, 323, 1979.
25. **Karnushina, I. L., Palacios, J. M., Barbin, G., Dux, E., Joó, F., and Schwartz, J. C.,** Studies on a capillary-rich fraction isolated from brain: histaminic components and characterization of the histamine receptors linked to adenylate cyclase, *J. Neurochem.,* 34, 1201, 1980.
26. **Robinson-White, A. and Beaven, M. A.,** Presence of histamine and histamine-metabolizing enzyme in rat and guinea-pig microvascular endothelial cells, *J. Pharmacol. Exp. Ther.,* 223, 440, 1982.
27. **Hollis, T. M. and Rosen, L. A.,** Histidine decarboxylase activity of bovine aortic endothelium and intima-media (36914), *Proc. Soc. Exp. Biol. Med.,* 141, 978, 1972.
28. **Oldendorf, W. H.,** Brain uptake of radiolabeled amino acids, amines, and hexoses after arterial injection, *Am. J. Physiol.,* 221, 1629, 1971.
29. **Finesinger, J. and Putnam, T. J.,** Cerebral circulation. XXIII. Induced variations in volume flow through the brain perfused at constant pressure, *Arch. Neurol. Psychiatry,* 30, 775, 1933.
30. **Karlsberg, P., Elliott, H. W., and Adams, J. E.,** Effect of various pharmacologic agents on cerebral arteries, *Neurology,* 13, 772, 1963.
31. **Anderson, W. D. and Kubicek, W. G.,** Effects of betahistine HCl, nicotinic acid, and histamine on basilar blood flow in anesthetized dogs, *Stroke,* 2, 409, 1971.
32. **Tindall, G. T. and Greenfield, J. C., Jr.,** The effects of intra-arterial histamine on blood flow in the internal and external carotid artery of man, *Stroke,* 4, 46, 1973.
33. **Saxena, P. R.,** The significance of histamine H_1 and H_2 receptors on the carotid vascular bed in the dog, *Neurology,* 25, 681, 1975.
34. **Lord, G. D. A., Mylecharane, E. J., Duckworth, J. W., and Lance, J. W.,** Effects of histamine H_1- and H_2-receptor antagonists in the cranial circulation of the monkey, *Clin. Exp. Pharmacol. Physiol.,* 8, 89, 1981.

35. **Gross, P. M., Harper, A. M., and Teasdale, G. M.,** Cerebral circulation and histamine. I. Participation of vascular H_1- and H_2receptors in vasodilatatory responses to carotid arterial infusion, *J. Cereb. Blood Flow Metab.,* 1, 97, 1981.
36. **Vesely, R., Hoffman, W. E., Gil, K. S. L., Albrecht, R. F., and Miletich, D. J.,** The cerebrovascular effects of curare and histamine in the rat, *Anesthesiology,* 66, 519, 1987.
37. **Shenkin, H. A.,** Effects of various drugs upon cerebral circulation and metabolism of man, *J. Appl. Physiol.,* 3, 465, 1951.
38. **Alman, R. W., Rosenberg, M., and Fazekas, F. F.,** Effects of histamine on cerebral hemodynamics and metabolism, *Arch. Neurol. Psychiat.,* 67, 354, 1952.
39. **Aebelholt-Krabbe, A. and Olesen, J.,** Effect of histamine on regional cerebral blood flow in man, *Cephalalgia,* 20, 15, 1982.
40. **Eidelman, B., Karanjia, P., Nemoto, E., and Singh, S.,** The effects of histamine on cerebral blood flow, *J. Cereb. Blood Flow Metab.,* 1(Suppl. 1), S365, 1981.
41. **Watters, J. W.,** The effects of bradykinin and histamine on cerebral arteries of monkeys, *Radiology,* 98, 299, 1971.
42. **Martins, A. N., Doyle, T. F., Wright, S. J., Jr., and Bass, B. G.,** Response of cerebral circulation to topical histamine, *Stroke,* 11, 469, 1980.
43. **DeLey, G., Weyne, J., Demeester, G., and Leusen, I.,** Response of local blood flow in the caudate nucleus of the cat to intraventricular administration of histamine, *Stroke,* 13, 499, 1982.
44. **Forbes, H. S., Wolff, H. G., and Cobb, S.,** The cerebral circulation, *Am. J. Physiol.,* 89, 266, 1929.
45. **Wahl, M. and Kuschinsky, W.,** The dilating effect of histamine on pial arteries of cats and its mediation by H_2 receptors, *Circ. Res.,* 44, 161, 1979.
46. **Gross, P. M., Harper, A. M., and Teasdale, G. M.,** Cerebral circulation and histamine. II. Responses of pial veins and arterioles to receptor agonists, *J. Cereb. Blood Flow Metab.,* 1, 219, 1981.
47. **Edvinsson, L., Gross, P. M., and Mohamed, A.,** Characterization of histamine receptors in cat cerebral arteries in vitro and in situ, *J. Pharmacol. Exp. Ther.,* 225, 168, 1983.
48. **Schilling, L., Ksoll, E., and Wahl, M.,** Effects of histamine on vasomotor response and permeability of extraparenchymal cerebral vessels, *J. Cereb. Blood Flow Metab.,* 7(Suppl. 1), S506, 1987.
49. **Mirro, R., Busija, D. W., Armstead, W. M., and Leffler, C. W.,** Histamine dilates pial arterioles of newborn pigs through prostanoid production, *Am. J. Physiol.,* 254, H1023, 1988.
50. **Gross, P. M., Harper, A. M., and Teasdale, G. M.,** Interaction of histamine with noradrenergic constrictory mechanisms in cat cerebral arteries and veins, *Can. J. Physiol. Pharmacol.,* 61, 756, 1983.
51. **Gross, P. M.,** Cerebral histamine: indications for neuronal and vascular regulation, *J. Cereb. Blood Flow Metab.,* 2, 3, 1982.
52. **Kamitani, T., Little, M. H., and Ellis, E. F.,** Effect of leukotrienes, 12-HETE, histamine, bradykinin, and 5-hydroxytryptamine on in vivo rabbit cerebral arteriolar diameter, *J. Cereb. Blood Flow Metab.,* 5, 554, 1985.
53. **Rosenblum, W. I., Nelson, G. H., and Weinbrecht, P.,** Histamine elicits competing endothelium-dependent constriction and endothelium-independent dilation in vivo in mouse cerebral arterioles, *Stroke,* 21, 305, 1990.
54. **Rosenblum, W. I. and Nelson, G. H.,** Tone regulates opposing endothelium-dependent and independent forces: resistance brain vessels in vivo, *Am. J. Physiol.,* 259, H243, 1990.
55. **Edvinsson, L. and Owman, C.,** A pharmacologic comparison of histamine receptors in isolated extracranial and intracranial arteries in vitro, *Neurology,* 25, 271, 1975.

56. **Shibata, S., Cheng, J. B., and Murakami, W.,** Reactivity of isolated human cerebral arteries to biogenic amines, *Blood Vessels,* 14, 356, 1975.
57. **Duckles, S. P. and Bevan, J. A.,** Responses of small rabbit pial arteries in vitro, *Blood Vessels,* 16, 80, 1979.
58. **Toda, N. and Hayashi, S.,** Age-dependent alteration in the response of isolated rabbit basilar arteries to vasoactive agents, *J. Pharmacol. Exp. Ther.,* 211, 716, 1979.
59. **Marco, E. J., Balfagon, G., Marin, J., Gómez, B., and Lluch, S.,** Indirect adrenergic effect of histamine in cat cerebral arteries, *Naunyn-Schmiedebergs Arch. Pharmakol.,* 312, 239, 1980.
60. **Lobato, R. D., Marin, J., and Salaices, M.,** Effect of subarachnoid hemorrhage on contractile responses and noradrenaline release evoked in cat cerebral arteries by histamine, *J. Neurosurg.,* 55, 543, 1981.
61. **Toda, N., Okamura, T., and Miyazaki, M.,** Heterogeneity in the response to vasoconstrictors of isolated dog proximal and distal middle cerebral arteries, *Eur. J. Pharmacol.,* 106, 291, 1984.
62. **Sercombe, R., Verrecchia, C., Philipson, V., Oudart, N., Dimitriadou, V., Bouchaud, C., and Seylaz, J.,** Histamine-induced constriction and dilatation of rabbit middle cerebral arteries in vitro: role of the endothelium, *Blood Vessels,* 23, 137, 1986.
63. **Ottoson, A., Jansen, I., and Edvinsson, L.,** Characterization of histamine receptors in isolated human cerebral arteries, *Br. J. Pharmacol.,* 94, 901, 1988.
64. **Chang, J.-Y., Hardebo, J. E., and Owman, C.,** Differential vasomotor action of noradrenaline, serotonin, and histamine in isolated basilar artery from rat and guinea-pig, *Acta Physiol. Scand.,* 132, 91, 1988.
65. **Usui, H., Kurahashi, K., Shirahase, H., Manabe, K., Shibata, S., and Fujiwara, M.,** Endothelium-dependent relaxation in monkey cerebral and contraction in canine cerebral arteries produced by histamine, *Med. Sci. Res.,* 17, 1035, 1989.
66. **Toda, N.,** Mechanism underlying responses to histamine of isolated monkey and human cerebral arteries, *Am. J. Physiol.,* 258, H311, 1990.
67. **van Riper, D. A. and Bevan, J. A.,** Selective variation of agonist and neurally mediated vasoconstriction with rabbit middle cerebral artery branch order, *J. Pharmacol. Exp. Ther.,* 257, 879, 1991.
68. **Miranda, F. J., Torregrosa, G., Salom, J. B., Alabadi, J. A., Alvarez, and Alborch, E.,** Direct and neuromodulatory effects of histamine on isolated goat cerebral arteries, *J. Autonom. Pharmacol.,* 12, 25, 1992.
69. **Berridge, M. J. and Irvine, R. F.,** Inositol trisphosphate, a novel second messenger in cellular signal transduction, *Nature,* 312, 315, 1984.
70. **Rembold, C. M. and Murphy, R. A.,** Histamine concentration and Ca^{2+} mobilization in arterial smooth muscle, *Am. J. Physiol.,* 257, C122, 1989.
71. **Hermsmeyer, K., Abel, P. W., and Harder, D. R.,** Membrane electrical responses to histamine in muscle cells of cat middle cerebral artery, in *Cerebral Blood Flow: Effects of Nerves and Neurotransmitters,* Heistad, D. D. and Marcus, M. L., Eds., Elsevier, New York, 1982, 3.
72. **Karashima, T. and Kuriyama, H.,** Electrical properties of smooth muscle cell membrane and neuromuscular transmission in the guinea-pig basilar artery, *Br. J. Pharmacol.,* 74, 495, 1981.
73. **Fallgren, B., Arlock, P., Jansen, I., and Edvinsson, L.,** Neuropeptide Y in cerebrovascular function: comparison of membrane potential changes and vasomotor responses evoked by NPY and other vasoconstrictors in the guinea pig basilar artery, *Neurosci. Lett.,* 114, 117, 1990.
74. **van Breemen, C. and Saida, K.,** Cellular mechanism regulating $[Ca^{2+}]_i$ smooth muscle, *Annu. Rev. Physiol.,* 51, 315, 1989.
75. **Karaki, H.,** Ca^{2+} localization and sensitivity in vascular smooth muscle, *Trends Pharmacol. Sci.,* 10, 320, 1989.

76. **Balfagon, G., Galvan, R., and Marco, E. J.,** Mechanism of the indirect adrenergic effects of histamine in cat cerebral arteries, *J. Pharm. Pharmacol.*, 36, 248, 1984.
77. **Marco, E. J. and Balfagon, G.,** Indirect adrenergic effect of compound 48/80 in cat cerebral arteries, *Agent Action,* 16, 310, 1985.
78. **Marco, E. J., Balfagon, G., and Conde, M. V.,** Indirect adrenergic effect of histamine in human cerebral arteries: influence of post-mortem period, *J. Pharm. Pharmacol.*, 36, 253, 1984.
79. **Hardebo, J. E., Kahrström, J., Owman, C., and Salford, L. G.,** Vasomotor effects of neurotransmitter and modulators on isolated human pial veins, *J. Cereb. Blood Flow Metab.*, 7, 612, 1987.
80. **Ea-Kim, L., Teste, J. F., Sercombe, R., and Oudart, N.,** Participation of vascular H_1-receptors in histaminergic relaxation of rabbit middle cerebral artery in vitro, *Arch. Int. Pharmacodyn. Ther.*, 283, 282, 1986.
81. **Dacey, R. G., Jr., and Bassett, J. E.,** Histaminergic vasodilation of intracerebral arterioles in the rat, *J. Cereb. Blood Flow Metab.*, 7, 327, 1987.
82. **Benedito, S., Prieto, D., and Nyborg, N. C. B.,** Influence of the endothelium on histamine-induced relaxation of rat middle cerebral arteries in vitro, *J. Cardiovasc. Pharmacol.*, 17, 90, 1991.
83. **Ea-Kim, L. and Oudart, N.,** A highly potent and selective H_3 agonist relaxes rabbit middle cerebral artery, in vitro, *Eur. J. Pharmacol.*, 150, 393, 1988.
84. **Ea-Kim, L., Javellaud, J., and Oudart, N.,** Endothelium-dependent relaxation of rabbit middle cerebral artery to a histamine H_3-agonist is reduced by inhibitors of nitric oxide and prostacyclin synthesis, *Br. J. Pharmacol.*, 105, 103, 1992.
85. **Ishikawa, S. and Sperelakis, N.,** A novel class (H_3) of histamine receptors on perivascular nerve terminals, *Nature,* 327, 158, 1987.
86. **Reinhardt, D. and Ritter, E.,** Hypothermia-induced potentiation of histamine H_2-receptor-mediated relaxation and cyclic AMP increase in the isolated mesenteric artery of the rabbit, *Agent Action,* 9, 9, 1979.
87. **Ksoll, E., Parsons, A. A., Mackert, J. R. L., Schilling, L., and Wahl, M.,** Analysis of cromakalim-, pinacidil-, and nicorandil-induced relaxation of the 5-hydroxytryptamine precontracted rat isolated basilar artery, *Naunyn-Schmiedebergs Arch. Pharmakol.*, 343, 377, 1991.
88. **Parsons, A. A., Ksoll, E., Mackert, J. R. L., Schilling, L., and Wahl, M.,** Comparison of cromakalim-induced relaxation of potassium pre-contracted rabbit, cat and isolated cerebral arteries, *Naunyn-Schmiedebergs Arch. Pharmakol.*, 343, 384, 1991.
89. **Schilling, L., Cremer, T., and Wahl, M.,** unpublished observation.
90. **Moncada, S., Palmer, R. M. J., and Higgs, E. A.,** The discovery of nitric oxide as the endogenous nitrovasodilator, *Hypertension,* 12, 365, 1988.
91. **Schilling, L., Parsons, A. A., Mackert, J. R. L., and Wahl, M.,** Is K^+ channel activation, EDRF, or cyclooxygenase products involved in acetylcholine-induced relaxation of rabbit isolated basilar artery, *J. Cereb. Blood Flow Metab.*, 11(Supp. 2), S256, 1991.
92. **Broman, T. and Lindberg-Broman, A. M.,** An experimental study of disorders in the permeability of the cerebral vessels (''the blood-brain-barrier'') produced by chemical and physico-chemical agents, *Acta Physiol. Scand.*, 10, 102, 1945.
93. **Gabbiani, G., Badonnel, M. C., and Majno, G.,** Intra-arterial injections of histamine, serotonin, or bradykinin: a topographic study of vascular leakage, *Proc. Soc. Exp. Biol. Med.*, 135, 447, 1970.
94. **Wolff, J. R., Schieweck, Ch., Emmenegger, H., and Meier-Ruge, W.,** Cerebrovascular ultrastructural alterations after intra-arterial infusions of ouabain, scillaglycosides, heparin and histamine, *Acta Neuropathol.*, 31, 45, 1975.
95. **Saria, A., Lundberg, J. M., Skofitsch, G., and Lembeck, F.,** Vascular protein leakage in various tissues induced by substance P, capsaicin, bradykinin, serotonin, histamine and by antigen challenge, *Naunyn-Schmiedebergs Arch. Pharmakol.*, 324, 212, 1983.

96. **Kilzer, P., Chang, K., Marvel, J., Kilo, C., and Williamson, J. R.,** Tissue differences in vascular permeability changes induced by histamine, *Microvasc. Res.*, 30, 270, 1985.
97. **Olesen, S.-P. and Crone, C.,** Substances that rapidly augment ionic conductance of endothelium in cerebral venules, *Acta Physiol. Scand.*, 127, 233, 1986.
98. **Watanabe, M. and Rosenblum, W. I.,** In vivo studies of pial vascular permeability to sodium fluorescein: absence of alterations by bradykinin, histamine, serotonin, or arachidonic acid, *Stroke,* 18, 1157, 1987.
99. **Hurst, E. W. and Davics, O. L.,** Studies on the blood-brain barrier. II. Attempts to influence the passage of substances into the brain, *Br. J. Pharmacol.*, 5, 147, 1950.
100. **Földes, I. and Kelentei, B.,** Studies on the haematoencephalic barrier. II. The effects of histamine with special reference to the passage of antibiotics, *Acta Physiol. Acad. Sci. Hung.*, 5, 149, 1954.
101. **Gross, P. M., Teasdale, G. M., Angerson, W. J., and Harper, A. M.,** H_2-receptors mediate increases in permeability of the blood-brain barrier during arterial histamine infusion, *Brain Res.*, 210, 396, 1981.
102. **Gross, P. M., Teasdale, G. M., Graham, D. I., Angerson, W. J., and Harper, A. M.,** Intra-arterial histamine increases blood-brain transport in rats, *Am. J. Physiol.*, 243, H307, 1982.
103. **Domer, F. R., Boertje, S. B., and Sweeney, S. A.,** Blockade of the acetylcholine- and histamine-induced changes in the permeability of the blood-brain barrier of normotensive and spontaneously hypertensive rats by atropine and pyrilamine, *Res. Commun. Chem. Pathol. Pharmacol.*, 42, 157, 1983.
104. **Gulati, A., Dhawan, K. N., Shukla, R., Srimal, R. C., and Dhawan, B. N.,** Evidence for the involvement of histamine in the regulation of blood-brain barrier permeability, *Pharmacol. Res. Commun.*, 17, 395, 1985.
105. **Dux, E., Temesvari, P., Joó, F., Adám, G., Clementi, F., Dux, L., Hideg, J., and Hossmann, K.-A.,** The blood-brain barrier in hypoxia: ultrastructural aspects and adenylate cyclase activity of brain capillaries, *Neuroscience,* 12, 951, 1984.
106. **Olesen, S.-P.,** Leakiness of rat brain microvessels to fluorescent probes following craniotomy, *Acta Physiol. Scand.*, 130, 63, 1987.
107. **Kawamura, S., Schürer, L., Goetz, A., Kempski, O., Schmücker, B., and Baethmann, A.,** An improved closed cranial window technique for investigation of blood-brain barrier function and cerebral vasomotor control in the rat, *Int. J. Microcirc. Clin. Exp.*, 9, 369, 1990.
108. **Butt, A. M. and Jones, H. C.,** Effect of histamine and antagonists on electrical resistance across the blood-brain barrier in rat brain-surface microvessels, *Brain Res.*, 569, 100, 1992.
109. **Wahl, M., Unterberg, A., and Baethmann, A.,** Intravital fluorescence microscopy for the study of blood-brain barrier function, *Int. J. Microcirc. Clin. Exp.*, 4, 3, 1985.
110. **Unterberg, A., Wahl, M., and Baethmann, A.,** Effects of bradykinin on permeability and diameter of pial vessels in vivo, *J. Cereb. Blood Flow Metab.*, 4, 574, 1984.
111. **Peroutka, S. J., Moskowitz, M. A., Reinhard, J. F., and Snyder, S. H.,** Neurotransmitter receptor binding in bovine cerebral microvessels, *Science,* 208, 610, 1980.
112. **O'Neill, C., Fowler, C. J., Marcusson, J. O., and Winblad, B.,** Adrenergic, serotoninergic, histaminergic, and imipramine binding sites in post-mortal human cerebral microvessel preparations, *J. Neural Transm.*, 73, 177, 1988.
113. **Dux, E. and Joó, F.,** Effects of histamine on brain capillaries. Fine structural and immunohistochemical studies after intracarotid infusion, *Exp. Brain Res.*, 47, 252, 1982.
114. **Schilling, L., Findling, A., and Wahl, M.,** unpublished observation.
115. **Joó, F., Rakonczay, R., and Wollemann, M.,** cAMP-mediated regulation of the permeability in the brain capillaries, *Experientia,* 31, 582, 1975.
116. **Palmer, G. C.,** Neurochemical coupled actions of transmitters in the microvasculature of the brain, *Neurosci. Neurobehav. Rev.*, 10, 79, 1986.

117. **Dux, E., Joó, F., Gecse, A., Mezei, Z., Dux, L., Hideg, J., and Telegdy, G.,** Histamine-stimulated prostaglandin synthesis in rat brain microvessels, *Agent Action,* 12, 146, 1982.
118. **Dux, E., Doczi, T., Joó, F., Szerdahelyi, P., and Siklos, L.,** Reverse pinocytosis induced in cerebral endothelial cells by injection of histamine into the cerebral ventricle, *Acta Neuropathol.,* 76, 484, 1988.
119. **Majno, G., Shea, S. M., and Leventhal, M.,** Endothelial contraction induced by histamine-type mediators. An electron microscopic study, *J. Cell Biol.,* 42, 617, 1969.
120. **Fox, J., Galey, F., and Wayland, H.,** Action of histamine on the mesenteric microvasculature, *Microvasc. Res.,* 19, 108, 1980.
121. **Orr, E. L.,** Cryogenic lesions induce a mast cell-dependent increase in cerebral cortical histamine levels in the mouse, *Neurochem. Pathol.,* 8, 43, 1988.
122. **Mohanty, S., Dey, P. K., Sharma, H. S., Singh, S., Chansouria, J. P. N., and Olsson, Y.,** Role of histamine in traumatic brain edema. An experimental study in the rat, *J. Neurol. Sci.,* 90, 87, 1989.
123. **Subramanian, N., Theodore, D., and Abraham, J.,** Experimental cerebral infarction in primates: regional changes in brain histamine content, *J. Neural Transm.,* 50, 225, 1981.
124. **Adachi, N., Itoh, Y., Oishi, R., and Saeki, K.,** Direct evidence for increased continuous histamine release in the striatum of conscious freely moving rats produced by middle cerebral artery occlusion, *J. Cereb. Blood Flow Metab.,* 12, 477, 1992.
125. **Saunier, C., Audibert, G., Hartemann, D., Sautegeau, A., Amend, P., Bigard, O., and Alvernhe, C.,** Preserved CO_2 response in cerebral and muscular blood vessels during cimetidine treatment, *Clin. Physiol.,* 11, 367, 1991.
126. **Dux, E., Temesvari, P., Szerdahelyi, P., Nagy, A., Kóvacs, J., and Joó, F.,** Protective effects of antihistamines on cerebral oedema induced by experimental pneumothorax in newborn piglets, *Neuroscience,* 22, 317, 1987.
127. **Joó, F., Szücs, A., and Csanda, E.,** Metiamide-treatment of brain oedema in animals exposed to ^{90}yttrium irradiation, *J. Pharm. Pharmacol.,* 28, 162, 1976.
128. **Csanda, E.,** Radiation brain edema, in *Brain Edema Advances in Neurology* 28, Cervos-Navarro, J. and Ferszt, R., Eds., Raven Press, New York, 1980, 125.
129. **Sztriha, L., Joó, F., and Szerdahelyi, P.,** Histamine H_2receptors participate in the formation of brain edema induced by kainic acid in rat thalamus, *Neurosci. Lett.,* 75, 334, 1987.
130. **Clasen, R. A., Cooke, P. M., Pandolfi, S., Carnecki, G., and Hass, G. M.,** Steroidantihistaminic therapy in experimental cerebral edema, *Arch. Neurol.,* 13, 584, 1965.
131. **Schilling, L. and Wahl, M.,** Effects of antihistaminics on experimental brain edema, *Acta. Neurochir. Suppl.,* in press.

Chapter 8

CHOLINERGIC CONTROL OF CEREBRAL BLOOD FLOW

Oscar U. Scremin

TABLE OF CONTENTS

I. Introduction 130

II. Historical Background 130

III. Histochemical and Biochemical Evidence 131

IV. Cholinergic Receptors in Blood Vessels 134

V. Effects of Cholinergic Agonists on Cerebral Blood Flow and Metabolism 134

VI. Observations on Isolated Cerebral Arteries 136

VII. Effects of Stimulation of Cholinergic Nerves on Cerebral Blood Flow 136

VIII. The Role of Central Pathways 137

IX. Functional Significance 137

References 140

0-8493-5096-0/93/$0.00 + $.50

I. INTRODUCTION

Research on cholinergic effects on the cerebral circulation embraces fields from molecular biology to intact animal research. This includes identification of specific receptors in vascular structures, the study of second messenger systems, evaluation of the effects of agonists in isolated cerebral arteries *in vitro,* anatomical investigation of the sources of cholinergic cerebrovascular innervation, and measurements of the rates of blood flow, metabolism, and electrical activity in the brains of anesthetized or conscious animals. It is very difficult to find parallels among these various approaches. Apparent contradictions stem from the fact that those blood vessels that make the greatest contribution to cerebrovascular resistance cannot be reached by neurotransmitters tested for effects on vascular smooth muscle without also affecting the glial and nerve cells that surround them. In the following sections an attempt is made to review the most salient facts at each of the levels mentioned above before attempting an interpretation of the possible functional significance of cholinergic mechanisms of the cerebral circulation.

II. HISTORICAL BACKGROUND

Baeyer synthesized acetylcholine (ACh) for the first time in 1867. Understanding of the physiological role of this molecule had to wait, however, until the present century. The cardiovascular effects of ACh and a number of other choline esters were described by Hunt and Taveau in 1906 following the demonstration by Mott and Halliburton that the blood pressure lowering effect of choline could be blocked by atropine.[1] Early observations with the Roy and Sherrington's brain oncometer by Müller[2] and with the cranial window technique by Wolff[3] suggested that systemically administered Ch or ACh, respectively, enhanced cerebral blood volume and dilated cerebral pial vessels. However, because of a large drop in blood pressure in those experiments, an autoregulatory noncholinergic mechanism could not be discarded as the explanation of the results. Many reports of similar effects in various species[4] including humans[5] followed. The ability of acetylcholine and other cholinergic agonists to dilate cerebral blood vessels and increase cerebral blood flow has been amply confirmed by modern experimentation.[6]

The first suggestion of a vasodilator role for cranial parasympathetic fibers originated from a collaboration between Cobb, Finesinger, and Penfield shortly before the definitive identification of ACh as a transmitter in sympathetic ganglia was established by Feldberg and Gaddum.[7] Cobb and Finesinger had developed a cranial window technique in monkeys and were dedicated to the study of pial vessels in animals in which Wilder Penfield had removed the cerebral sympathetic supply. In the words of the authors,[8] "In one of these monkeys, Penfield exposed the medulla oblongata and stimulated the different cranial nerves. To our surprise, no dilatation of the pial artery occurred when the trigeminal root was stimulated close to the medulla, but dilatation was observed when the facial root was stimulated, and when the vagus was stimulated. This experiment was done because ever since the work of Forbes and Wolff, which showed that pial arteries dilate if the vagus nerve in the neck is stimulated we had been curious to know what the pathway of the dilator impulses might be.'' These findings were published simultaneously in two papers. In one of them,[8] Cobb and Finesinger described the effects of stimulation of cranial nerves and of the cervical sympathetic on pial arteries. In the other,[9] Chorobski and Penfield examined the anatomy and described a bundle of small myelinated and nonmyelinated nerve fibers that they identified as a portion of the nervus intermedius of Wrisberg. This bundle, in their description, passed without interruption through the geniculate ganglion and into the superficial petrosal nerve from which it reached the carotid plexus after relaying in small ganglia and scattered cells. Stimulation at any point along this pathway elicited pial arterial dilatation in about 70% of the cases. These apparently straightforward experiments have been repeated in numerous laboratories with a variety of techniques over a 60-year span with a balanced number of confirmations and denials of the phenomenon, as discussed in detail below, and, therefore, the question of whether there is a parasympathetic influence on cerebral blood flow has yet to be settled.

III. HISTOCHEMICAL AND BIOCHEMICAL EVIDENCE

A cholinergic innervation of cerebral vessels was earlier suggested by the persistence of nerve fibers after cervical sympathetic ganglionectomy that were classified as cholinergic based on morphological (fiber profiles with small agranular vesicles that do not accumulate 6-hydroxydopamine)[10] or histochemical (presence of acetylcholinesterase activity)[11] criteria. These presumed cholinergic fibers were described to run alongside the adrenergic fibers, and structures described as neurovascular contacts were identified.[12,13] Cholinesterase is known to be present in noncholinergic fibers, however.[14] More positive histochemical identification was possible with the availability of monoclonal antibodies to choline-acetyltransferase (ChAT), a specific marker of cholinergic nerve terminals, which also revealed the presence of ChAT immunoreactive fibers in cerebral arteries.[15]

Cerebral blood vessels are known to express much greater ChAT activity than most extracerebral ones[16] (Figure 1), and this correlates with ACh contents.[17] The functional nature of this cerebral cholinergic innervation is supported by the work of Duckles, who was able to detect an enhanced release of tritium during electrical stimulation of segments of the rabbit basilar and cat middle cerebral arteries prelabeled with tritiated choline[17] (Figure 2).

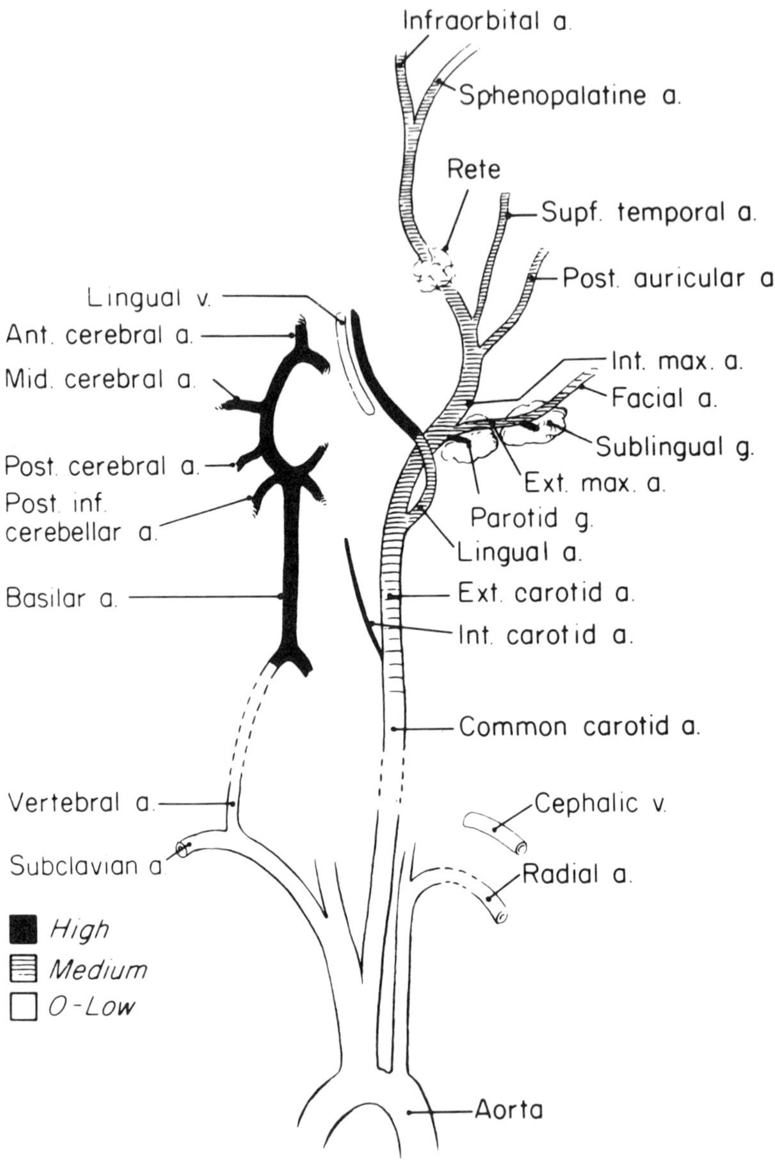

FIGURE 1. Anatomical representation of ChAT levels in cranial arterial system and some other blood vessels of the cat. (From Bevan, J., et al., *Circ. Res.*, 50, 470, 1982. With permission.)

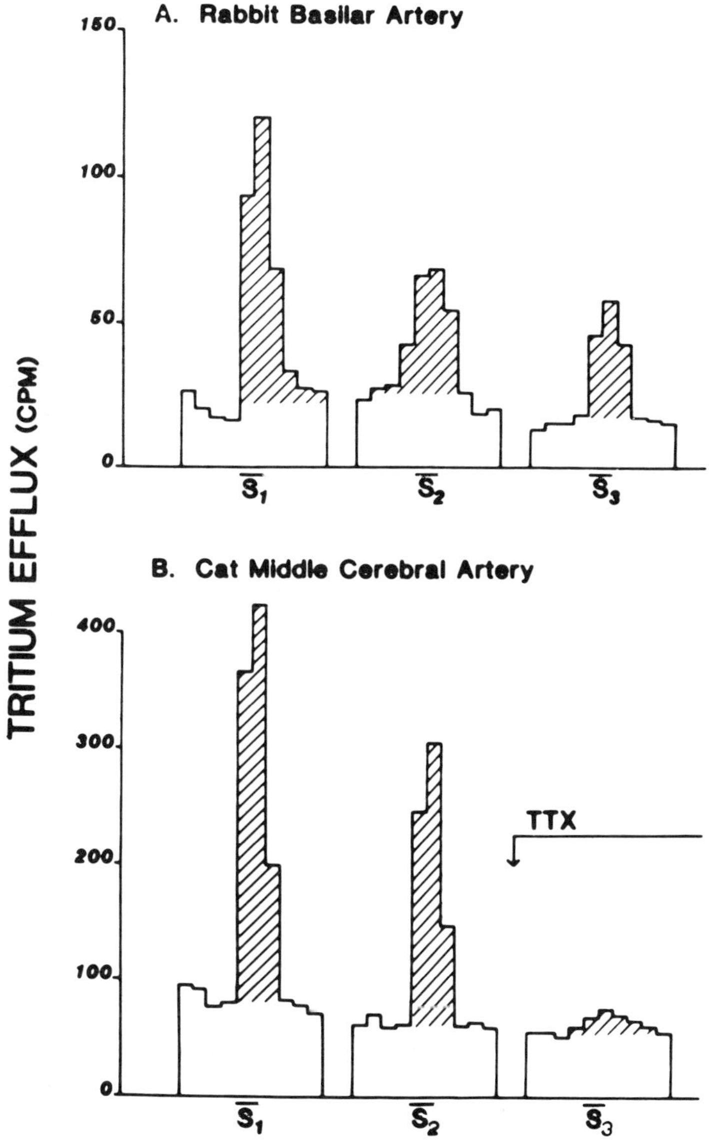

FIGURE 2. Tritium efflux from vessel segments prelabeled with ^3H-choline. Transmural electrical stimulation (8 Hz, 120 s) was administered for three successive stimulation periods labeled S_1, S_2, and S_3. Tetrodotoxin (TTX, 10^{-6} *M*) was added to the superfusion solution as indicated. Hatched areas indicate stimulation-evoked tritium efflux. (From Duckles, S. P., *J. Pharmacol. Exp. Ther.*, 217, 544, 1981. With permission.)

IV. CHOLINERGIC RECEPTORS IN CEREBRAL VESSELS

Muscarinic receptors in association with cerebral microvessels have been identified by use of QNB binding.[18,19] Estrada et al. have reported that cerebral endothelial cells, isolated by treating capillaries with collagenase, bound QNB to the same extent as did cerebral capillaries, a fact that supports the endothelial localization of capillary muscarinic receptors.[19]

Muscarinic receptors can be differentiated into subtypes according to their drug affinity, and, in the case of the M1, M2, and M3 receptors, there seems to be a correspondence with the cloned m1, m2, and m3 receptors.[20] These, in addition to M4 receptors, can be found in membranes from smooth muscle cells and endothelial cells of cerebral arterioles, cerebral capillaries, and cerebrovascular nerve terminals. Conclusions about the distribution of muscarinic receptor subtypes among the structural elements mentioned above is complicated by difficulties in obtaining pure preparations devoid of contamination from cerebral parenchymal membranes. The picture at the moment is far from clear, but some generalizations seem to be emerging. Muscarinic receptors in endothelial cells mediating endothelium-dependent relaxation of the feline middle cerebral artery[21] and rabbit basilar artery[20] have been identified as M3. M1 receptors, coupled to endothelium-independent phosphoinositide hydrolysis, have been identified in smooth muscle cells[20] and are associated with contraction in feline[22] and porcine[23] but not in bovine[20] arteries. M2 receptors seem to be predominant in vascular smooth muscle from bovine[20] and cat but not human[24] pial vessels, and these receptors have been associated also with contraction of pig basilar arteries.[25] M4 receptors have been described in "microvessel" preparations.[20] It is still perhaps premature to make associations between the different receptor types and the cholinergic cerebrovascular responses that can be demonstrated *in vivo*. A systematic study of receptor characterization for cerebrovascular cholinergic responses *in vivo* is still lacking.

V. EFFECTS OF CHOLINERGIC AGONISTS ON CEREBRAL BLOOD FLOW AND METABOLISM

Cholinergic agonists induce a significant increase in CBF *in vivo*,[26-30] an effect blocked by atropine[26] but not by dihydro-β-erythroidine.[31] This phenomenon can be demonstrated by topical application of ACh, carbachol, arecoline, or pilocarpine to the exposed cerebral cortex[26] or by systemic administration of cholinergic agonists or cholinesterase inhibitors that cross the bloodbrain barrier such as pilocarpine,[32,33] oxotremorine,[34] arecoline,[35] physostigmine,[36-38] eptastigmine,[39] and soman.[40] These vascular changes are accompanied by changes in arterial blood pressure (AP) for most cholinergic agonists administered systemically, but there is no correlation between these

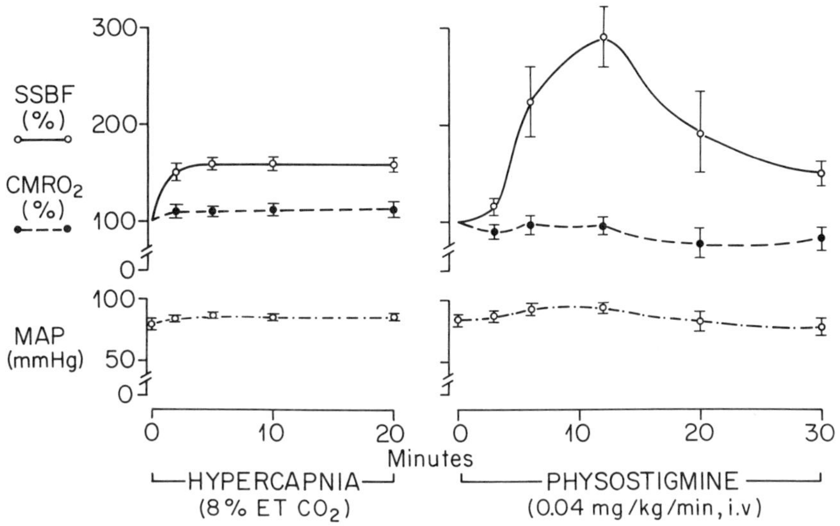

FIGURE 3. (Right) Sagittal sinus blood flow (SSBF) and the calculated O_2 uptake ($CMRO_2$) during I.V. infusion of physostigmine in six rabbits under normocapnia. Values are means and SE (vertical bars) of normalized SSBF and $CMRO_2$. **(Left)** For comparison, the effect of hypercapnia in the same animals before physostigmine administration is shown. (From Scremin, O. U. et al., *J. Cereb. Blood Flow Metab.*, 2, 241, 1982. With permission.)

two effects. Thus at doses that enhance CBF, pilocarpine induces a transient pronounced drop followed by a sustained increase in AP,[32] physostigmine, an increase,[41] eptastigmine, a small drop at low and no changes at higher nontoxic doses,[39] and soman, no change at nontoxic doses.[40] Blockade of the rise in AP does not prevent the cholinergic increase in CBF.[41]

At the doses that enhance CBF by systemic administration, physostigmine, eptastigmine and oxotremorine do not affect cerebral oxygen consumption or glucose utilization (CGU)[27,31,34,39] (Figure 3). An exception to this rule is the superficial gray layer of the superior colliculus, where metabolic activation is observed following central cholinesterase inhibition.[27,42] Thus the cholinergic cerebral vasodilatation is not secondary to activation of metabolism.

There are two factors that have a major effect on the ability of cholinesterase inhibitors to enhance CBF: anesthesia and blood PCO_2. Both effects may be related to the level of ACh release.[43] Pentobarbital is known to depress ACh release and it completely blocks the cerebrovascular effects of physostigmine, leaving that of a direct cholinergic agonist intact.[32] The slope of the regression of CBF on arterial blood PCO_2 is enhanced by physostigmine.[37,44] Interventions that decrease ACh release also decrease the value of this slope and prevent the effect of cholinesterase inhibition on CBF.[37] Moreover, ACh release is enhanced by hypercapnia.[43,45]

A number of drugs may act on CBF through activation of the cholinergic vasodilator system, such as amphetamine,[46] vincamine,[47] ketamine,[48] cismethrin,[49] and thyrotrophin-releasing hormone.[50]

VI. OBSERVATIONS ON ISOLATED CEREBRAL ARTERIES

The discovery by Furchgott and Zawadski[51] of the obligatory role of the endothelium for the vasodilator effects of acetylcholine on extracerebral arteries was also found to apply to cerebral vessels and provided an explanation for the inconsistent results obtained until then. It is now clear that the cholinergic dilatation of isolated cerebral arteries requires an intact endothelium and, that after its destruction, ACh induces only constriction.[52] A report on monkey cerebral arteries has found no consistent effects of ACh on vascular tone, however.[53] Transmural electrical stimulation can also relax precontracted cerebral arteries. This phenomenon is diminished or abolished by atropine in cat[16] and rabbit[54] cerebral arteries, although atropine-resistant vasodilatation to transmural stimulation has also been demonstrated.[52]

VII. EFFECTS OF STIMULATION OF CHOLINERGIC NERVES ON CEREBRAL BLOOD FLOW

The parasympathetic outflow to the head and neck consists of preganglionic fibers from nuclei cf cranial nerves 3rd, 7th, and 9th. Postganglionic fibers originate from the ciliary (3rd), sphenopalatine (7th), submandibular (7th), and otic (9th) ganglia as well as from several microscopic ganglia and scattered cells. All of these sources are known to supply fibers to cerebral blood vessels or to contribute to the internal carotid plexus, a meshwork of nerve fibers that surrounds the internal carotid arteries.[9,55,56] There is therefore a potential role of the autonomic efferent component in these nerves in the control of cerebral circulation. In addition, visceral afferent fibers from the 9th and 10th nerves have been postulated to participate in responses of the cerebral blood vessels to direct or receptor mediated stimulation of these nerves.[57] Cobb and Finesinger[8] stimulated the 3rd, 5th, 7th, 8th, 9th, 10th, 11th, and 12th and reported dilatation of pial arteries only in response to stimulation of the peripheral stump of the 7th and the central stump of the 10th. Other studies suggested the existence of cerebral vasodilator fibers in the 3rd cranial nerve.[58,59] These early experiments examined changes in the size of pial vessels, and it is difficult to infer from these results the impact of these interventions on cerebral blood flow (CBF). When quantitative techniques for the estimation of regional or global CBF were applied to this problem, the results proved to be absent in the case of nerves 3rd, 9th, and 10th.[32] Some authors have reported a small increase in CBF following stimulation of the 7th nerve, superficial petrosal nerve, or sphenopalatine ganglion that in some cases could be blocked by atropine[57,60-63] while others have failed to detect any changes.[32,64-66] The magnitude of the CBF responses that could be blocked by atropine is small compared with the effects of cholinergic agonists reviewed above (Section V), and this fact suggests that even if an influence of cholinergic nerves on CBF exists, it fails to account for the totality of the well-known cholinergic pharmacological actions. This could be interpreted as evidence for a nonparasympathetic innervation of cerebral blood vessels or for the existence of noninnervated cholinergic receptors.

VIII. THE ROLE OF CENTRAL PATHWAYS

Stimulation of certain sites within the central nervous system is known to enhance CBF. This has been shown for brainstem[64,67-69] and basal forebrain[70-73] locations. Some of these responses can be blocked by scopolamine[69,73] or atropine[72] or enhanced by cholinesterase inhibition with physostigmine.[69,73] The evidence for direct cholinergic projections from the brain stem to the cerebral cortex is not very strong.[74] It is therefore possible that stimulation of brain stem sites may indirectly activate cholinergic cells at still unknown locations, projecting to cerebral vessels. The basal forebrain is different, however, since this area is the source of a large number of cortical cholinergic fibers projecting to the cerebral cortex and hippocampus.[75] There are difficulties in the interpretation of CBF changes elicited by stimulation of the basal forebrain since a number of fibers of passage and nearby structures might be also stimulated in such experiments. This is particularly true in rats that lack an anatomically well-defined basal nucleus of Meynert. In this species, cholinergic cells of the basal nucleus are scattered along the border of the internal capsule[76] making extremely difficult a selective stimulation of such cells without concomitant activation of noncholinergic structures. Furthermore, the cholinergic cells of the basal forebrain are also key structures in cortical arousal,[77] and any stimulation that elicits this response will also generate, as mentioned below, a cholinergic vasodilatation. Thus CBF responses elicited from the basal nucleus may induce an indirect cholinergic vasodilatation by this mechanism and do not necessarily impute that structure as the source of the cholinergic innervation of cortical blood vessels. Experiments in which discrete lesions of the basal nucleus were performed have revealed no change in CBF and persistence of the cerebral vasodilator effect of physostigmine,[78,79] casting doubts on the role of this area in cerebrovascular control.

IX. FUNCTIONAL SIGNIFICANCE

One of the best established functional characteristics of the cerebral circulation is the correlation between the rates of glucose or oxygen utilization and the rate of cerebral blood flow. This phenomenon has two main

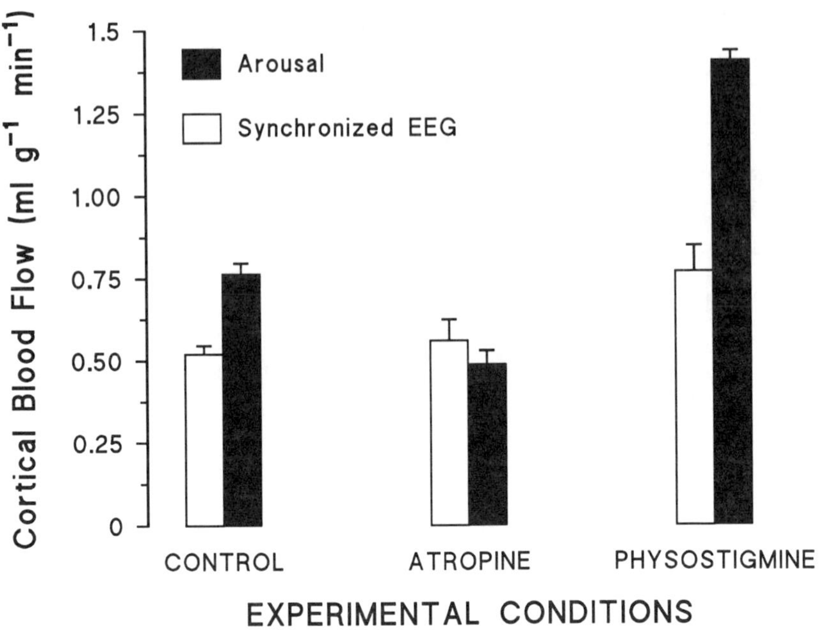

FIGURE 4. Blood flow of the somatosensory cerebral cortex of rats, measured with the hydrogen clearance technique (means, SE). EEG fluctuated spontaneously between a state of high voltage with predominance of slow waves (synchronized EEG) and a state resembling arousal (low voltage EEG with theta rhythm in hippocampus and rhythmic movements of vibrissa). A cortical cup over the exposed cortex was used to apply synthetic CSF by itself (control) or with atropine (0.4 mg/ml) or physostigmine (0.5 mg/ml). Data from Scremin, O. U. et al., *Stroke,* 4, 232, 1973.

manifestations: (1) when neuronal activity increases, an accompanying increase in the rate of cerebral blood flow is observed[80] and (2) when paired measurements of metabolic rate and blood flow are performed in multiple regions of the central nervous system, a close correlation can be found between these variables. A quantitative estimate of the dependence of blood flow on metabolism in brain tissue is given by the slope of the regression of CBF on CGU.[81] Both phenomena are affected by interventions on the cholinergic system. Exposure of the cerebral cortex to a cholinesterase inhibitor potentiates the increase in cortical blood flow associated with spontaneous arousal, while local atropinization blocks it[26] (Figure 4). The slope of the regression of CBF (ml g^{-1} min^{-1}) on CGU (μmol g^{-1} min^{-1}) calculated from autoradiographic measurements of these variables in conscious rats is enhanced from 1 to 2.9 in the presence of eptastigmine, a long acting cholinesterase inhibitor that is effective by intravenous administration.[39] Thus it seems that endogenous ACh is capable of enhancing CBF and that this phenomenon occurs under physiological circumstances.

Another well-established characteristic of the cerebral circulation is the dependence of CBF on the partial pressure of carbon dioxide in blood (CO_2 reactivity of CBF).[82] This phenomenon was believed to provide the coupling mechanism between brain tissue metabolism and blood flow. Many sources of evidence, however, have seriously questioned this assumption. It is difficult to demonstrate local acidosis in the presence of enhanced neuronal activity and in fact local tissue pH may increase during cerebral hyperemia.[83] Moreover, interventions that do not interfere with metabolism can modify the CO_2 reactivity of CBF.[84-86] It is more likely that the enhancement of CBF induced by hypercapnia may be an adaptation to asphyxia. This phenomenon is also altered by interventions on the cholinergic system. Systemic administration of atropine decreases the CO_2 reactivity of CBF, and central cholinesterase inhibition enhances it.[36-38,73,87,88] These phenomena are in line with the well-known ability of CO_2 to enhance ACh release in brain tissue[89,90] and the recent observation by Iadecola[91] who reports blockade of CO_2 reactivity of CBF by arginine competitive analogues, implying a role of NO in this phenomenon. It is then possible that hypercapnia may trigger ACh release in cerebral tissue that may act on endothelial cells to release NO and dilate cerebral vessels.

Acetylcholine metabolism is profoundly altered in ischemia. In moderate ischemia, the increased choline tissue content acts by a precursor loading effect to autoregulate ACh levels.[92] The fact that increased availability of ACh induced by cholinesterase inhibition enhances CBF in areas of moderate ischemia in animals[41] and humans[93] suggests that blood vessels in these areas are susceptible to the dilator effect of ACh. In severe ischemia (CBF lower than 0.2 ml g^{-1} min^{-1}), on the other hand, decreases in ACh contents,[94] synthesis,[95] and release[96] are known to occur. It is likely that these phenomena may also be present in neurovascular structures. This is a potential source of a vicious circle, since impairment of cholinergic vasodilatation may further aggravate ischemia induced by embolism or thrombosis. The finding of impairment of cholinergic vasodilatation because of decreased EDRF production induced by arachidonic acid[97] is also of significance in this regard since this fatty acid is known to be released in severe ischemia.[98] Thus cholinergic vasodilatation may be impaired by multiple mechanisms in the ischemic brain and may play a role in the pathogenesis of this condition that deserves to be investigated further.

Although the role of CBF in the pathogenesis of Alzheimer's disease is largely considered only of historical interest, it seems clear that in this condition there is a decrease in CBF, particularly in the temporal cortex, of a magnitude greater than expected from the effect of age alone.[99] A deficit of cerebral ACh is a prominent finding in Alzheimer's disease, and it has been reported recently that physostigmine, which induces a modest symptomatic improvement in some patients, also reverses the decrease in CBF.[100]

In summary, although it is not always possible to correlate findings from various methodological approaches, it seems clear that endogenous acetylcholine can significantly affect the level of CBF. This action may be mediated through muscarinic cholinergic receptors, possibly related to the release of NO or nitroso compounds by ACh released from still unknown sources. The physiological role of the cerebral cholinergic vasodilator system may be associated with generalized increases in CBF associated with behavioral arousal and hypercapnia. These responses of CBF could be viewed as adaptations in which this variable adjusts in anticipation of an enhanced cerebral energy consumption (arousal) or a decrease in pulmonary ventilation (hypercapnia). A role of cholinergic vascular mechanisms in the regional adjustment of CBF to metabolic activity is suggested by the ability of prolonged cholinesterase inhibition to enhance the coupling of CBF to CGU throughout the brain.

REFERENCES

1. **Hunt, R. and Taveau, R. M.,** On the physiological action of certain cholin derivatives and new methods for detecting cholin, *Br. Med. J.*, ii, 1788, 1906.
2. **Müller, F.,** Beitrage zur analyse der cholinwirkung, *Pfluegers Arch. Gesamte. Physiol.*, 134, 289, 1910.
3. **Wolff, H. G.,** The cerebral circulation: XIa. The action of acetylcholine, *Arch. Neurol. Psychiatry,* 22, 686, 1929.
4. **Sokoloff, L.,** The action of drugs on the cerebral circulation, *Pharmacol. Rev.*, 11, 1, 1959.
5. **Michelazzi, M.,** Sull' Innervazione vasomotrice dell'encefalo. Influenze farmacologiche, *Arch. Fisiol,* 33, 472, 1934.
6. **Scremin, O. U.,** Pharmacological Control of the Cerebral Circulation, *Annu. Rev. Pharmacol. Toxicol.*, 31, 229, 1991.
7. **Feldberg, W. and Gaddum, J. H.,** The chemical transmitter at synapses in a sympathetic ganglion, *J. Physiol. (London),* 81, 305, 1934.
8. **Cobb, S. and Finesinger, J. E.,** Cerebral circulation. XIX. The vagal pathway of the vasodilator impulses, *Arch. Neurol. Psychiatry,* 28, 1243, 1932.
9. **Chorobski, J. and Penfield, W.,** Cerebral vasodilator nerves and their pathway from the medulla oblongata, *Arch. Neurol. Psychiatry,* 28, 1257, 1932.
10. **Iwayama, T., Furness, J. B., and Burnstock, G.,** Dual adrenergic and cholinergic innervation of the cerebral arteries of the rat, *Circ. Res.*, 26, 635, 1970.
11. **Lavrentieva, N. B., Mchedlishvili, G. I., and Plechkova, E. K.,** Distribution and activity of cholinesterase in the nervous structures of the pial arteries (a histochemical study), *Bull. Biol. Med. Exp. URSS,* 64, 110, 1968.
12. **Edvinsson, L., Nielsen, K. C., Owman, C., and Sporrong, B.,** Cholinergic mechanisms in pial vessels: histochemistry, electron microscopy and pharmacology, *Z. Zellforsch.*, 134, 311, 1972.
13. **Nelson, E. and Rennels, M.,** Innervation of intracranial arteries, *Brain,* 93, 475, 1970.
14. **Lehmann, J. and Fibiger, H. C.,** Minireview: acetylcholinesterase and the cholinergic neuron, *Life Sci.*, 25, 1939, 1979.
15. **Miao, F. J. and Lee, T. J.,** VIP-ergic and cholinergic innervations in internal carotid arteries of the cat and rat, *J. Cardiovasc. Pharmacol.*, 18, 369, 1991.
16. **Bevan, J. A., Buga, G. M., Florence, V. M., Gonsalves, A., and Snowden, A.,** Distribution of choline acetyltransferase in cerebral and extracerebral cranial arteries of the cat, *Circ. Res.*, 50, 470, 1982.

17. **Duckles, S. P.,** Evidence for a functional cholinergic innervation of cerebral arteries, *J. Pharmacol. Exp. Ther.,* 200, 117, 1977.
18. **Grammas, P., Diglio, C. A., Marks, B. H., Giacomelli, F., and Wiener, J.,** Identification of muscarinic receptors in rat cerebral cortical microvessels, *J. Neurochem.,* 40, 645, 1983.
19. **Estrada, C., Hammel, E., and Krause, D. N.,** Biochemical evidence for cholinergic innervation of intracerebral blood vessels, *Brain Res.,* 266, 261, 1983.
20. **Garcia-Villalon, A. L., Krause, D. N., Ehlert, F. J., and Duckles, S. P.,** Heterogeneity of muscarinic receptor subtypes in cerebral blood vessels, *J. Pharmacol. Exp. Ther.,* 258, 304, 1991.
21. **Dauphin, F. and Hamel, E.,** Muscarinic receptor subtype mediating vasodilation feline middle cerebral artery exhibits M3 pharmacology, *Eur. J. Pharmacol.,* 178, 203, 1990.
22. **Dauphin, F., Ting, V., Payette, P., Dennis, M., and Hamel, E.,** Vasocontractile muscarinic M1 receptors in cat cerebral arteries: pharmacological identification and detection of mRNA, *Eur. J. Pharmacol.,* 207, 319, 1991.
23. **Armstead, W. M., Mirro, R., Leffler, C. W., and Busija, D. W.,** Acetylcholine produces cerebrovascular constriction through activation of muscarinic-1 receptors in the newborn pig, *J. Pharmacol. Exp. Ther.,* 247, (3), 926, 1988.
24. **Dauphin, F. and Hamel, E.,** Identification of multiple muscarinic binding site subtypes in cat and human cerebral vasculature, *J. Pharmacol. Exp. Ther.,* 260, 660, 1992.
25. **Van Charldorp, K. J., Davidesko, D., and Zwieten, P. A.,** Selectivity of methoctramine for muscarinic receptors in porcine cerebral arteries, *Eur. J. Pharmacol.,* 150 (Abstr.), 197, 1988.
26. **Scremin, O. U., Rovere, A. A., Raynald, A. C., and Giardini, A.,** Cholinergic control of blood flow in the cerebral cortex of the rat, *Stroke,* 4, 232, 1973.
27. **Scremin, O. U., Allen, K., Torres, C. D., and Scremin, A. M. E.,** Physostigmine enhances blood flow metabolism ratio in neocortex, *Neuropsychopharmacology,* 1 (4), 297, 1988.
28. **Aubineau, P., Sercombe, R., Edvinsson, L., and Owman, C.,** Cholinergic influence on the cerebrovascular bed mediated through actions on the vascular smooth musculature and on the perivascular sympathetic nerves, in *Neurogenic Control of the Brain Circulation,* Owman, C. and Edvinsson, L., Eds., Pergamon Press, New York, 1977, 331.
29. **Triguero, D., López de Pablo, A. L., Gómez, B., and Estrada, C.,** Regional differences in cerebrovascular cholinergic innervation in goats, *Stroke,* 19, 736, 1988.
30. **Dora, E. and Kovach, A. G. B.,** Role of hypoxia and acetylcholine in the regulation of cerebral blood flow, *Adv. Exp. Med. Biol.,* 215, 237, 1987.
31. **Scremin, O. U., Sonnenschein, R. R., and Rubinstein, E. H.,** Cholinergic cerebral vasodilatation in the rabbit: absence of concomitant metabolic activation, *J. Cereb. Blood Flow Metab.,* 2, 241, 1982.
32. **Scremin, O. U., Sonnenschein, R. R., and Rubinstein, E. H.,** Cholinergic cerebral vasodilatation: lack of involvement of cranial parasympathetic nerves, *J. Cereb. Blood Flow Metab.,* 3, 362, 1983.
33. **Scremin, A. M. E., Allen, K., and Scremin, O. U.,** Regional distribution of the cerebral vasodilatation induced by a cholinergic agonist, *FASEB J.,* 2 (Abstr.), A722, 1988.
34. **Pelligrino, D. A., Miletich, D. J., and Albrecht, R. F.,** Diminished muscarinic receptor-mediated cerebral blood flow response in steptozotocin-treated rats, *Am. J. Physiol.,* 262, E447, 1992.
35. **Maiese, K., Holloway, H. W., Larson, D. M., Reis, D. J., and Soncrant, T. T.,** Coupling of regional cerebral metabolism and blood flow in the conscious rat is maintained after treatment with the muscarinic agonist arecoline, *Soc. Neurosci. Abstr.,* 17 (Abstr.), 26, 1991.
36. **Rovere, A. C., Scremin, O. U., Beresi, M. R., Raynald, A. C., and Giardini, A.,** Cholinergic mechanism in the cerebrovascular action of carbon dioxide, *Stroke,* 4, 969, 1973.

37. **Scremin, O. U., Rubinstein, E. H., and Sonnenschein, R. R.,** Cerebrovascular CO_2 reactivity: role of a cholinergic mechanism modulated by anesthesia, *Stroke,* 9, 160, 1978.
38. **Molnar, L., Hegedus, K., and Fekete, I.,** Difference between the cerebrovascular effect of purinergic Co-ATP and that of the cholinesterase inhibitor, physostigmine, in vivo, *Eur. J. Pharmacol.,* 209, 81, 1991.
39. **Scremin, A. M. E., Scremin, O. U., Heuser, D., Hudgell, R., Romero, E., and Imbimbo, B.,** Effects of eptastigmine on cerebral blood flow and metabolism in rats, *FASEB J.,* 6, A1770, 1992.
40. **Scremin, O. U., Shih, T.-M., and Corcoran, K. D.,** Cerebral blood flow-metabolism coupling after administration of soman at non-toxic levels, *Brain Res. Bull.,* 260, 353, 1991.
41. **Scremin, O. U. and Scremin, A. M. E.,** Physostigmine induced reversal of ischemia following middle cerebral artery occlusion in the rat, *Stroke,* 17, 1004, 1986.
42. **Dam, M. and London, E. D.,** Effects of cholinomimetics on glucose utilization in rat brain optic systems, *Eur. J. Pharmacol.,* 87, 137, 1983.
43. **Hudson, D. M., Jenden, D. J., Scremin, O. U., and Sonnenschein, R. R.,** Cortical acetylcholine efflux with hypercapnia and nociceptive stimulation, *Brain Res.,* 338, 267, 1985.
44. **Scremin, O. U., Rubinstein, E. H., and Sonnenschein, R. R.,** Cholinergic modulation of the cerebrovascular response to CO_2 in the rabbit, in *Neurogenic Control of Brain Circulation,* Owman, C. and Edvinsson, L., Eds., Pergamon Press, New York, 1977, 471.
45. **Metz, B.,** Correlation between the electrical activity and acetylcholine release from the cerebral cortex and medulla during hypercapnia, *Can. J. Physiol. Pharmacol.,* 49, 331, 1971.
46. **Rovere, A. C., Raynald, A. C., and Scremin, O. U.,** On the mechanism of amphetamine induced vasodilatation of the rat's cerebral cortex, *Experientia,* 33, 1461, 1977.
47. **Rovere, A. A.,** A cholinergic participation in the increase of cerebral cortical blood flow induced by vincamine, *Acta Physiol. Lat. Am.,* 26, 206, 1976.
48. **Reicher, D., Bhalla, P., and Rubinstein, E. H.,** Cholinergic cerebral vasodilator effect of ketamine in rabbits, *Stroke,* 18, 445, 1987.
49. **Lister, T. and Ray, D. E.,** The role of basal forebrain in the primary cholinergic vasodilation in rat neocortex produced by systemic administration of cismethrin, *Brain Res.,* 450, 364, 1988.
50. **Inanami, O., Meguro, K., Ohno, K., and Sato, A.,** Contribution of cholinergic vasodilators on the increase in cerebral cortical blood flow responses to the intravenous administration of thyrotropin releasing hormone in anesthetized rats, *Neurosci. Lett.,* 88, 184, 1988.
51. **Furchgott, R. F. and Zawadzki, J. V.,** The obligatory role of endothelial cells in the relaxation of arterial smooth muscle by acetylcholine, *Nature,* 288, 373, 1980.
52. **Lee, T. J. F.,** Sympathetic and nonsympathetic transmitter mechanisms in cerebral vasodilation and constriction, in *Neural Regulation of Brain Circulation,* Owman, C. and Hardebo, J. E., Eds., Elsevier, New York, 1986, 285.
53. **Toda, N., Kawakami, M., Yamazaki, M., and Okamura, T.,** Comparison of endothelium-dependent responses of monkey cerebral and temporal arteries, *Br. J. Pharmacol.,* 102, 805, 1991.
54. **Van Riper, D. A. and Bevan, J. A.,** Electrical field stimulation-mediated relaxation of rabbit middle cerebral artery. Evidence of a cholinergic endothelium-dependent component, *Circ. Res.,* 70, 1104, 1992.
55. **Mitchell, G. A. G.,** *Anatomy of the Autonomic Nervous System,* Livingstone, Edimburgh, 1953, 147.
56. **Suzuki, N.,** Origins, Pathways and Effects of Electrical Stimulation on Dilatory Peptidergic Vascular Nerves in Rat Brain, Ph.D. Thesis, University of Lund, Sweden, 1989.

57. **James, I. M., Millar, R. A., and Purves, M. J.,** Observations on the extrinsic neural control of cerebral blood flow in the baboon, *Circ. Res.,* 25, 77, 1969.
58. **Klosovskii, B. N.,** Blood circulation in the brain, Israel Program for Scientific Translations, Jerusalem, 1963.
59. **Kameyama, S.,** Cholinergic innervation of the cerebral blood vessels in the dog- the effect of electrical stimulation of the ciliary ganglion, *No To Shinkei,* 32, 539, 1980.
60. **D'Alecy, L. G. and Rose, C. J.,** Parasympathetic cholinergic control of cerebral blood flow in dogs, *Circ. Res.,* 41, 324, 1977.
61. **Pinard, E., Purves, M. J., Seylaz, J., and Vasquez, J. V.,** The cholinergic pathway to cerebral blood vessels. II. Physiological studies, *Pfluegers Arch.,* 379, 165, 1979.
62. **Goadsby, P. J.,** Effect of stimulation of facial nerve on regional cerebral blood flow and glucose utilization in cats, *Am. J. Physiol.,* 257, R517, 1989.
63. **Seylaz, J., Hara, H., Pinard, E., Mraovitch, S., MacKenzie, E. T., and Edvinsson, L.,** Effect of stimulation of the sphenopalatine ganglion on cortical blood flow in the rat, *J. Cereb. Blood Flow Metab.,* 8, 875, 1988.
64. **Meyer, J. S., Teraura, T., Sakamoto, K., and Kondo, A.,** Central neurogenic control of cerebral blood flow, *Neurology,* 21, 247, 1971.
65. **Busija, D. W. and Heistad, D. D.,** Effects of cholinergic nerves on cerebral blood flow in cats, *Circ. Res.,* 48, 62, 1981.
66. **Linder, J.,** Effects of facial nerve section and stimulation on cerebral and ocular blood flow in hemorrhagic hypotension, *Acta Physiol. Scand.,* 112, 185, 1981.
67. **Langfitt, T. W. and Kassell, N. P.,** Cerebral vasodilatation produced by brain stem stimulation: neurogenic control vs autoregulation, *Am. J. Physiol.,* 215, 90, 1968.
68. **Molnár, L.,** *Sur le Contrôle Nerveux de la Circulation Sanguine Regionale des Centres Cerebraux,* Akademiai Kiado, Budapest, 1967, 1.
69. **Scremin, O. U., Rubinstein, E. H., and Sonnenschein, R. R.,** Role of central pathways and cranial nerves in cerebral cholinergic vasodilatation, in *Advances in Physiological Sciences, Vol. 9, Cardiovascular Physiology, Neural Control Mechanisms,* Kovach, A. G. B., Sandor, P., and Kollai, M., Eds., Pergamon Press, New York, 1980.
70. **Lacombe, P., Sercombe, R., Verrecchia, C., Philipson, V., MacKenzie, E. T., and Seylaz, J.,** Cortical blood flow increases induced by stimulation of the substantia innominata in the unanesthetized rat, *Brain Res.,* 491, 1, 1989.
71. **Linville, D. G. and Arneric, S. P.,** Cortical cerebral blood flow governed by the basal forebrain: age-related impairments, *Neurobiol. Aging,* 12, 503, 1991.
72. **Biesold, D., Inanami, O., Sato, A., and Sato, Y.,** Stimulation of the nucleus basalis of Meynert increases cerebral cortical blood flow in rats, *Neurosci. Lett.,* 98, 39, 1989.
73. **Dauphin, F., Lacombe, P., Sercombe, R., Hamel, E., and Seylaz, J.,** Hypercapnia and stimulation of the substantia innominata increase rat frontal cortical blood flow by different cholinergic mechanisms, *Brain Res.,* 553, 75, 1991.
74. **Fibiger, H. C.,** The organization and some projections of cholinergic neurons of the mammalian forebrain, *Brain Res. Rev.,* 4, 327, 1982.
75. **Cuello, A. C. and Sofroniew, M. V.,** The anatomy of the CNS cholinergic neurons, *Trends Neurosci.,* 7, 74, 1984.
76. **Sofroniew, M. V., Pearson, R. C. A., and Powell, T. P. S.,** The cholinergic nuclei of the basal forebrain of the rat: normal structure, development and experimentally induced degeneration, *Brain Res.,* 411, 310, 1987.
77. **Buzsàki, G. and Gage, F. H.,** The cholinergic nucleus basalis: a key structure in neocortical arousal, in *Central Cholinergic Synaptic Transmission,* Frotscher, M., and Misgeld, U., Eds., Birkhauser Verlag, Basel, 1989, 159.
78. **Scremin, O. U., Torres, C. D., Scremin, A. M. E., O'Neal, M., Heuser, D., and Blisard, K. S.,** The role of the nucleus basalis in cholinergic control of cortical blood flow, *J. Neurosci. Res.,* 28, 382, 1991.

79. **Namba, H., Irie, T., Fukushi, K., Yamasaki, T., Tateno, Y., and Hasegawa, S.,** Lesion of the nucleus basalis magnocellularis does not affect cerebral cortical blood flow in rats, *Neurosci. Res.*, 12, 463, 1991.
80. **Sokoloff, L.,** Circulation and energy metabolism of the brain, in *Basic Neurochemistry,* Siegel, G. J., Agranoff, B. W., Albers, R. W., and Molinoff, P., Eds., Raven Press, New York, 1989, 565.
81. **Sokoloff, L.,** Localization of functional activity in the central nervous system by measurement of glucose utilization with radioactive deoxyglucose, *J. Cereb. Blood Flow Metab.*, 1, 7, 1981.
82. **Heistad, D. D. and Kontos, H. A.,** Cerebral circulation, in *The Cardiovascular System, Vol. 3, Peripheral Circulation and Organ Blood Flow,* Shepherd, J. T. and Abboud, F. M., Eds., American Physiological Society, Bethesda, MO, 1983, 137.
83. **Siesjö, B. K.,** Cerebral circulation and metabolism, *J. Neurosurg.*, 60, 883, 1984.
84. **Aoyagi, M., Deshmukh, V. D., Meyer, J. S., Kawamura, Y., and Tagashira, Y.,** Effect of beta-adrenergic blockade with propranolol on cerebral blood flow, autoregulation and CO_2 responsiveness, *Stroke,* 7, 291, 1976.
85. **Kawamura, Y., Meyer, J. S., Hiromoto, H., Aoyagi, M., and Hashi, K.,** Neurogenic control of cerebral blood flow in the baboon. Effects of alpha adrenergic blockade with phenoxybenzamine on cerebral autoregulation and vasomotor reactivity to changes in $PaCO_2$, *Stroke,* 5, 747, 1974.
86. **Pickard, J. D. and McKenzie, E. T.,** Inhibition of prostaglandin synthesis and the response of baboon cerebral circulation to carbon dioxide, *Nature (New Biol.),* 245, 187, 1973.
87. **Aoyagi, M., Meyer, J. S., Deshmukh, V. D., Ott, E. O., Tagashira, Y., Kawamura, Y., Matsuda, M., Amrit, A., and Chee, A. N. C.,** Central cholinergic control of cerebral blood flow in the baboon: effect of cholinesterase inhibition with neostigmine on autoregulation and CO_2 responsiveness, *J. Neurosurg.*, 43, 689, 1975.
88. **Kawamura, Y., Meyer, J. S., Hiromoto, H., Aoyagi, M., Tagashira, Y., and Ott, E. O.,** Neurogenic control of cerebral blood flow in the baboon: effects of the cholinergic inhibitory agent, atropine, on cerebral autoregulation and vasomotor reactivity to changes in $PaCO_2$, *J. Neurosurg.*, 43, 676, 1975.
89. **Szerb, J. C.,** Cortical acetylcholine release and electroencephalographic arousal, *J. Physiol.*, 192, 329, 1967.
90. **Hudson, D. M., Jenden, D. J., Scremin, O. U., and Sonnenschein, R. R.,** Cortical acetylcholine efflux with hypercapnia and nociceptive stimulation, *Brain Res.*, 338, 267, 1985.
91. **Iadecola, C.,** Does nitric oxide mediate the increases in cerebral blood flow elicited by hypercapnia?, *Proc. Natl. Acad. Sci. U.S.A.*, 89, 3913, 1992.
92. **Scremin, O. U. and Jenden, D. J.,** Effects of middle cerebral artery occlusion on cerebral cortex choline and acetylcholine in rats, *Stroke,* 20, 1524, 1989.
93. **Scremin, A. M. E., Kunkel, C. F., Eisenberg, B., Elliot, T., and Scremin, O. U.,** Physostigmine improves cerebral blood flow in human focal cerebral ischemia, *J. Stroke Cerebrovasc. Dis.*, 2, 87, 1992.
94. **Scremin, O. U. and Jenden, D. J.,** Time-dependent changes in cerebral choline and acetylcholine induced by transient global ischemia in rats, *Stroke,* 22, 643, 1991.
95. **Kumagae, Y. and Matsui, Y.,** Output, tissue levels, and synthesis of acetylcholine during and after transient forebrain ischemia in the rat, *J. Neurochem.*, 56, 1169, 1991.
96. **Scremin, O. U. and Jenden, D. J.,** Focal ischemia enhances choline output and decreases acetylcholine output from rat cerebral cortex, *Stroke,* 20, 92, 1989.
97. **Kontos, H. A., Wei, E. P., Povlishock, J. T., Kukreja, R. C., and Hess, M. L.,** Inhibition by arachidonate of cerebral arteriolar dilation from acetylcholine, *Am. J. Physiol.*, 256, H665, 1989.
98. **Bazán, N. G.,** Effects of ischemia and electroconvulsive shock on free fatty acid pool in the brain, *Biochim. Biophys. Acta,* 218, 1, 1970.

99. **Rogers, R. L., Meyer, J. S., Mortel, K. F., Mahurin, R. K., and Judd, B. W.,** Decreased cerebral blood flow precedes multi-infarct dementia, but follows senile dementia of Alzheimer type, *Neurology,* 36, 1, 1986.
100. **Geaney, D. P., Soper, N., Shepstone, B. J., and Cowen, P. J.,** Effect of central cholinergic stimulation on regional cerebral blood flow in Alzheimer disease, *Lancet,* 335, 1484, 1990.

Chapter 9

NEUROPEPTIDE Y AND THE CEREBRAL CIRCULATION

U.I. Tuor

TABLE OF CONTENTS

I. Introduction 148
- A. Historical Perspective 148
- B. NPY and the Cerebral Circulation 148

II. Localization of NPY in Cerebral Vessels 148
- A. Distribution of NPY in Perivascular Nerve Fibers: Immunohistochemical Studies 148
- B. Distribution of NPY in Perivascular Nerve Fibers: Radioimmunoassay Studies 149
- C. NPY Innervation During Development and Aging 150
- D. Colocalization of NPY with Noradrenaline (NA) 150
- E. Colocalization of NPY with Acetylcholine and Vasoactive Intestinal Peptide (VIP) 151
- F. Origin of NPY Containing Nerves 151

III. Effects of NPY on Cerebral Vessels 152
- A. Vasomotor Actions *In Vitro* and *In Situ* 152
- B. Receptors for NPY 154
- C. Modification of Other Neurotransmitter Effects 155
- D. Endothelial Dependence 155
- E. Signal Transduction 156

IV. Effect of NPY on Cerebral Blood Flow 157
- A. Introduction 157
- B. Intravenous Administration of NPY 159
- C. Intraarterial Administration of NPY 159
- D. Intracerebral Administration of NPY 160
- E. Potential Physiological or Pathological Significance 160

Acknowledgments 161

References 161

0-8493-5096-0/93/$0.00 + $.50

I. INTRODUCTION

A. HISTORICAL PERSPECTIVE

Two different peptides, which were originally isolated from the pancreas, avian pancreatic peptide (aPP), and bovine pancreatic peptide (bPP), were subsequently also observed to be present in nerve fibers as indicated by their immunocytochemical staining of various neural elements. However, attempts to extract these peptides from the tissues were unsuccessful, suggesting that the immunoreactive staining was a cross-reaction to an alternate peptide. This was confirmed to be the case following the isolation in 1982 of two new peptides from the porcine gut and brain — peptide YY (PYY) and neuropeptide Y (NPY), respectively.[1-4]

The peptides — NPY, PYY, and PP — form a family of neurohormonal peptides with considerable sequence homology between their 36 amino acid residues (Table 1). Tyrosine moieties are located at one or both ends with the C terminal being aminated. Based on conformational X-ray studies of aPP, the amino acids of these peptides are considered to form two antiparallel helices with a PP fold. An N terminal polyproline helix and a long amphiphilic alpha-helix are held together by a core of interdigitating hydrophobic residues.[6] Concerning their respective anatomical distributions, PP is localized to the pancreas whereas PYY is primarily, but not exclusively, found in endocrine cells of the gut. NPY is abundant in both central and peripheral neural elements of both mammals and vertebrates. The amino acid sequence for NPY is remarkably conserved between species, being unchanged during a major part of vertebrate evolution.[7]

B. NPY AND THE CEREBRAL CIRCULATION

Following the discovery of NPY, several laboratories demonstrated its presence within a plexus of nerve fibers on the cerebral vessels.[4,8,9] NPY has since been extensively investigated as a putative transmitter involved in the neurogenic control of the cerebral circulation. The present chapter will concentrate on reviewing the literature most directly concerned with NPY and the cerebrovasculature. However, the influence of NPY on local cerebral metabolism is also of importance, since NPYinduced changes in flow could be secondary to alterations in neuronal activity. For details concerning the distribution of NPY in the CNS and its effects on brain function, the reader is referred to a recent extensive review by Dumont et al.[5]

II. LOCALIZATION OF NPY IN CEREBRAL VESSELS

A. DISTRIBUTION OF NPY IN PERIVASCULAR NERVE FIBERS: IMMUNOHISTOCHEMICAL STUDIES

A dense plexus of NPY-like immunoreactive (NPY-IR) nerve fibers has been observed on a variety of blood vessels from various organs.[5,10,11] In the brain, NPY-IR nerve fibers have been demonstrated on blood vessels for all

TABLE 1
Amino Acid Sequences for Neuropeptide Y (NPY) and Related Peptides

Peptide	Residue: 1 5 10 15 20 25 30 35
pNPY	YPSKPDNPGEDAPAEDLARYYSALRHYINLITRQRY[a]
rNPY	================M===================
hNPY	================M===================
pPYY	==A==EA=====SP=E=S===AS====L==V=====
aPP	G==Q=TY==D===V===I=F=DN=QQ=L=VV==H==
bPP	A=LE=EY==DA=TP=QM=Q=AAE==R===ML==P==

Note: pNPY, porcine neuropeptide Y; rNPY, rat neuropeptide Y; hNPY, human neuropeptide Y; pPYY, porcine peptide YY; aPP, avian pancreatic peptide; bPP, bovine pancreatic peptide.

[a] Amidation of Y terminus.

species examined including mouse, rat, guinea pig, gerbil, cat, and man.[3,8,10,12,13] In cross-section, these fibers can be seen to be located within the adventitia or at the adventitia-media layer. The fibers are most dense on the large arteries at the base of the brain, and smaller branches of the large pial arteries have fewer NPY-IR fibers. A sparse number of fibers also surround small cortical pial arterioles and have been observed to follow penetrating arterioles such as the lenticulostriate arteries into the parenchyma.[10,14] NPY-IR fibers also surround cerebral veins, but the density of these fibers is less than that on arteries of similar size.[10] Detailed studies examining the distribution of fibers within the circle of Willis of the rabbit and guinea pig have demonstrated a greater density of innervation in the rostral than caudal portion of the circle of Willis.[10,15]

B. DISTRIBUTION OF NPY IN PERIVASCULAR NERVE FIBERS: RADIOIMMUNOASSAY STUDIES

Several laboratories have also examined the distribution and species differences in NPY immunoreactivity measured with radioimmunoassays (Table 2). These studies confirm a high content of NPY in the cerebral vessels — often in amounts comparable to that observed in certain regions of the CNS. There is a large interspecies variation in NPY concentration — the levels in pig, rabbit, and guinea pig cerebral arteries exceeding those in cat, rat, or human.

The distribution of NPY has also been examined by measuring NPY concentrations in different cerebral vascular segments. In one study of human arteries from the circle of Willis, the concentration of NPY was rather uniform, whereas in another study the concentration of NPY varied regionally, with

TABLE 2
Comparison of Concentration of NPY within Cerebral Arteries and the CNS

	Concentration of NPY (pmol/g)				
		CNS			
Species	Cerebral arteries	Cerebral cortex	Caudate nucleus	Cerebellum	Refs.
Pig	649 ± 290	517–1100	134–149	<1–8	12, 4
Rabbit	412 ± 29;85 ± 10	—	—	—	16
Guinea pig	78 ± 20	—	—	—	10
Cat	19 ± 3	—	—	—	10
Rat	117 ± 11	179 ± 24	313 ± 69	27 ± 5	10, 17
Human	47 ± 11;4 ± 3;2.7 ± 0.5	120 ± 13	534 ± 170	1.3 ± .2	9, 10, 17

Note: Data presented as mean ± SEM.

the lowest amounts occurring in the basilar and inferior cerebellar arteries and the highest amounts at the bifurcations of the major vessels and in the anterior cerebral artery.[9,10] In the rabbit, the concentration of NPY in large cerebral arteries from the circle of Willis (i.e., those most densely innervated) exceeds that in smaller pial arteries.[16] Thus, studies of NPY content in cerebral vessels overall confirm a degree of regional heterogeneity in the distribution of NPY.

C. NPY INNERVATION DURING DEVELOPMENT AND AGING

During development, NPY innervation becomes more dense. The number of NPY-IR nerve fibers surrounding the major arteries at the base of the brain is low in rats 4 to 6 weeks of age and increases approximately twofold between 6 to 8 weeks of age, stabilizing thereafter.[15] Similarly, the density of perivascular nerve fibers containing NA also changes, but the increase precedes that of NPY by 2 weeks.[15] With old age, there is a reduction in the concentration of NPY observed in human cerebral arteries suggesting a decline in the density of innervation later in life.[18]

D. COLOCALIZATION OF NPY WITH NORADRENALINE (NA)

Studies of NPY-IR nerve fibers on peripheral blood vessels have provided extensive evidence that NPY and NA coexist in these fibers.[5,10,11,19] Similar evidence is available to support the fact that many of the NPY-containing fibers on cerebral vessels also contain NA. An initial indication of such co-localization was the resemblance of the ground plexus of NPY-IR fibers on the cerebral vessels to that of the NA-containing sympathetic innervation. Subsequent studies have also shown that many of the NPY fibers are sympathetic in origin (see Section II.F). The coexistence of NPY with NA is further supported by experiments using sequential immunostaining methods. These studies have demonstrated that NPY-IR is co-localized with either dopamine-β-hydroxylase (DBH) or tyrosine hydroxylase (TH) (enzymes involved in catecholamine synthesis).[10,13,20] For example, in guinea pig cerebral arteries, 86% of the varicosities with TH also contained NPY-IR whereas only a few fibers contained TH or NPY alone.[13]

Studies of peripheral tissues have examined the intracellular localization and release of NPY. Subcellular fractionation experiments suggest that NA is contained in small dense-cored vesicles, whereas both NPY and NA are co-localized in the same large dense-cored vesicles.[21,22] Stimulation conditions likely control the release of transmitter, with high frequency or strong stimuli favoring the release of NPY (and NA) and low frequency or weak stimuli favoring the release of NA.[5,22-24]

E. COLOCALIZATION OF NPY WITH ACETYLCHOLINE AND VASOACTIVE INTESTINAL PEPTIDE (VIP)

Recent studies have demonstrated that a population of NPY containing nerve fibers around the pial vessels also coexist with VIP and/or choline acetyltransferase (ChAT).[13,25] In guinea pig cerebral arteries, 18% of VIP immunoreactive axons contained NPY-like immunoreactivity and, similarly, approximately 40% of those in rat arteries contained NPY.[13,20] Furthermore, approximately 23% of NPY positive fibers contained acetylcholine as indicated by the presence of ChAT.[20]

There appears to be a plasticity regarding the expression of these peptides within the perivascular nerves. Following cranial sympathectomy the number of NPY and VIP positive nerves is enhanced.[13,20] Furthermore, following neonatal sympathectomy, although one would expect some reduction in the number of NPY-IR fibers (see next section), the abundance of NPY fibers is similar to controls with most of the remaining fibers containing both NPY and VIP.[26]

F. ORIGIN OF NPY CONTAINING NERVES

Available evidence indicates that the majority of fibers containing NPY-IR originate in the superior cervical sympathetic ganglia with a population of fibers also originating from cranial parasympathetic ganglia. Following bilateral removal of the superior cervical ganglion in the cat, rat, or guinea pig, there is a substantial loss of NPY-IR in nerve fibers on cerebral vessels.[3,10,13,20,27] One to two weeks following cranial sympathectomy, NPY content of pial arteries decreases approximately 60% in rat and 70% in rabbit and the number of NPY containing fibers around pial arteries is reduced approximately 50% in guinea pig and 60% in rat.[10,13,16,20] Similarly, chemical sympathectomy with 6-OHDA or reserpine results in a substantial reduction in NPY within rat cerebral vessels.[10] When both the origins of sympathetic and parasympathetic fibers are removed by bilateral removal of the superior cervical ganglia and bilateral section of the postganglionic fibers of the sphenopalatine ganglia, all NPY-IR nerve fibers disappear in the anterior part of

TABLE 3
Effect of NPY on Isolated Blood Vessels *In Vitro*

Species	Type of cerebral vessel	Maximal contraction	EC_{50} ($\times 10^{-8}M$)	Reference
Cat	MCA	47 (% K$^+$)	13 ± 15	10
	MCA	Variable	7.6 ± 2.5	30
Rabbit	Basilar	5 (%K$^+$)	50–100	10
	MCA	21 (% of Histamine)	22 ± 2	31
	Internal carotid	21 (?)	32 ± 1	31
Guinea pig	Basilar	76 ± 10 (%K$^+$)	81 ± 20	32
	Basilar	35 ± 15 (%K$^+$)	8	33
Rat	Basilar	19.2 ± 8.2 (%K$^+$)	50–100	10
	Basilar	—	—	27
	MCA	6 (%K$^+$)	21 ± 8.0	14
	MCA	70 ± 13 mg	72 ± 1	27
	ACA	134 ± 11 mg	83 ± 2	27
	Intracerebral	19 (% control)	.62	62
Dog	MCA	50 (%K$^+$)	2	37
	Basilar	29 (%K$^+$)	2	37
	Vertebral/common carotid	Nil	—	37
Man	Pial (temporal)	Variable	70	30
	Pial	30 (%K$^+$)	~10	10

Note: Values presented as mean ± SEM; MCA, middle cerebral artery; ACA, anterior cerebral artery.

the circle of Willis, although a few NPY positive fibers remain in the posterior circle of Willis.[20]

Recent studies also indicate that cranial parasympathetic ganglia contain NPY/VIP/ChAT, TH/VIP/ChAT, or DBH/VIP/ChAT.[28,29] Furthermore, VIP/ChAT containing neurons that project to the cerebral vessels have also been observed to contain DBH.[28] Although these results indicate that the presence of DBH or TH within nerve fibers does not necessarily signify that the fibers are adrenergic and of sympathetic origin, the number of fibers on the cerebral vessels containing both TH or DBH and NPY, which are not sympathetic, are likely to be sparse. Cervical sympathectomy results in a loss of most or all DBH, TH, and TH/NPY positive perivascular nerve fibers.[13]

III. EFFECTS OF NPY ON CEREBRAL VESSELS

A. VASOMOTOR ACTIONS *IN VITRO* AND *IN SITU*

Many studies have demonstrated that NPY administration elicits a constriction of isolated blood vessels from a number of different organ systems.[5,10,11,19] Cerebral arteries are one of the most sensitive types of vessels, with NPY being a potent vasoconstrictor in most species examined (Table 3). Pial arterioles *in situ* have also been shown to vasoconstrict in response to the perivascular application of NPY.[3] Although rather less potent, NPY also elicits a constriction of pial veins *in situ.*[3]

The vasomotor response to NPY has been extensively characterized, primarily using isolated cerebral arteries. As the concentration of NPY increases above a threshold, cerebral arteries contract in a dose-dependent manner. The contraction is associated with a corresponding depolarization of the smooth muscle, at least in guinea pig and rabbit, if not rat, cerebral arteries.[27,31,33] The concentration of NPY producing a half maximal response (EC_{50}) varies widely from 2 to 600 $\times$ 10^{-8} *M*. The maximal response to NPY also varies markedly between species and the type of artery examined (Table 3). Differential densities of NPY innervation do not readily explain these variations as there is no strong correspondence between the density of NPY containing fibers and the maximal response observed. For example, some of the highest densities of NPY-IR fibers are in the rabbit and lowest in human, yet both have similar vasomotor responses to NPY. Similarly, the density of NPY immunoreactive nerve fibers surrounding middle cerebral arteries is much greater than that on arterioles penetrating the parenchyma; yet, in the rat, intracerebral arterioles are the most sensitive to NPY (Table 3).

Despite the large variability in the response of the cerebrovasculature to NPY, this neuropeptide is still one of the most potent vasoconstrictor peptides/neurotransmitters present within the cerebral perivascular nerve fibers. When comparing NA and NPY, rat cerebral arteries contract in response to the application of NPY whereas they are unaffected by the application of NA.[10,14,27,34,35] Similarly, cat and guinea pig cerebral arteries *in vitro* and feline cerebral arteries *in situ* are more sensitive to NPY than NA.[33,36] An exception is rabbit cerebral arteries for which the opposite is true.[31]

In addition to its relatively high potency, NPY also has a relatively prolonged action on cerebral vessels of several species. Constriction in response to NPY of feline pial arteries *in situ* is of long duration (5 min) when compared to that produced by NA (1 min).[3] *In vitro,* the contraction produced by NPY applied to guinea pig basilar arteries is also relatively long lasting when compared to that for NA.[33] In dog cerebral arteries the contraction with NPY is not only prolonged but also relatively slow to start.[37] In contrast, the contraction of rat pial arteries is sustained longer with the application of NA than NPY.[10] The long-lasting action of NPY observed in select cerebral arteries may be due to both a slow local degradation/diffusion of peptide within the synaptic cleft and a depolarization of smooth muscle cells which would allow a continual refilling of calcium stores.[22,33]

Examinations of the effect of sympathectomy on the responsiveness of isolated cerebral arteries to NPY have shown little effect. Rat middle cerebral, rat basilar, or rabbit basilar arteries had equivalent responses to NPY irrespective of whether or not they were innervated by sympathetic nerve fibers.[10,27,31] Denervation supersensitivity may not have occurred in these vessels due to the incomplete loss of NPY containing nerve fibers following removal of the cervical sympathetic ganglia (Section II.F).

Clearly, there is a large variation in the sensitivity of isolated cerebral arteries to NPY. Several factors may account for this variability. First, the response to NPY may be substantially dependent on experimental conditions. Evidence from peripheral arteries demonstrate that a degree of preconstriction may be essential in order to observe a contractile effect of NPY. In addition, substances in the bathing medium such as NA or histamine can influence the constriction evoked by NPY.[38,39] Second, it is possible that the distributions and types of receptors for NPY differ markedly within different cerebrovascular segments and in different species resulting in differential responsiveness in these vessels (see next section). Finally, the response to NPY may also be affected by the rate of degradation or diffusion of the peptide from the synapse which may be variable. Note that endogenous NPY is likely resupplied to the nerve terminal exclusively by axonal transport.[22]

B. RECEPTORS FOR NPY

Studies which have examined the specificity of the vasoconstrictor effects of NPY indicate that the contraction elicited by NPY is specific for this peptide and thus likely mediated by receptors for NPY on the vascular smooth muscle. Indeed, the cerebrovascular constriction induced by NPY is not inhibited either by alpha or beta receptor blockade with phentolamine, rauwolscine, or propranolol or by a blockade of serotonin receptors with ketanserin.[3,8,37] Similarly, the cerebral vasomotor response to NPY is unaffected by adding cocaine, a blocker of amine reuptake, to the bathing medium.[3,8]

Investigation of the binding characteristics of radiolabeled NPY to membrane preparations of the CNS and other tissues initially demonstrated the presence of specific binding sites for NPY.[5,11] The subsequent demonstration that various fragments or analogues of NPY bind with differing affinities and possess differing physiological potencies indicated the existence of more than one type of NPY receptor. Based on the original classification proposed by Wahlestedt et al.,[40] there are now three or more known NPY receptor types potentially present in blood vessels.[5,11,41,42] The first receptor, the Y_1-receptor, is a postsynaptic receptor which has been shown to mediate the direct vasoconstrictor effect of NPY in a number of different systems. Regarding the agonist selectivity of this receptor, the peptides NPY, PYY, or the specific Y_1 agonist [Leu31, Pro34]NPY bind with much greater affinity and are more potent than C terminal fragments of NPY. The second receptor, the Y_2 receptor, is either a presynaptic or postsynaptic receptor. Presynaptic effects in blood vessels include the inhibition of the release of neurotransmitters such as NA and may explain the reduction in the contractile response to NA by NPY in dog cerebral arteries.[37] Postsynaptic mediated effects of Y_2 include vasoconstriction as indicated by the pressor effects induced with C terminal NPY fragments. Regarding the agonist selectivity of the Y_2 receptor, the peptides PYY, NPY, and C terminal fragments bind with greater affinity and are more potent than the specific Y_1 agonist [Leu31, Pro34]NPY. A third type of receptor (Y_3) has been proposed to be present in tissues such as chromaffin cells where the receptor is activated by NPY but not PYY. Finally, an NPY receptor cloned recently is neither a Y_1 nor Y_2 receptor and thus may indicate the existence of yet a fourth type of NPY receptor.[43] Whether the newer receptors exist in the cerebral circulation is not presently known. Also, most of our knowledge concerning receptor subtypes in vascular smooth muscle has been obtained from peripheral vessels so that the relative concentrations of receptors and their synaptic localization in different cerebrovascular segments has yet to be elucidated.

C. MODIFICATION OF OTHER NEUROTRANSMITTER EFFECTS

In peripheral vessels, NPY has been demonstrated to potentiate the vasoconstriction and inhibit the relaxation induced by a variety of other neurotransmitters.[11] Although similar results are available for some cerebral vessels, a modulatory role for NPY (1 to 10 n*M*) has not been universally demonstrable. For example, the contractile responses of rat or human cerebral arteries to either NA or serotonin are not modified by NPY.[10,18,27,30] In contrast to these negative studies, rabbit cerebral arteries exposed to NPY have a threefold potentiation of the contractile response to NA.[44] In addition, exposure of rabbit cerebral arteries to NPY results in a potentiation of the constrictor response to histamine and an inhibition of the relaxation produced by adenosine and acetylcholine.[31] Similarly, in rat basilar arteries, the relaxation elicited by calcitonin gene related peptide is reduced by preexposure to 10 n*M* NPY.[10]

The mechanism by which NPY modulates the responses of other neurotransmitters in some cerebral vessels is not certain. However, as in peripheral vessels, the diversity of substances which are enhanced or inhibited by NPY suggest a nonspecific postreceptor effect.[11] One such nonspecific mechanism would be a threshold synergism phenomenon between NA and NPY such as occurs with a converging stimulation of phospholipase C and subsequent phosphoinositol hydrolysis in rabbit pulmonary arteries.[39] NPY could also lower the threshold for muscle contraction by opening voltage-dependent channels. In rabbit cerebral arteries this is the most likely mechanism, since the potentiation of the response to NA is associated with a depolarization of the smooth muscle.[31]

D. ENDOTHELIAL DEPENDENCE

Most studies which have examined the role of the endothelial cell in mediating the direct vasomotor response of NPY agree that this effect is independent of the endothelium. Except for rat tail artery, most peripheral arteries (rabbit central ear artery, human skeletal artery, and pig splenic artery) do not alter their contractile response to NPY following removal of the endothelium.[38,45,46] Similarly, in the cerebrovasculature, the response of the guinea pig basilar artery to NPY is unaffected by removal of the endothelium.[33]

The role of the endothelium in potentiating the effects of NPY has been examined in peripheral arteries and the results are inconclusive. In several studies, the enhancement by NPY of the constriction observed in response to electrical field stimulation or NA was dependent on an intact endothelium.[45,47] In contrast, several other studies have reported that the potentiation was not affected by removal of the endothelium.[48-50]

E. SIGNAL TRANSDUCTION

Although our knowledge concerning the molecular mechanisms involved in mediating the cellular actions of NPY is expanding rapidly, generalization concerning the types of receptors involved and their localization in the cerebral circulation is difficult since there is considerable diversity within tissues and species concerning NPY receptors and their potential second messenger systems.[5,41] Furthermore, it remains unclear at present whether specific signaling mechanisms are linked to distinct receptor subtypes. Irrespective of the intermediary steps, the final process linking NPY receptor activation and contraction of the smooth muscle cell is an increased concentration of free calcium in the vicinity of the contractile proteins (Figure 1). This increase in intracellular calcium may be achieved in several ways.

First, multiple lines of evidence indicate that most known NPY effects are mediated by receptors which are coupled to G proteins. In various systems studied, the effects of NPY can usually be blocked by pertussis toxin — a substance which inactivates various G proteins. In addition, the binding to NPY receptors in most systems is inhibited by analogues of GTP or pertussis toxin.[5,41,51] The G proteins may be further coupled to Ca^{2+} channels or to adenyl cyclase which can then mobilize intracellular calcium via other messenger systems which are either dependent or independent of inositol phosphate turnover.[41] In feline cerebral arteries, NPY has been shown to inhibit the accumulation of adenosine 3′5′ cyclic monophosphate (cAMP) stimulated by forskolin — a response mediated via an inhibitory G protein.[41,52] The systems subsequently affected by reductions in cAMP have yet to be identified.

Extracellular calcium plays an important role in the contractile response of blood vessels to NPY. Activation of NPY receptors in various culture systems is associated directly with an increased influx of extracellular calcium.[51] In addition, binding of NPY to the receptor on porcine aorta is enhanced by elevated levels of extracellular calcium.[53] In cerebral arteries, contraction is inhibited by the calcium channel antagonists diltiazem and nimodipine.[3,8] Furthermore, the contractile response to NPY of feline cerebral arteries is markedly reduced but not abolished in a calcium-free medium. Thus, in feline pial arteries at least, NPY appears able to elevate free cytosolic concentration of Ca^{2+} by two mechanisms — via an increase in the influx of extracellular Ca^{2+} via voltage sensitive calcium channels and via the mobilization of intracellular Ca stores.[33,36]

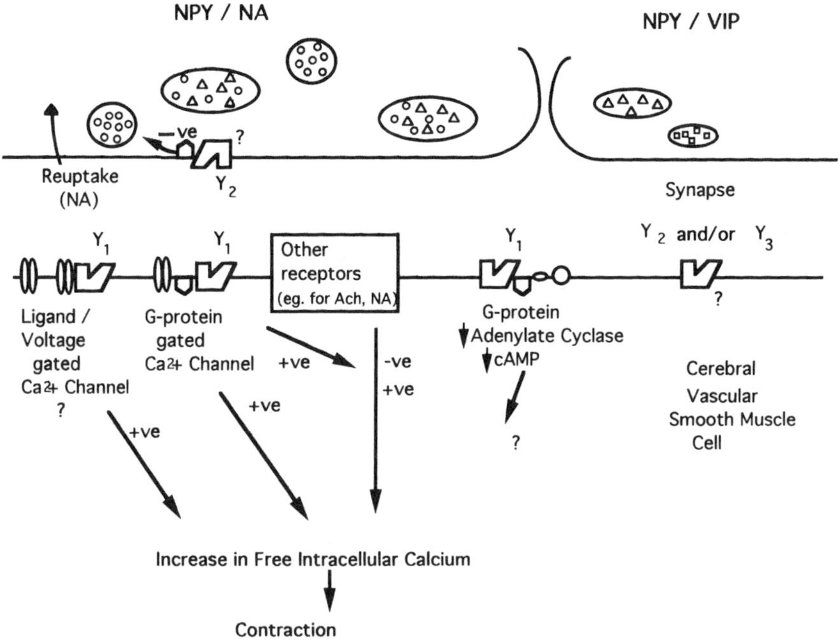

FIGURE 1. Schematic diagram of potential mechanisms of action of NPY released from nerve fibers surrounding the cerebrovascular smooth muscle. NPY can be co-localized in nerve fibers containing either noradrenaline (NA) or vasoactive intestinal peptide (VIP). Receptors for NPY, located postsynaptically (Y_1) and presynaptically (Y_2), have been identified in peripheral blood vessels. In cerebral blood vessels their relative distribution may vary according to species or type of vessel segment. In general, Y_1 mediates the direct vasoconstrictor effect of NPY whereas Y_2 is involved in the inhibition of the presynaptic release of NA. Other receptors for NPY have been identified, but their presence on cerebral vessels is unknown. The receptors for NPY are considered to be coupled to G proteins which are further coupled to Ca^{2+} channels or to adenylate cyclase. In feline cerebral arteries, NPY inhibits adenylate cyclase and the accumulation of cAMP. NPY also appears able to elevate free cytosolic concentration of Ca^{2+} by both an increase in the influx of extracellular Ca^{2+} via voltage-sensitive calcium channels and via the mobilization of intracellular Ca^{2+} stores. In some cerebral vessels, NPY enhances or inhibits the effects of other vasoconstrictor or vasodilator neurotransmitters. A nonspecific postsynaptic effect of NPY, such as a decrease in the threshold for contraction, is likely the mechanism involved.

IV. EFFECT OF NPY ON CEREBRAL BLOOD FLOW

A. INTRODUCTION

The demonstration that NPY-IR fibers are abundant on cerebral vessels and that exogenous NPY is a potent contractile agent *in vitro* provides strong evidence favoring an important role for NPY in the control of the cerebral circulation *in vivo*. Several laboratories have examined whether NPY is active in the intact cerebrovasculature by measuring the effect of NPY on cerebral blood flow (Table 4). Considering the fact that most peptides cross the blood-

TABLE 4
Effect of NPY on Cerebral Blood Flow (CBF)

Administration	Species	NPY[a] dose	MABP increase (mmHg)	Flow measurement method	CBF decrease (time max./measurement effect)	Ref.
Intravenous	Cat	0.01 nmol/kg/min	6	Microspheres	No change at 5 min	54
		0.1 nmol/kg/min	37	Microspheres	No change total CBF, 5 min	
Intravenous	Rabbit	0.12 nmol/kg/min	Nil	Microspheres	No change total CBF, 2 or 10 min	55
Intravenous	Rat	0.05 nmol/kg/min[d]	15	^{14}C-IAP	No change most regions, 15 min	56
Intracarotid[b]	Rat	2 nmol	Nil	^{14}C-IAP	No change at 15 min	14
Intracarotid[b]	Rat	2.23 nmol/min (total) (6.6 nmol)	45	^{14}C-IAP	30–90% at 2 min	57
Intracarotid[c]	Rat	2 nmol	Nil	H_2 Clearance	95% in cortex, 15 min–2 h	9
Intracarotid[b]	Rat	1 nmol	Nil	H_2 Clearance	15–20% in striatum, 30–60 min	25
		5 nmol	Nil	H_2 Clearance	40–50% in striatum, 30 min–2 h	
Intravertebral	Dog	1 nmol	—	Electromagnetic flow meter	20% at 1 min, ns[e] at 10 min	37
		5 nmol	—		30–25%, 1–10 min	
Intrastriatal	Rat	0.2 nmol	Nil	^{14}CIAP	45% in striatum, 20–55 min	14

[a] Bolus injection unless otherwise indicated.
[b] External carotid artery (Retrograde).
[c] Internal carotid artery.
[d] PYY instead of NPY was administered.
[e] ns, not significant

brain barrier poorly, it is unsurprising that the magnitude of the effect of NPY on cerebral blood flow depends on the route of NPY administration.

B. INTRAVENOUS ADMINISTRATION OF NPY

Studies examining the effect of the systemic administration of NPY on the cerebral circulation have observed no major influence of this peptide on cerebral blood flow (Table 4). NPY infused at concentrations ranging from 0.01 to 0.12 nmol/kg/min did not alter cerebral blood flow in cats, rabbits, or rats despite elevating mean arterial blood pressure 0 to 37 mmHg.[54-56] However, in two of these studies, subregional analysis of blood flow indicates that there may be a slight effect of NPY, particularly when it is administered at high concentrations or for more prolonged periods.[54,55]

C. INTRAARTERIAL ADMINISTRATION OF NPY

In contrast to intravenous infusion, injection of NPY directly into cerebral supply arteries results in the selective application of high concentrations of NPY, thereby minimizing potential systemic effects such as hypertension (Table 4). When administered in this way, there are reductions in cerebral blood flow which vary greatly in their magnitude and time of onset. In general, lower concentrations of NPY (1 to 2 nmol) injected intraarterially produce a modest (<20%) reduction in cerebral blood flow with the exception of one study in which cortical flow decreased up to 95%.[14,25,37,57] Higher concentrations of NPY (5 nmol or more) are consistently more effective in influencing the cerebral circulation, with reductions in cerebral blood flow of 30 to 90% being reported.[25,37,57] Thus, the bulk of the evidence indicates that the administration of rather high concentrations of NPY directly into arteries supplying blood to the brain elicits a reduction in cerebral blood flow.

A unique characteristic of the response of the cerebral circulation to intraarterial NPY is that the flow reduction, although usually prolonged, has a delay in the time to onset which varies substantially, from 1 to 30 min.[25,37] These delays in the CBF response to NPY exceed those for the contractile response *in vitro* and make the measurement of the effect of NPY in any one system highly dependent on the time after NPY administration. The mechanism involved in mediating the delay is unknown, but the time period to the onset of a response may depend on anesthesia or other conditions which affect resting vessel tone or smooth muscle cell depolarization.

The site of action of NPY in mediating these blood flow decreases is not known, although most investigators have interpreted their results as indicative of a vasoconstriction of cerebral vessels by NPY *in vivo*. In isolated cerebral vessels, the site of action of NPY-mediated contraction is the vascular smooth muscle; however, when administering NPY intraarterially, one must consider that the blood-brain barrier is likely to restrict the simple diffusion of NPY across the endothelium. An increased permeability of the blood-brain barrier is associated with hypertension which would increase accessibility of NPY to the cerebral smooth muscle, but marked hypertension occurs in very few of these studies (Table 4). Another possible site of action is that the effects of NPY are mediated by the cerebral endothelium. However, the majority of the *in vitro* studies indicate that the direct constrictor effect, and often even the modification of the responses of other transmitters by NPY, is independent of the endothelium (Section III.D). This suggests that, with the high concentrations of NPY administered intraarterially, sufficient amounts of NPY diffuse or are transported across the endothelium to activate NPY receptors on cerebral arterioles. Alternatively, NPY may be acting primarily on large pial arteries, which are generally more permeable than cerebral capillaries. In either case, NPY would also have access to neurons within the CNS and could thereby affect blood flow indirectly via primary alterations in cerebral metabolism. Although the local metabolic rate of oxygen or glucose metabolism were not measured in these intra-arterial studies, intracerebral administration of NPY has been shown to have only minor effects on local cerebral glucose utilization.[14] This suggests that the increases in cerebrovascular resistance observed with intra-arterial injection of NPY are due to a direct vasoconstriction of the cerebral vessels.

D. INTRACEREBRAL ADMINISTRATION OF NPY

Only one study has examined the vasoactive effects of NPY when administered directly into the brain.[14] The injection of NPY (2 to 200 pmol) into the caudate nucleus results in a pronounced local reduction in cerebral blood flow in proximity to the injection site. Since there is no corresponding change in glucose utilization in a similar group of rats, these reductions in flow are indicative of a direct local vasoconstriction by NPY of intracerebral arterioles.

E. POTENTIAL PHYSIOLOGICAL OR PATHOLOGICAL SIGNIFICANCE

The existence of NPY in perivascular sympathetic nerve fibers suggests that it is released during sympathetic activation. Furthermore, the fact that NPY is often a more potent constrictor than NA in cerebral arteries indicates that NPY may be the predominant neurotransmitter within these fibers. Although the sympathetic nerve fibers on the cerebral vessels have rather a modest influence on the cerebral circulation under normal conditions, one important putative function is their protection of the cerebral circulation from hyperemia and blood-brain barrier disruption during severe hypertension.[58,59] Indeed, additional protection against high blood pressure may be provided by the increased density of both NPY and NA containing nerve fibers on the pial arteries of hypertensive rats.[15] The importance of NPY in other nerve fibers such as those which originate in parasympathetic ganglia has yet to be determined.

NPY may also play role in pathophysiological conditions such as subarachnoid hemorrhage. Following experimentally induced subarachnoid hemorrhage in rats and dogs, there is a marked decrease in the number of NPY immunoreactive fibers.[60,61] The reduction in NPY-IR fibers has been proposed to be due to a massive release of transmitter which may contribute to the reductions in cerebral blood flow or vasospasm associated with subarachnoid hemorrhage. The influence of NPY on cerebral vessels may also have relevance in other clinical conditions such as migraine with aura.

To conclude, evidence from the bulk of the anatomical, pharmacological, and physiological studies supports the fact that NPY is a perivascular peptide with the capability of exerting an important regulatory influence on the cerebral circulation. A better understanding of the mechanisms of action of endogenous NPY awaits the development of potent, competitive, and selective NPY antagonists with which to further investigate the importance of NPY in the cerebral circulation.[41]

ACKNOWLEDGMENTS

U.I.T is supported by a scholarship from the Canadian Heart Foundation. The author thanks C. Frater for assisting in the preparation of the manuscript.

REFERENCES

1. **Tatemoto, K.,** Neuropeptide Y: complete amino acid sequence of the brain peptide, *Proc. Natl. Acad. Sci. U.S.A.*, 79, 5485, 1982.
2. **Tatemoto, K., Carlquist, M., and Mutt, V.,** Neuropeptide Y — a novel brain peptide with structural similarities to peptide YY and pancreatic polypeptide, *Nature,* 296, 659, 1982.
3. **Edvinsson, L., Emson, P., McCulloch, J., Tatemoto, K., and Uddman, R.,** Neuropeptide Y: immunocytochemical localization to and effect upon feline pial arteries and veins in vitro and in situ, *Acta Physiol. Scand.*, 122, 155, 1984.
4. **Lundberg, J. M., Terenius, J. G., Hökfelt, T., and Tatemoto, K.,** Comparative immunohistochemical and biochemical analysis of pancreatic polypeptide-like peptides with special references to presence of neuropeptide Y in central and peripheral neurons, *J. Neurosci.*, 4, 2376, 1984.
5. **Dumont, Y., Martel, J.C., Fournier, A., St-Pierre, S., and Quirion, R.,** Neuropeptide Y and neuropeptide Y receptor subtypes in brain and peripheral tissues, *Prog. Neurobiol.*, 38, 125, 1992.
6. **Glover, I. D., Barlow, D. J., Pitts, J. E., et al.,** Conformational studies on the pancreatic polypeptide hormone family, *Eur. J. Biochem.*, 142, 379, 1985.
7. **Blomqvist, A. G., Söderberg, C., Lundell, I., Milner, R. J., and Larhammar, D.,** Strong evolutionary conservation of neuropeptide Y: sequences of chicken, goldfish, and *Torpedo marmorata* DNA clones, *Proc. Natl. Acad. Sci. U.S.A.*, 89, 2350, 1992.
8. **Edvinsson, L., Emson, P., McCulloch, J., Tatemoto, K., and Uddman, R.,** Neuropeptide Y: cerebrovascular innervation and vasomotor effects in the cat, *Neurosci. Lett.*, 43, 79, 1983.

9. **Allen, J. M., Schon, F., Todd, N., Yeats, J. C., Crockard, H. A., and Bloom, S. R.,** Presence of neuropeptide Y in human circle of Willis and its possible role in cerebral vasospasm, *Lancet,* 1, 550, 1984.
10. **Edvinsson, L., Copeland, J. R., Emson, P. C., McCulloch, J., and Uddman, R.,** Nerve fibres containing neuropeptide Y in the cerebrovascular bed: immunocytochemistry, radioimmunoassay, and vasomotor effects, *J. Cereb. Blood Flow Metab.,* 7, 45, 1987.
11. **Walker, P., Grouzmann, E., Burnier, M., and Waeber, B.,** The role of neuropeptide Y in cardiovascular regulation, *Trends Pharmacol. Sci.,* 12, 111, 1991.
12. **Lundberg, J. M., Terenius, L., Hökfelt, T., and Goldstein, M.,** High levels of neuropeptide Y in peripheral noradrenergic neurons in various mammals including man, *Neurosci. Lett.,* 42, 167, 1983.
13. **Gibbins, I. L. and Morris, J. L.,** Co-existence of immunoreactivity to neuropeptide Y and vasoactive intestinal peptide in non-noradrenergic axons innervating guinea pig cerebral arteries after sympathectomy, *Brain Res.,* 444, 402, 1988.
14. **Tuor, U. I., Kelly, P., Edvinsson, L., Tatemoto, K., and McCulloch, J.,** Neuropeptide Y and the cerebral circulation, *J. Cereb. Blood Flow Metab.,* 10, 591, 1990.
15. **Dhital, K. K., Gerli, R., Lincoln, J., et al.,** Increased density of perivascular nerves to the major cerebral vessels of the spontaneously hypertensive rat: differential changes in noradrenaline and neuropeptide Y during development, *Brain Res.,* 444, 33, 1988.
16. **Duverger, D., Edvinsson, L., MacKenzie, E. T., et al.,** Concentrations of putative neurovascular transmitters in major cerebral arteries and small pial vessels of various species, *J. Cereb. Blood Flow Metab.,* 7, 497, 1987.
17. **Allen, Y. S., Adrian, T. E., Allen, J. M., et al.,** Neuropeptide Y distribution in the rat brain, *Science,* 221, 877, 1983.
18. **Edvinsson, L., Ekman, R., Jansen, I., Ottosson, A., and Uddman, R.,** Peptide-containing nerve fibers in human cerebral arteries: immunocytochemistry, radioimmunoassay, and in vitro pharmacology, *Ann. Neurol.,* 21, 431, 1987.
19. **Tuor, U. I., Edvinsson, L., and McCulloch, J.,** Neuropeptide Y and the control of the cerebral circulation, in *Peptidergic Mechanisms in the Cerebral Circulation,* Edvinsson, L. and McCulloch, J., Eds., Ellis Horwood Ltd., Chichester, 1987, 75.
20. **Suzuki, N., Hardebo, J. E., Kåhrström, J., and Owman, C.,** Neuropeptide Y coexists with vasoactive intestinal polypeptide and acetylcholine in parasympathetic cerebrovascular nerves originating in the sphenopalatine, otic, and internal carotid ganglia of the rat, *Neuroscience,* 36, 507, 1990.
21. **Fried, G., Terenius, L., Hökfelt, T., and Goldstein, M.,** Evidence for differential localization of noradrenaline and neuropeptide Y in neuronal storage vesicles isolated from rat vas deferens, *J. Neurosci.,* 5, 450, 1985.
22. **Lundberg, J. M., Rudehill, A., Sollevi, A., Fried, G., and Wallin, G.,** Co-release of neuropeptide Y and noradrenaline from pig spleen in vitro: importance of subcellular storage, nerve impulse frequency and pattern, feedback regulation and resupply by axonal transport, *Neuroscience,* 28, 475, 1989.
23. **Öhlen, A., Persson, M. G., Lindbom, L., Gustafsson, L. E., and Hedqvist, P.,** Nerve-induced nonadrenergic vasoconstriction and vasodilation in skeletal muscle, *Am. J. Physiol.,* 258, H1334, 1990.
24. **Lundberg, J. M., Rudehill, A., Sollevi, A., TheodorssonNorheim, E., and Hamberger, B.,** Frequency- and reserpine-dependent chemical coding of sympathetic transmission: differential release of noradrenaline and neuropeptide Y from pig spleen, *Neurosci. Lett.,* 63, 96, 1986.
25. **Suzuki, Y., Satoh, S.-I., Ikegaki, I., et al.,** Effects of neuropeptide Y and calcitonin gene-related peptide on local cerebral blood flow in rat striatum, *J. Cereb. Blood Flow Metab.,* 9, 268, 1989.
26. **Suzuki, N., Hardebo, J. E., Kåhrström, J., and Owman, C.,** New aspects on cerebrovascular NPY: coexistence with VIP and acetylcholine in parasympathetic nerves and increase after sympathectomy, *J. Cereb. Blood Flow Metab.,* 9, S677, 1989.

27. **Brayden, J. E. and Conway, M. A.,** Neuropeptide Y and vasoactive intestinal polypeptide in cerebral arteries of the rat: relationships between innervation pattern and mechanical response, *Regul. Pept.,* 22, 253, 1988.
28. **Hardebo, J. E., Suzuki, N., Ekblad, E., and Owman, C.,** Vasoactive intestinal polypeptide and acetylcholine coexist with neuropeptide Y, dopamine-β-hydroxylase, tyrosine hydroxylase, substance P or calcitonin gene-related peptide in neuronal subpopulations in cranial parasympathetic ganglia of rat, *Cell Tissue Res.,* 267, 291, 1992.
29. **Leblanc, G. C., Trimmer, B. A., and Landis, S. C.,** Neuropeptide Y-like immunoreactivity in rat cranial parasympathetic neurons: coexistence with vasoactive intestinal peptide and choline acetyltransferase, *Proc. Natl. Acad. Sci. U.S.A.,* 84, 3511, 1987.
30. **Hanko, J. H., Törnebrandt, K., Hardebo, J. E., Kåhrström, J., Nobin, A., and Owman, C.,** Neuropeptide Y induces and modulates vasoconstriction in intracranial and peripheral vessels of animals and man, *J. Auton. Pharmacol.,* 6, 117, 1986.
31. **Abel, P. W. and Han, C.,** Effects of neuropeptide Y on contraction, relaxation, and membrane potential of rabbit cerebral arteries, *J. Cardiovasc. Pharmacol.,* 13, 52, 1989.
32. **Edvinsson, L., Adamsson, M., and Jansen, I.,** Neuropeptide Y antagonistic properties of D-myo-inositol 1.2.6-trisphosphate in guinea pig basilar arteries, *Neuropeptides,* 17, 99, 1990.
33. **Fallgren, B., Arlock, P., Jansen, I., and Edvinsson, L.,** Neuropeptide Y in cerebrovascular function: comparison of membrane potential changes and vasomotor responses evoked by NPY and other vasoconstrictors in the guinea pig basilar artery, *Neurosci. Lett.,* 114, 117, 1990.
34. **Hirst, G. D. S., Neild, T. O., and Silverberg, G. D.,** Noradrenaline receptors on the rat basilar artery, *J. Physiol.,* 328, 351, 1982.
35. **Dacey, R. G., Jr. and Duling, B. R.,** Effect of norepinephrine on penetrating arterioles of rat cerebral cortex, *Am. J. Physiol.,* 264, H380, 1984.
36. **Edvinsson, L.,** Characterization of the contractile effect of neuropeptide Y in feline cerebral arteries, *Acta Physiol. Scand.,* 125, 33, 1985.
37. **Suzuki, Y., Shibuya, M., Ikegaki, I., Satoh, S.-I., Takayasu, M., and Asano, T.,** Effects of neuropeptide Y on canine cerebral circulation, *Eur. J. Pharmacol.,* 146, 271, 1988.
38. **MacLean, M. R. and McGrath, J. C.,** Effects of pre-contraction with endothelin-1 on α_2-adrenoceptor-and (endothelium-dependent) neuropeptide Y-mediated contractions in the isolated vascular bed of the rat tail, *Br. J. Pharmacol.,* 101, 205, 1990.
39. **Wahlestedt, C., Håkanson, R., Vaz, C. A., and Zukowska-Grojec, Z.,** Norepinephrine and neuropeptide Y: vasoconstrictor cooperation in vivo and in vitro, *Am. J. Physiol.,* 258, R736, 1990.
40. **Wahlestedt, C., Yanaihara, N., and Håkanson, R.,** Evidence for different pre- and post-junctional receptors for neuropeptide Y and related peptides, *Regul. Pept.,* 13, 307, 1986.
41. **Michel, M. C.,** Receptors for neuropeptide Y: multiple subtypes and multiple second messengers, *Trends Pharmacol. Sci.,* 12, 389, 1991.
42. **Sheikh, S. P.,** Neuropeptide Y and peptide YY: major modulators of gastrointestinal blood flow and function, *Am. J. Physiol.,* 261, G701, 1991.
43. **Rimland, J., Xin, W., Sweetnam, P., Saijoh, K., Nestler, E. J., and Duman, R. S.,** Sequence and expression of a neuropeptide Y receptor cDNA, *Mol. Pharmacol.,* 40, 869, 1991.
44. **Abel, P. W., Han, C., Noe, B. D., and McDonald, J. K.,** Neuropeptide Y: vasoconstrictor effects and possible role in cerebral vasospasm after experimental subarachnoid hemorrhage, *Brain Res.,* 463, 250, 1988.
45. **Daly, R. N. and Hieble, J. P.,** Neuropeptide Y modulates adrenergic neurotransmission by an endothelium dependent mechanism, *Eur. J. Pharmacol.,* 138, 445, 1987.
46. **Pernow, J. and Lundberg, J. M.,** Neuropeptide Y induces potent contraction of arterial vascular smooth muscle via an endothelium-independent mechanism, *Acta Physiol. Scand.,* 134, 157, 1988.

47. **Hieble, J. P., Duesler, J. G., Jr., and Daly, R. N.,** Effects of neuropeptide Y on the response of isolated blood vessels to norepinephrine and sympathetic field stimulation, *J. Pharmacol. Exp. Ther.*, 250, 523, 1989.
48. **Small, D. L., Bolzon, B. J., and Cheung, D. W.,** Endothelium-independent potentiating effects of neuropeptide Y in the rat tail artery, *Eur. J. Pharmacol.*, 210, 131, 1992.
49. **Budai, D., Vu, H. Q., and Duckles, S. P.,** Endothelium removal does not affect potentiation by neuropeptide Y in rabbit ear artery, *Eur. J. Pharmacol.*, 168, 97, 1989.
50. **Adamsson, M., Fallgren, B., and Edvinsson, L.,** Inhibition of neuropeptide Y-induced potentiation of noradrenaline-induced vasoconstriction by PP56 (D-*myo*-inositol 1,2,6-trisphosphate), *Br. J. Pharmacol.*, 105, 93, 1992.
51. **Wahlestedt, C., Regunathan, S., and Reis, D. J.,** Identification of cultured cells selectively expressing Y1-, Y2-, or Y3-type receptors for neuropeptide Y/peptide YY, *Life Sci.*, 50, PL7, 1992.
52. **Fredholm, B. B., Jansen, I., and Edvinsson, L.,** Neuropeptide Y is a potent inhibitor of cyclic AMP accumulation in feline cerebral blood vessels, *Acta Physiol. Scand.*, 124, 467, 1985.
53. **Shigeri, Y., Mihara, S.-I., and Fujimoto, M.,** Neuropeptide Y receptor in vascular smooth muscle, *J. Neurochem.*, 56, 852, 1991.
54. **Granstam, E. and Nilsson, S. F. E.,** Effects of cervical sympathetic nerve stimulation and neuropeptide Y (NPY) on cranial blood flow in the cat, *Acta Physiol. Scand.*, 142, 21, 1991.
55. **Nilsson, S. F. E.,** Neuropeptide Y (NPY): a vasoconstrictor in the eye, brain and other tissues in the rabbit, *Acta Physiol. Scand.*, 141, 455, 1991.
56. **Tuor, U. I., Kondysar, M. H., and Harding, R. K.,** Effect of angiotensin II and peptide YY on cerebral and circumventricular blood flow, *Peptides*, 9, 141, 1988.
57. **Okazaki, S., Sako, K., and Yonemasu, Y.,** Effects of intracarotid infusion of neuropeptide Y on cerebral blood flow in rats, *Brain Res.*, 575, 347, 1992.
58. **Tuor, U. I.,** Local distribution of the effects of sympathetic stimulation on cerebral blood flow in the rat, *Brain Res.*, 529, 224, 1990.
59. **Tuor, U. I.,** Acute hypertension and sympathetic stimulation: local heterogenous changes in cerebral blood flow, *Am. J. Physiol.*, 263, H511, 1992.
60. **Uemura, Y., Sugimoto, T., Okamoto, S., Handa, H., and Mizurio, N.,** Changes of neuropeptide immunoreactivity in cerebrovascular nerve fibres after experimentally produced SAH. Immunohistochemical study in the dog, *J. Neurosurg.*, 66, 741, 1987.
61. **Jackowski, A., Crockard, A., Burnstock, G., and Lincoln, J.,** Alterations in serotonin and neuropeptide Y content of cerebrovascular sympathetic nerves following experimental subarachnoid hemorrhage, *J. Cereb. Blood Flow Metab.*, 9, 271, 1989.
62. **Dacey, R. G., Jr., Bassett, J. E., and Takayasu, M.,** Vasomotor responses of rat intracerebral arterioles to vasoactive intestinal peptide, substance P, neuropeptide Y, and bradykinin, *J. Cereb. Blood Flow Metab.*, 8, 254, 1988.

Chapter 10

NEURAL REGULATION OF CEREBRAL BLOOD FLOW: VASOACTIVE INTESTINAL PEPTIDE (VIP)

Jan Fahrenkrug

TABLE OF CONTENTS

I. Introduction 166

II. Immunocytochemical Localization of Cerebrovascular VIP 166

III. Cerebrovascular Responsiveness to VIP 169

IV. VIP as Cerebrovascular Neurotransmitter 173

Acknowledgments 174

References 174

0-8493-5096-0/93/$0.00 + $.50

I. INTRODUCTION

Vasoactive intestinal polypeptide (VIP) was isolated from the porcine small intestine by Said and Mutt.[1] The peptide has derived its name from the profound and long-lasting vasodilatory action seen upon systemic administration.[2,3] By subsequent amino acid sequence analysis, porcine VIP was found to be a highly basic, single-chain linear polypeptide.[4,5] VIP contains 28 amino acid residues in its sequence and has a C terminal asparagine amide. It has, however, been shown that carboxyamidation of VIP is not critical for the biological activity.[6] The primary structure of VIP is closely related to that of secretin, PHI (peptide with N terminal histidine and C terminal isoleucine amide), helodermin, PACAP (pituitary adenylate cyclase activating polypeptide), and to a lesser extent to pancreatic glucagon, gastric inhibitory polypeptide (GIP), and growth hormone-releasing factor (GHRF). VIP of mammalian origin has a remarkably constant structure, since the sequences of bovine, human, ovine, goat, canine, rabbit, and rat have been shown to be identical to that of the porcine peptide.[7-12] Guinea pig VIP, however, differs in four amino acid residues from VIP in the other mammalian species.[13]

VIP is derived from a precursor, prepro-VIP, consisting of 170 amino acid residues.[14] The precursor contains, besides VIP, another biologically active peptide PHM (peptide with N terminal histidine and C terminal methionine amide) in its sequence (Figure 1). PHM (human form; PHI in rat and pig) is structurally related to VIP[15] and shares many of its biological actions, although generally less potent than VIP.[16-20] Other peptide sequences which are found during the proteolytic cleavage of the VIP precursor are prepro-VIP 22–79 (N terminal flanking peptide), prepro-VIP 111–122 (bridging peptide), and prepro-VIP 156–170 (C terminal flanking peptide).[21,22] The processing of VIP precursor can follow an alternative pathway in which the dibasic cleavage site after PHM is uncleaved resulted in a C terminally extended form of PHM (Figure 1). This peptide, designated PHV-42 (peptide with N terminal histidine and C terminal valine) is found to be just as potent as VIP in relaxing smooth muscle activity.[23,24]

By immunohistochemistry VIP has been localized to nerve cell bodies and nerve fibers of both the central and peripheral nervous system.[25] VIP fibers are associated with smooth muscle, blood vessels, glands, and surface epithelia and there is evidence that the peptide plays a transmitter role controlling motility, blood flow, and secretion.[26]

II. IMMUNOCYTOCHEMICAL LOCALIZATION OF CEREBROVASCULAR VIP

The presence of VIP and other prepro-VIP derived peptides has been demonstrated in cerebrovascular tissues of a variety of mammalian species including man by immunohistochemical procedures, and in some instances

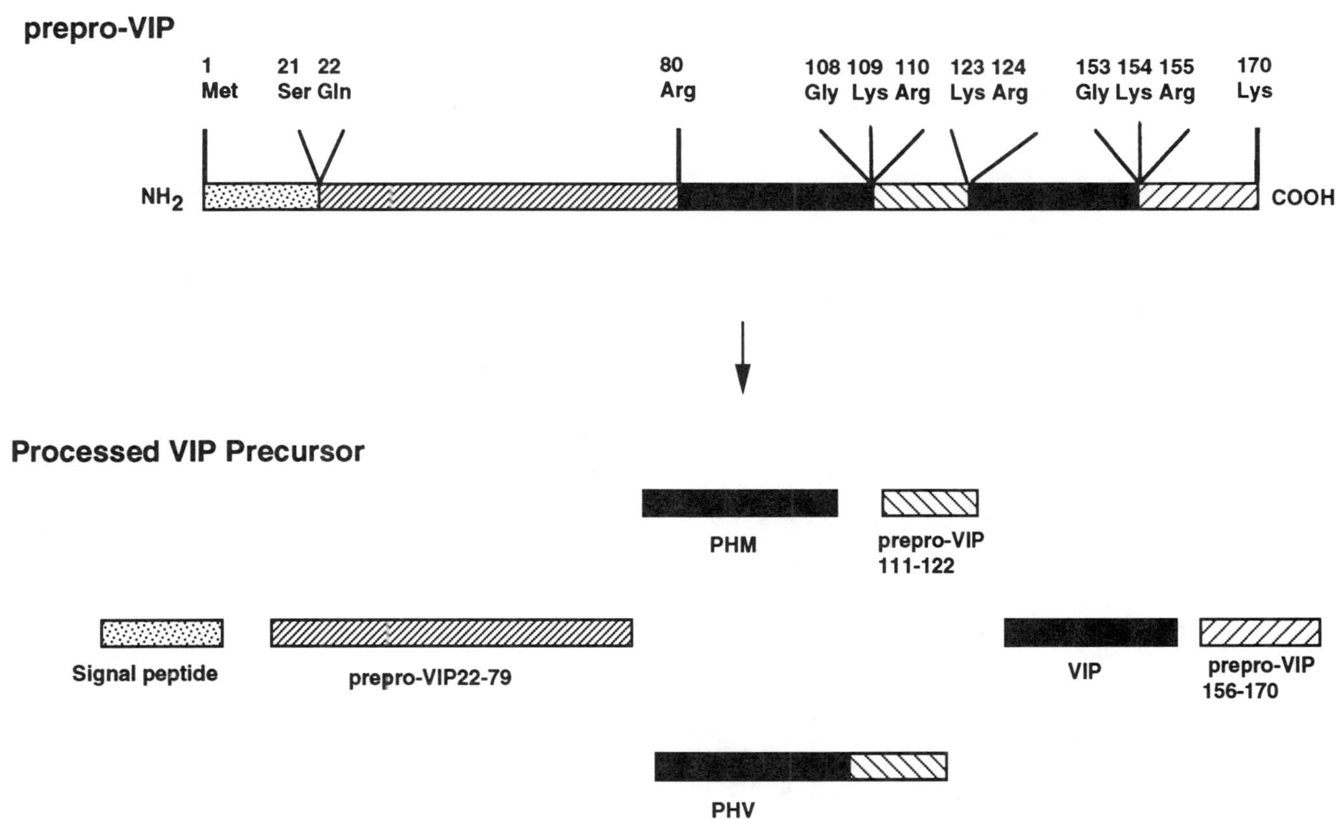

FIGURE 1. Schematic representation of the proteolytic processing of human vasoactive intestinal polypeptide precursor (prepro-VIP). Amino acid residues at putative posttranslational processing sites are shown.

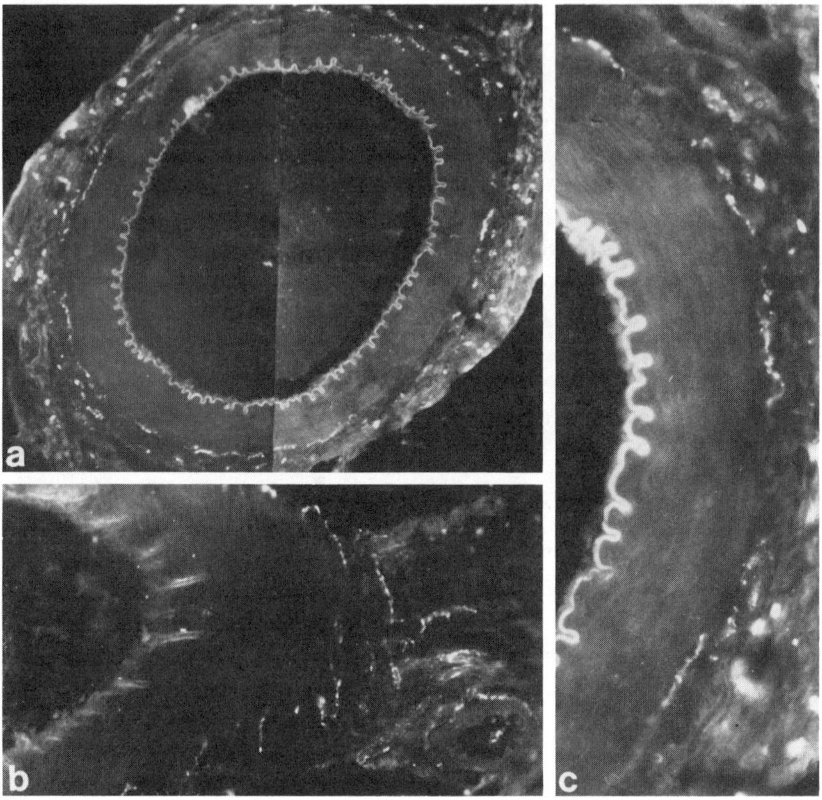

FIGURE 2. VIP immunoreactivity in anterior cerebral arteries of the cat. (a) The picture is composed of two adjacent cross-sections and shows numerous VIP nerves enclosing the vessel (×200). (b) Oblique section through the vessel wall. Several delicate VIP-containing nerves with a beaded appearance run in the wall and also enclose an adjacent small arteriole in the lower right corner (×450). (c) Cross-section of the vessel demonstrating that the VIP nerves run at the surface of the smooth muscle layer (×450). The internal elastic membrane is autofluorescent in all pictures. (From Larsson, L.-I., et al., *Brain Res.*, 113, 400, 1976. With permission.)

the peptide content in the vessels has been measured by radioimmunoassay. When observations were made on the same vessel, radioimmunoassay and immunohistochemical findings seem to agree.[27] Nerve fibers displaying VIP immunoreactivity in the wall of pial arteries were first identified in 1976.[28] The VIP fibers are located in the adventitia and at the border between adventitia and media (Figure 2). The distribution of VIP fibers is variable among cerebrovascular regions and between different species.[27-33] Pial arteries from the pig, cat, and rat have a particularly dense innervation while cow, dog, guinea pig, and hamster have a moderate number of VIP nerve fibers. Only few fibers are found in pial arteries from the monkey, rabbit, gerbil, and mouse. In most species VIP nerves are most abundant in the circle of Willis and around the major cerebral arteries with their proximal branches supplying the ventral areas of the brain. The density of the nerve plexuses tends to be highest in the carotid system of vessels and diminishes in the caudal direction. No evidence is found for VIP innervation of the spinal cord blood vessels as studied in rabbits and cats,[27] while the choroid plexus of several mammalian species receives a moderate number of VIP immunoreactive nerve fibers.[34] Well-developed plexuses of perivascular nerve fibers, containing in addition to VIP immunoreactive material for each of the other prepro-VIP derived peptides, are observed in the walls of all major cerebral arteries of the rat (Figure 3), but not around veins or capillaries.[35] Using sequential incubation of the vessel preparations with PHI followed by VIP antisera, evidence for coexistence of the two peptides in perivascular fibers has been provided,[36] in accordance with the fact that the peptides arise from the same precursor. Also extracranial vessels on the arterial and venous sides are found to have VIP nerve fibers located in the adventitia close to the smooth muscle cells of the media.[37]

By electronmicroscopy, VIP immunoreactivity is found in about 30% of the large vesicles (90 mm in diameter) in a varicosity.[38] The nonreactive vesicles may contain too low a concentration of VIP to react or possibly store other transmitter substances. In this context it is worth mentioning that there are findings indicating that neuropeptide Y and acetylcholine are costored with VIP in some populations of cerebrovascular nerves.[39,40]

The origin of the perivascular VIP innervation of cerebral arteries has been clarified to some extent. The majority of the VIP fibers, at least those belonging to the rostral part of the circle of Willis, are contained within the cerebrovascular parasympathetic innervation derived from the sphenopalatine ganglion.[33,41-43] This is supported by retrograde tracing with horseradish peroxidase[44] and true blue,[43,45] showing a considerable supply also from the otic ganglion. It has, in addition, been suggested that at least some of the VIP fibers to cerebral arteries have a more dispersed origin; some fibers derive from local microganglia in the vicinity of e.g., the cavernous plexus, close to bifurcation of large basal arteries, and the external rete.[31,43,46] Besides the multiple sites of origin of VIP fibers, there seems to be some degree of bilateral innervation.[45] Finally, it has been shown that VIP and PHI immunoreactive fibers from neocortical neurons on some occasions penetrate the cortical surface to enter the pial membrane and make contacts with cerebral blood vessels (Figure 4).[35,47-48]

III. CEREBROVASCULAR RESPONSIVENESS TO VIP

Considerable evidence is available describing dilatory actions of VIP upon cerebral vessels both *in vitro*[28,36,38,49,50] and *in situ*.[51-53] In appropriate intact animal preparations, these actions of VIP are manifested, as might be

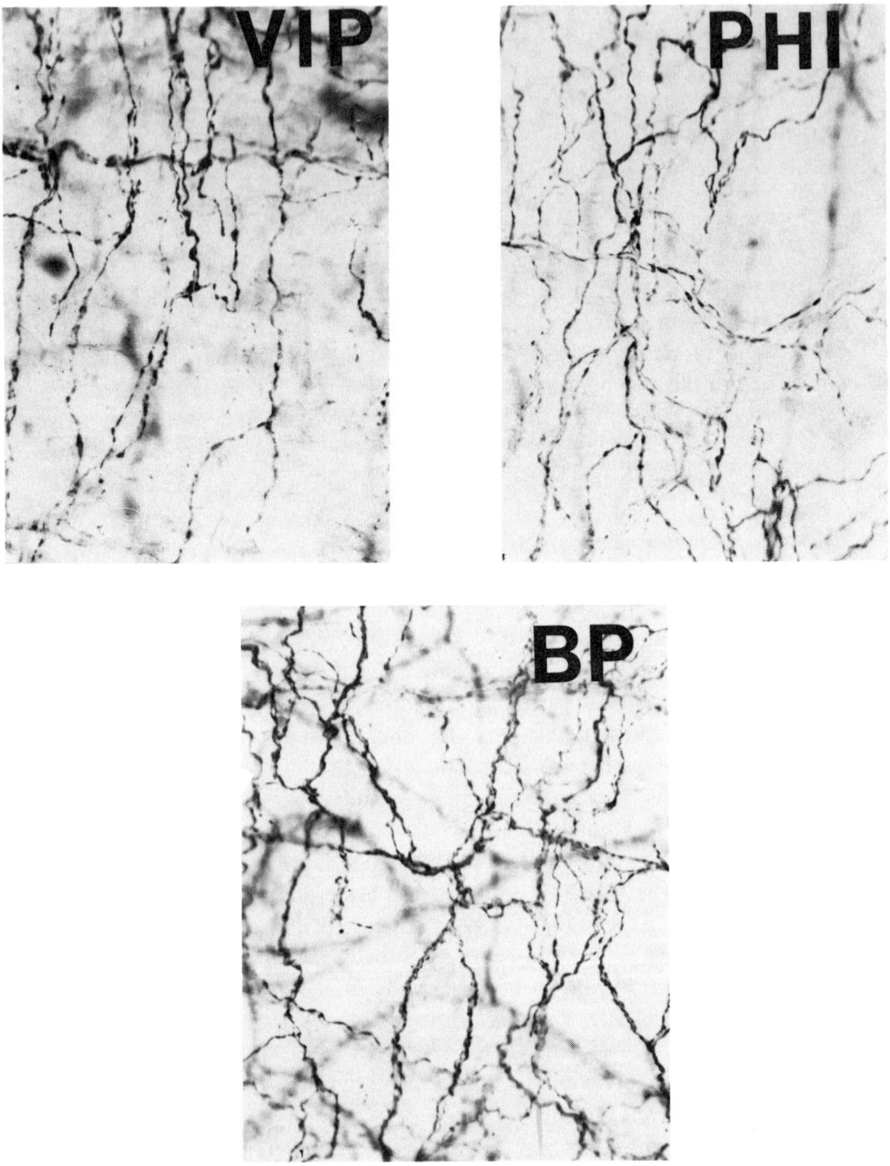

FIGURE 3. Photomicrographs of whole mount preparations of the rat basilar arteries reacted with antisera against the following sequences of prepro-VIP: vasoactive intestinal polypeptide (VIP), peptide histidine isoleucine amide (PHI), and prepro-VIP 111–122 or the bridging peptide (BP) (×460).

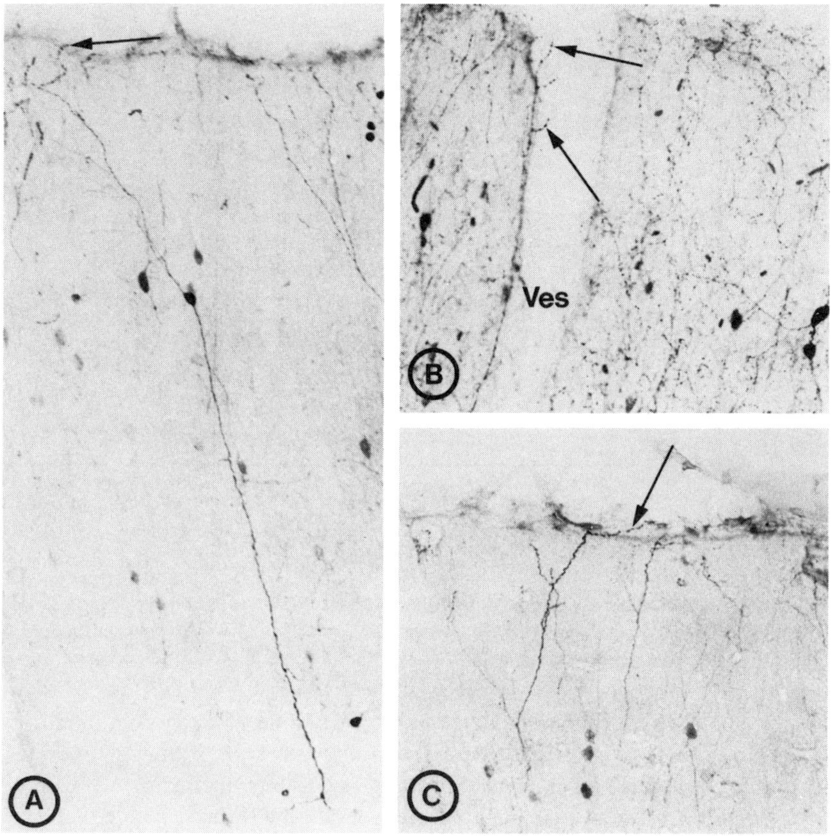

FIGURE 4. (A) Rat neocortex showing PHI immunoreactive neurons of bipolar type. Processes from the immunoreactive perikarya can be followed into the pial tissue (arrow) covering the surface (×180). (B) PHI immunoreactive processes (arrows) originating from an intracortical perikarya extending to a pial vessels (Ves.) (×460). (C) PHI immunoreactive processes extending into the pial layer (arrow) (×460).

expected, as an increased cerebral blood flow.[52,54,55] *In vitro* VIP is without obvious effect on isolated blood vessels during resting conditions. VIP induces, however, relaxation on isolated cerebral arteries to which prostaglandin $F_{2\alpha}$ ($PGF_{2\alpha}$) has been given to produce an active tone of the vessel.[36] VIP causes a concentration dependent vasodilation with a mean effective concentration varying between 1×10^{-9} and 3×10^{-8} *M* depending on the type of vessels examined. VIP is able to relax isolated vascular preparation by about 50% of the tone induced by $PGF_{2\alpha}$ (Figure 5), and relaxation is also obtained after precontraction with other agents such as norepinephrine, 5-hydroxytryptamine, and potassium (120 m*M*). The VIP-induced relaxation is independent of the endothelial cells[38,56] and unaffected by β-adrenoreceptor

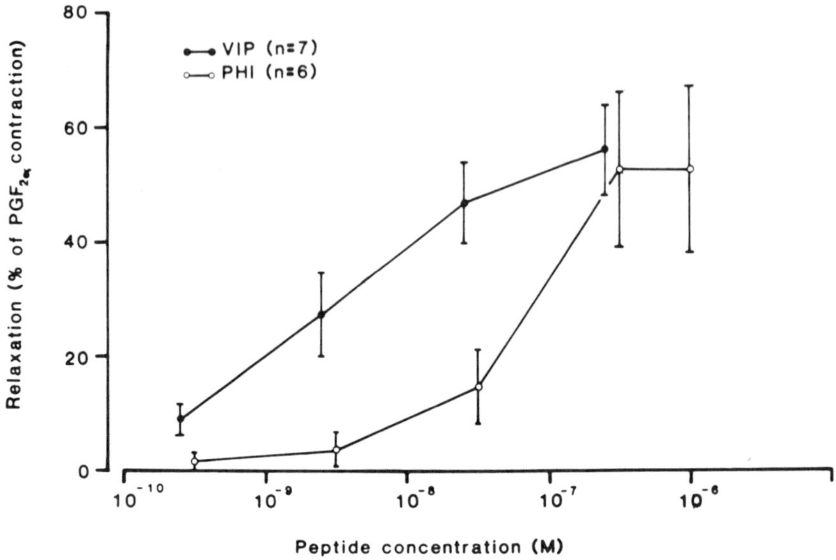

FIGURE 5. Concentration-response curves for the dilatory effects of VIP and PHI on isolated cat middle cerebral arteries precontracted by the addition of 3×10^{-6} *M* of prostaglandin $F_{2\alpha}$. (From Edvinsson, L. and McCulloch, J., *Regul. Pept.*, 10, 345, 1985. With permission.)

blockade, cholinoceptor blockade, or the histamine antagonist burimamide. PHI is also able to relax isolated cerebral arteries, but 25 times more PHI is required to produce an equal dilatory response to that elicited by VIP (Figure 5). Vessels responding normally to either PHI or VIP are capable of further dilation in response to papaverine, while the administration of PHI to vessels already dilated in response to VIP shows no further effect and vice versa. Thus, it appears that both PHI and VIP act upon vascular smooth muscle at a common receptor site or via a common mechanism.

Receptors for VIP have been characterized in cerebral arteries by studying the interaction of radiolabeled VIP with brain vessel membrane preparations.[57] The binding data suggest the presence of both high and low affinity binding sites for VIP and the results correlate well with the concentrations of the peptide mediating dilation. By light microscopic autoradiography, binding sites for VIP have been localized to the medial layer of circle of Willis and pial arteries.[58,59] The adenylate cyclase system appears to act as a second messenger since the dose response curves for VIP binding are similar to those for cAMP formation and functional smooth muscle vasodilation.[57] The ability of PHI to increase cellular cAMP levels appear also to be mediated via interaction with the VIP receptor.[60]

Application *in vivo* of VIP into the perivascular space surrounding individual pial arteries and also veins increases vessel diameter in a concentration-dependent manner.[61] The response of smaller arteries (less than 60 μm prior to the injection) is found to be proportionally greater than that of larger vessels (initial size more than 150 μm). The preinjection resting caliber of the arterioles has no measurable effect upon the magnitude of the response. In accordance with the *in vitro* findings, PHI also increases arteriolar caliber, but with a much lower potency than VIP.[36] The maximal responses to the two peptides are, however, indistinguishable. A diffusion barrier for VIP between the vascular lumen of the cerebral circulation, on the one hand, and the arterial wall as well as the brain parenchyma, on the other, seems to exist. Thus intracarotid infusions of a small VIP dose into baboons are found to be without significant effects on cerebral blood flow and metabolism (cerebral oxygen consumption) as well as on the EEG under normal conditions.[52] In contrast, if the same concentration of VIP is administered following hypertonic opening of the blood-brain barrier, flow and metabolism are significantly increased. The metabolic stimulation and rise in blood flow are accompanied by an increase in the low voltage fast activity of the EEG. Infusions into the baboon internal carotid artery of a greater concentration of VIP, when the barrier is intact, consistently result in a small increase in cerebral blood flow and metabolism. This indicates that VIP under these circumstances has reached the cerebral tissue in a concentration high enough to activate VIP-sensitive neurons, thereby masking direct relaxant effects on the arterial wall. In agreement with this, ventriculo-cisternal perfusion with cerebrospinal fluid containing VIP, circumventing the blood-brain barrier, has been shown to produce cerebral vasodilation.[55] Furthermore, local injection of VIP, either into the striatum or into the anterior cingulate cortex, elicits complex neuronatomically organized patterns of metabolic activation with increases in local glucose consumption both ipsi- and contralaterally.[62,63]

IV. VIP AS CEREBROVASCULAR NEUROTRANSMITTER

VIP can be released upon activation of cerebrovascular nerves,[64,65] which in connection with its potent vasodilator action in the brain makes it a putative transmitter in nonadrenergic, noncholinergic cerebral vasodilation. This has been corroborated by flow studies in which the postganglionic VIP fibers have been stimulated selectively.[66] A crucial link in the evidence for effective transmission is the demonstration of blockade of nerve-induced responses by a specific antagonist. Specific VIP antagonists in the usual pharmacological sense are not available, although some peptide analogues have been claimed to be antagonists in receptor binding studies. However, a VIP-specific antibody has been successfully used *in vitro* to antagonize neurogenic vasodilation.[67] It has been shown in the middle cerebral artery of the cat that antibody selectively inhibits atropine-resistant neurovasodilation in the guanethidine-treated artery. Blockade is related to the concentration of the antibody and inversely to the frequency of nerve activation.

Although the physiological function of cerebrovascular VIP innervation is not yet fully understood, the findings summarized above may suggest that the peptide could be involved in the maintenance of the interrelation between neuronal activity, energy generation, and local blood flow.

ACKNOWLEDGMENTS

Supported by the Danish Biotechnology Center for Signal Peptide Research.

REFERENCES

1. **Said, S. I. and Mutt, V.,** Polypeptide with broad biological activity: isolation from small intestine, *Science,* 169, 1217, 1970.
2. **Said, S. I. and Mutt, V.,** Potent peripheral and splanchnic vasodilator peptide from normal gut, *Nature,* 225, 863, 1970.
3. **Said, S. I. and Mutt, V.,** Isolation from porcine-intestinal wall of a vasoactive octacosapeptide related to secretin and to glucagon, *Eur. J. Biochem.,* 28, 199, 1972.
4. **Mutt, V. and Said, S. I.,** Structure of the porcine vasoactive intestinal octacosapeptide. The amino-acid sequence. Use of kallikrein in its determination, *Eur. J. Biochem.,* 42, 581, 1974.
5. **Bodanszky, M., Klausner, U. S., Lin, C. Y., Mutt, V., and Said, S. I.,** Synthesis of the vasoactive intestinal peptide (VIP), *J. Am. Chem. Soc.,* 96, 4973, 1974.
6. **Fahrenkrug, J., Ottesen, B., and Palle, C.,** Non amidated forms of VIP (glycine-extended VIP and VIP-free acid) have full bioactivity on smooth muscle, *Regul. Pept.,* 26, 235, 1989.
7. **Carlquist, M., McDonald, T. J., Go, V. L. W., Bataille, D., Johansson, C., and Mutt, V.,** Isolation and amino acid composition of human vasoactive intestinal polypeptide (VIP), *Horm. Metab. Res.,* 14, 28, 1982.
8. **Dimaline, R., Reeve, J. R., Shively, J. E., and Hawke, D.,** Isolation and characterization of rat vasoactive intestinal peptide, *Peptides,* 5, 183, 1984.
9. **Wang, S. C., Du, B. H., Eng, J., Chang, M., Hulmes, J. D., Pan, Y.-C. E., and Yalow, R. S.,** Purification of dog VIP from a single animal, *Life Sci.,* 37, 979, 1985.
10. **Bounjoua, Y., Vandermeers, A., Robberecht, P., Vandermeers-Piret, M.-C., and Christophe, J.,** Purification and amino acid sequence of vasoactive intestinal peptide, peptide histidine isoleucinamide and secretin from the ovine small intestine, *Regul. Pept.,* 32, 169, 1991.
11. **Gafvelin, G.,** Isolation and primary structure of VIP from sheep brain, *Peptides,* 11, 703, 1990.
12. **Gossen, D., Buscail, L., Cauvin, A., Gourlet, P., de Neef, P., Rathe, J., Robberecht, P., Vandermeers-Piret, M.-C., Vandermeers, A., and Christophe, J.,** Amino acid sequence of VIP, PHI and secretin from the rabbit small intestine, *Peptides,* 11, 123, 1990.
13. **Du, B.-H., Eng, J., Hulmes, J. D., Chang, M., Pan, Y.-C. E., and Yalow, R. S.,** Guinea pig has a unique mammalian VIP, *Biochem. Biophys. Res. Commun.,* 128, 1093, 1985.

14. **Itoh, N., Obata, K.-I., Yanaihara, N., and Okamoto, H.,** Human preprovasoactive intestinal polypeptide contains a novel PHI27-like peptide, PHM-27, *Nature,* 304, 547, 1983.
15. **Tatemoto, K. and Mutt, V.,** Isolation and characterization of the intestinal peptide porcine PHI (PHI-27), a new member of the glucagon-secretin family, *Proc. Natl. Acad. Sci. U.S.A.,* 78, 6603, 1981.
16. **Bataille, D., Gespach, C., Laburthe, M., Amiranoff, B., Tatemoto, K., Vauclin, N., Mutt, V., and Rosselin, G.,** Porcine peptide having *N*-terminal histidine and *C*-terminal isoleucine amide (PHI): vasoactive intestinal peptide (VIP) and secretin-like effects in different tissues from the rat, *FEBS Lett.,* 114, 240, 1980.
17. **Lundberg, J. M. and Tatemoto, K.,** Vascular effects of the peptides PYY and PHI: comparison with APP and VIP, *Eur. J. Pharmacol.,* 83, 143, 1982.
18. **Anagnostides, A. A., Manolas, K., Christofides, N. D., Yiangou, Y., Welbourn, R. G., Bloom, S. R., and Chadwick, V. S.,** Peptide histidine isoleucine (PHI). A secretagogue in porcine intestine, *Dig. Dis. Sci.,* 28, 893, 1983.
19. **Lundberg, J. M., Fahrenkrug, J., Hökfelt, T., Martling, C.-R., Larsson, O., Tatemoto, K., and Änggård, A.,** Coexistence of peptide HI (PHI) and VIP in nerves regulating blood flow and bronchial smooth muscle tone in various mammals including man, *Peptides,* 5, 593, 1984.
20. **Suzuki, Y., McMaster, D., Lederis, K., and Rorstad, O. P.,** Characterization of the relaxant effects of vasoactive intestinal peptide (VIP) and PHI on isolated brain arteries, *Brain Res.,* 322, 9, 1984.
21. **Fahrenkrug, J. and Emson, P.,** Characterization and regional distribution of peptides derived from the VIP-precursor in the normal human brain, *J. Neurochem.,* 53, 1142, 1989.
22. **Bredkjaer, H. E., Rønnov-Jessen, D., Fahrenkrug, L., Ekblad, E., and Fahrenkrug, J.,** Expression of prepro-VIP-derived peptides in the human gastrointestinal tract: a biochemical and immunocytochemical study, *Regul. Pept.,* 33, 145, 1991.
23. **Yiangou, Y., Di Marzo, V., Spokes, R. A., Panico, M., Morris, H. R., and Bloom, S. R.,** Isolation, characterization and pharmacological actions of peptide histidine valine 42, a novel preprovasoactive intestinal peptide-derived peptide, *J. Biol. Chem.,* 262, 14010, 1987.
24. **Palle, C., Ottesen, B., and Fahrenkrug, J.,** Peptide histidine valine (PHV) is present and biologically active in the human female genital tract, *Regul. Pept.,* 38, 101, 1992.
25. **Hökfelt, T., Schultzberg, M., Lundberg, J. M., Fuxe, K., Mutt, V., Fahrenkrug, J., and Said, S. I.,** Distribution of vasoactive intestinal polypeptide in the central and peripheral nervous systems as revealed by immunocytochemistry, in *Advances in Peptide Hormone Research. Vasoactive Intestinal Polypeptide,* Said, S. I., Ed., Raven Press, New York, 1982, 65.
26. **Fahrenkrug, J.,** VIP and autonomic transmission, *Pharmacol. Ther.,* 41, 515, 1989.
27. **Edvinsson, L., Fahrenkrug, J., Hanko, J., Owman, C., Sundler, F., and Uddman, R.,** VIP (vasoactive intestinal polypeptide) containing nerves of intracranial arteries in mammals, *Cell Tissue Res.,* 208, 135, 1980.
28. **Larsson, L.-I., Edvinsson, L., Fahrenkrug, J., Håkanson, R., Owman, C., Schaffalitzky de Muckadell, O., and Sundler, F.,** Immunohistochemical localization of a vasodilatory polypeptide (VIP) in cerebrovascular nerves, *Brain Res.,* 113, 400, 1976.
29. **Della, N. G., Papka, R. E., Furness, J. B., and Costa, M.,** Vasoactive intestinal peptide-like immunoreactivity in nerves associated with the cardiovascular system of guinea-pigs, *Neuroscience,* 9, 605, 1983.
30. **Edvinsson, L. and Ekman, R.,** Distribution and dilatory effect of vasoactive intestinal polypeptide (VIP) in human cerebral arteries, *Peptides,* 5, 329, 1984.
31. **Gibbins, I. L., Brayden, J. E., and Bevan, J. A. C.,** Perivascular nerves with immunoreactivity to vasoactive intestinal polypeptide in cephalic arteries of the cat: Distribution, possible origins and functional implications, *Neuroscience,* 13, 1327, 1984.

32. **Itakura, T., Okuno, T., Nakakita, K., Kamei, I., Naka, Y., Nakai, K., Imai, H., Komai, N., Kimura, H., and Maeda, T.,** A light and electron microscopic immunohistochemical study of vasoactive intestinal polypeptide and substance P-containing nerve fibers along the cerebral blood vessels: comparison with aminergic and cholinergic nerve fibers, *J. Cereb. Blood Flow Metab.*, 4, 407, 1984.
33. **Hara, H., Hamill, G. S., and Jacobowitz, D. M.,** Origin of cholinergic nerves to the cat major cerebral arteries: coexistence with vasoactive intestinal polypeptide, *Brain Res. Bull.*, 14, 179, 1985.
34. **Lindvall, M., Alumets, J., Edvinsson, L., Fahrenkrug, J., Håkanson, R., Hanko, J., Owman, C., Schaffalitzky de Muckadell, O. B., and Sundler, F.,** Peptidergic (VIP) nerves in the mammalian choroid plexus, *Neuroscience Lett.*, 9, 77, 1978.
35. **Zhang, E.-T., Mikkelsen, J. D., Fahrenkrug, J., Møller, M., Kronborg, D., and Lauritzen, M.,** Prepro-vasoactive intestinal polypeptide-derived peptide sequences in cerebral blood vessels of rats: on the functional anatomy of metabolic autoregulation, *J. Cereb. Blood Flow Metab.*, 11, 932, 1991.
36. **Edvinsson, L. and McCulloch, J.,** Distribution and vasomotor effects of peptide HI (PHI) in feline cerebral blood vessels *in vitro* and *in situ*, *Regul. Pept.*, 10, 345, 1985.
37. **Uddman, R., Alumets, J., Edvinsson, L., Håkanson, R., and Sundler, F.,** VIP nerve fibers around peripheral blood vessels, *Acta Physiol. Scand.*, 112, 65, 1981.
38. **Lee, T. J.-F., Saito, A., and Berezin, I.,** Vasoactive intestinal polypeptide-like substance: the potential transmitter for cerebral vasodilation, *Science*, 224, 898, 1984.
39. **Gibbins, I. L. and Morris, J. L.,** Co-existence of immunoreactivity to neuropeptide Y and vasoactive intestinal peptide in non-noradrenergic axons innervating guinea pig cerebral arteries after sympathectomy, *Brain Res.*, 444, 402, 1988.
40. **Suzuki, N., Hardebo, J. E., Kåhrström, J., and Owman, C.,** Neuropeptide Y coexists with vasoactive intestinal polypeptide and acetylcholine in parasympathetic cerebrovascular nerves originating in the sphenopalatine, otic, and internal carotid ganglia of the rat, *Neuroscience*, 2, 507, 1990.
41. **Hara, H., Jansen, I., Ekman, R., Hamel, E., MacKenzie, E. T., Uddman, R., and Edvinsson, L.,** Acetylcholine and vasoactive intestinal peptide in cerebral blood vessels: effect of extirpation of the sphenopalatine ganglion, *J. Cereb. Blood Flow Metab.*, 9, 204, 1989.
42. **Hara, H. and Weir, B.,** Pathway of acetylcholinesterase-containing nerves to the major cerebral arteries, *J. Comp. Neurol.*, 250, 245, 1986.
43. **Suzuki, N., Hardebo, J. E., and Owman, C.,** Origins and pathways of cerebrovascular vasoactive intestinal polypeptide-positive nerves in rat, *J. Cereb. Blood Flow Metab.*, 8, 697, 1988.
44. **Walters, B. B., Gillespie, S. A., and Moskowitz, M. A.,** Cerebrovascular projections from the sphenopalatine and otic ganglia to the middle cerebral artery of the cat, *Stroke*, 17, 488, 1986.
45. **Edvinsson, L., Hara, H., and Uddman, R.,** Retrograde tracing of nerve fibers to the rat middle cerebral artery with true blue: co-localization with different peptides, *J. Cereb. Blood Flow Metab.*, 9, 212, 1989.
46. **Hara, H. and Kobayashi, S.,** Vasoactive intestinal polypeptide (VIP)-like immunoreactive cells in the skull base of rats: a combined study using acetylcholinesterase histochemistry, *Histochemistry*, 87, 217, 1987.
47. **Eckenstein, F. and Baughman, R. W.,** Two types of cholinergic innervation in cortex, one co-localized with vasoactive intestinal polypeptide, *Nature*, 309, 153, 1984.
48. **Lorén, I., Emson, P. C., Fahrenkrug, J., Björklund, A., Alumets, J., Håkanson, R., and Sundler, F.,** Distribution of vasoactive intestinal polypeptide in the rat and mouse brain, *Neuroscience*, 4, 11953, 1979.
49. **Duckles, S. P. and Said, S. I.,** Vasoactive polypeptide as a neurotransmitter in the cerebral circulation, *Eur. J. Pharmacol.*, 78, 371, 1982.

50. **Bevan, J. A., Buga, G. M., Moskowitz, M. A., and Said, S. I.,** *In vitro* evidence that vasoactive intestinal peptide is a transmitter of neuro-vasodilation in the head of the cat, *Neuroscience,* 19, 597, 1986.
51. **Edvinsson, L., McCulloch, J., and Uddman, R.,** Feline cerebral veins and arteries: comparison of autonomic innervation and vasomotor responses, *J. Physiol.,* 325, 161, 1982.
52. **McCulloch, J. and Edvinsson, L.,** Cerebral circulatory and metabolic effects of vasoactive intestinal polypeptide, *Am. J. Physiol.,* 239, H449, 1980.
53. **Wei, E. P., Kontos, H. A., and Said, S. I.,** Mechanism of action of vasoactive intestinal polypeptide on cerebral arterioles, *Am. J. Physiol.,* 239, H765, 1980.
54. **Heistad, D. D., Marcus, M. L., Said, S. I., and Gross, P. M.,** Effect of acetylcholine and vasoactive intestinal peptide on cerebral blood flow, *Am. J. Physiol.,* 239, H73, 1980.
55. **Wilson, D. A., O'Neill, J. T., Said, S. I., and Traystman, R. J.,** Vasoactive intestinal polypeptide and the canine cerebral circulation, *Circ. Res.,* 48, 138, 1981.
56. **Edvinsson, L., Fredholm, B. B., Hamel, E., Jansen, I., and Verrecchia, C.,** Perivascular peptides relax cerebral arteries concomitant with stimulation of cyclic adenosine monophosphate accumulation or release of an endothelium-derived relaxing factor in the cat, *Neurosci. Lett.,* 58, 213, 1985.
57. **Suzuki, Y., McMaster, D., Huang, M., Lederis, K., and Rorstad, O. P.,** Characterization of functional receptors for vasoactive intestinal peptide in bovine cerebral arteries, *J. Neurochem.,* 45, 890, 1985.
58. **Amenta, F., Cavalotti, C., De Michele, M., De Vincentis, G., Rossodivita, A., and Rossodivita, I.,** Vasoactive intestinal polypeptide receptors in rat cerebral vessels: an autoradiographic study, *J. Auton. Pharmacol.,* 11, 285, 1991.
59. **Poulin, P., Suzuki, Y., Lederis, K., and Rorstad, O. P.,** Autoradiographic localization of binding sites for vasoactive intestinal peptide (VIP) in bovine cerebral arteries, *Brain Res.,* 381, 382, 1986.
60. **Huang, M. and Rorstad, O. P.,** Cerebral vascular adenylate cyclase: evidence for coupling to receptors for vasoactive intestinal peptide and parathyroid hormone, *J. Neurochem.,* 43, 849, 1984.
61. **Edvinsson, L., Fahrenkrug, J., Hanko, J., McCulloch, J., Owman, C., and Uddman, R.,** Vasoactive intestinal polypeptide: distribution and effects on cerebral blood flow and metabolism, in *Cerebral Microcirculation and Metabolism,* Cervós-Navarro, J. and Fritschka, E., Eds., Raven Press, New York, 1981, 147.
62. **McCulloch, J. and Kelly, P. A. T.,** A functional role for vasoactive intestinal polypeptide in anterior cingulate cortex, *Nature,* 304, 438, 1983.
63. **McCulloch, J., Kelly, P. A. T., Uddman, R., and Edvinsson, L.,** Functional role for vasoactive intestinal polypeptide in the caudate nucleus: A 2-deoxy (^{14}C) glucose investigation, *Proc. Natl. Acad. Sci. U.S.A.,* 80, 1472, 1983.
64. **Levitt, B. and Duckles, S. P.,** Potassium-evoked release of vasoactive intestinal polypeptide (VIP) from cat cerebral arteries, *Pharmacologist,* 25, 204, 1983.
65. **Bevan, J. A., Moskowitz, M., Said, S. I., and Buga, C.,** Evidence that vasoactive intestinal polypeptide is a dilator transmitter to some cerebral and extracerebral cranial arteries, *Peptides,* 5, 385, 1984.
66. **Suzuki, N., Hardebo, J. E., Kåhrström, J., and Owman, C.,** Selective electrical stimulation of postganglionic cerebrovascular parasympathetic nerve fibers originating from the sphenopalatine ganglion enhances cortical blood flow in the rat, *J. Cereb. Blood Flow Metab.,* 10, 383, 1990.
67. **Brayden, J. E. and Bevan, J. A.,** Vasoactive intestinal polypeptide (VIP) is a cerebral vasodilator transmitter, *Stroke,* 16, 136, 1985.

Chapter 11

CALCITONIN GENE-RELATED PEPTIDE (CGRP)

Yoshio Suzuki

TABLE OF CONTENTS

I. Introduction 180

II. Vascular Sensory Fibers 180

III. Vasodilatory Activity of CGRP 182
A. *In Vitro* Studies 182
B. *In Vivo* Studies 182

IV. Release of CGRP from Sensory Nerve Fibers 185

V. Influence of Sensory Fibers on Cerebral Blood Flow 187

VI. Structure-Function Relationship 187

VII. Pathologic Conditions 188
A. Migraine 188
B. Subarachnoid Hemorrhage 189
C. Cerebral Hyperperfusion Syndromes 190

References 190

0-8493-5096-0/93/$0.00 + $.50

I. INTRODUCTION

Calcitonin gene-related peptide (CGRP), a 37 amino acid peptide, is widely distributed throughout the central and peripheral nervous system. It is particularly abundant in perivascular sensory fibers. Sensory fibers which form networks in intracranial vessels contain CGRP, in some cases colocalized with tachykinins such as substance P (SP) and neurokinin A. The main function of these nerve fibers appears to be the transmission of nociceptive signals from the blood vessels, dura, or arachnoid membranes to the central nervous system. In addition to this sensory function, stimulation of sensory fibers leads to vasodilation by antidromic activation or axon reflex, thereby playing a role in the regulation of regional hemodynamics. CGRP is the most potent vasodilator released from sensory fibers in cerebral arteries.

II. VASCULAR SENSORY FIBERS

The sensory fibers that innervate cerebral blood vessels are predominantly unmyelinated C fibers derived from the trigeminal ganglion, in particular from the ophthalmic division of the ganglion.[1,2] These fibers have been called the trigeminovascular system. The level C_2 dorsal ganglion contributes to the posterior circulation.[3] Innervation derives not only from the ipsilateral ganglion but also, to a minor degree, from the contralateral ganglion.[4] In primates, fibers pass directly from the trigeminal nerve to the internal carotid artery through the cavernous sinus.[5,6] In addition to blood vessels, the pia, arachnoid membrane, and dura are innervated by sensory fibers and fibers containing CGRP. These fibers are found in the adventitia or at the adventitia-media border of blood vessels, where they form both meshwork and spiral patterns.[7,8] (Figure 1) The concentration of CGRP in the major cerebral arteries at the base of the human brain at autopsy is higher than that of vasoactive intestinal peptide (VIP) or SP. CGRP concentration varies between 2.6 and 5.5 pmol/g, showing a gradual decline with increasing age. The proximal arteries of the circle of Willis exhibit higher levels of CGRP than do more distal blood vessels. Electron microscopic studies have demonstrated the presence of CGRP in nerve terminals lacking granular vesicles and have shown that, while most of the SP terminals were some distance from the arterial muscle cells, some of the CGRP fiber terminals existed relatively close to the arterial smooth muscle cells.[9]

Whereas the abundant SP fibers also innervate cerebral veins, including the cortical veins, deep cerebral veins, and dural sinuses, CGRP, VIP, and neuropeptide Y (NPY) fibers are found in extremely low density only in the cortical veins. This morphologic difference has been interpreted as indicating that SP fibers obtain information on the entire brain vasculature. Other peptidergic vasomotor neurons apparently function less actively in cerebral veins than cerebral arteries because of their extremely low density.

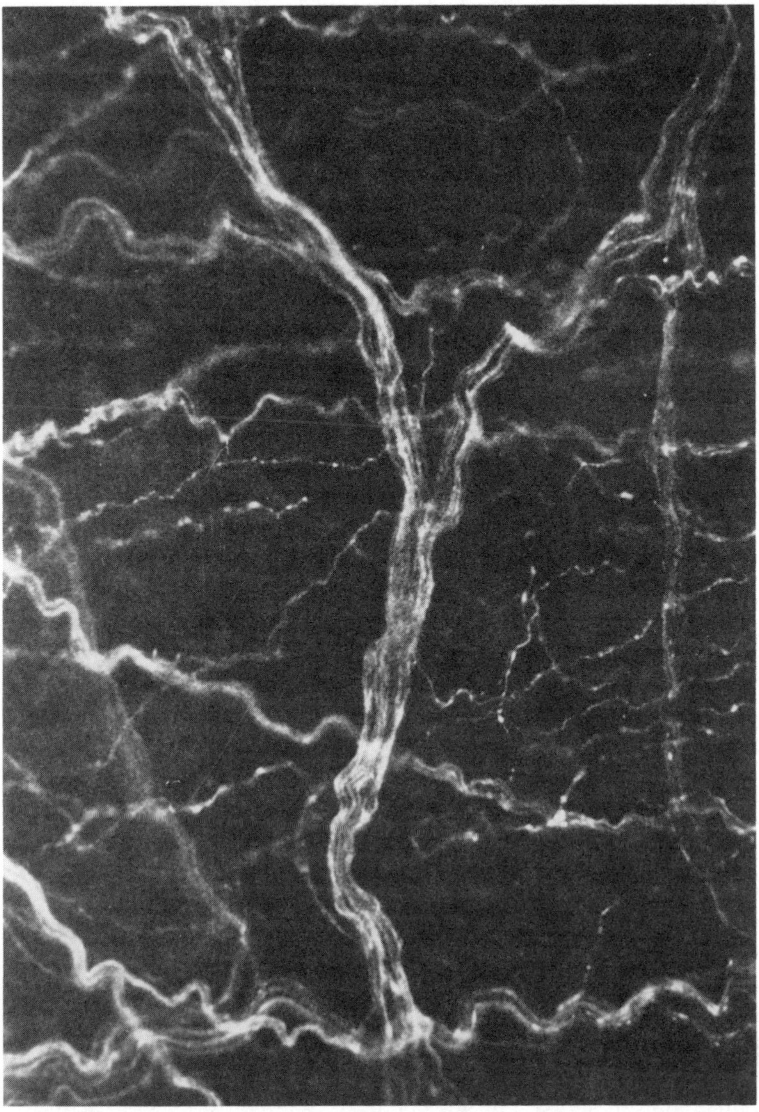

FIGURE 1. Whole-mount preparation of the canine basilar artery showing numerous CGRP-immunoreactive nerve fibers (×40).

III. VASODILATORY ACTIVITY OF CGRP

A. *IN VITRO* STUDIES

CGRP is a potent vasodilator of isolated pial arteries from humans, dogs, cats, pigs, rabbits, and rats and of parenchymal cerebral arterioles from rats.[10,11,12,13,14] CGRP applied perivascularly to the convexity pial arterioles of cats has been shown to produce vasodilation with a potency superior to that of SP, VIP, neurokinin A, or peptide histidine isoleucine (PHI).[15] This vasodilation is not an endothelium-dependent mechanism, as the response to CGRP does not require the presence of an intact endothelium. It is not antagonized by propranolol, atropine, methysergide, indomethacin, tetrodotoxin, VIP, or SP antagonist, suggesting that its action does not involve adrenergic, cholinergic, histaminergic, serotoninergic, SP, or VIP receptors, and that it does not stimulate either the arachidonic cascade or other neurogenic factors. The vasodilatory response of pial veins to CGRP or VIP is weaker than of pial arteries.[16]

The presence of specific binding sites for CGRP has been demonstrated by ^{125}I-CGRP binding and autoradiography studies in the rat heart, aorta, coronary arteries, and heart valves.[17] The CGRP receptor in the cat and rat cerebral blood vessels and the VIP receptor in bovine cerebral arteries[18,19] appear to be coupled to adenylate cyclase but not guanylate cyclase.[20] Cyclic AMP is, therefore, probably a second messenger in CGRP-mediated vasodilation in vascular smooth muscle. Notably, cyclic AMP is thought to mediate the actions of other vasodilatory peptides including VIP, PHI, and parathyroid hormone or forskolin.[21,22] The CGRP fragment human $CGRP_{8-37}$ has been shown to inhibit both CGRPstimulated adenylate cyclase activity and CGRP-induced vasorelaxation in a noncompetitive manner.[23] Recent evidence has shown that CGRP activates an ATP-sensitive K^+ channel in rabbit mesenteric artery muscle cells.[24] Further studies will elucidate whether this phenomen is mediated by cyclic AMP.

The response to SP, unlike that of CGRP or VIP, has been found to depend on the presence of an intact endothelium. SP released from the nerve terminals probably has to diffuse through the wall of the smooth muscle in order to reach the endothelium and produce its vasorelaxation effect. As this seems unlikely to occur in intact animals, the main action of SP on the vascular wall *in vivo* may be different from the endothelium-dependent vasodilation observed *in vitro*.

B. *IN VIVO* STUDIES

Administration of CGRP into the canine vertebral artery causes a dose-dependent, long-lasting increase in blood flow. The duration of this increase is significantly longer than that produced by either VIP or SP, but the maximal blood flow is not as high as that achieved with VIP or SP (Figures 2 and 3). Bolus injection of CGRP into the internal carotid artery also produces a long-

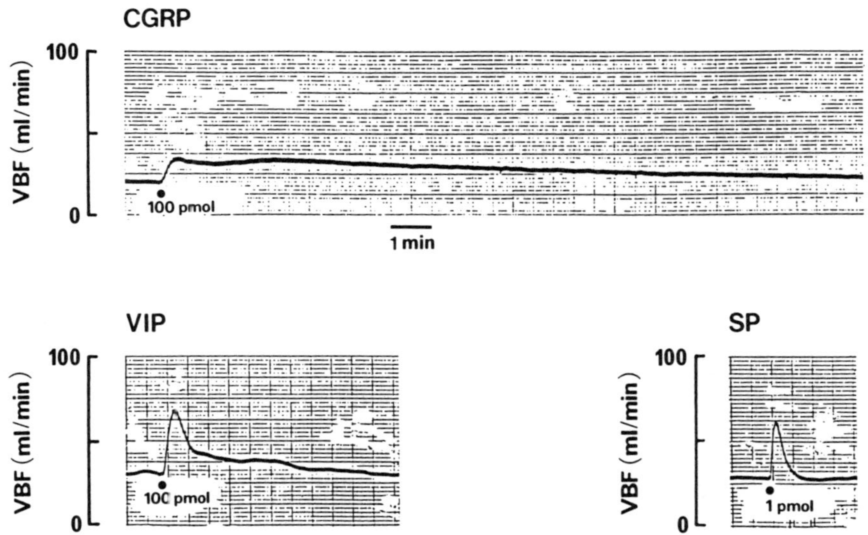

FIGURE 2. Vasodilatory responses induced by CGRP, VIP, and SP on canine vertebral blood flow. Each peptide was injected into the vertebral artery as a bolus. Vertebral blood flow was measured by means of an electromagnetic flow meter.

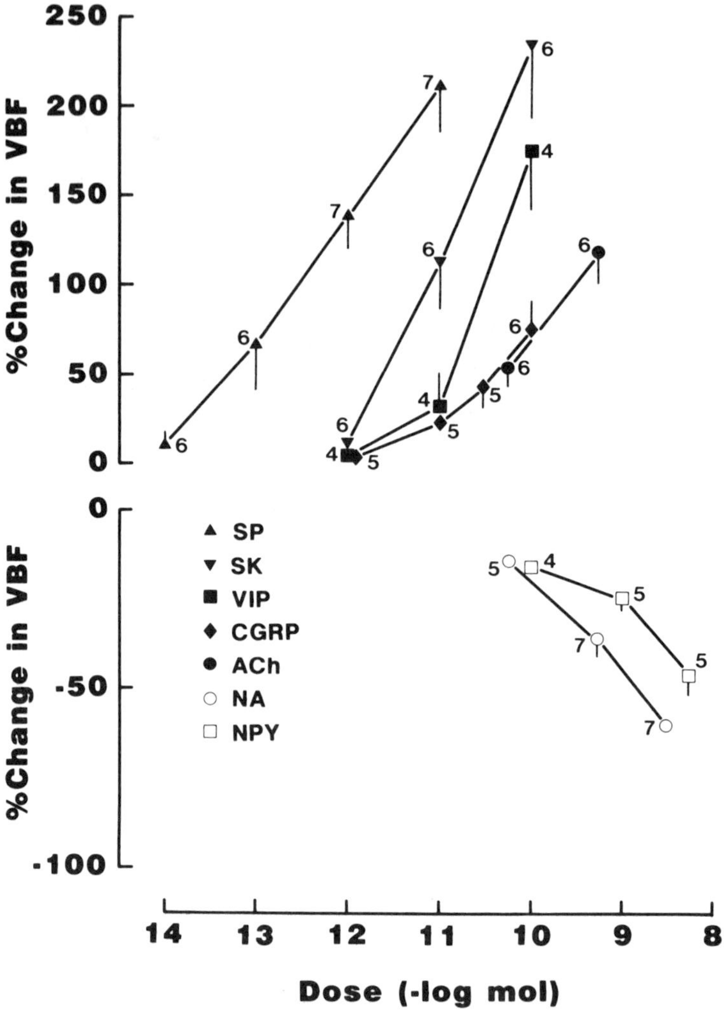

FIGURE 3. Comparison of the effects of vasoactive substances on canine vertebral blood flow. Maximum effect at each concentration was plotted as the mean ± SE obtained from the number of animals indicated beside each point. SK, substance K (neurokinin A); ACh, acetylcholine; NA, noradrenaline.

lasting increase in local cerebral blood flow (CBF) in rat striatum, without affecting mean systemic arterial pressure.[25] CGRP in low concentrations increases CBF, while CGRP in concentrations above 100 nmol induces a decrease in CBF, probably by influencing systemic blood pressure and heart function. Intravenous infusion of CGRP has been shown to increase internal carotid blood flow and cardiac output in human volunteers.[26] While *in vitro* studies clearly demonstrate a dose-dependent vasorelaxation by CGRP, other factors affecting general and local circulation may contribute to results obtained from *in vivo* studies. The amount of CGRP necessary to produce an increase in regional CBF *in vivo* appears to be very low. The half-life of CGRP in plasma has been reported to be biexponential, with a fast decay of less than 10 min and a slow decay of 26 min.[27] Its half-life is relatively long compared to that of VIP, which is probably one of the reasons why CGRP-mediated vasodilation lasts so long.

In recent studies, we demonstrated that intracisternal injection of CGRP dilates canine major cerebral arteries, including the vertebral and basilar arteries, and the circle of Willis and its main branches (Figure 4).[28] Vasodilatory stimulation from the adventitial side of vessels may be more physiologically relevant. Pretreatment with N^G-monomethyl-L-arginine (L-NMMA), which inhibits the formation of nitric oxide from L-arginine, did not affect CGRP-induced vasodilation, while vasopressin or SP-induced vasodilation was inhibited by L-NMMA and recovered by L-arginine. These results are consistent with previous *in vitro* results which show that the vasodilatory action of CGRP is not dependent on nitric oxide formation.

IV. RELEASE OF CGRP FROM SENSORY NERVE FIBERS

Most newly synthesized peptides are transported from ganglial cell bodies to afferent nerve fibers, where depolarization induced by nerve stimulation leads to release of neurotransmitter from nerve terminals in the wall of the cerebral blood vessels. Extracellular SP has been found in pial vessels after depolarization of sensory fibers *in vitro,* suggesting a similar mechanism of release to that of CGRP and other peptides, or indicating corelease of these peptides.[29] In fact, depolarization has been demonstrated to induce the release of CGRP from cultured trigeminal ganglion cells,[30] and the corelease of CGRP, SP, and tachykinins in spinal cord,[31] and perivascular electrical stimulation has been shown to induce the release of CGRP in peripheral arteries.[32] Also supporting such a mechanism of release, neurogenic vasodilation in cat cerebral artery has been found to be attenuated after incubation with tetrodotoxin or capsaicin. Capsaicin, a pungent agent found in hot peppers, leads to release of CGRP and SP from trigeminal nerve terminals. Furthermore, thermocoagulation of trigeminal ganglion in the treatment of trigeminal neuralgia in humans, and electrical stimulation of trigeminal ganglion in cats, is known to markedly increase the level of both SP and CGRP in the external jugular vein,[33,34] but not in peripheral veins.[35] Neurogenic vasodilation of extracephalic blood vessels following stimulation of the trigeminal ganglion usually increases extracerebral blood flow with facial flushing[36] and an elevation in skin temperature in the distribution of the stimulated divisions. These findings support the idea that CGRP-induced vasodilation is mediated by antidromic activation of trigeminal nerves.

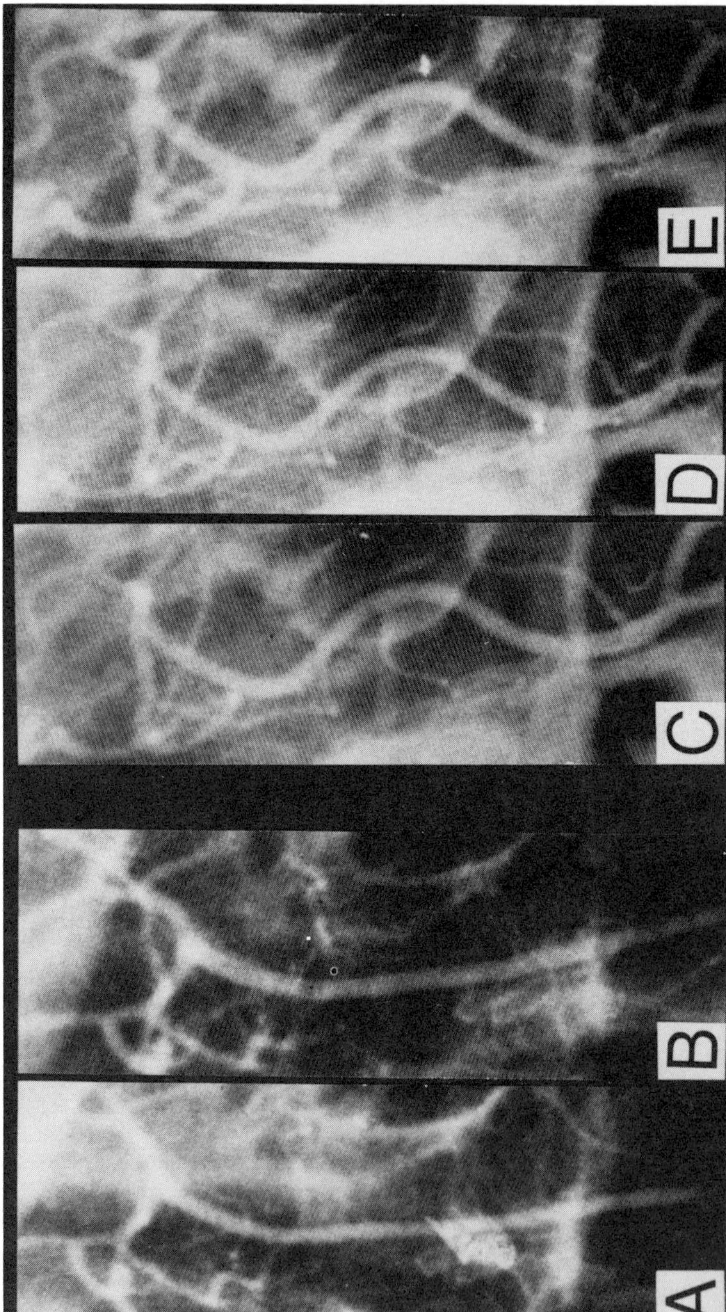

FIGURE 4. Vertebral angiograms showing the effect of CGRP and L-NMMA on the internal diameter of the canine basilar artery: (A) Control (before injection of CGRP); (B) 15 min after intracisternal injection of 1 nmol CGRP; (C) Control (before injection of L-NMMA); (D) 30 min after intracisternal injection of 10 μmol L-NMMA; (E) 15 min after intracisternal injection of 1 nmol CGRP following injection L-NMMA.

V. INFLUENCE OF SENSORY FIBERS ON CEREBRAL BLOOD FLOW

In addition to pain transmission, the trigeminovascular system is known to monitor luminal blood pressure and/or vessel wall tension, and thus may influence neurogenic adjustment of the local perfusion pressure or permeability by the stimulation of pial arteries. Denervation experiments help us understand the function of sensory fibers. Trigeminal ganglionectomy depletes the ipsilateral circle of Willis of SP and CGRP, but leaves the noradrenaline or NPY containing sympathetic and the VIP or PHI containing parasympathetic systems of innervation intact.

Neither the basal CBF nor the vasodilatory response to hypercapnia is influenced by deafferentation of sensory fibers.[37] Chronic denervation of the ipsilateral trigeminal nerve in cats increases the vasocontraction induced by noradrenaline, prostaglandin $F_{2\alpha}$, and alkaline CSF. Thus, the effects of vasoconstrictors are enhanced in the absence of sensory nerves. The increases in cortical gray matter blood flow induced both by acute severe hypertension ($190 <$ mean arterial pressure < 210 mmHg, which is beyond the limits of autoregulation) and by generalized seizures is reduced by 20 to 30% by trigeminal ganglionectomy in cats. Attenuation of flow was observed only within regions adjacent to pial arteries receiving innervation from the trigeminal nerve. Deep gray matter nuclei (thalamus. caudate) supplied by the posterior and middle cerebral arteries are minimally innervated by the trigeminal nerve and do not manifest significant differences in the blood flow between the deafferented and the intact side. Trigeminal ganglionectomy has also been found to diminish the extravasation of radiolabeled albumin which results from disruption of the blood-brain barrier.[38]

Sensory fibers may protect the brain circulation from severe vasocontraction by secreting stored CGRP and tachykinins, which restore normal vascular diameter.

VI. STRUCTURE-FUNCTION RELATIONSHIP

On the basis of the binding and bioassay studies using various CGRP fragments, analogue and homologues,[39,40] the N terminal portion of the molecule, which contains a disulfide bridge at positions 2 and 7, has been shown to be unnecessary for the binding of the ligand to the CGRP receptor. Whereas N terminal fragments lack biological and binding activity, C terminal fragments, including hCGRP,$_{12\text{-}27}$ bind with a relatively high affinity. A number of modifications of N terminal, including (Cys [ACM]^{2,7})hCGRP, cyclo^{2,7} (Asp,^{2} Lys^{7})hCGRP did not alter the binding affinity. Using the analogue DesAla deamino(Asu^{2,7})hCGRP to replace the S–S bond at positions 2 and 7 with a C–C bond did not detectably alter canine vertebral blood flow (Figure 5). These findings suggest that the C terminal contains the active site. A

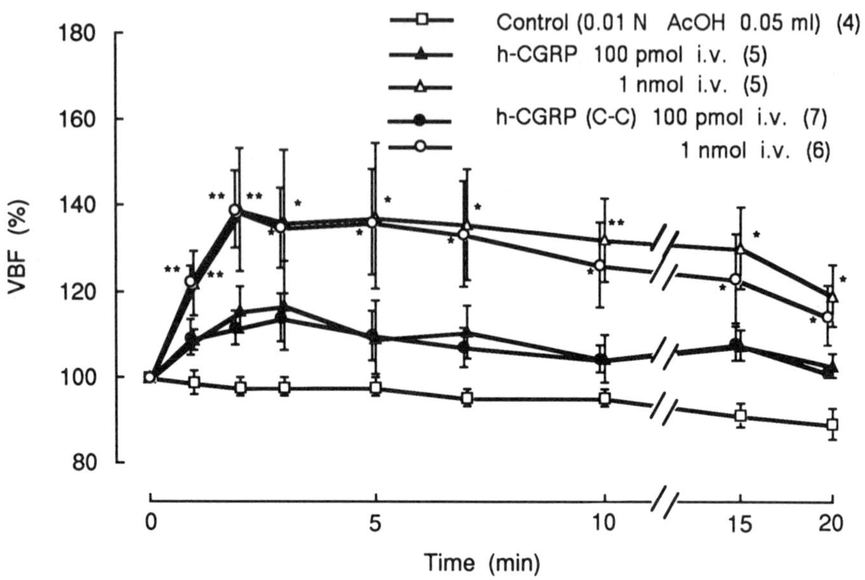

FIGURE 5. Effects of DesAla deamino (Asu^{2,7})hCGRP on canine vertebral blood flow.

recent study revealed that $CGRP_{8\text{-}37}$ displaced ^{125}I-Tyr^0 hCGRP binding and inhibited CGRP-induced cAMP accumulation in rat liver plasma membranes, suggesting that $CGRP_{8\text{-}37}$ is a CGRP receptor antagonist.[41] The authors of this study proposed that CGRP receptors sensitive to the antagonist activity of $CGRP_{8\text{-}37}$ be designated $CGRP_1$ receptors while those insensitive to $CGRP_{8\text{-}37}$ be designated $CGRP_2$. $CGRP_{8\text{-}37}$ antagonized both the vasorelaxant effect of CGRP and the CGRP-induced stimulation of adenylate cyclase in the rat cerebral arterioles, indicating that the receptor present on cerebral blood vessels is of the $CGRP_1$ subtype.

VII. PATHOLOGIC CONDITIONS

A. MIGRAINE

Nociceptive information from cranial blood vessels is conveyed to the central nervous system via sensory nerve fibers and is expressed as migraine or vascular headaches. Neurogenic inflammation (vasodilation and plasma protein extravasation) within cephalic tissues has been proposed as a possible mechanism of headache pathogenesis.[42] Neurogenic inflammation is mediated by the release of vasoactive neuropeptides, including SP, neurokinin A, and

CGRP, from sensory fibers. Large pial arteries with dense sensory innervations are more sensitive to stimulation of the proximal segments, but become progressively less sensitive over the hemispheric convexities. Vascular pain in humans is usually referred to the ipsilateral temporal, retro-orbital, and frontal region, and is expressed as throbbing, aching, burning, or crushing. The decline in CGRP concentration with age corresponds well with the reduced frequency and intensity of migraine attacks noted with advancing age. In all patients suffering from either classical or common migraines, CGRP is elevated in the cranial but not in the peripheral blood during migraine attacks.[43] The increase of CGRP levels in the external jugular vein is greater in classic migraine than in common migraine.

B. SUBARACHNOID HEMORRHAGE

A reduction of CGRP has been demonstrated in perivascular nerves of cerebral arteries during the acute stage of subarachnoid hemorrhage (SAH).[44-48] The reduction in CGRP appears to be greater than that of SP. Subarachnoid blood may stimulate the secretion of peptides from the nerve terminals, ultimately leading to their depletion. CGRP levels were found to be increased in the external jugular vein following SAH in man.[49] While increased levels of CGRP in plasma or in CSF after SAH may serve as a defense system protecting the brain from acute vasospasm, depletion of CGRP or tachykinins from sensory fibers during the chronic stage may promote the prolonged vasospasm which often causes ischemic brain damage. Since there is no mechanism for reuptake of peptides into nerve terminals, the replenishment of the terminal stores requires new synthesis in nerve cell bodies and therefore depletion following SAH usually persists for several weeks.

Not all experimental animals exhibit an alteration in the responsiveness and sensitivity of cerebral arteries to exogenous CGRP after SAH. For example, CGRPinduced relaxation is unaltered in rabbit cerebral arteries[50] but is increased in the rat basilar artery and is slightly decreased in the canine basilar artery.

In a preliminary clinical trial, systemic infusion of CGRP was given to patients with neurological deficits following intracranial aneurysm surgery for SAH.[51] Improvements in neurological evaluation and in blood flow velocity in the middle cerebral artery as detected by transcranial Doppler were found in the group treated with CGRP. Since CGRP significantly modified cardiac function and peripheral circulation, it was not possible to use high doses of CGRP without causing severe hypotension with a probable decrease in CBF.

Data from canine studies suggest that a different therapeutic approach, intracisternal injection of CGRP, might reverse cerebral arterial spasm after SAH. It is highly likely that high concentrations of CGRP are maintained around the major cerebral arteries following intracisternal injection of CGRP, accompanied by a slight increase in mean arterial blood pressure and heart rate. When injected into the ventricles or cisterns, CGRP may, in addition to its direct effect on the vascular smooth muscle, have a variety of effects due to stimulation of the brain parenchyma. It may, for example, cause a rise in plasma noradrenaline levels, a rise in mean arterial blood pressure, or a suppression of the gastrointestinal tract.[52]

C. CEREBRAL HYPERPERFUSION SYNDROMES

Reactive hyperemia occurs during reperfusion following acute or chronic vascular occlusion of tissues. It is characterized by cerebral blood flow exceeding the metabolic needs of the brain and is accompanied by acute increases in systemic blood pressure, vasodilation, and breakdown of the blood-brain barrier, all of which may complicate the original insult by exacerbating cerebral edema or intraparenchymal hemorrhage. Pathologic conditions which can result in reactive hyperemia include embolic stroke, carotid endarterectomy, seizures, head trauma, and excision of large arteriovenous malformations. Recent experimental evidence has demonstrated that postocclusive hyperemia in cortical gray matter is significantly attenuated by either trigeminal ganglionectomy or by pretreatment with capsaicin.[53,54] The attenuation was, however, insignificant in regions with minimal trigeminal innervation. It has been suggested that the vasodilatory sensory neuropeptides mediated by reflex mechanisms contribute significantly to the generation of hyperperfusion. CGRP rather than SP or neurokinin A appeared to be the most important mediator of the neurogenic component of cortical hyperemia. Other neurogenic contribution would include parasympathetic VIP-containing innervations, and nonneurologenic factors would include a variety of substances such as free oxygen radicals, adenosine, nitric oxide, and arachidonic metabolites. The finding that neuropeptides released from sensory fibers contribute to reactive hyperemia indicates the utility of therapeutic approaches based on the inactivation of sensory innervation or neuropeptides.

REFERENCES

1. **Mayberg, M. R., Langer, R. S., Zervas, N. T., and Moskowitz, M. A.,** Perivascular meningeal projections from cat trigeminal ganglia: possible pathway for vascular headache in man, *Science,* 213, 228, 1981.
2. **Mayberg, M. R., Zervas, N. T., and Moskowitz, M. A.,** Trigeminal projections to supratentorial pial and dural blood vessels in cats demonstrated by horseradish peroxidase histochemistry, *J. Comp. Neurol.,* 223, 46, 1984.
3. **Saito, K. and Moskowitz, M. A.,** Contributions from the upper cervical dorsal roots and trigeminal ganglia to the feline circle of Willis, *Stroke,* 20, 524, 1989.
4. **Edvinsson, L., Hara, H., and Uddman, R.,** Retrograde tracing of nerve fibers to the rat middle cerebral artery with true blue: colocalization with different peptides, *J. Cereb. Blood Flow Metab.,* 9, 212, 1989.

5. **Hardebo, J. E., Arbab, M., Suzuki, N., and Svendgaard, N. A.,** Pathways of parasympathetic and sensory cerebrovascular nerves in monkeys, *Stroke,* 122, 331, 1991.
6. **Ruskell, G. L. and Simons, T.,** Trigeminal nerve pathways to the cerebral arteries in monkey, *J. Anat.,* 155, 23, 1987.
7. **Nakakita, K.,** Peptidergic innervation in the cerebral blood vessels of the guinea pig: an immunohistochemical study, *J. Cereb. Blood Flow Metab.,* 10, 819, 1990.
8. **Uddman, R., Edvinsson, L., Ekman, R., Kingman, T., and McCulloch, J.,** Innervation of the feline cerebral vasculature by nerve fibers containing calcitonin gene-related peptide: trigeminal origin and co-existence with substance P, *Neurosci. Lett.,* 62, 131, 1985.
9. **Saito, A., Masaki, T., Uchiyama, Y., Lee, T. J-F., and Goto, K.,** Calcitonin gene-related peptide and vasodilator nerves in large cerebral arteries of cats, *J. Pharmacol. Exp. Ther.,* 248, 455, 462, 1989.
10. **Edvinsson, L., Ekman, R., Jansen, I., Ottosson, A., and Uddman, R.,** Peptide-containing nerve fibers in human cerebral arteries: Immunocytochemistry, radioimmunoassay, and in vitro pharmacology, *Ann. Neurol.,* 21, 431, 1987.
11. **Hanko, J., Hardebo, J. E., Kahrstrom, J., Owman, C., and Sundler, F.,** Calcitonin gene-related peptide is present in mammalian cerebrovascular nerve fibers and dilates pial and peripheral arteries, *Neurosci. Lett.,* 57, 91, 1985.
12. **Ikegaki, I., Suzuki, Y., Satoh, S., Asano, T., Shibuya, M., and Sugita, K.,** Effects of calcitonin gene-related peptide on canine cerebral arterial strips and the in-vivo vertebral blood flow in dogs, *Naunyn-Schmiedebergs Arch. Pharmakol.,* 340, 431, 1989.
13. **Mejia, J. A., Pernom, J., von Holst, H., Rudehill, A., and Lundberg, J. M.,** Effects of neuropeptide Y, calcitonin gene-related peptide, substance P, and capsaicin on cerebral arteries in man and animals, *J. Neurosurg.,* 69, 913, 1988.
14. **Nozaki, K., Uemura, Y., Okamoto, S., Kikuchi, H., and Mizuno, N.,** Relaxant effect of calcitonin gene-related peptide on cerebral arterial spasm induced by experimental subarachnoid hemorrhage in dogs, *J. Neurosurg.,* 71, 558, 1989.
15. **McCulloch, J., Uddman, R., Kingman, T. A., and Edvinsson, L.,** Calcitonin gene-related peptide: functional role in cerebrovascular regulation, *Proc. Natl. Acad. U.S.A.,* 83, 5731, 1986.
16. **Edvinsson, L., McCulloch, J., and Uddman, R.,** Feline cerebral veins and arteries: comparison of autonomic innervation and vasomotor responses, *J. Physiol.,* 325, 161, 1982.
17. **Sigrist, S., Franco-Cereceda, A., Muff, R., Henke, H., Lundberg, J. M., and Fischer, J. A.,** Specific receptor and cardiovascular effects of calcitonin gene-related peptide, *Endocrinology,* 119, 381, 1986.
18. **Poulin, P., Suzuki, Y., Lederis, K., and Rorstad, O. P.,** Autoradiographic localization of binding sites for vasoactive intestinal peptide (VIP) in bovine cerebral arteries, *Brain Res.,* 381, 382, 1986.
19. **Suzuki, Y., McMaster, D., Huang, M., Lederis, K., and Rorstad, O.,** Characterization of functional receptors for vasoactive intestinal peptide in bovine cerebral arteries, *J. Neurochem.,* 45, 890, 1985.
20. **Kubota, M., Moseley, J. M., Butera, L., Dusting, G. J., MacDonald, P. S., and Martin, T. J.,** Calcitonin gene-related peptide stimulates cyclic AMP formation in rat aortic smooth muscle cells, *Biochem. Biophys. Res. Commun.,* 132, 88, 1985.
21. **Huang, M. and Rorstad, O. P.,** Cerebral vascular adenylate cyclase: evidence for coupling to receptors for vasoactive intestinal peptide and parathyroid hormone, *J. Neurochem.,* 43, 849, 1984.
22. **Suzuki, Y., Huang, M., Lederis, K., and Rorstad, O.,** The role of adenylate cyclase in relaxation of brain arteries: studies with forskolin, *Brain Res.,* 457, 241, 1988.
23. **Edwards, R. M., Stack, E. J., and Trizna, W.,** Calcitonin gene-related peptide stimulates adenylate cyclase and relaxes intracerebral arterioles, *J. Pharmacol. Exp. Ther.,* 257, 1020, 1991.

24. **Nelson, M. T., Huang, Y., Brayden, J. E., Hescheler, J., and Standen, N.,** Arterial dilations in response to calcitonin generelated peptide involve activation of K^+ channels, *Nature,* 344, 770, 1990.
25. **Suzuki, Y., Satoh, S., Ikegaki, I., Okada, T., Shibuya, M., Sugita, K., and Asano, T.,** Effects of neuropeptide Y and calcitonin gene-related peptide on local cerebral blood flow in rat striatum, *J. Cereb. Blood Flow Metab.,* 9, 268, 1989.
26. **Struthers, A. D., Brown, M. J., MacDonald, D. W. R., Beacham, J. L., Stevenson, J. C., Morris, H. R., and MacIntyre, I.,** Human calcitonin gene related peptide: a potent endogenous vasodilator in man, *Clin. Sci.,* 70, 389, 1986.
27. **Kraenzlin, M. E., Ch'ng, J. L. C., Mulderry, P. K., Ghatei, M. A., and Bloom, S. R.,** Infusion of a novel peptide, calcitonin gene-related peptide (CGRP) in man. Pharmacokinetics and effects on gastric acid secretion and on gastrointestinal hormones, *Regul. Pept.,* 10, 189, 1985.
28. **Suzuki, Y., Satoh, S., Kimura, M., Oyama, H., Asano, T., Shibuya, M., and Sugita, K.,** Effects of vasopressin and oxytocin on canine cerebral circulation *in vivo, J. Neurosurg.,* 77, 424, 1992.
29. **Moskowitz, M. A., Brody, M. R., and Liu-Chen, L-Y.,** In vitro release of immunoreactive substance P from putative afferent nerve endings in bovine pia arachnoid, *Neuroscience,* 9, 809, 1983.
30. **Mason, R. T., Peterfreund, R. A., Sawchenko, P. F., Corrigan, A. Z., Rivier, J. E., and Vale, W. W.,** Release of the predicted calcitonin gene-related peptide from cultured rat trigeminal ganglion cells, *Nature,* 308, 653, 19.
31. **Saria, A., Gamse, R., Petermann, J., Fischer, J. A., Theodorsson-Norheim, E., and Lundberg, J. M.,** Simultaneous release of several tachykinins and calcitonin gene-related peptide from rat spinal cord slices, *Neurosci. Lett.,* 63, 310, 1986.
32. **Fujimori, A., Saito, A., Kimura, S., Watanabe, T., Uchiyama, Y., Kawasaki, H., and Goto, K.,** Neurogenic vasodilation and release of calcitonin gene-related peptide (CGRP) from perivascular nerves in the rat mesenteric artery, *Biochem. Biophys. Res. Commun.,* 165, 1391, 1989.
33. **Goadsby, P. J., Lambert, G. A., and Lance, J. W.,** Stimulation of the trigeminal ganglion increases flow in the extracerebral but not the cerebral circulation of the monkey, *Brain Res.,* 381, 63, 1986.
34. **Goadsby, P. J., Edvinsson, L., and Ekman, R.,** Vasoactive peptide release in the extracerebral circulation of humans during migraine headache, *Ann. Neurol.,* 28, 183, 1990.
35. **Schon, F., Thomas, D. T., Jewkes, D. A., Ghatei, M. A., Mulderry, P. K., and Bloom, S. R.,** Failure to detect plasma neuropeptide release during trigeminal thermocoagulation, *J. Neurol. Neurosurg. Psychiatry,* 50, 642, 1987.
36. **Lambert, G. A., Bogduk, N., Goadsby, P. J., Duckworth, J. W., and Lance, J. W.,** Decreased carotid arterial resistance in cats in response to trigeminal stimulation, *J. Neurosurg.,* 61, 307, 1984.
37. **Sakas, D. E., Moskowitz, M. A., Wei, E. P., Kontos, H. A., Kano, M., and Ogilvy, C. S.,** Trigeminovascular fibers increase blood flow in cortical gray matter by axon reflex-like mechanisms during acute severe hypertension or seizures, *Proc. Natl. Acad. Sci. U.S.A.,* 86, 1041, 1989.
38. **Moskowitz, M. A., Sakas, D. E., Wei, E. P., Kano, M., Buzzi, M. G., Ogilvy, C., and Kontos, H. A.,** Postocclusive cerebral hyperemia is markedly attenuated by chronic trigeminal ganglionectomy, *Am. J. Physiol.,* 257, H1736, 1989.
39. **Dennis, T., Fournier, A., Pierre, S. S., and Quirion, R.,** Structure-activity profile of calcitonin gene-related peptide in peripheral and brain tissues. Evidence for receptor multiplicity, *J. Pharmacol. Exp. Ther.,* 251, 718, 1989.

40. **Dennis, T., Fournier, A., Cadieux, A., Pomerleau, F., Jolicoeur, F. B., Pierre, S. S., and Quirion, R.,** hCGRP8-37, a calcitonin gene-related peptide antagonist revealing calcitonin gene-related peptide receptor heterogeneity in brain and periphery, *J. Pharmacol. Exp. Ther.*, 254, 123, 1990.
41. **Chiba, T., Yamaguchi, A., Yamatani, T., Nakamura, A., Morishita, T., Inui, T., Fukase, M., Noda, T., and Fujita, T.,** Calcitonin gene-related peptide receptor antagonist human CGRP-(8-37), *Am. J. Physiol.*, 256, E331, 1989.
42. **Moskowitz, M. A.,** The neurobiology of vascular head pain, *Ann. Neurol.*, 16, 157, 1984.
43. **Olesen, J. and Edvinsson, L.,** Migraine: a research field matured for the basic neurosciences, *TINS*, 14, 3, 1991.
44. **Ariente, C., Balbi, S., Caroli, M., and Fumagalli, G.,** Depletion of calcitonin gene-related peptide in perivascular nerves during acute phase of posthemorrhagic vasospasm in the rabbit, *Brain Res. Bull.*, 27, 605, 1991.
45. **Edvinsson, L., Uddman, R., and Juul, R.,** Peptidergic innervation of the cerebral circulation. Role in subarachnoid hemorrhage in man, *Neurosurg. Rev.*, 13, 265, 1990.
46. **Edvinsson, L., Delgado-Zygmunt, T., Ekman, R., Jansen, I., Svendgaard, N. A., and Uddman, R.,** Involvement of perivascular sensory fibers in the pathophysiology of cerebral vasospasm following subarachnoid hemorrhage, *J. Cereb. Blood Flow Metab.*, 10, 602, 1990.
47. **Hara, H. and Edvinsson, L.,** Perivascular innervation of the cerebral circulation: involvement in the pathophysiology of subarachnoid hemorrhage, *Neurosurg. Rev.*, 10, 171, 1987.
48. **Nozaki, K., Okamoto, S., Uemura, Y., Kikuchi, H., and Mizuno, N.,** Erythrocytes suppress calcitonin gene-related peptide- and vasoactive intestinal polypeptide-like immunoreactivies in cerebrovascular nerve fibers after subarachnoid hemorrhage, *Neurosci. Lett.*, 110, 22, 1990.
49. **Juul, R., Edvinsson, L., Gisvold, S. E., Ekman, R., Brubakk, A. O., and Fredriksen, T. A.,** Calcitonin gene-related peptide-LI in subarachnoid hemorrhage in man. Signs of activation of the trigemino-cerebrovascular system? *Br. J. Neurosurg.*, 4, 171, 1990.
50. **Hongo, K., Tsukahara, T., Kassell, N., and Ogawa, H.,** Effect of subarachnoid hemorrhage on calcitonin gene-related peptide-induced relaxation in rabbit basilar artery, *Stroke*, 20, 100, 1989.
51. **Johnston, F. G., Bell, B. A., Robertson, I. J. A., Miller, J. D., Haliburn, C., O'Shaughnessy, D., Riddell, A. J., and O'Laorie, S. A.,** Effect of calcitonin gene-related peptide on postoperative neurological deficits after subarachnoid hemorrhage, *Lancet*, 335, 869, 1990.
52. **Fisher, L. A., Kikkawa, D. O., Rivier, J. E., Amara, S. G., Evans, R. M., Rosenfeld, M. G., Vale, W. W., and Brown, M. R.,** Stimulation of noradrenergic sympathetic outflow by calcitonin gene-related peptide, *Nature*, 305, 534, 1983.
53. **Macfarlane, R., Moskowitz, M. A., Tasdemiroglu, E., Wei, E. P., and Kontos, H. A.,** Postischemic cerebral blood flow and neuroeffector mechanisms, *Blood Vessels*, 28, 46, 1991.
54. **Macfarlane, R., Tasdemiroglu, E., Moskowitz, M. A., Uemura, Y., Wei, E. P., and Kontos, H. A.,** Chronic trigeminal ganglionectomy or tropical capsaicin application to pial vessels attenuates postocclusive cortical hyperemia but does not influence postischemic hypoperfusion, *J. Cereb. Blood Flow Metab.*, 11, 261, 1991.

Chapter 12

TACHYKININS AND CEREBRAL BLOOD FLOW

Toru Itakura and Takashi Okuno

TABLE OF CONTENTS

I. Introduction 196

II. General Considerations 196

III. Morphology of Tachykinin Nerves in the Cerebral Blood Vessels 199
- A. Substance P-Containing Nerve Fibers 199
  - 1. Distribution and Running Pattern 199
  - 2. Origin of SP Nerve Fibers 200
- B. Neurokinin A 202
- C. Neurokinin B 202
- D. Neuropeptide K 202

IV. Pharmacology of Tachykinins in the Cerebral Blood Vessels 204
- A. Substance P 204
- B. Neurokinin A and B 204
- C. Neuropeptide K 204

V. Clinical Considerations 204
- A. Migraine 204
- B. Cerebral Vasospasm after Subarachnoid Hemorrhage (SAH) 205

References 206

0-8493-5096-0/93/$0.00 + $.50

I. INTRODUCTION

Aminergic,[1-4] cholinergic,[5-7] and some peptidergic nerve fibers have been demonstrated in cerebral blood vessels. Among the peptidergic nerve fibers, those containing vasoactive intestinal polypeptide (VIP), neuropeptide Y (NPY), calcitonin gene-related peptide (CGRP), and substance P (SP) are densely located in cerebral blood vessels.[8-15] Recent investigations have also demonstrated that gamma-aminobutyric acid (GABA), one of the main inhibitory amino acid neurotransmitters in the central nervous system (CNS), also occurs in cerebral arteries.[16,17] Pharmacological studies have shown that relaxation induced by isoproterenol is inhibited by the exogenous application of GABA in tissue bath experiments.[18] Thus, cerebral blood vessels are innervated in a complex manner by a considerable number of vasodilator and vasoconstrictor nerves that contain various neurotransmitters.

SP-containing nerve fibers densely innervate not only cerebral arteries[19-22] but also cerebral veins[23] as a vasodilator or a sensory nerve. In addition, neurokinin A (NKA)[24] and neurokinin B (NKB),[24] which are classified into the tachykinin group with SP, have been shown to play important roles in cerebral blood flow (CBF).[24,25] The aim of this review is to summarize the role of the tachykinins on CBF from morphological and pharmacological aspects.

II. GENERAL CONSIDERATIONS

A family of tachykinins, which literally means fast acting, is a group of vasoactive peptides sharing Phe–X–Gly–Leu–Met–NH2 in the carboxyl terminal.[26] SP, NKA, NKB, neuropeptide K (NPK), and neuropeptide gamma (NPG) have been demonstrated in mammals,[27-32] while the similar tachykinin peptides physalaemin, kassinin, and eledoisin exist in amphibians and molluscans[33-37] (Figure 1). These tachykinins induce hypotension, salivary secretion, and constriction of smooth muscles in the gastrointestinal, urogenital, and respiratory tracts.[26]

SP was first extracted from the equine brain by von Euler and Gaddum in 1931[27] and was demonstrated to be widely distributed in both the CNS and the peripheral nervous system, being regarded as a transmitter mediating nociceptive stimuli.[38] SP-immunoreactive nerve fibers have been demonstrated by immunohistochemistry in human, pig, cat, rabbit, guinea pig, and rat cerebral arteries.[39-45] For many years, SP was thought to be the only tachykinin in the mammalian brain. However, recent studies demonstrated that several homologues of SP can be extracted from amphibian and molluscan tissues.[33-37] NKA and NKB, members of another tachykinin group, were isolated from the porcine spinal cord[29] and the existence of the two tachykinins in the CNS was established. The distribution of NKA is quite similar to that of SP in the brain, which is densely distributed in the substantia nigra,

Tachykinin in Mammals

Arg — Pro — Lys — Pro — Gln — Gln — Phe — Phe — Gly — Leu — Met — NH2 ***Substance P***

His — Lys — Thr — Asp — Ser — Phe — Val — Gly — Leu — Met — NH2

Neurokinin A

Asp — Met — His — Asp — Phe — Phe — Val — Gly — Leu — Met — NH2

Neurokinin B

Asp — Ala — Asp — Ser — Ser — Ile — Glu — Lys — Gln — Val — Ala — Leu — Leu — Lys — Ala — Leu — Tyr — Gly — His — Gly — Gln — Ile — Ser — His — Lys — Arg — His — Lys — Thr — Asp — Ser — Phe — Val — Gly — Leu — Met — NH2

Neuropeptide K

Asp — Ala — Gly — His — Gly — Gln — Ile — Ser — His — Lys — Arg — His — Lys — Thr — Asp — Ser — Phe — Val — Gly — Leu — Met — NH2

Neuropeptide G

Tachykinin in Amphibians

pGlu — Ala — Asp — Pro — Asn — Lys — PPhe — Tyr — Gly — Leu — Met — NH2

Physalaemin

Asp — Val — Pro — Lys — Ser — Asp — Gln — Phe — Val — Gly — Leu — Met — NH2

Kassinin

FIGURE 1. Tachykinin groups in mammals and amphibians.

habenular nucleus, and nucleus tractus solitarius.[46,47] NKB is distributed in the globus pallidus and the hypothalamus,[47] unlike SP. The difference in the distribution of these tachykinins is based on different expression of genes. SP and NKA are expressed from the same SP/NKA gene[48-50] (Figure 2), but NKB is expressed from a different gene.[51,52] NPK is a prolonged form of NKA that is expressed from the SP/NKA gene and has potent effects at low doses on the salivation response of rats.[53]

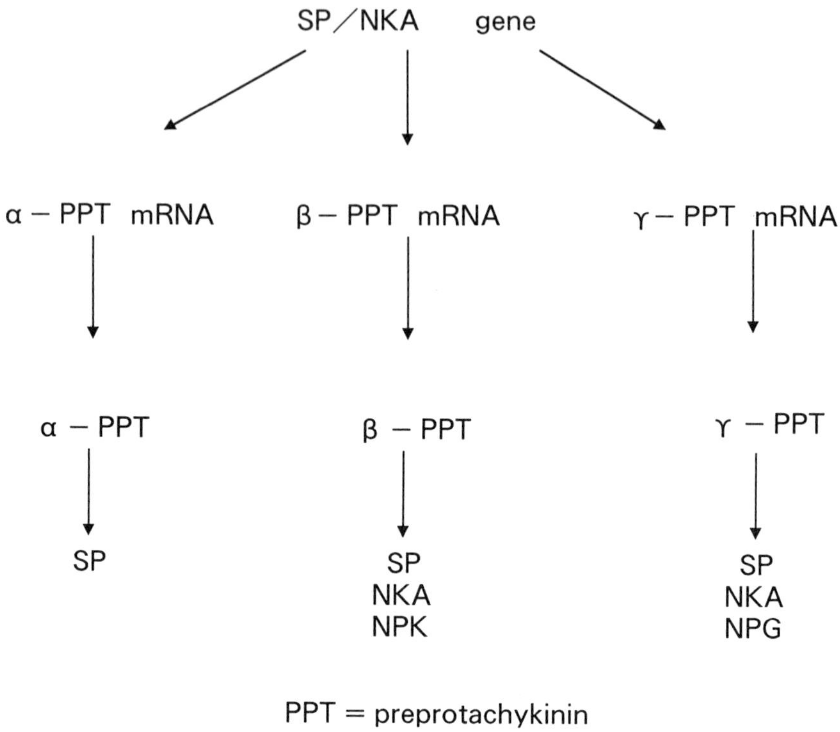

FIGURE 2. Schematic representation of the preprotachykinin gene.

There are three kinds of tachykinin receptors: NK1, NK2, and NK3.[54-56] The ligand specificity is SP=1 > NKA=0.06 > NKB=0.01 in NK1, NKA > NKB > SP in NK2, and NKB > NKA > SP in NK3.[57] NK1 receptor (for SP) is expressed in the brain, duodenum, and colon. NK2 (for NKA) is in the stomach, duodenum, and colon but not in the brain, which shows a mismatch of the peptide and the receptor, because high concentrations of NKA have been measured in the brain, but no NK2 receptors for NKA have been found in the brain. NK3 (for NKB) receptors have been found primarily in the CNS, especially in the deep layer of the cerebral cortex.[58]

Mechanisms underlying the vasodilative effects of tachykinins are still unknown. Tachykinins (e.g., SP) bind to the NK1 receptor on the surface of the endothelium, which opens the C^{2+} channel and induces Ca^{2+} influx into the endothelium. Ca^{2+} produces EDRF (endothelium-derived relaxing factor), nitric oxide(NO), from L-arginine. Then NO stimulates guanylate cyclase producing cyclic GMP in the vascular smooth muscle, which results in muscle relaxation[59] (Figure 3).

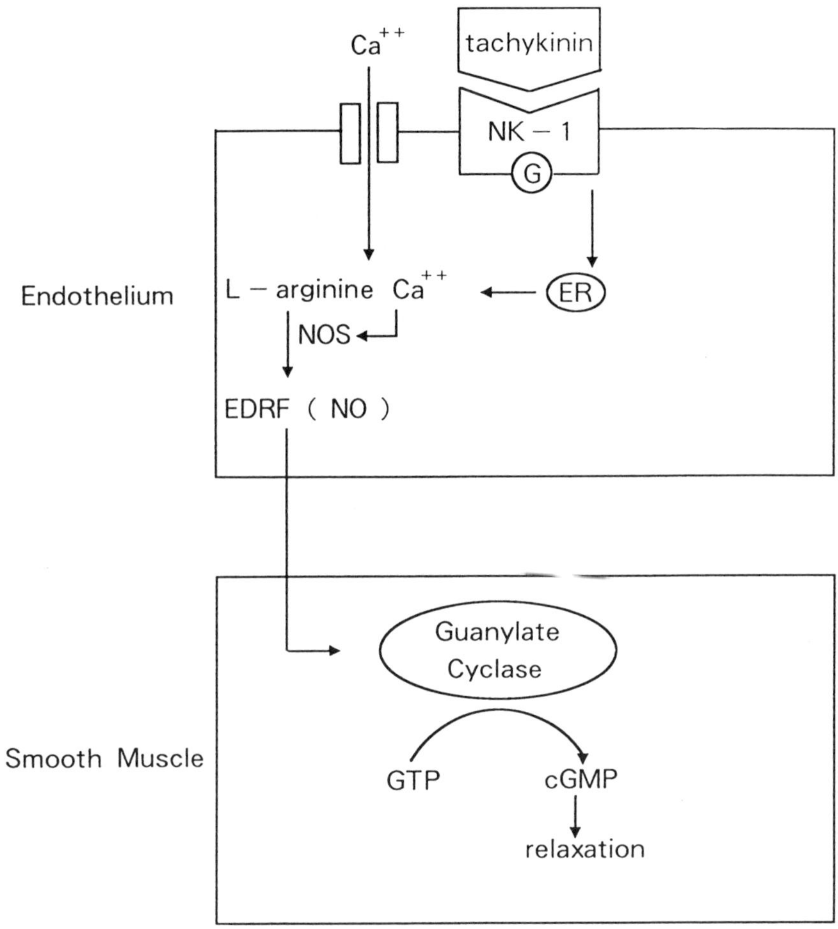

FIGURE 3. Mechanism of the action of the tachykinin in the blood vessel.

III. MORPHOLOGY OF TACHYKININ NERVES IN THE CEREBRAL BLOOD VESSELS

A. SUBSTANCE P-CONTAINING NERVE FIBERS

1. Distribution and Running Pattern

High concentrations of SP were measured in cerebral blood vessels by high performance liquid chromatography.[60,61] Immunohistochemical techniques have demonstrated SP-immunopositive nerve fibers in cerebral arteries and veins. In the cerebral artery, the anterior portion of the Willis ring is most densely innervated by this nerve, whereas SP fibers are sparsely found in the vertebrobasilar system[45] as well as other perivascular nerve fibers.

Cerebral veins also show dense innervation by SP-immunoreactive nerve fibers, although the density of the fibers is slightly less in the veins than in the cerebral arteries.[23] Among the cerebral veins, these fibers are densest in the deep cerebral veins such as the internal cerebral vein[62] and are sparsest in the superficial cortical veins. In the nerve fibers along the cerebral veins, only norepinephrine (NE)- and SP-containing nerve fibers are densely observed.[62] The running pattern of the SP-immunoreactive nerve fibers is a meshwork in both the artery (Figure 4a) and vein, which contrasts with a spiral running pattern in other vasoactive cerebral nerves.[21,62] For example, NE- or VIP-containing nerve fibers show a spiral running pattern similar to that of vascular smooth muscle cells[21] (Figure 4b). This unique running pattern of SP-containing nerve fibers suggests that the perivascular SP nerve may contribute to nonvasomotor activity such as sensory or trophic actions. The application of capsaicin, a neurotoxic agent, to the C-type (unmyelinated) fibers in the afferents[63] induces a decrease in SP-containing nerve fibers in cerebral arteries,[50,64] which indicates that perivascular SP fibers are axon nerve fibers in the sensory neurons. Edvinsson et al. demonstrated that SP-immunoreactive nerve fibers run in the same manner as CGRP-immunoreactive fibers in the cerebral artery, and colocalization of these two peptides is shown in the cerebrovascular nerves by the double immunolabeling method.[65-68] Ultrastructural studies demonstrated that SP-immunoreactive nerve terminals are found in the adventitial layer of the blood vessels. SP-immunoreactive terminal boutons have been observed slightly apart from the muscle cells.[21] The distance between the nerve terminal and vascular smooth muscle cell is longer than that of NE- and VIP-immunoreactive terminal boutons, which are observed very close to the smooth muscle cell.[21,62,69] These ultrastructural findings support the hypothesis of a nonvasomotor action of SP nerve fibers on the cerebral blood vessel, although *in vitro* tissue bath studies showed a potent vasodilative effect of SP on the cerebral artery.[19,41]

2. Origin of SP Nerve Fibers

Sympathectomy does not induce the disappearance of perivascular SP-immunoreactive nerves,[7] while NE- and NPY-containing nerve fibers are lost after sympathectomy.[70] In contrast,[71] trigeminal ganglionectomy produces a loss of SP fibers around cerebral blood vessels and reduces the SP content in the Willis ring to less than half.[61,65] This suggests that most SP-containing nerves in the cerebral blood vessels originated from the trigeminal ganglion, but some may have originated from ganglia other than the trigeminal. Furthermore, retrograde dye tracers, such as horseradish peroxidase (HRP) and true blue, injected around the middle cerebral artery are transported to the nerve cells in the trigeminal ganglion, the dorsal root ganglion of the spinal

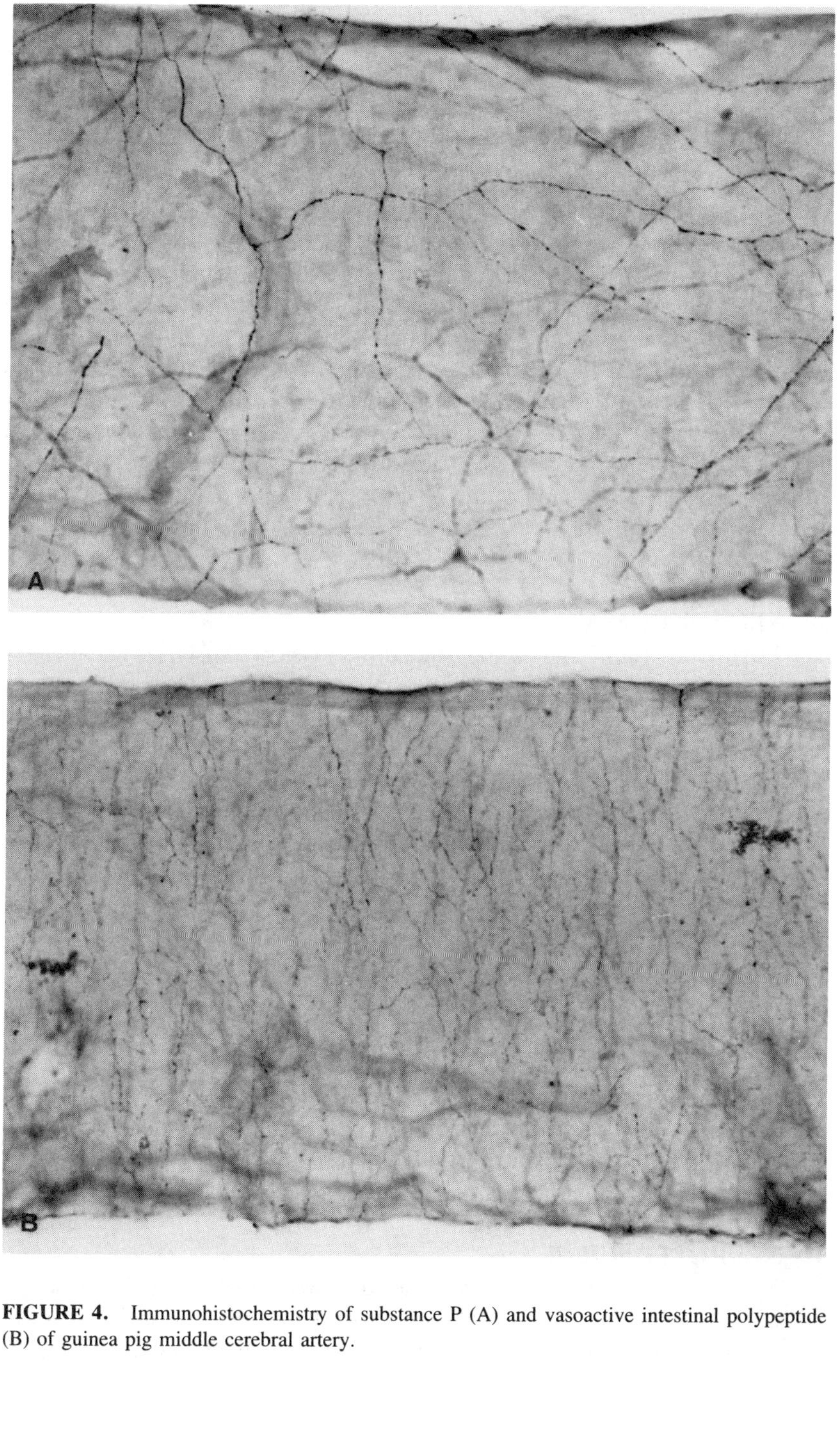

FIGURE 4. Immunohistochemistry of substance P (A) and vasoactive intestinal polypeptide (B) of guinea pig middle cerebral artery.

cord (C2 level),[72,73] and the miniganglia around the internal carotid artery (IC).[74] Of the three trigeminal nerve divisions, the ophthalmic division sends SP-immunopositive fibers to the brain vessels, as evidenced by the fact that HRP applied to the cerebral arteries is transported only to neurons in the ophthalmic division of the trigeminal ganglion.[75] These results suggest that the origin of SP fibers in the cerebral blood vessels is mainly from the trigeminal ganglion, although some arise from the dorsal root ganglion and the miniganglia around the IC.[76] In the trigeminal ganglion, SP immunoreactivity is found in cell bodies showing CGRP immunoreactivity, which suggests colocalization of SP and CGRP, not only in nerve terminals in the cerebral blood vessels, but also in the trigeminal ganglion.[67,73,77-79] Hardebo et al.[80] studied the detailed pathways of trigeminocerebrovascular nerves and showed that these nerves originated from the trigeminal ganglion and reached the anterior part of the Willis ring via the nasociliary nerve through the ethmoid foramen. SP fibers originating from the IC miniganglia, in contrast, ran along the IC and were distributed in the anterior part of the Willis ring. The vertebrobasilar system was innervated by SP fibers from the C2 level of the spinal dorsal root ganglion.[57,58]

B. NEUROKININ A

Edvinsson et al.[24] first demonstrated the existence of NKA nerve fibers around cerebral blood vessels by immunohistochemistry. These nerve fibers were found in the cerebral arteries of the cat, guinea pig, and rat, showing a meshwork fashion of distribution similar to that of perivascular SP fibers (Figure 5a). The coexistence of NKA, SP, and CGRP was demonstrated by Edvinsson et al.[24] in some nerve bundles in the cerebral artery. NKA immunoreactivity found medium-sized nerve cells in the trigeminal ganglion (Figure 5b), which also colocalized with SP and CGRP immunoreactivity.[24] This finding suggests that the origin of NKA nerve fibers is also the trigeminal ganglion. NKA coexists with SP and CGRP in both nerve terminals in the blood vessels and the trigeminal ganglion.

C. NEUROKININ B

So far, the existence of NKB fibers in cerebral blood vessels has not been shown by immunohistochemistry, probably because no specific antibodies against NKB are available. Since the exogenous application of NKB to the cerebral artery produces vasodilation of the artery,[24,25] the existence of NKB or NKB receptors is also suggested in cerebral blood vessels.

D. NEUROPEPTIDE K

Since specific NPK antibody is not available, there is no evidence of NPK immunopositive nerve fibers around cerebral blood vessels, although the exogenous application of NPK induced vasodilation of a cerebral artery.[24]

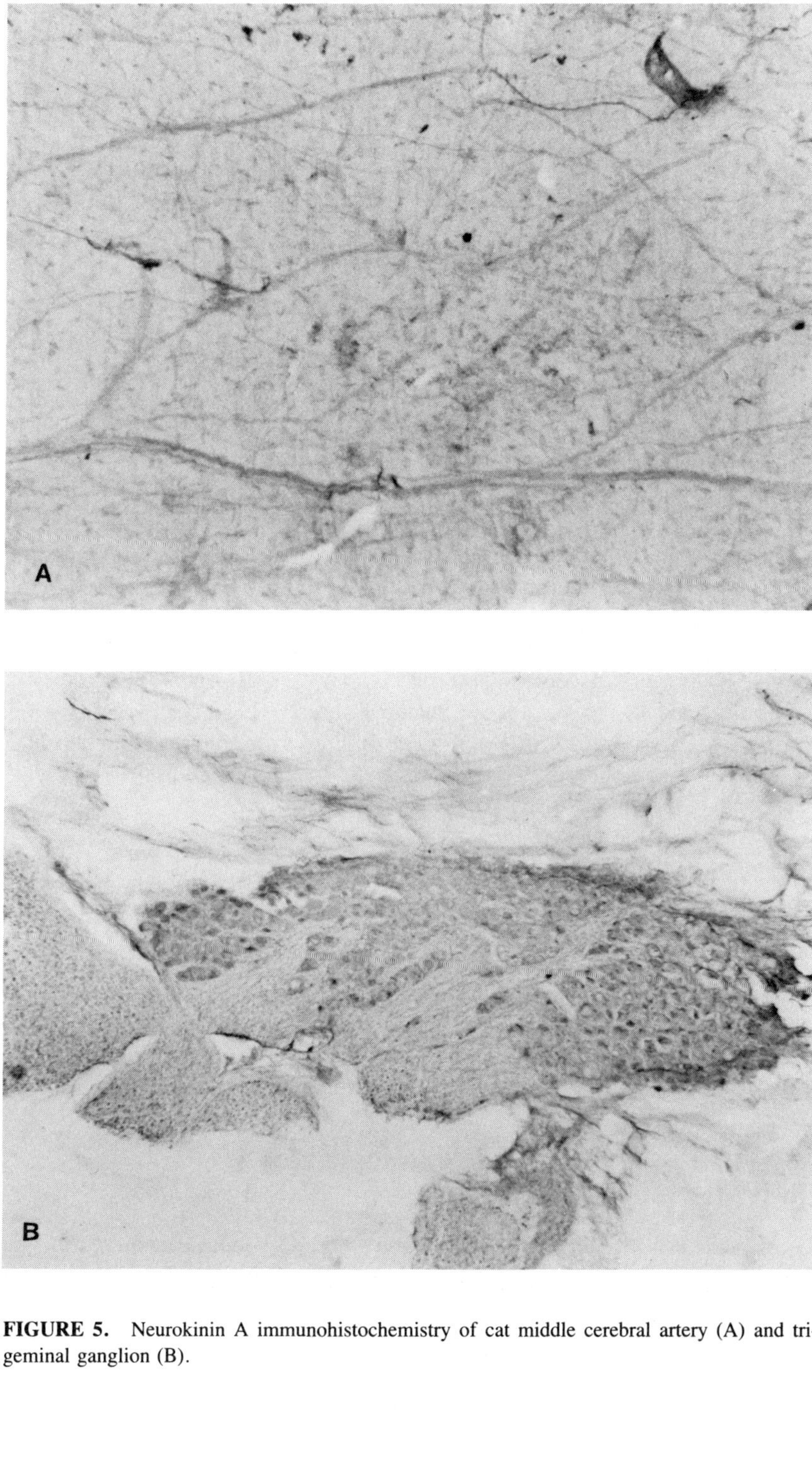

FIGURE 5. Neurokinin A immunohistochemistry of cat middle cerebral artery (A) and trigeminal ganglion (B).

IV. PHARMACOLOGY OF TACHYKININS IN THE CEREBRAL BLOOD VESSELS

A. SUBSTANCE P

In vitro studies using the tissue bath technique have shown dose-dependent vasodilator effects of SP on cerebral arteries and veins.[25,81-83] The vasodilative action of SP was long-lasting but less potent than that of CGRP.[81,83,84] The vasodilator action of SP is more potent in the cerebral artery than in the cerebral vein. Its action is dependent on the endothelium,[82,83,85] while vasodilations induced by VIP and CGRP are independent of the endothelium.[83] The exogenous application of the SP antagonist spantide resulted in a parallel shift to the right of the concentration-dependent curve of SP.[25,86]

Subarachnoid administration of SP also produced a slight increase in local CBF due to vasodilation. However, the intraparenchymal administration of SP did not change local CBF measured by the hydrogen clearance method.

B. NEUROKININ A AND B

In vitro administration of NKA in the cerebral artery produced endothelium-dependent vasodilation.[25,87] The degree of vasodilator action of tachykinins differs between species. In human and cat cerebral arteries, SP is the most potent vasodilator and NKA is less potent than SP and NKB (SP > NKB > NKA).[25] In contrast, the order of potency for tachykinin is SP > NKA > NKB in the guinea pig basilar artery.[25] These results suggest that tachykinin receptors are NK1 in the guinea pig basilar artery, but a non-NK1 receptor or a combination with NK1 and NK2 subtypes are in the human and cat cerebral arteries.

In vivo microapplication of NKB into the subarachnoid spaces produced an increase in arterioler caliber (vasorelaxation).[25]

C. NEUROPEPTIDE K

Jansen et al.[25] studied the vasomotor response of NPK in *in vitro* and *in vivo* experiments. *In vitro* studies showed potent endothelium-dependent vasodilator effects of NPK on the cerebral artery. The potency of the dilation was quite different between species. For example, NPK had a stronger vasodilator effect on human and guinea pig arteries than on cat and pig arteries.

V. CLINICAL CONSIDERATIONS

A. MIGRAINE

Headache is generally classified into vascular, muscle contraction, and traction headache and other headaches related to disorders of the nose, teeth, and ears.[88] Migraine, which is classified as a vascular headache, is a unilateral, pulsatile, severe headache associated with, or without, aura such as visual and gastrointestinal disturbances. The pathogenesis of migraine is unknown, but excessive amounts of serotonin released into the blood stream is a probable cause. Recent investigations[89] suggest that innervation of the face and the dura mater by the trigeminal nerve is involved in the occurrence of migraine, because headaches during migraine attacks sometimes refer to the forehead, which the trigeminal nerves innervate. Neurotransmitters found in the trigeminal ganglion can be putative vasoactive substances eliciting migraine. Among these transmitters, craniovascular levels of CGRP markedly increase during attacks of migraine, but no change has been demonstrated in the levels of SP and NKB.[90] These findings suggest that CGRP released from the trigeminocerebrovascular nerve system produces vasodilation of the cerebral blood vessel, which results in a vascular headache.

Lembeck et al.[91] demonstrated that antidromic stimulation of the peripheral nerves produces inflammatory phenomena such as vasodilation and extravasation of plasma and that these phenomena were blocked by a substance P antagonist. Moskowitz et al.[92] demonstrated these phenomena in the blood vessels in the dura mater of the cranium, in which antidromic stimulation of the trigeminal nerve resulted in vasodilation and extravasation of plasma in the dura mater in association with the release of SP. They suggested that the inflammatory response of the dura mater and migraine are due to SP released from nerve endings of the trigeminal nerve innervating the dura. Ergot alkaloids, such as ergotamine and dihydroergotamine that relieve classic and common migraine, decrease neurogenic plasma extravasation by blocking tachykinin release from the trigemino-cerebrovascular nerves.[93]

B. CEREBRAL VASOSPASM AFTER SUBARACHNOID HEMORRHAGE (SAH)

SAH occurring after the rupture of cerebral aneurysms may induce cerebral vasospasm after 1 to 2 weeks, which produces neurological deficits such as hemiplegia and aphasia due to cerebral ischemia. This ischemic event is one of the most important factors determining the prognosis of patients with SAH. The mechanism underlying the occurrence of vasospasm is unknown, and an effective treatment for vasospasm remains to be found. Cerebral vasospasm after SAH is caused by prolonged contact of blood clots with the cerebral artery. Breakdown products of the blood clots may act as vasoconstrictors and may induce postsynaptic changes after SAH. Edvinsson et al.[94] showed that injection of blood into the subarachnoid space of rats resulted in a 50% reduction in CGRP and a slight reduction in SP. They also demonstrated that the sensitivity of the rat basilar artery to CGRP increased from 50 to 80%, which suggested that pre- and postsynaptic modulation of CGRP and SP occurs after SAH. Onoue et al.[95] showed that oxyhemoglobin suppressed the relaxation of the dog middle cerebral artery caused by either nicotine or SP. They suggested that subarachnoid hemorrhage induced the impairment of vasodilator intervention by factors such as vasodilator nerves.

REFERENCES

1. **Nielsen, K. C. and Owman, C.,** Adrenergic innervation of pial arteries related to the circle of Willis in the cat, *Brain Res.*, 6, 773, 1967.
2. **Nelson, E. and Rennels, M.,** Innervation of intracranial arteries, *Brain Res.*, 93, 475, 1970.
3. **Iwayama, T., Furness, J. B., and Burnstock, G.,** Dual adrenergic and cholinergic innervation of the cerebral arteries of the rat, *Circ. Res.*, 26, 635, 1970.
4. **Itakura, T.,** Aminergic innervation of the cerebral veins shown by catecholamine histofluorescence, DBH immunohistochemistry, and electron microscopy, in *Neural Regulation of Brain Circulation,* Owman, C. and Hardebo, J. D., Eds. Elsevier, New York, 1986, 451.
5. **Borodulya, A. V. and Pletchkova, E. K.,** Distribution of cholinergic and adrenergic nerves in the internal carotid artery: a histochemical study, *Acta Anat.*, 86, 410, 1973.
6. **Edvinsson, L., Nielsen, K. C., Owman, C., and Sporrong, B. L.,** Cholinergic mechanisms in pial vessels. Histochemistry, electron microscopy and pharmacology, *Z. Zellforsch. Mikroskop. Anat.*, 134, 311, 1972.
7. **Saito, A., Wu, J. Y., and Lee, T. JF.,** Evidence for the presence of cholinergic nerves in cerebral arteries: an immunohistochemical demonstration of choline acetyltransferase, *J. Cereb. Blood Flow Metab.*, 5, 327, 1985.
8. **Itakura, T. and Imai, H.,** Origin of cerebrovascular peptide containing nerve fibers, in *Neurotransmission and Cerebrovascular Function II,* Seylaz, J. and Sercombe, R., Eds. Elsevier, Amsterdam, 1989, 211.
9. **Edvinsson, L., McCulloch, J., and Uddman, R.,** Substance P: immunocytochemical localization and effect upon pial arteries in vitro and in situ, *J. Physiol. (London)* 318, 251, 1981.
10. **Furness, J., Papka, R. E., Della, N. G., Costa, M., and Eskay, R. L.,** Substance P-like immunoreactivity in nerves associated with the vascular system of guinea pigs, *Neuroscience,* 7, 447, 1982.
11. **Kobayashi, S., Koshiyama, K., Olschowka, J. A., and Jacobowitz, D. M.,** Vasoactive intestinal polypeptide immunoreactive and cholinergic nerves in the whole mount preparation of the major cerebral arteries of the rat, *Histochemistry,* 79, 377, 1983.
12. **Itakura, T., Okuno, T., Nakakita, K., Kamei, I., Naka, Y., Imai, H., Nakai, K., and Komai, N.,** A light and electron microscopic immunohistochemical study of vasoactive intestinal polypeptide- and substance P-containing fibers along the cerebral blood vessels: comparison with aminergic and cholinergic nerve fibers, *J. Cereb. Blood Flow Metab.*, 4, 407, 1984.
13. **Edvinsson, L., Emson, P., McCulloch, J., Tatemoto, K., and Uddman, R.,** Neuropeptide Y: cerebrovascular innervation and vasomotor effects in the cat, *Neurosci. Lett.*, 43, 79, 1983.
14. **Hanko, J., Hardebo, J. E., Kåhrström, J., Owman, C., and Sundler, F.,** Calcitonin gene-related peptide is present in mammalian cerebrovascular nerve fibers and dilates pial and peripheral arteries, *Neurosci. Lett.*, 57, 91, 1985.
15. **Uddman, R., Edvinsson, L., Eckman, R., Kingman, T., and McCulloch, J.,** Innervation of the feline cerebral vasculature by nerve fibers containing calcitonin gene-related peptide: trigeminal origin and co-existence with substance P, *Neurosci. Lett.*, 62, 131, 1985.
16. **Imai, H., Okuno, T., Wu, J.-Y., and Lee, T. J-F.,** GABAergic innervation in cerebral blood vessels: an immunohistochemical demonstration of L-glutamic acid decarboxylase and GABA transaminase, *J. Cereb. Blood Flow Metab.*, 11, 129, 1991.
17. **Okuno, T. and Lee, T. J-F.,** GABAergic and other autonomic innervation in cerebral arteries of the cat: a sequential double labelling immunohistochemical study, *J. Cereb. Blood Flow Metab.*, in press.

18. **Okuno, T. and Lee, T. J-F.,** Neuromodulatory effects of GABA in cerebral pial arterial innervations: a pharmacological study, (unpublished observations.)
19. **Edvinsson, L., McCulloch, J., and Uddman, R.,** Substance P: immunocytochemical localization and effect upon pial arteries in vitro and in situ, *J. Physiol. (London),* 318, 251, 1981.
20. **Furness, J. B., Papka, R. E., Della, N. G., Costa, M., and Eskay, R. L.,** Substance P-like immunoreactivity in nerves associated with the vascular system of guinea pigs, *Neuroscience,* 7, 447, 1982.
21. **Itakura, T., Okuno, T., Nakakita, K., Kamei, I., Naka, Y., Nakai, K., Imai, H., Komai, N., Kimura, H., and Maeda, T.,** A light and electron microscopic immunohistochemical study of vasoactive intestinal polypeptide- and substance P-containing nerve fibers along the cerebral blood vessels: comparison with aminergic and cholinergic fibers, *J. Cereb. Blood Flow Metab.,* 4, 407, 1984.
22. **Itakura, T., Nakakita, K., Imai, H., Nakai, K., Kamei, I., Naka, Y., Okuno, T., Komai, N., Hirai, T., Arai, T., and Komi, H.,** Three dimensional observation of the nerve fibers along the cerebral blood vessels, *Histochemistry,* 84, 217, 1986.
23. **Itakura, T., Nakakita, K., and Kamei, I.,** Immunohistochemical studies of peptidergic nerve fibers in the cerebral vein, in *Peptidergic Mechanisms in the Cerebral Circulation,* Edvinsson, L. and McCulloch, J., Eds., VCH Publishers, Weinheim, 1987.
24. **Edvinsson, L., Brodin, E., Jansen, I., and Uddman, R.,** Neurokinin A in cerebral vessels: characterization, localization and effects in vitro, *Regul. Pept.,* 20, 181, 1988.
25. **Jansen, I., Alafaci, C., McCulloch, J., Uddman, R., and Edvinsson, L.,** Tachykinins (substance P, Neurokinin A, Neuropeptide K, and Neurokinin B) in the cerebral circulation: vasomotor responses in vitro and in situ, *J. Cereb. Blood Flow Metab.,* 11, 567, 1991.
26. **Erspamer, V.,** The tachykinin peptide family, *Trends Neurosci.,* 4, 267, 1981.
27. **von Euler, U. S. and Gaddum, J. H.,** An unidentified depressor substance in certain tissue extracts, *J. Physiol. (London),* 72, 74, 1931.
28. **Chang, M. M. and Leeman, S. E.,** Isolation of a sialogic peptide from bovine hypothalamic tissue and its characterization as SP, *J. Biol. Chem.,* 245, 4784, 1970.
29. **Kimura, S., Okada, M., Sugita, Y., Kanazawa, I., and Munekata, E.,** Novel neuropeptides, neurokinin α and β, isolated from porcine spinal cord, *Proc. Jpn. Acad.,* 59, 101, 1983.
30. **Kangawa, K., Minamino, N., Fukuda, A., and Matsuo, H.,** Neuromedin K: a novel mammalian tachykinin identified in porcine spinal cord, *Biochem. Biophys. Res. Commun.,* 114, 533, 1983.
31. **Tatemoto, K., Lundberg, J. M., Jornvall, H., and Mutt, V.,** Neuropeptide K: isolation, structure, and biological activities of a novel brain tachykinin, *Biochem. Biophys. Res. Commun.,* 128, 947, 1985.
32. **Kage, R., McGregor, G. P., Thim, L., and Conlon, J. M.,** Neuropeptide γ: a peptide isolated from rabbit intestine that is derived from γ-preprotachykinin, *J. Neurochem.,* 50, 1412, 1988.
33. **Anastasi, A., Erspamer, V., and Cei, J. M.,** Isolation and amino acid sequence of physalaemin, the main active polypeptide of the skin of *Physalemus Fuscumaculatus, Arch. Biochem. Biophys.,* 108, 341, 1964.
34. **Erspamer, V., Anastasi, A., Bertaccini, G., and Cei, J. M.,** Structure and pharmacological actions of physalaemin, the main active polypeptide of the skin of *Physalaemus fuscumaculatus, Experientia,* 20, 489, 1964.
35. **Anastasi, A., Montecacci, P., Erspamer, V., and Visser, J.,** Amino acid composition and sequence of Kassinin, a tachykinin dodecapeptide from the skin of the Africa frog, *Kassina senegalesis, Experientia,* 33, 857, 1977.
36. **Erspamer, V. and Melchiorri, P.,** Active polypeptides from amphibian skin to gastrointestinal tract and brain of mammals, *Trends Pharmacol. Sci.,* 1, 391, 1980.

37. **Erspamer, V. and Anastasi, A.,** Structure and pharmacological actions of eledoisin, the active endecapeptide of the posterior salivary glands of eledone, *Experientia,* 18, 58, 1962.
38. **Pernow, B.,** Substance P, *Pharmacol. Rev.,* 35, 85, 1983.
39. **Chan-Palay, V.,** Innervation of cerebral blood vessels by norepinephrine, indoleamine, substance P and neurotensin fibers and leptomeningeal indoleamine axons: their roles in vasomotor activity and local alterations of brain blood compositions, in *Neurogenic Control of Brain Circulation,* Owman, C. and Edvinsson, L., Eds., Pergamon Press, Oxford, 1977, 39.
40. **Uddman, R., Edvinsson, L., Owman, C., and Sundler, F.,** Perivascular substance P: occurrence and distribution in mammalian pial vessels, *J. Cereb. Blood Flow Metab.,* 1, 227, 1981.
41. **Edvinsson, L. and Uddman, R.,** Immunohistochemical localization and dilatory effect of substance P on human cerebral vessels, *Brain Res.,* 232, 466, 1982.
42. **Hanko, J., Hardebo, J. E., Kåhrström, J., Owman, C., and Sundler, F.,** Existence and coexistence of calcitonin gene-related peptide (CGRP) and substance P in cerebrovascular nerves and trigeminal ganglion cells, *Acta Physiol. Scand.,* 127(Suppl.), 552, 29, 1986.
43. **Hara, H. and Weir, B.,** Different distribution of substance P and vasoactive intestinal polypeptide in the cerebral arterial innervation in rat and guinea pig, *Anat. Anz.,* 163, 19, 1987.
44. **Liu-Chen, L. Y., Mayberg, M. Y., and Moskowitz, M. A.,** Immunohistochemical evidence for a substance P-containing trigeminovascular pathway to pial arteries in cats, *Brain Res.,* 268, 162, 1983.
45. **Yamamoto, K., Matsuyama, T., Shiosaka, S., Inagaki, S., Senba, E., Shimizu, Y., Ishimoto, I., Hayakawa, T., Matsmoto, M., and Tohyama, M.,** Overall distribution of substance P-containing nerves in the wall of the cerebral arteries of the guinea pig and its origins, *J. Comp. Neurol.,* 215, 421, 1983.
46. **Takano, Y., Nagashima, A., Masui, H., Kuromizu, K., and Kamiya, H.,** Distribution of substance K (neurokinan A) in the brain and peripheral tissues of rats, *Brain Res.,* 369, 400, 1986.
47. **Nagashima, A., Takano, Y., Tateishi, K., Matsuoka, Y., Hamaoka, T., and Kamiya, H.,** Central pressor actions of neurokinin B: increases in neurokinin B contents in discrete nuclei in spontaneously hypertensive rats, *Brain Res.,* 499, 198, 1989.
48. **Nawa, H., Hirose, T., Takashima, H., Inayama, S., and Nakanishi, S.,** Nucleotide sequences of cloned cDNAs for two types of bovine brain substance P precursor, *Nature (London),* 306, 32, 1983.
49. **Nawa, H., Kotani, H., and Nakanishi, S.,** Tissue specific generation of two preprotachykinin mRNAs from one gene by alternative RNA splicing, *Nature (London),* 312, 729, 1984.
50. **Krause, J. E., Chirgwin, J. M., Carter, M. S., Xu, Z. S., and Hershey, A. D.,** Three rat preprotachykinin mRNAs encode the neuropeptides substance P and neurokinin A, *Proc. Natl. Acad. Sci. U.S.A.,* 84, 881, 1984.
51. **Kotani, H., Hoshimaru, M., Nawa, H., and Nakanishi, H.,** Structure and gene organization of bovine neuromedin K precursor, *Proc. Natl. Acad. Sci. U.S.A.,* 83, 7074, 1986.
52. **Booner, T. I., Affolter, H. U., Young, A. C., and Youg, W. S., III,** A cDNA encoding the precursor of the rat neuropeptide, neurokinin B, *Mol. Brain Res.,* 2, 243, 1987.
53. **Takeda, Y. and Kruse, J. E.,** Neuropeptide K potently stimulates salivary gland secretion and potentiates substance P-induced salivation, *Proc. Natl. Acad. Sci. U.S.A.,* 86, 392, 1989.
54. **Watson, S. P., Sandberg, B. E. B., Hanely, R. R., and Iversen, L. L.,** Tissue selectivity of substance P alkyl esters: suggesting multiple receptors, *Eur. J. Pharmacol.,* 87, 77, 1983.

55. **Laufer, R., Worsmer, V., Freidman, Z. Y., Glian, C., Chorev, M., and Selinger, Z.,** Neurokinin B is a preferred agonist for a neuronal substance P receptor and this action is antagonized by enkephalin, *Proc. Natl. Acad. Sci. U.S.A.*, 82, 7447, 1985.
56. **Lee, C., Campbell, N., Williams, B. J., and Iversen, L. L.,** Multiple tachykinin binding sites in peripheral tissues and in brain, *Eur. J. Pharmacol.*, 130, 209, 1986.
57. **Saffroy, M., Beaujouan, J. C., Torrens, Y., Besseyre, J., Begstrom, L., and Glowinski, J.,** Localization of tachykinin binding sites (NK1, NK2, NK3 ligands) in the rat brain, *Peptides*, 9, 237, 1988.
58. **Mantyh, P. W., Gates, T. S., Mantyh, C. R., and Maggio, J. E.,** Autoradiographic localization and characterization of tachykinin receptor binding sites in the rat brain and peripheral tissues, *J. Neurosci.*, 9, 258, 1989.
59. **Ignarro, L. J.,** Biological actions and properties of endothelium-derived nitric oxide formed and released from artery and vein, *Circ. Res.*, 65, 1, 1989.
60. **Edvinsson, L., Rosendahl-Helgesen, S., and Uddman, R.,** Substance P: localization, concentration and release in cerebral arteries, choroid plexus, and dura mater, *Cell Tissue Res.*, 234, 1, 1983.
61. **Norregaard, T. V. and Moskowitz, M. A.,** Substance P and the sensory innervation of intracranial and extracranial feline cephalic arteries, *Brain*, 108, 517, 1985.
62. **Nakakita, K., Imai, H., Kamei, I., Naka, Y., Nakai, K., Itakura, T., and Komai, N.,** Innervation of the cerebral veins as compared with cerebral arteries: a histochemical and electron microscopic study, *J. Cereb. Blood Flow Metab.*, 3, 127, 1983.
63. **Bevan, S. and Szolcsanyl, J.,** Sensory neuron-specific actions of capsaicin: mechanisms and applications, *Trend Pharmacol. Sci.*, 11, 330, 1990.
64. **Duckles, P. and Buck, S. H.,** Substance P in the cerebral vasculature: depletion by capsaicin suggests a sensory role, *Brain Res.*, 245, 171, 1982.
65. **Uddman, R., Edvinsson, L., Eckman, R., Kingman, T., and McCulloch, J.,** Innervation of the feline cerebral vasculature by nerve fibers containing calcitonin gene-related peptide: trigeminal origin and co-existence with substance P, *Neurosci. Lett.*, 62, 131, 1985.
66. **Hanko, J., Hardebo, J. E., Kåhrström, J., Owman, C., and Sundler, F.,** Calcitonin gene-related peptide is present in mammalian cerebrovascular nerve fibers and dilates pial and peripheral arteries, *Neurosci. Lett.*, 57, 91, 1985.
67. **McCulloch, J., Uddman, R., Kingman, T. A., and Edvinsson, L.,** Calcitonin gene-related peptide: functional role in cerebrovascular regulation, *Proc. Natl. Acad. Sci. U.S.A.*, 83, 5731, 1986.
68. **Edvinsson, L., Ekman, R., Jansen, I., McCulloch, J., and Uddman, R.,** Calcitonin gene-related peptide and cerebral blood vessels: distribution and vasomotor effects, *J. Cereb. Blood Flow Metab.*, 7, 720, 1987.
69. **Liu-Chen, L. Y., Liszczak, T. M., King, J. C., and Moskowitz, M. A.,** Immunoelectron microscopic study of substance P-containing fibers in feline cerebral arteries, *Brain Res.*, 360, 12, 1986.
70. **Edvinsson, L., Emson, P., McCulloch, J., Tatemoto, K., and Uddman, R.,** Neuropeptide Y: immunocytochemical localization to and effect upon feline pial arteries and veins *in vitro* and *in situ*, *Acta Physiol. Scand.*, 122, 155, 1984.
71. **Yamamoto, K., Matsuyama, T., Shiosaka, S., Inagaki, S., Senba, S., Shimizu, Y., Ishimoto, I., Hayakawa, T., Matsumoto, M., and Tohyama, M.,** Overall distribution of substance P-containing nerves in the wall of the cerebral arteries of the guinea pig and its origin, *J. Comp. Neurol.*, 215, 421, 1983.
72. **Arbab, M. A. R., Wiklund, L., and Svendggard, N. A.,** Origin and distribution of cerebral vascular innervation from superior cervical, trigeminal and spinal ganglia investigated with retrograde and anterograde WGA-HRP tracing in the rat, *Neuroscience*, 19, 695, 1986.

73. **Edvinsson, L., Hara, H., and Uddman, R.,** Retrograde tracing of nerve fibers to the rat middle cerebral artery with true blue: co-localization with different peptides, *J. Cereb. Blood Flow Metab.*, 9, 212, 1989.
74. **Suzuki, N., Hardebo, J. E., and Owman, C.,** Origins and pathways of cerebrovascular nerves storing substance P and calcitonin gene-related peptide in rat, *Neuroscience,* 31, 427, 1989.
75. **Mayberg, M. R., Zervas, N. T., and Moskowitz, M. A.,** Trigeminal projections to supratentorial pial and dural blood vessels in cat demonstrated by horseradish peroxidase histochemistry, *J. Comp. Neurol.*, 223, 46, 1984.
76. **Suzuki, N., Hardebo, J. E., and Owman, C.,** Origins and pathways of cerebrovascular nerves storing substance P and calcitonin gene-related peptide in rat, *Neuroscience,* 31, 427, 1989.
77. **Gibbins, I. L., Furness, J. B., Costa, M., MacIntyre, I., Hillyard, C. J., and Girgis, S.,** Co-localization of calcitonin gene-related peptide-like immunoreactivity with substance P in cutaneous, vascular and visceral sensory neurons of guinea pig, *Neurosci. Lett.*, 57, 125, 1985.
78. **Lee, T., Kawai, Y., Shiosaka, S., Takami, K., Kiyama, H., Hillyard, C. J., Girgis, S., MacIntyre, I., Emson, P. C., and Tohyama, M.,** Coexistence of calcitonin gene-related peptide and substance P-like peptide in single cells of the trigeminal ganglion of the rat: immunohistochemical analysis, *Brain Res.*, 330, 194, 1985.
79. **Sundler, F., Brodin, E., Ekblad, E., Håkanson, R., and Uddman, R.,** Sensory nerve fibers: distribution of substance P, neurokinin A and calcitonin gene-related peptide, in *Tachykinin Antagonists,* Håkanson, R. and Sundler, F., Eds., Fernström Symp. Vol. 6, Elsevier, Amsterdam, 1985, 3.
80. **Hardebo, J. E., Arbab, M., Suzuki, N., and Svendgaard, N. A.,** Pathways of parasympathetic and sensory cerebrovascular nerves in monkeys, *Stroke,* 22, 331, 1991.
81. **Edvinsson, L. and Jansen, I.,** Characterization of tachykinin receptors in isolated cerebral arteries of the guinea pig, *Br. J. Pharmacol.*, 90, 553, 1987.
82. **Furchgott, R. F.,** Role of endothelium in responses of vascular smooth muscle, *Circ. Res.*, 53, 557, 1983.
83. **Edvinsson, L., Fredholm, B. B., Hamel, E., Jansen, I., and Verrecchia, C.,** Perivascular peptides relax cerebral arteries concomitant with stimulation of cyclic adenosine monophosphate accumulation or release of endothelium-derived relaxing factor, *Neurosci. Lett.*, 58, 213, 1985.
84. **Brain, S. D., Williams, T. J., Tippins, J. R., Morris, H. R., and MacIntyre, I.,** Calcitonin gene-related peptide is a potent vasodilator, *Nature (London),* 313, 54, 1985.
85. **Mejia, J. A., Pernow, J., von Holst, H., Rudehill, A., and Lundberg, J. M.,** Effects of neuropeptide Y, calcitonin gene-related peptide, substance P and capsaicin on cerebral arteries in man and animals, *J. Neurosurg.*, 69, 913, 1988.
86. **Edvinsson, L., McCulloch, J., Rosell, S., and Uddman, R.,** Antagonism by (D-Pro2, DTrp7,9)-substance P of the cerebrovascular dilatation induced by substance P, *Acta Physiol. Scand.*, 116, 411, 1982.
87. **Macfarlane, R., Moskowitz, M. A., Tasdemiroglu, E., Wei, E. P., and Kontos, H. A.,** Postischemic cerebral blood flow and neuroeffector mechanisms, *Blood Vessels,* 28, 46, 1991.
88. Ad hoc committee on the classification of headache, Classification of headache, *JAMA,* 179, 717, 1962.
89. **Moskowitz, M. A., Mayberg, M. R., and Chen, L.,** Biochemical and histochemical observations on the fifth cranial nerve and its relationship to meninges and its blood vessels, *Stroke,* 12, 125, 1981.
90. **Goadsby, P. J., Edvinsson, L., and Ekman, R.,** Vasoactive peptide release in the extracerebral circulation of human during migraine headache, *Ann. Neurol.*, 28, 183, 1990.

91. **Lembeck, F., Donnerer, J., and Bartho, L.,** Inhibition of neurogenic vasodilation and plasma extravasation by substance P antagonists, somatostatin and (D-MET2-PRO5) enkephalinamide, *Eur. J. Pharmacol.*, 85, 171, 1982.
92. **Markowitz, S., Saito, K., and Moskowitz, M. A.,** Neurogenically mediated plasma extravasation in dura mater: effect of ergot alkaloids. A possible mechanism of action in vascular headache, *Cephalalgia,* 8, 83, 1988.
93. **Saito, K., Markowitz, S., and Moskowitz, M. A.,** Ergot alkaloids block neurogenic extravasation in dura mater: proposed action in vascular headaches, *Ann. Neurol.*, 24, 732, 1988.
94. **Edvinsson, L., DelgadoZygmunt, T., Ekman, R., Jansen, I., Svendgaard, N. A., and Uddman, R.,** Involvement of perivascular sensory fibers in the pathophysiology of cerebral vasospasm following subarachnoid hemorrhage, *J. Cereb. Blood Flow Metab.*, 16, 602, 1990.
95. **Onoue, H., Nakamura, N., and Toda, N.,** Prolonged exposure to oxyhemoglobin modifies the response of isolated dog middle cerebral arteries to vasoactive substances, *Stroke,* 20, 657, 1989.

Chapter 13

VASOPRESSIN RECEPTORS IN CEREBRAL ARTERIES

M. C. Martínez, J. M. Vila, M. Aldasoro, and S. Lluch

TABLE OF CONTENTS

I. Introduction 214

II. Experiments *In Vivo* 215

III. Experiments *In Vitro* 217
  A. V_1 Receptors 217
  B. V_2 Receptors 220

IV. Summary and Conclusions 222

References 222

0-8493-5096-0/93/$0.00 + $.50

I. INTRODUCTION

In addition to exerting antidiuretic effects, arginine vasopressin (AVP) has been shown to play an important role in cardiovascular homeostasis and in the pathogenesis of hypertension.[1-3] The vasopressin receptor designated V_1 seems to mediate all the cardiovascular actions of the peptide whereas its antidiuretic action is mediated by V_2 cyclic adenosine monophosphate-dependent receptors.[4-6] Some cardiovascular actions of vasopressin are mediated by V_2-like receptors in both humans[7] and dogs.[8] A common finding in the vascular effects of vasopressin is the heterogeneity of responsiveness depending on regional and species differences.[9,10] With respect to the cerebral vasculature, the debate goes on whether pharmacologic studies of vasopressin in various animal species can be extrapolated to humans.[11]

Kozniewska et al.[12] reported that cerebral blood flow, measured by injecting ^{133}Xe into the carotid artery in anesthetized cats, is increased in response to intracarotid infusion of vasopressin. These results were later confirmed in experiments on normotensive and hypertensive rats.[13] The increase in the cerebral blood flow was particularly evident in the hypertensive rats in which increases in cerebral blood flow up to 83% were recorded after injections of 10 mU of vasopressin into the internal carotid artery. These potent effects were ascribed to the passage of vasopressin through the blood-brain barrier due to the increase in arterial blood pressure. Lassoff and Altura[14] showed that local application of vasopressin failed to exert any measurable effects on the vascular diameter of rat pial arterioles and concluded that smooth muscle cells of this vascular bed might be the only resistance microvessels which lack receptor sites for this neuropeptide.

Charocopos et al.[15] found that stimulation of endogenous vasopressin by sodium and fluid load in anephric rats produced elevations of vascular resistance in the gastrointestinal tract, the muscle, and the skin. However, cerebral blood flow actually increased during stimulation of vasopressin, indicating small or no change in vascular resistance of this organ. On the other hand, intravenous infusion of vasopressin in conscious dogs produced small reductions[16] or no significant change[17] in cerebral blood flow. In the light of these findings, it has been proposed that vasopressin might selectively constrict some vascular beds (skeletal muscle, skin, splanchnic) while maintaining blood flow to brain tissue and the heart.

Only a few investigations on the effects of vasopressin on isolated cerebral arteries have been performed during recent years, and the results further support the hypothesis that regional and species differences may be determinant factors in the vascular responsiveness to this neuropeptide. Hanko et al.[18] showed that vasopressin exerts dose-dependent constrictor effects on isolated cat pial arteries. The pial vasoconstriction seemed to require extracellular calcium since treatment with calcium uptake inhibitors nimodipine or nifedipine considerably reduced the contraction. On the other hand, vasopressin caused concentration-dependent relaxation in rings of canine basilar arteries, which was abolished by endothelium removal or by previous treatment with the V_1 vasopressinergic antagonist $d(CH_2)_5Tyr(Me)AVP$.[19] Thus it was concluded that the endothelial cells of the basilar artery appear to have V_1vasopressinergic receptors which mediate smooth muscle relaxation.

The conflicting observations referred to above would imply a situation for cerebral vessels far removed from that clearly established in other vascular regions in which vasopressin produces severe vasoconstriction. With the development of sensitive radioimmunoassays, it has been shown that vasopressin is present not only in blood but also in normal cerebrospinal fluid,[20,21] and it has been suggested that cerebrospinal fluid may be a transport system whereby neurohypophysial secretion can reach various parts of the brain.[22] Furthermore, immunocytochemical studies have provided strong evidence for a role of arginine vasopressin as a putative neurotransmitter or neuromodulator within the brain.[23,24] These considerations suggest that vasopressin may be involved in the regulation of blood supply to the brain.

The next section gives a brief account of our experience concerning the *in vivo* and *in vitro* effects of arginine vasopressin on the cerebral circulation. The experiments *in vivo* were carried out in the unanesthetized goat, using an experimental preparation that permits the effects on cerebral blood flow of various interventions to be assessed on a beat-to-beat basis in normal states.[25,26] The experiments *in vitro* were accomplished in cerebral vessels obtained from humans (during autopsy of patients who died 3 to 12 h before). Special attention is focused upon endothelium-dependent responses of human cerebral arteries to selective vasopressin receptor agonists and antagonists.

II. EXPERIMENTS *IN VIVO*

Infusion of 1 to 12 mU of vasopressin into the internal maxillary artery of unanesthetized goats causes dose-dependent reductions in cerebral blood flow without detectable changes in systemic arterial pressure or heart rate (Table 1). These effects on total hemispheric blood flow were confirmed when blood supply to a relatively small region of the brain was measured in a pial artery. Figure 1 shows the decrease in blood flow in a small branch of the middle cerebral artery after injection of 10 mU of vasopressin into the internal maxillary artery.

We also studied the dose-response relationship of the cerebral vessels to vasopressin after treatment with (1-deaminopenicillamine 4-valine)-8-D-arginine-vasopressin (dPVDAVP), a compound that antagonizes in a competitive way the vasopressor effects of exogenously administered vasopressin[28-30] and reduces the increased blood pressure resulting from sodium-induced vasopressin release.[31,32] Infusion of dPVDAVP in doses of 3 to 6 μg/min does not appreciably modify resting values of cerebral blood flow, arterial pressure, or heart rate, but markedly diminishes the cerebral blood flow reduction

TABLE 1
Changes in Cerebral Blood Flow (CBF), Mean Arterial Pressure (MAP), and Heart Rate (HR) Induced by Infusion of Vasopressin into the Internal Maxillary Artery of Unanesthetized Goats

		Vasopressin infusion (mU/min)			
	Control	1	3	6	12
CBF (ml/min/100 g)	112 ± 4.6[a]	104 ± 5.7	89 ± 5.8[b]	82 ± 2.4[b]	72 ± 7.4[b]
MAP (mmHg)	95 ± 3.8	94 ± 3.3	95 ± 3.5	96 ± 3.3	95 ± 3.5
HR (beats/min)	67 ± 3.8	70 ± 4.1	72 ± 4.2	68 ± 3.5	67 ± 4.1

[a] Values are means ± SE obtained from six goats
[b] Statistically different from control ($p < 0.05$). Based on data from Lluch et al.[27]

From Lluch, S. et al., *J. Pharmacol. Exp. Ther.*, 228, 749, 1984. With permission.

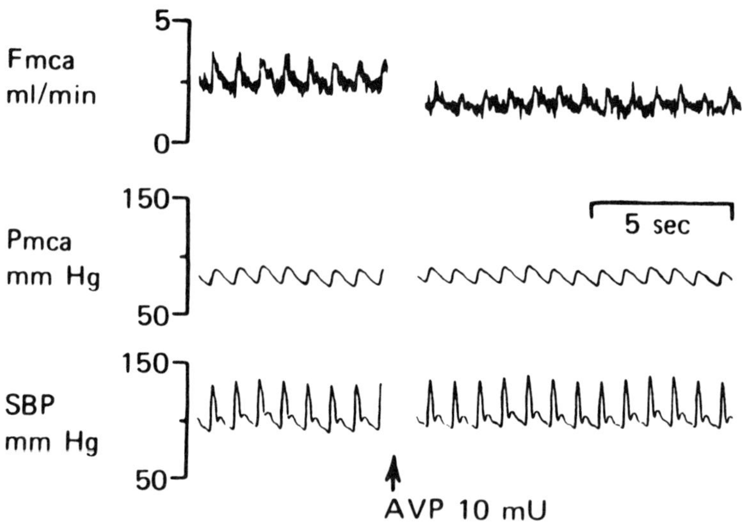

FIGURE 1. Effects of arginine vasopressin (AVP) injected into the internal maxillary artery on middle cerebral artery blood flow (Fmca) and pressure (Pmca) and systemic blood pressure (SBP) in one anesthetized goat. Fmca was measured with an electromagnetic flow probe (0.75 mm). Pmca was measured in a branch of the middle cerebral artery with a polyvinyl catheter. (From Lluch, S. and Gómez, B., *Peptidergic Mechanisms in the Cerebral Circulation,* Ellis Horwood, Chichester, 1987, 152. With permission of Ellis Horwood Ltd.)

induced during the response to vasopressin (Figure 2). The reduction of cerebral blood flow caused by norepinephrine (0.3 to 9 μg) or 5-hydroxytryptamine (0.1 to 9 μg) was not altered during administration of the vasopressin antagonist. These experiments in unanesthetized goats indicate that the decrease in cerebral blood flow is due to a direct action of vasopressin

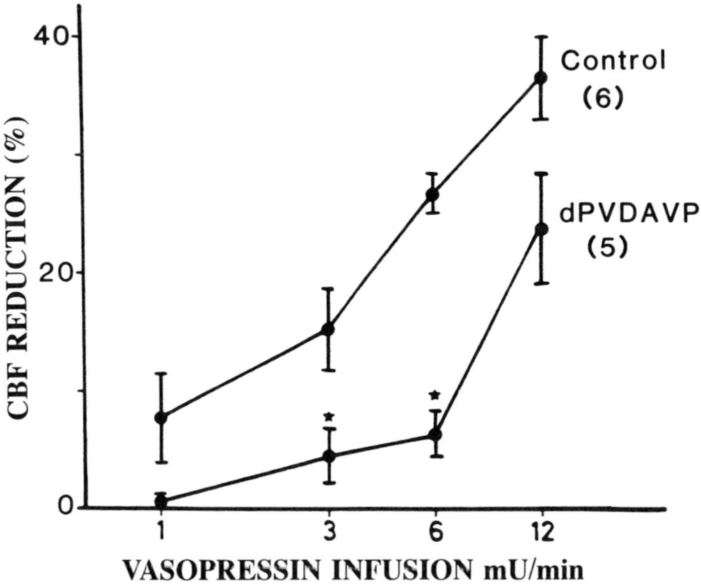

FIGURE 2. Effects of infusion of vasopressin before and during prolonged infusion of dPVDAVP in unanesthetized goats. Values are means ± SE. Number of experiments are indicated within parentheses. * Statistically significant ($p < 0.05$) compared with corresponding control values. (From Lluch, S. et al., *J. Pharmacol. Exp. Ther.*, 228, 749, 1984. With permission.)

on cerebral vessels rather than a consequence of changes in systemic variables. The results also indicate that the reduction of cerebral blood flow is mediated through the activation of V_1 vasopressinergic receptors.

III. EXPERIMENTS *IN VITRO*

A. V_1 RECEPTORS

Human cerebral arteries were obtained during the autopsy of patients who had died 3 to 12 h before. Outside diameter of the segments ranged from 500 to 700 μm. In approximately 50% of the arterial segments, the endothelium was removed mechanically by inserting a roughened stainless steel wire into the lumen.

Cumulative application of vasopressin produced a constrictor response that was concentration-dependent. The maximum tension developed as well as the EC_{50} were similar ($p > 0.05$) in arterial segments with and without endothelium (Table 2). There was no significant difference in the contraction of segments with and without endothelium to the addition of 60 m*M* KCl (904 ± 325 vs. 805 ± 207 mg, $p > 0.05$).

The presence of $10^{-8}M$ $d(CH_2)_5Tyr(Me)AVP$, a selective V_1 receptor antagonist, displaced the control curve for vasopressin to the right, but

TABLE 2
EC_{50} Values and Maximal Responses of Vasopressin in Human Cerebral Artery Segments

	Numb.	$EC_{50}(M)$ Geometric mean	$EC_{50}(M)$ 95% Confidence interval	Maximal response (mg)
With endothelium	11	7.0×10^{-10}	2.6×10^{-10} to 1.8×10^{-9}	821 ± 142
Without endothelium	12	4.2×10^{-10}	1.9×10^{-10} to 9.2×10^{-9}	830 ± 84
With $d(CH_2)_5Tyr(Me)AVP$				
10^{-8} *M*	11	3.2×10^{-8}*	1.5×10^{-8} to 6.8×10^{-8}	972 ± 119
10^{-6} *M*	7	1.9×10^{-6}**	1.0×10^{-6} to 3.5×10^{-6}	954 ± 75

*, ** $p < 0.05$, 0.001, respectively, different from segments with or without endothelium by Student's *t* test. Based on data from Martín de Aguilera et al.[33]

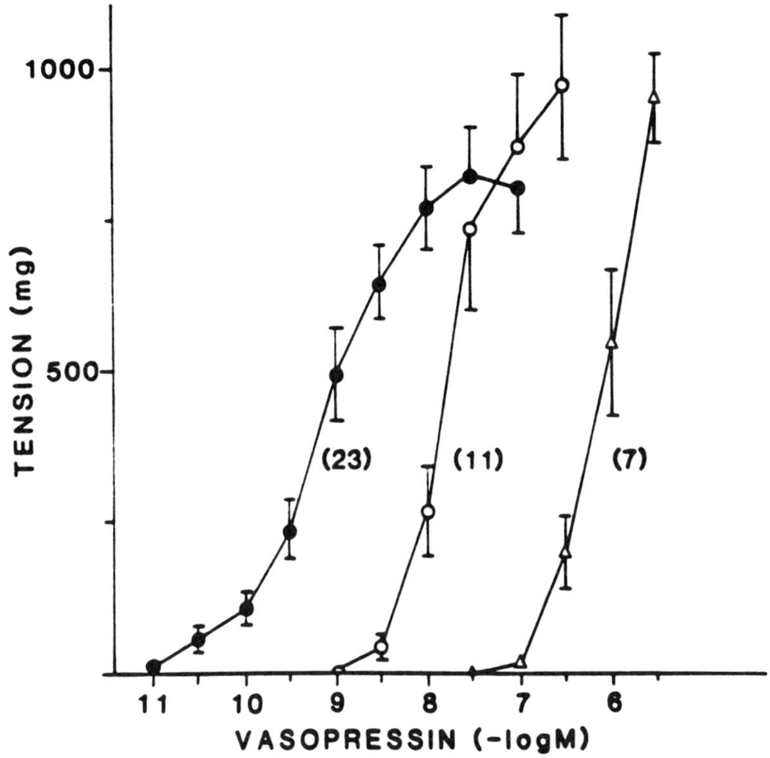

FIGURE 3. Concentration-response curves for vasopressin determined in human cerebral arterial segments in the absence (closed circles) and presence of $d(CH_2)_5Tyr(Me)AVP$ (open circles, 10^{-8} *M,* triangles, 10^{-6} *M*). Values are means ± SE. Number of experiments are indicated within parentheses. (From Martín de Aguilera, E., et al., *Stroke,* 21, 1689, 1990. With permission.)

differences in the maximal tensions developed were not significant ($p > 0.05$). Increasing the concentration of $d(CH_2)_5Tyr(Me)AVP$ to $10^{-6}M$ further displaced the control curve for vasopressin (Figure 3, Table 2).

With respect to human cerebral arteries, vasopressin appears to be a much more potent constrictor, both in terms of lower EC_{50} and maximum response, than is either angiotensin II, norepinephrine, 5-hydroxytryptamine, or tyramine.[34,35]

Our data also show that the vasopressin-induced contraction is not linked to the presence of an intact endothelium, thus indicating that vasodilator substances secreted by endothelial cells under basal, spontaneous conditions[36] do not counteract the potent contractile effects of vasopressin on smooth muscle cells. In agreement with our results, previous experiments have shown that vasopressin causes endothelium-independent contraction in human mesenteric arteries[37] and in the aorta and renal and carotid arteries of rats.[38]

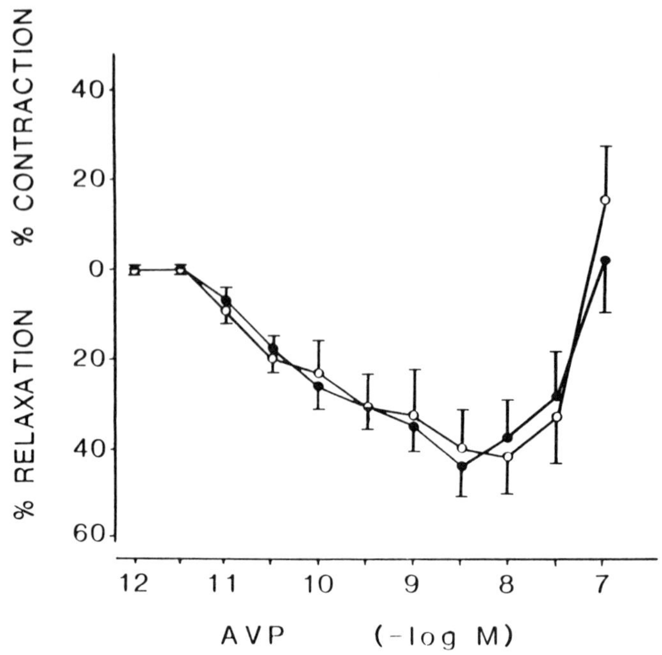

FIGURE 4. Effects of arginine vasopressin (AVP) on human cerebral arterial segments in the presence of the V_1 antagonist d(CH_2)$_5$Tyr(Me)AVP (closed circles, n = 11) and in the presence of the mixed V_1/V_2 antagonist d(CH_2)$_5$D-Tyr(Et)^2-Val^{4}desGly^9 AVP (open circles, n = 12). Values are means ± SE.

B. V_2 RECEPTORS

Further studies of the physiologic effects of vasopressin have implicated a possible role of V_2 receptors in mediating vasodilation in some vascular beds. Administration of either V_2 agonists or vasopressin during V_1 receptor blockade decreases systemic vascular resistance and increases cardiac output.[39-41] In particular, desmopressin (1-deamino-8-D-arginine vasopressin, DDAVP), a very selective antidiuretic agonist, induces forearm vasodilation in normal humans.[42] Intracarotid administration of 1-deamino,4-valine,8-D-arginine vasopressin (dVDAVP), another V_2 receptor agonist, increases cerebral blood flow in anesthetized rats.[43] These responses have been interpreted to suggest the existence of V_2 receptors mediating vasodilation.[42]

In our experiments in human cerebral arteries, we have observed only constriction in response to AVP even when the arterial segments were precontracted with KCl or $PGF_{2\alpha}$.[33] However, application of vasopressin during V_1 receptor blockade induces concentration-dependent relaxations in precontracted arteries (Figure 4). Furthermore, DDAVP, a highly specific V_2 receptor agonist, induces similar concentration-dependent relaxations to those observed in response to AVP (Figure 5).

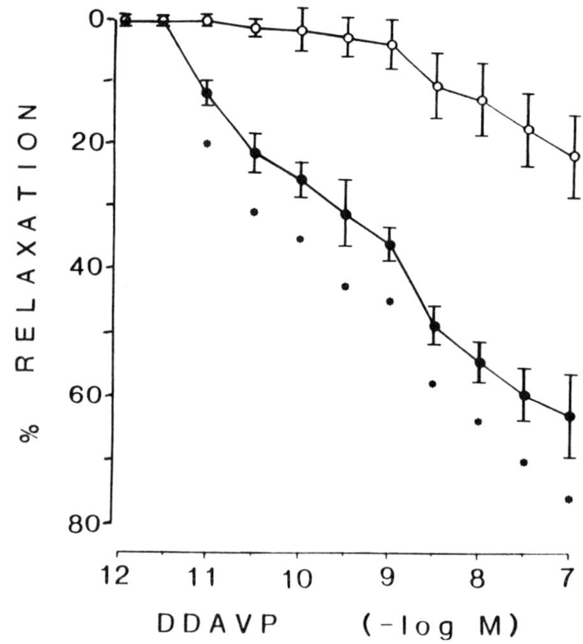

FIGURE 5. Effects of 1-deamino-8-D-arginine vasopressin (DDAVP) on human cerebral arterial segments in the absence (closed circles, n = 10) and in the presence of the mixed V_1/V_2 antagonist $d(CH_2)_5$D-Tyr(Et)^2-Val^{4}desGly^9 AVP (open circles, n = 12). Values are means ± SE.

Efforts to develop a specific V_2 antagonist have been unsuccessful (for review see László et al.[44]) The mixed V_1/V_2 antagonist $d(CH_2)_5$D–Tyr(Et)^{2}Val^{4}desGly^9 AVP appears to be the most potent antagonist of AVP stimulated antidiuresis in conscious water-loaded rats.[45] In our experiments in human cerebral arteries we have observed that $d(CH_2)_5$D–Tyr(Et)^{2}Val^{4}desGly^9 AVP is a potent antagonist of the DDAVP mediated relaxation (Figure 5). In contrast, this antagonist did not show a significant effect on vasopressin-induced relaxation of precontracted arteries (Figure 4). Therefore it seems unlikely that the vasodilating action of AVP and that of DDAVP are mediated by similar receptor sites. Definitive confirmation of the existence of another receptor subtype in smooth muscle mediating vasodilation different than the antidiuretic V_2 needs further experimental support. Other mechanisms could account for the observed vasodilation in response to AVP or DDAVP. For example, both DDAVP and AVP stimulate prostacyclin production in rabbit aortic rings.[46] Vasodilation might also result from augmented release of endothelial relaxant factors. From our previous experiments it is apparent that vasoconstriction due to V_1 receptor stimulation is endothelium independent;[33] this does not, however, rule out a significant role of these endothelial factors in cerebral vasodilation.

IV. SUMMARY AND CONCLUSIONS

It appears that vasopressin may constrict, dilate, or have no effect on cerebral vessels. Possibly a number of physiological, pharmacological, and experimental factors might determine the vascular action of vasopressin. In view of the results from our laboratory, vasopressin exerts powerful constrictor action on isolated human cerebral arteries and decreases cerebral blood flow in the unanesthetized goat by direct stimulation of V_1 vasopressin receptors predominantly located on smooth muscle cells. It appears that in human cerebral arteries the contractile response to vasopressin is not modulated by the presence of an intact endothelium.

The selective V_2 receptor agonist DDAVP causes concentration-dependent relaxation of human cerebral arteries which is blocked by the vasopressin antagonist $d(CH_2)_5$D–Tyr(Et)^{2}Val^{4}desGly^9 AVP. These results may be consistent with the existence of vasodilator V_2-like receptors in human cerebral arteries.

Vasopressin induces relaxation of human cerebral arteries in the presence of V_1 blockade; this relaxation, however, was not affected by the V_2 antagonist $d(CH_2)_5$D–Tyr(Et)^{2}Val^{4}desGly^9 AVP. Therefore the mechanisms responsible for AVP-induced relaxation appears to be different from those elicited by V_2 receptor stimulation.

REFERENCES

1. **Andrews, C. E., Jr. and Brenner, B. M.,** Relative contributions of arginine vasopressin and angiotensin II to maintenance of systemic arterial pressure in the anaesthetized water-deprived rat, *Circ. Res.*, 48, 254, 1981.
2. **Cowley, A. W.,** Vasopressin and cardiovascular regulation, in *International Review of Physiology,* Vol. 26, Guyton, A. C. and Hall, J. E., Eds., University Park Press, Baltimore, 1982, 190.
3. **Nakano, J.,** Cardiovascular actions of vasopressin, *Jpn. Circ. J.*, 37, 363, 1973.
4. **Michell, R. H., Kirk, C. J., and Billah, M. M.,** Hormonal stimulation of phosphatidylinositol breakdown, with particular reference to the hepatic effects of vasopressin, *Biochem. Soc. Trans.*, 7, 861, 1979.
5. **Penit, J., Faure, M., and Jard, S.,** Vasopressin and angiotensin II receptors in rat aortic muscle cells in culture, *Am. J. Physiol.*, 244, E72, 1983.
6. **Liard, J. F.,** Effects of arginine vasopressin on regional circulations, in *Vasopressin,* Schrier, R. W., Ed., Raven Press, New York, 1985, 59.
7. **Bichet, D. G., Razi, M., Lonergan, M., Arthus, M. F., Papukna, V., Kortas, C., and Barjon, J. N.,** Hemodynamic and coagulation responses to 1-desamino 8-D-arginine vasopressin in patients with congenital nephrogenic diabetes insipidus, *N. Engl. J. Med.*, 318, 881, 1988.
8. **Liard, J. F.,** Peripheral vasodilatation induced by a vasopressin analogue with selective V_2-agonism in dogs, *Am. J. Physiol.*, 256, H1621, 1989.

9. **Schmid, P. G., Abboud, F. M. Wendling, M. G., Ramberg, E. S., Mark, A. L., Heistad, D. D., and Eckstein, J. W.,** Regional vascular effects of vasopressin: plasma levels and circulatory response, *Am. J. Physiol.*, 227, 998, 1974.
10. **Altura, B. M. and Altura, B. T.,** Actions of vasopressin, oxytocin, and synthetic analogs on vascular smooth muscle, *Fed. Proc.*, 43, 80, 1984.
11. **Share, L.,** Role of vasopressin in cardiovascular regulation, *Physiol. Rev.*, 68, 1248, 1988.
12. **Kozniewska, E., Rap, Z., and Skolasinska, K.,** Cerebrovascular effect of vasopressin, *Acta Neurol. Scand.*, 72(Suppl.), 602, 1979.
13. **Kozniewska, R., Ostenda, M., and Skolasinska, K.,** The effect of vasopressin on cerebral blood flow in normotensive and spontaneously hypertensive rats, in *Cerebral Microcirculation and Metabolism,* Cervós-Navarro, J. and Fristschka, E., Eds., Raven Press, New York, 1981, 163.
14. **Lassoff, S. and Altura, B. M.,** Do pial terminal arterioles respond to local perivascular application of the neurohypophyseal peptide hormones, vasopressin and oxytocin?, *Brain Res.*, 196, 266, 1980.
15. **Charocopos, F., Hatzinikolaou, P., North, W. G., and Gavras, H.,** Systemic and regional hemodynamic effects of endogenous vasopressin stimulation in rats, *Am. J. Physiol.*, 243, H560, 1982.
16. **Liard, J. F., Dériaz, O., Schelling, P., and Thibonnier, M.,** Cardiac output distribution during vasopressin infusion or dehydration in conscious dogs, *Am. J. Physiol.*, 243, H663, 1982.
17. **Moursi, M. M., Van Wylen, D. G. L., and D'Alecy, L. G.,** Regional blood flow changes in response to mildly pressor doses of triglycyl desamino lysine and arginine vasopressin in the conscious dog, *J. Pharmacol. Exp. Ther.*, 232, 360, 1985.
18. **Hanko, J., Hardebo, J. E., and Owman, C.,** Vasomotor effects of some neuropeptides on isolated pial arteries of the cat, in *Cerebral Microcirculation and Metabolism,* Cervós-Navarro, J. and Fristschka, E., Eds., Raven Press, New York, 1981, 157.
19. **Katusic, Z. S., Shepherd, J. T., and Vanhoutte, P. M.,** Vasopressin causes endothelium-dependent relaxation of the canine basilar artery, *Circ. Res.*, 55, 575, 1984.
20. **Luerssen, T. G., Shelton, R. L., and Robertson, G. L.,** Evidence for separate origin of cerebrospinal fluid vasopressin, *Clin. Res.*, 25, 14A, 1977.
21. **Jenkins, S. J., Mather, H. M., and Ang, V.,** Vasopressin in human cerebrospinal fluid, *J. Clin. Endocrinol. Metab.*, 50, 364, 1980.
22. **Rodríguez, E. M.,** The cerebrospinal fluid as a pathway in neuroendocrine integration, *J. Endocrinol.*, 71, 407, 1976.
23. **Buijs, R. M.,** Intra-and extrahypothalamic vasopressin and oxytocin pathways in the rat, *Cell. Tissue Res.*, 192, 523, 1978.
24. **Buijs, R. M.,** Immunocytochemical demonstration of vasopressin and oxytocin in the rat brain by light and electronmicroscopy, *J. Histochem. Cytochem.*, 28, 357, 1980.
25. **Reimann, C. V., Lluch, S., and Glick, G.,** Development and evaluation of an experimental model for the study of the cerebral circulation in the unanesthetized goat, *Stroke,* 3, 322, 1972.
26. **Lluch, S., Gómez, B., Alborch, E., and Urquilla, P. R.,** Adrenergic mechanisms in cerebral circulation of the goat, *Am. J. Physiol.*, 228, 985, 1975.
27. **Lluch, S., Conde, M. V., Diéguez, G., López de Pablo, A. L., González, M. C., Estrada, C., and Gómez, B.,** Evidence for the direct effect of vasopressin on human and goat cerebral arteries, *J. Pharmacol. Exp. Ther.*, 228, 749, 1984.
28. **Manning, M., Lowbridge, J., Stier, C. T., Jr., Haldar, J., and Sawyer, W. H.,** (1-Deaminopenicillamine,4-valine-8-D-arginine)-vasopressin, a highly potent inhibitor of the vasopressor response to arginine-vasopressin, *J. Med. Chem.*, 20, 1228, 1977.

29. **Lowbridge, J., Manning, M., Haldar, J., and Sawyer, W. H.,** (1-(- Mercapto-cyclopentamethylenepropionic acid), 4-valine,-8-D-arginine) vasopressin, a potent and selective inhibitor of the vasopressor response to arginine-vasopressin, *J. Med. Chem.*, 21, 313, 1978.
30. **Pang, C. C. Y., McNeil, J. R., Wilcox, W. C., Manning, M., Sawyer, W. H.,** (1-Deaminopenicillamine,4-valine-8-D-arginine)vasopressin antagonizes the mesenteric vasoconstrictor response to arginine vasopressin in cats, *Proc. Soc. Exp. Biol. Med.*, 161, 41, 1979.
31. **Crofton, J. T., Shade, R. E., Lee-Kwon, W. J., Manning, M., and Sawyer, W. H.,** The importance of vasopressin in the development and maintenance of DOC-salt hypertension in the rat, *Hypertension (Dallas)*, 1, 31, 1979.
32. **Hatzinikolaou, P., Gavras, H., Brunner, H. R., and Gavras, I.,** Sodium-induced elevation of blood pressure in the anephric state, *Science (Washington, D.C.)*, 209, 935, 1980.
33. **Martín de Aguilera, E., Vila, J. M., Irurzun, A., Martínez, M. C., Martínez Cuesta, M. A., and Lluch, S.,** Endothelium-independent contractions of human cerebral arteries in response to vasopressin, *Stroke*, 21, 1689, 1990.
34. **Lluch, S. and Gómez, B.,** Vasopressin and the cerebral circulation, in *Peptidergic Mechanisms in the Cerebral Circulation*, Edvinsson, L. and McCulloch, J., Eds., Ellis Horwood, Chichester, 1987, 152.
35. **Conde, M. V., Gómez, B., and Lluch, S.,** Contractile responses of isolated human middle cerebral artery to vasoactive agents, *J. Cereb. Blood Flow Metab.*, 1, S350, 1981.
36. **Martin, W., Furchgott, F., Villani, M., and Jothianandan, D.,** Depression of contractile responses in rat aorta by spontaneously released endothelium-derived relaxing factor, *J. Pharmacol. Exp. Ther.*, 237, 529, 1986.
37. **Ohlstein, E. H. and Berkowitz, B. A.,** Human vascular vasopressin receptors: analysis with selective vasopressin receptor antagonists, *J. Pharmacol. Exp. Ther.*, 239, 737, 1986.
38. **Katusic, Z. S. and Krstic, M. K.,** Vasopressin causes endothelium-independent contractions of the rat arteries, *Pharmacology*, 35, 264, 1987.
39. **Schwartz, J., Liard, J. F., Ott, C., and Cowley, A. W.,** Hemodynamic effects of neurohypophyseal peptides with antidiuretic activity in dogs, *Am. J. Physiol.*, 249, H1001, 1985.
40. **Walker, B. R.,** Evidence for a vasodilatory effect of vasopressin in the conscious rat, *Am. J. Physiol.*, 251, H34, 1986.
41. **Liard, J. F. and Spadone, J. C.,** Hemodynamic effects of antagonists of the vasoconstrictor action of vasopressin in conscious dogs, *J. Cardiovasc. Pharmacol.*, 6, 713, 1984.
42. **Hirsch, A. T., Dzau, V. J., Majzoub, J. A., and Creager, M. A.,** Vasopressin-mediated forearm vasodilation in normal humans, *J. Clin. Invest.*, 84, 418, 1989.
43. **Kozniewska, E. and Szczepanska-Sadowska, E.,** V_2-like receptors mediate cerebral blood flow increase following vasopressin administration in rats, *J. Cardiovasc. Pharmacol.*, 15, 579, 1990.
44. **László, F. A., László, F., Jr. and De Wied, D.,** Pharmacology and clinical perspectives of vasopressin antagonists, *Pharmacol. Rev.*, 43, 73, 1991.
45. **Kinter, L. B., Dytko, G., Ashton, D., McDonald, J., Huffman, W., and Stassen, F. L.,** Discovery and therapeutical utility of vasopressin antagonists in rats, *J. Cardiovasc. Pharmacol.*, 7(Suppl.), S36, 1986.
46. **Belch, J. J. F., Small, M., McKenzie, F., Hill, P. A., Lowe, G. D. O., McIntyre, D. E., Forbes, C. D., and Prentice, C. R. M.,** DDAVP stimulates prostacyclin production, *Thromb. Haemostasis*, 47, 122, 1982.

Chapter 14

PURINERGIC TRANSMISSION IN CEREBRAL ARTERIES

Ikunobu Muramatsu

TABLE OF CONTENTS

I. Introduction 226

II. Neurogenic Purinergic Response 226

III. Purinergic Receptor Subtypes 228

IV. Conclusion 229

Acknowledgments 230

References 230

0-8493-5096-0/93/$0.00 + $.50

I. INTRODUCTION

Adenosine has been considered as a potential candidate for metabolic regulation of cerebral blood flow, because the nucleoside is rapidly formed from ATP under ischemic conditions and produces a potent cerebrovascular dilatation.[1,2] However, not only adenosine, but also adenine nucleotides were recently found to be released from many tissues such as vascular smooth muscle, perivascular nerves, and endothelial cells.[3-6] For example, ATP or related nucleotides are released from cerebral blood vessels, which receive a rich supply of sympathetic, parasympathetic, and sensory nerves, producing purinergic responses.[7,8] Cerebral blood vessels are highly sensitive to adenine nucleoside and nucleotides,[9,10] and different purinergic receptor subtypes are involved in the purinergic responses of cerebral vessels.[2,11] Therefore, it appears that purinergic mechanisms in the regulation of cerebral blood flow are important, but complex. In this chapter recent developments of purinergic transmission in the cerebral arteries will be described.

II. NEUROGENIC PURINERGIC RESPONSE

Purinergic nerves were originally considered as nerves which selectively release ATP, or a related substance, as their neurotransmitter.[12] However, other kinds of nerves have recently been demonstrated to release this purine, producing purinergic responses.[11] For example, in the dog mesenteric artery, sympathetic nerve stimulation produces a purinergic contraction in addition to an adrenergic contraction.[13,14] The purinergic response is associated with an excitatory junctional potential and is resistant to adrenergic receptor blocking agents, but is completely inhibited by adrenergic neuron blocking agents such as guanethidine or tetrodotoxin or by desensitization of P_{2X}-purinergic receptors.

Such purinergic responses were also found in dog cerebral arteries.[7,8] Figure 1 shows a representative recording of neurogenic responses in the isolated dog basilar artery, where electrical transmural stimulation was applied repeatedly. A transient contraction followed by a relaxation is evoked upon electrical stimulation. The contraction, but not relaxation, is abolished after desensitization of the P_{2X}-purinergic receptor with α,β-methylene ATP or by treatment with adrenergic neuron blocking agents such as guanethidine. In basilar arteries isolated from the dogs in which both superior cervical ganglia were removed beforehand, the transient contraction cannot be produced by electrical transmural stimulation. Prazosin, propranolol, and atropine have no effect on the contractile responses to electrical stimulation. These results strongly suggest that the transient contraction of dog basilar artery induced by electrical stimulation is sympathetic in origin but purinergic in nature.

Cerebral arteries of dog and other species receive a dense innervation of sympathetic adrenergic fibers,[15,16] and norepinephrine has been demonstrated

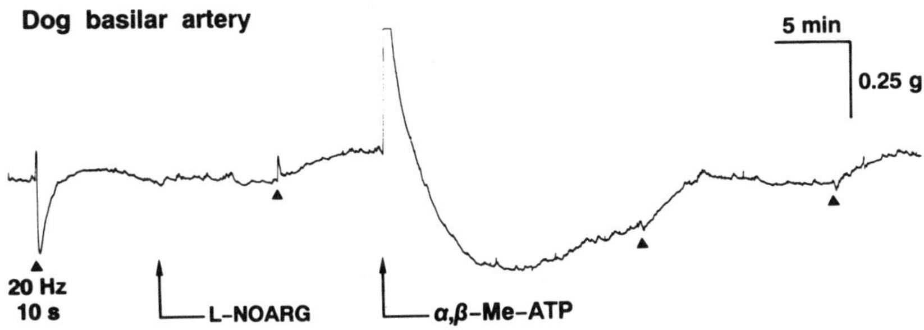

FIGURE 1. Representative neurogenic responses to electrical transmural stimulation in isolated dog basilar artery (endothelium rubbed preparation). L-NOARG: 5×10^{-6} *M* (N^G-nitro-L-arginine), α,β-Me-ATP: 10^{-5} *M* (α,β-methylene-ATP).

to be released from the nerve terminals.[7,18] Therefore, it is natural to question why an adrenergic contraction is not evoked in response to electrical stimulation in the dog cerebral artery. We have examined the postjunctional responsiveness to various drugs of the dog cerebral artery and found that the α-adrenergic receptors are of the α_2, but not α_1, subtype.[19,20] Furthermore, the contractile response mediated through the α_2-adrenergic receptors was much less than that to ATP or other contractile substances. These findings may account for the absence of a sympathetic adrenergic contraction in the dog cerebral artery. In contrast, both norepinephrine release and the transient contraction induced by electrical stimulation are enhanced by phentolamine and yohimbine.[7,8] Therefore, it is likely that norepinephrine acts as a neuromodulator (via prejunctional α_2-adrenergic receptors) rather than as a neurotransmitter in the dog cerebral artery.[8]

Sympathetic nervous system induced contractions, which are antagonized by adrenergic neuron blocking agents but are resistant to α-adrenergic receptor blocking agents, have been also reported in cerebral arteries isolated from monkey[21] and rabbit.[22] In contrast, sympathetic nervous system-evoked contractions of human and sheep cerebral arteries are potently inhibited by phentolamine,[21,23] indicating that the adrenergic component is predominant in these arteries.

In addition, the cerebral arteries of many species, including dog, are known to produce nonadrenergic, noncholinergic relaxations.[7,8,21,23,24] Such relaxation in dog cerebral arteries is resistant to α,β-methylene ATP, guanethidine, chronic reserpinization, and bilateral superior cervical ganglionectomy.[7,8] These results indicate that sympathetic nerves are not involved in the nonadrenergic, noncholinergic relaxation. Recently, the relaxing response was found to be completely inhibited by NO-synthase inhibitors and this inhibition was reversed by further addition of L-arginine, suggesting that the nonadrenergic, noncholinergic response is NOergic.[24,25] Figure 1 shows the selective inhibition by the NO-synthase inhibitor L-NOARG

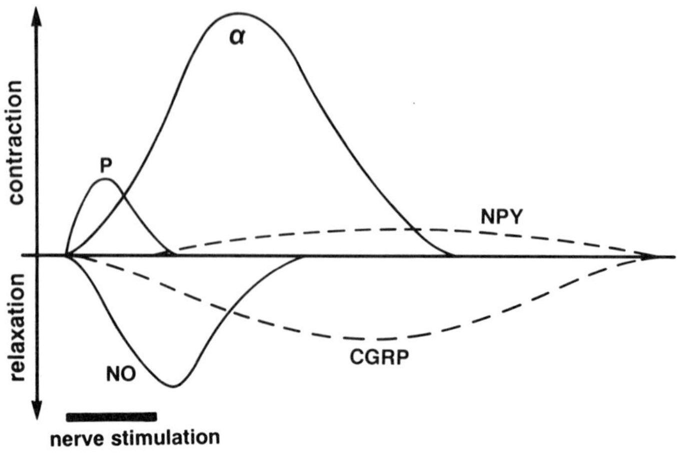

FIGURE 2. Schematic comparison of possible neurogenic components in the cerebral arteries. P, purinergic; α, α-adrenergic; NPY, NPYergic; NO, NOergic; CGRP, CGRPergic.

(N^G-nitro-L-arginine) of the nonadrenergic, noncholinergic relaxation, revealing a residual purinergic contraction. Dog basilar artery thus appears to be innervated reciprocally by purinergic and NOergic nerves.

In general, the purinergic contraction is transient and undergoes a gradual decline during continuous stimulation of the nerve[13] (Figure 2). This feature is due to a rapid desensitization of P_{2X}-purinergic receptors, indicating that the purinergic response is caused predominantly through P_{2X}-purinergic receptors. If other types of stronger and longer lasting responses were to be evoked simultaneously in the cerebral artery, the transient purinergic contraction would be easily masked. Heterogeneity or species differences in the neurogenic responses of cerebral arteries may reflect a variability in the components involved in the neurogenic response (Figure 2).

III. PURINERGIC RECEPTOR SUBTYPES

Since the initial classification of purinergic receptors into P_1 and P_2,[26] several subtypes have been proposed.[11] The distribution and some of the functions of these subtypes are listed in Table 1.

P_{2X}-purinergic receptors exist on cerebrovascular smooth muscle cells. α,β-Methylene ATP is a selective agonist for the P_{2X}-purinergic receptor, activation of which produces a contraction of cerebral blood vessels and a decrease in cerebral blood flow.[27,28] However, continuous treatment with this compound at high concentrations produces a desensitization of P_{2X}-purinergic receptors, after an initial stimulation (Figure 1). On the other hand, P_{2Y}-purinergic receptors are distributed on both endothelial and smooth muscle cells of cerebral arteries.[27] Stimulation of P_{2Y}-purinergic receptors on the

TABLE 1
Purinergic Receptor Subtypes in Cerebral Arteries

Subtype	Distribution	Response
P_1 (A_2)	Smooth muscle	Relaxation
(A_1)	Sympathetic nerve terminals	Inhibition of transmitter release
P_{2X}	Smooth muscle	Contraction
P_{2Y}	Smooth muscle	Relaxation
	Endothelial cell	Release of EDRF or EDCF

Note: EDRF, Endothelium derived relaxing factor; EDCF, Endothelium derived contracting factor.

endothelial cells releases EDRF (presumably NO) or EDCF (thromboxane A_2, etc.), while the receptors on smooth muscle are associated with the direct relaxation response. *In vivo,* administration of ATP produces cerebral vasodilation which is mediated through both of these P_{2Y}-purinergic receptors in addition to P_1-purinergic receptors on the smooth muscle cells.[28]

Adenosine, topically applied to exposed pial arterioles of the cat or infused to the intracarotid or internal maxillary arteries of the rabbit[29] or goat,[30] dilates the arterioles and increases cerebral blood flow. Adenosine and its analogues elicit relaxations of isolated dog, rabbit, cat, and human cerebral blood vessels through P_1-purinergic receptors on the smooth muscle, which are blocked by methylxanthines.[9,10,31] The rank order of potency for several adenosine analogues is adenosine 5′-N-ethylcarboxamide (NECA) $>$ 2-chloroadenosine $\geq$ adenosine $>$ L-N^6-phenylisopropyl adenosine (L-PIA). Adenosine and related agonists activate adenylate cyclase in the rat, rabbit, cat, and guinea pig cerebral microvessels, resulting in an accumulation of cAMP. The order of potency is the same as that in eliciting relaxations mentioned above.[31,32] These results, together with binding data for [^{3}H]-NECA or 2-chloro-[^{3}H]adenosine, reveal that the P_1-purinergic receptors of cerebral blood vessels are of the A_2 subtype (adenylate cyclase stimulating site) rather than A_1(inhibitory site).[33]

P_1-purinergic receptors also occur at prejunctional sites. In the dog and cat cerebral arteries preincubated with ^{3}H-norepinephrine, ^{3}H-release from sympathetic nerve terminals evoked by electrical stimulation or high K^+ is inhibited by adenosine, ATP, or L-PIA (A_1-receptor agonist) and these inhibitions are antagonized by methylxanthines.[7,8,18] In contrast, NECA (A_2-receptor agonist) and α,β-methylene ATP are without effect on the ^{3}H-release. These results indicate that transmitter release from sympathetic nerve terminals in the cerebral arteries may be regulated by prejunctional P_1-purinergic receptors (A_1-subtype).

IV. CONCLUSION

Adenosine and adenine nucleotides are released from many cerebral sources (glia cells, vascular smooth muscle, perivascular nerves, endothelial cells).

Since the different purinergic receptor subtypes are widely distributed in cerebral blood vessels, it seems that cerebral blood flow may be regulated not only by purinergic neurogenic and metabolic systems but also by purinergic paracrine and/or autocrine systems.

ACKNOWLEDGMENTS

The author thanks Ms. N. Aoki for secretarial assistance. This work was supported in part by a grant from the Suzuken Memorial Foundation, Japan.

REFERENCES

1. **Berne, R. M., Rubio, R., and Curnish, R. R.,** Release of adenosine from ischemic brain: effect on cerebral vascular resistance and incorporation into cerebral adenine nucleotides, *Circ. Res.*, 35, 262, 1974.
2. **Phillis, J. W.,** Adenosine in the control of the cerebral circulation, *Cereb. Brain Metab. Rev.*, 1, 26, 1989.
3. **Pearson, J. and Gordon, J.,** Vascular endothelial and smooth muscle cells in culture selectively release adenine nucleotides, *Nature,* 281, 384, 1979.
4. **Su, C.,** Extracellular functions of nucleotides in heart and blood vessels, *Annu. Rev. Physiol.*, 47, 665, 1985.
5. **White, T. D.,** Role of adenine compounds in autonomic neurotransmission, *Pharmacol. Ther.*, 38, 129, 1988.
6. **Sedaa, K. O., Bjur, R. A., Shinozuka, K., and Westfall, D. P.,** Nerve and drug-induced release of adenine nucleotides and nucleotides from rabbit aorta, *J. Pharmacol. Exp. Ther.*, 252, 1060, 1990.
7. **Muramatsu, I., Fujiwara, M., Miura, A., and Sakakibara, Y.,** Possible involvement of adenine nucleotides in sympathetic neuroeffector mechanisms of dog basilar artery, *J. Pharmacol. Exp. Ther.*, 216, 401, 1981.
8. **Muramatsu, I. and Kigoshi, S.,** Purinergic and non-purinergic innervation in the cerebral arteries of the dog, *Br. J. Pharmacol.*, 92, 901, 1987.
9. **Muramatsu, I., Fujiwara, M., Miura, A., and Shibata, S.,** Reactivity of isolated canine cerebral arteries of adenine nucleotides and adenosine, *Pharmacology,* 21, 198, 1980.
10. **Hardebo, J. E., Kåhrström, J., and Owman, C.,** P_1- and P_2-purine receptors in brain circulation, *Eur. J. Pharmacol.*, 144, 343, 1987.
11. **Burnstock, G.,** Purinergic mechanisms, *Ann. N.Y. Acad. Sci.*, 603, 1, 1990.
12. **Burnstock, G.,** Purinergic nerves, *Pharmacol. Rev.*, 24, 509, 1972.
13. **Muramatsu, I., Ohmura, T., and Oshita, M.,** Comparison between sympathetic adrenergic and purinergic transmission in the dog mesenteric artery, *J. Physiol.*, 411, 227, 1989.
14. **MacHaly, M., Dalziel, H. H., and Sneddon, P.,** Evidence for ATP as a cotransmitter in dog mesenteric artery, *Eur. J. Pharmacol.*, 147, 83, 1988.
15. **Owman, C., Edvinsson, L., and Nielsen, K. C.,** Autonomic neuroeffector mechanisms in brain vessels, *Blood Vessels,* 11, 2, 1974.
16. **Marín, J. and Rivilla, F.,** Nerve endings and pharmacological receptors in cerebral vessels, *Gen. Pharmacol.*, 13, 361, 1982.

17. **Muramatsu, I., Fujiwara, M., Osumi, Y., and Shibata, S.,** Vasoconstrictor and dilator actions of nicotine and electrical transmural stimulation of isolated dog cerebral arteries, *Blood Vessels,* 15, 110, 1978.
18. **Rivilla, F., Güemes, M., SanchezFerrer, C. F., Ibãnez, C., Salaices, M., and Marin, J.,** Role of presynaptic purinoceptors and cyclic AMP on the noradrenaline release in cat cerebral arteries, *J. Pharm. Pharmacol.,* 42, 481, 1990.
19. **Sakakibara, Y., Fujiwara, M., and Muramatsu, I.,** Pharmacological characterization of the alpha adrenoceptors of the dog basilar artery, *Naunyn-Schmiedebergs Arch. Pharmakol.,* 319, 1, 1982.
20. **Fujiwara, M., Tsukahara, T., and Taniguchi, T.,** α-Adrenoceptors in human and animal cerebral arteries: alterations after sympathetic denervation and subarachnoid hemorrhage, *Trends Pharmacol. Sci.,* 8, 329, 1989.
21. **Usui, H., Fujiwara, M., Tsukahara, T., Taniguchi, T., and Kurahashi, K.,** Differences in contractile responses to electrical stimulation and α-adrenergic binding sites in isolated cerebral arteries of humans, cows, dogs and monkeys, *J. Cardiovasc. Pharmacol.,* 7, S47, 1985.
22. **Lee, T. J.-F., Su, C., and Bevan, J. A.,** Neurogenic sympathetic vasoconstriction of the rabbit basilar artery, *Circ. Res.,* 39, 120, 1976.
23. **Duckles, S. P.,** Neurogenic dilator and constrictor responses of pial arteries in vitro, *Circ. Res.,* 44, 482, 1979.
24. **Lee, T. J.-F., Fang, Y. X., and Nickols, G. A.,** Cyclic nucleotide and cerebral neurogenic vasodilation, in *Neurotransmission and Cerebrovascular Function,* Seylaz, J. and Mackenzie, E. T., Eds., Elsevier, Amsterdam, 1989, 277.
25. **Toda, N. and Okamura, T.,** Role of nitric oxide in neurally induced cerebroarterial relaxation, *J. Pharmacol. Exp. Ther.,* 258, 1027, 1991.
26. **Burnstock, G.,** A basis for distinguishing two types of purinergic receptor, in *Cell Membrane Receptors for Drugs and Hormones: A Multidisciplinary Approach,* Bolis, L. and Staub, R. W., Eds., Raven Press, New York, 1978, 107.
27. **Shirahase, H., Usui, H., Shimaji, H., Kurahashi, K., and Fujiwara, M.,** Endothelium-independent and endothelium-dependent contractions mediated by P_{2X}- and P_{2Y}-purinoceptors in canine basilar arteries, *J. Pharmacol. Exp. Ther.,* 256, 683, 1991.
28. **Torregrosa, G., Miranda, F. J., Salom, J. B., Alabadí, J. A., Alvarez, C., and Alborch, E.,** Heterogeneity of P_2-purinoceptors in brain circulation, *J. Cereb. Blood Flow Metab.,* 10, 572, 1990.
29. **Heistad, D. D., Marcus, M. L., Gourley, J. K., and Busija, D. W.,** Effect of adenosine and dipyridamole on cerebral blood flow, *Am. J. Physiol.,* 240, H775, 1981.
30. **Torregrosa, G., Terrasa, J. C., Salom, J. B., Miranda, F. J., Campos, V., and Alborch, E.,** P_1-purinoceptors in the cerebrovascular bed of the goat in vivo, *Eur. J. Pharmacol.,* 149, 17, 1988.
31. **Edvinsson, L. and Fredholm, B. B.,** Characterization of adenosine receptors in isolated cerebral arteries of cat, *Br. J. Pharmacol.,* 80, 631, 1983.
32. **Li, Y.-O. and Fredholm, B. B.,** Adenosine analogues stimulate cyclic AMP formation in rabbit cerebral microvessels via adenosine A_2-receptors, *Acta Physiol. Scand.,* 124, 253, 1985.
33. **Kalaria, R. N. and Harik, S. I.,** Adenosine receptors of cerebral microvessels and choroid plexus, *J. Cereb. Blood Flow Metab.,* 6, 463, 1986.

Chapter 15

ROLE OF NITRIC OXIDE IN CEREBROARTERIAL RELAXATION

Noboru Toda and Tomio Okamura

TABLE OF CONTENTS

I. Introduction 234

II. Relaxation Mediated by EDRF or NO in Isolated Cerebral Arteries 234

III. Modification of Relaxation Mediated by EDRF or NO 237

IV. Arteriolar Dilatation Mediated by EDRF or NO *In Vivo* 238

V. Relaxation Mediated by NO Released from Vasodilator Nerves 239

VI. Conclusion 241

References 242

0-8493-5096-0/93/$0.00 + $.50

I. INTRODUCTION

Since the epoch-making discovery by Furchgott and Zawadzki (1980)[1] of endothelium-derived relaxing factor (EDRF), numerous studies have been carried out to chemically identify this substance. However, it was difficult to achieve success in this, because of its instability. The effect of EDRF is abolished by hemoglobin (Hb), which binds EDRF to its heme moiety, methylene blue, a guanylate cyclase inhibitor, and antioxidants (pyrogallol, hydroquinone, etc.), but is potentiated by treatment with superoxide dismutase (SOD).[2] EDRF activates guanylate cyclase, as do nitroglycerin and sodium nitroprusside. EDRF released from the endothelium stimulates the synthesis of cyclic GMP in smooth muscle, resulting in its relaxation. Palmer et al.,[3] Furchgott,[4] and Ignarro et al.[5] have independently demonstrated that the biological and chemical natures of EDRF are quite similar to those of nitric oxide (NO) and hypothesized that EDRF is NO. Despite some discrepancy in the evidence supporting this hypothesis, NO or an S-nitroso compound that liberates the NO radical is widely accepted to be EDRF. NO is synthesized from L-arginine,[6] and this synthesis is inhibited by L-arginine derivatives,[7] such as N^G-monomethyl-L-arginine (L-NMMA), N^G-nitro-L-arginine (L-NA), L-NA methylester (L-NAME), etc.

Recent studies have demonstrated that relaxations mediated by EDRF, although not always, are usually identical to those mediated by NO. Literature on EDRF in cerebral blood vessels became available only a couple of years ago; analyses of responses mediated by endothelium-derived NO are quite limited. In this chapter, we describe the ability of cerebral arteries to liberate EDRF or NO, its action *in vitro* and *in vivo,* and the role of NO released from vasodilator nerves innervating the cerebrovascular wall.

II. RELAXATION MEDIATED BY EDRF OR NO IN ISOLATED CEREBRAL ARTERIES

Acetylcholine (ACh) is a representative in releasing relaxing substances from the endothelium in a variety of blood vessels obtained from different mammals.[1] This is true in isolated human (Figure 1),[8-10] cat,[11] rabbit,[12] and rat cerebral arteries.[13] ACh-induced relaxations are abolished by endothelium denudation but are not influenced by treatment with cyclooxygenase inhibitors. Although the effectiveness of inhibitors, including Hb, methylene blue, and NO synthase inhibitors, has not been determined, the induced responses are suggested to derive from mediation by an EDRF, possibly NO, but not from prostaglandin (PG) I_2. In cat arteries, an involvement of M_3 muscarinic receptor subtypes is postulated. ACh hyperpolarizes rabbit middle cerebral arteries.[14] The hyperpolarization is abolished in the arteries without their endothelium and in the presence of K^+ channel inhibitors. ACh-induced relaxations are not inhibited by these K^+ channel inhibitors but are diminished

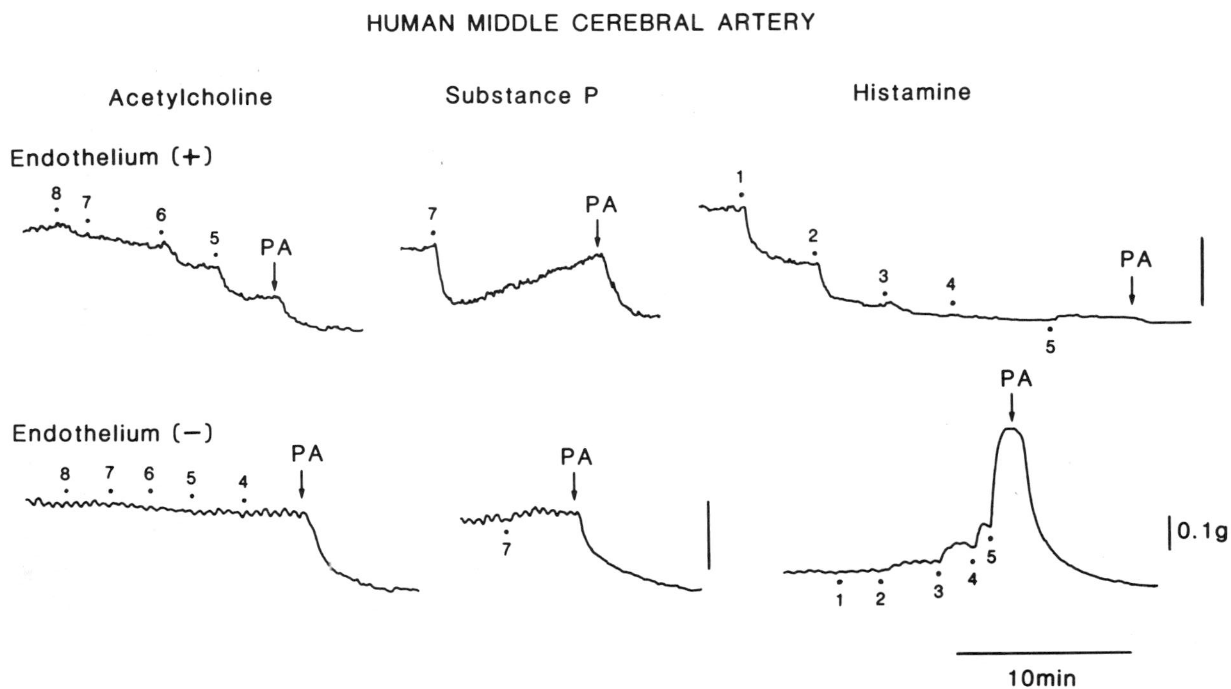

FIGURE 1. Responses to acetylcholine, substance P, and histamine of a human middle cerebral artery strip with intact and damaged endothelium. The strip was partially contracted with prostaglandin $F_{2\alpha}$. Concentrations of acetylcholine from 8 to 5 = 10^{-8}, 10^{-7}, 10^{-6}, and 10^{-5} *M*, respectively; concentration of substance P = 10^{-7} *M;* concentrations of histamine from 1 to 5 = 2×10^{-8}, 10^{-7}, 5×10^{-7}, 2×10^{-6}, and 10^{-5} *M*, respectively. PA = 10^{-4} *M* papaverine. (From Toda, N., *Am. J. Physiol.*, 258, H311, 1990. With permission.)

by methylene blue. NO relaxes, but does not hyperpolarize, the smooth muscle cells. On the other hand, cerebral arteries from dogs[15,16] and monkeys[17] do not respond to ACh consistently with relaxations, and even though slight relaxations are induced, endothelium dependency cannot always be observed. Despite such a slight responsiveness to ACh, the same preparations relax in response to other agents liberating EDRF, such as histamine, ATP, substance P, vasopressin, etc., to a marked or moderate extent. These findings indicate that although cerebral arteries have an ability to release EDRF, the distribution or/and sensitivity of muscarinic receptors in the endothelium responsible for its release varies in different animal species.

Bradykinin relaxes human,[8,18] dog,[19] and porcine cerebral arteries,[20] the relaxation being dependent on the endothelium and not associated with cyclooxygenase products. In the human arteries, a B_2 receptor subtype seems to be involved.[8] In dog arteries, the response is potentiated by treatment with SOD plus catalase and inhibited by methylene blue, Hb, and LY83583, a cyclic GMP lowering agent.[19] These authors compared the responses to bradykinin and NO and concluded, from the similarities of their actions, that EDRF is NO, as postulated in other blood vessels. Arginine vasopressin and oxytocin also produce endothelium-dependent relaxations of dog basilar arteries[21] that are mediated possibly by V_1 receptors.[22] In the dog, basilar and posterior cerebral arteries respond with a greater relaxation than middle cerebral arteries.[23] Whether this variability is due to differences in the EDRF-mediated relaxation or to an additional direct constrictor action on smooth muscle has not been determined. Substance P-induced relaxations in human (Figure 1)[10] and dog cerebral arteries[23] are also endothelium-dependent. The dog artery relaxation is not influenced by indomethacin, but is markedly suppressed by methylene blue, suggesting the involvement of EDRF. Thrombin relaxes human[18] and dog basilar arteries;[12] the relaxations are endothelium-dependent, but tachyphylaxis developed rapidly in the human arteries. The Ca^{2+} ionophore A23187 elicits an endothelium-dependent relaxation in human,[9] monkey,[17] and dog cerebral arteries.[16] The response is not associated with a stimulation of specific pharmacological receptors but possibly with an increase in Ca^{2+} influx into endothelial cells, which stimulates the synthesis of EDRF.

Concentration-related relaxations caused by histamine are reversed to contractions by endothelial denudation in human cerebral arteries (Figure 1)[10] and are significantly suppressed in the monkey arteries. Evidence for the involvement of an H_1 receptor subtype in the relaxation has been presented. The relaxation of monkey arteries is abolished by treatment with methylene blue, suggesting that EDRF is involved. In addition, our recent study showed that phasic relaxations caused by histamine in arteries treated with cimetidine were reversed to a contraction by treatment with L-NA, an NO synthase inhibitor, and that the relaxation was restored by the addition of L-arginine. Therefore, NO liberated from the endothelium by a stimulation of an H_1 histaminergic receptor subtype evokes the transient relaxation.

Relaxations induced by ATP and ADP in monkey cerebral arteries are partially dependent on the endothelium, whereas those in monkey temporal arteries are totally abolished by endothelium denudation.[17] ADP also produces relaxations, which are partially dependent on the endothelium, in porcine basilar arteries.[20]

Cd^{2+}, a nonselective Ca^{2+} entry blocker, suppresses the relaxant response to substance P in dog cerebral arteries but does not influence the relaxation caused by NO.[24] Ca^{2+} appears to be prerequisite in releasing EDRF in cerebral arteries, as evidenced in peripheral blood vessels. Participation of NO in the endothelium-dependent relaxation caused by substance P[25] and vasopressin has been revealed in dog basilar arteries. Treatment with L-NA abolishes the substance P-induced relaxation and reverses the vasopressin-induced relaxation to a contraction (Toda et al., unpublished data), suggesting that an EDRF, distinct from NO, is not involved. The release of EDRF by vasopressin and bradykinin from dog basilar arteries has been detected by a bioassay system, using a coronary artery ring denuded of the endothelium as a bioassay tissue.[26] The content of cyclic GMP in dog cerebral arteries is increased by the addition of substance P.[24] Therefore, as hypothesized in other blood vessels, Ca^{2+} introduced, by stimulation of drug receptors, into cerebral artery endothelial cells activates NO synthase and releases NO (EDRF), resulting in an activation of soluble guanylate cyclase in smooth muscle, an increased production of cyclic GMP and a relaxation.

III. MODIFICATION OF RELAXATION MEDIATED BY EDRF OR NO

Endothelium-dependent relaxations by thrombin in human basilar arteries are related inversely to increasing age, but those caused by bradykinin are not age-dependent.[18] Hypoxia inhibits the thrombin-induced relaxation of dog basilar arteries.[12] The mechanism underlying the decreased response has not been determined.

Relaxations induced by ACh in basilar arteries isolated from normotensive rats are not different from those in coarctation hypertensive rats.[13] In contrast, responses mediated by EDRF *in vivo* are impaired in spontaneously hypertensive rats, as described in the next section.

In basilar arteries isolated from dogs or rabbits with vasospasm experimentally induced by intracisternal injections of autologous blood, endothelium-dependent relaxations caused by bradykinin, vasopressin, ACh, or A23187 are reduced, compared to the responses of the arteries from intact dogs.[26-29] The mechanism of the decreased responsiveness is postulated not to be due to an impaired release of EDRF[26] but possibly to a depressed production of cyclic GMP in smooth muscle.[29] On the other hand, cerebral arteries from dogs with subarachnoid hemorrhage respond to substance P and Ca^{2+} ionophore A23187 with relaxations to a similar extent to those obtained from intact dogs.[30] Even though the endothelium-dependent relaxations are unaffected in isolated preparations, Hb produced by a lysis of blood clots in the subarachnoid space would be expected to suppress the response.[31] Thus, an attenuated relaxation mediated by EDRF would be involved in the pathogenesis of vasospasm after subarachnoid hemorrhage.

IV. ARTERIOLAR DILATATION MEDIATED BY EDRF OR NO *IN VIVO*

In anesthetized mice, rats, and cats, the effects of agents topically applied on cerebral arteriolar diameter have been investigated. ACh applied to the perivascular perfusion fluid dilates the arterioles; the dilatation is suppressed in association with endothelial damage induced by applications of laser/dye,[32] arachidonic acid, or hydrogen peroxide[33] and after treatment with methylene blue, Hb, or L-NMMA.[33-39] The release of EDRF is determined by an *in vivo* bioassay system in cat brain microvessels.[35] EDRF is produced in the donor window by ACh, and the superfusate is conducted to the assay window, in which the effect of ACh has been abolished by atropine. Treatment of the donor window with indomethacin does not alter the dilatation in the assay window, but it is inhibited by endothelial damage, methylene blue, or Hb. Wei and Kontos[33] postulated the involvement of S-nitrosothiol, instead of NO, since hydrogen peroxide inhibits the dilatation caused by NO and sodium nitroprusside but does not alter the responses to EDRF released by ACh and to S-nitroso-L-cysteine. Choline acetyltransferase has been immunocytochemically demonstrated to be localized in endothelial cells of small vessels in the rat brain.[40] These authors suggest the release of ACh following damage of endothelial cells during ischemia.

Bradykinin produces endothelium-dependent dilatation of cerebral arterioles in mice, rats, and cats.[34,37,41-43] In contrast to the response to ACh, bradykinin-induced dilatations in the mouse and cat brain are eliminated by deferoxamine, an agent that scavenges iron and thereby inhibits the production of hydroxyl radical,[41,42] and by cyclooxygenase inhibitors.[42] Therefore, the peptide-induced arteriolar dilatation is considered to derive from oxygen radicals, including hydroxyl radical, generated in association with arachidonate metabolism. As described previously,[19] bradykinin-induced, endothelium-dependent relaxations in isolated dog cerebral arteries are mediated by NO. Whether the involvement of different radicals (NO vs. oxygen radical) is due to animal species (dog vs. mouse and cat) or to the vascular size (artery vs. arteriole) remains to be elucidated.

Apart from the data obtained in isolated cerebral arteries, endothelium-dependent dilatation in the mouse brain by Ca^{2+} ionophore is abolished by treatment with indomethacin and aspirin, suggesting the response to be cyclooxygenase-dependent.[44] Topical application of angiotensin II and III to the rabbit brain surface produces an arteriolar dilatation that is eliminated by methylene blue but not by cyclooxygenase inhibitors.[45] Whether the response is endothelium-dependent has not been determined.

Topical application of L-NMMA constricts all the arterioles tested in the mouse brain, and L-arginine dilates the microvessels. Both the constriction and dilatation are abolished by endothelial damage by laser/dye application.[38] Basal release of endothelium-derived NO appears to participate in the vasodilator regulation of resistance vessel tone in the mouse brain *in vivo*. However, in the piglet[46] and rat brain,[47] L-NMMA does not constrict the arterioles.

Impairment of endothelium-dependent, L-NMMA-sensitive dilatation by ACh and bradykinin of the basilar artery is observed during the chronic stage of spontaneously hypertensive rats.[47,48] ACh-induced, endothelium-dependent, arteriolar dilatation is reduced in cats after fluid-percussion brain injury.[49] Endothelium-dependent dilatation of cerebral arterioles in response to ADP and serotonin is profoundly impaired in diabetic rats.[50]

V. RELAXATION MEDIATED BY NO RELEASED FROM VASODILATOR NERVES

The idea of vasodilator innervation in cerebral blood vessels originated from a report that nicotine elicits relaxations of dog cerebral artery strips in a nonadrenergic and noncholinergic fashion.[51] Treatment with the pharmacological antagonists so far available does not attenuate the response to nicotine or to electrical neural stimulation. Similar results were also obtained in human,[52] monkey,[53] cat,[54] and bovine cerebral arteries.[55] Cerebral vasodilator peptides, including substance P, vasoactive intestinal peptide, calcitonin gene-related peptide, and atrial natriuretic peptide, are excluded from consideration as candidates for the responsible chemical transmitter, since arteries made insensitive to these peptides by repeated applications still respond to the stimulation with similar magnitude of relaxations.[53,56,57] Methylene blue and Hb abolish the relaxation or reverse it to a contraction, suggesting that the vasodilator transmitter increases smooth muscle cyclic GMP.[58] L-NMMA or L-NA abolished the relaxant response to electrical or chemical stimulation of nerves in dog and monkey cerebral arteries (Figure 2).[59-62] D-enantiomers are ineffective. L-, but not D-, arginine reverses the inhibition by NO synthase inhibitors. The response is not dependent on the endothelium. Transmural electrical stimulation applied to superfused dog cerebral artery strips significantly increases the output of nitroxy compounds (NO_x) into the superfusate, the effect being diminished by treatment with tetrodotoxin and L-NA.[60] In addition, nicotine and electrical stimulation increase the content of cyclic GMP in cerebral arteries, and treatment with L-NA abolishes the stimulating effect.[25] Immunohistochemical studies have visualized perivascular nerves containing NO synthase[63] or NADPH diaphorase in cerebral arteries. These findings indicate the following possibilities:

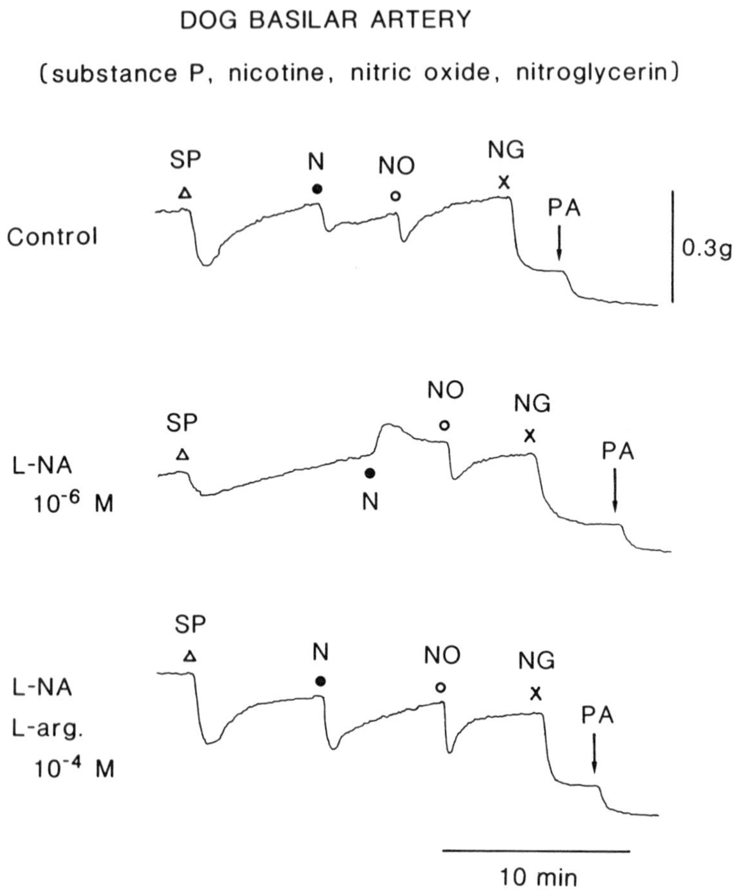

FIGURE 2. Responses to substance P (SP, 10^{-8} *M*), nicotine (N, 10^{-4} *M*), NO (10^{-7} *M*), and nitroglycerin (NG, 10^{-8} *M*) of a dog basilar artery strip with the endothelium, before (control) and after treatment with L-NA and L-NA plus L-arginine (L-arg.). The strip was treated with 10^{-6} *M* indomethacin and partially contracted with prostaglandin $F_{2\alpha}$. PA = 10^{-4} *M* papaverine. (From Toda, N. and Okamura, T., *J. Pharmacol. Exp. Ther.*, 258, 1027–1032, 1991. With permission of ©American Society for Pharm. & Exper. Ther.)

1. NO is synthesized in nerve terminals in association with electrical or chemical neural stimulation and liberated as a neurotransmitter that acts on soluble guanylate cyclase to increase cyclic GMP in smooth muscle,
2. NO synthesized in nerve terminals initiates and enhances the release of an unidentified transmitter that acts on guanylate cyclase in smooth muscle, and
3. An unidentified transmitter is released and acts on postjunctional receptors responsible for activation of NO synthase in smooth muscle.[61]

The second alternative is ruled out, since the suppression of neural function by NO synthase inhibitors is not reversed by the addition of exogenous NO. As the production of NO has been demonstrated in rat and bovine blood vessels denuded of endothelium,[64] the third alternative appeared possible. In fact, excitatory responses via NMDA receptors in the brain are considered to be provoked by the mediation of NO produced in postjunctional effector cells.[65] However, a recent study proved that NO synthase in vascular smooth muscle is of the inducible type;[66] therefore, a rapid, Ca^{2+}-dependent NO synthesis cannot be considered. Further, immunohistochemical studies with an antibody made to the constitutive type of NO synthase from brain demonstrated staining only in perivascular nerves and endothelium in the cerebral artery.[63] On the basis of the findings so far obtained, the first possibility that NO synthesized and released from vasodilator nerve acts as neurotransmitter in cerebral arteries is most likely.

VI. CONCLUSION

The regulation, by NO released from the endothelium (EDRF), of cerebral arterial and arteriolar tone *in vitro* and *in vivo* is summarized. As shown in Figure 3, agonist-induced receptor activation results in the increased influx of Ca^{2+} that stimulates the synthesis of NO from L-arginine. Released NO activates intracellular guanylate cyclase and increases production of the cyclic GMP that is responsible for muscle relaxation. There are variations in the response mediated by EDRF or NO in primate and subprimate mammals and in brain regions or vessels of different sizes. In addition, we introduced our idea on the role of NO released from vasodilator nerves (Figure 3; nitroxidergic nerve) in the control of cerebroarterial tone. Smooth muscle and macrophages are also sites of NO production, although NO synthases in these cells are different from those in the endothelium and nerve (inducible vs. constitutive). Therefore, care has to be taken to determine the source of NO released by chemical and physical stimuli.

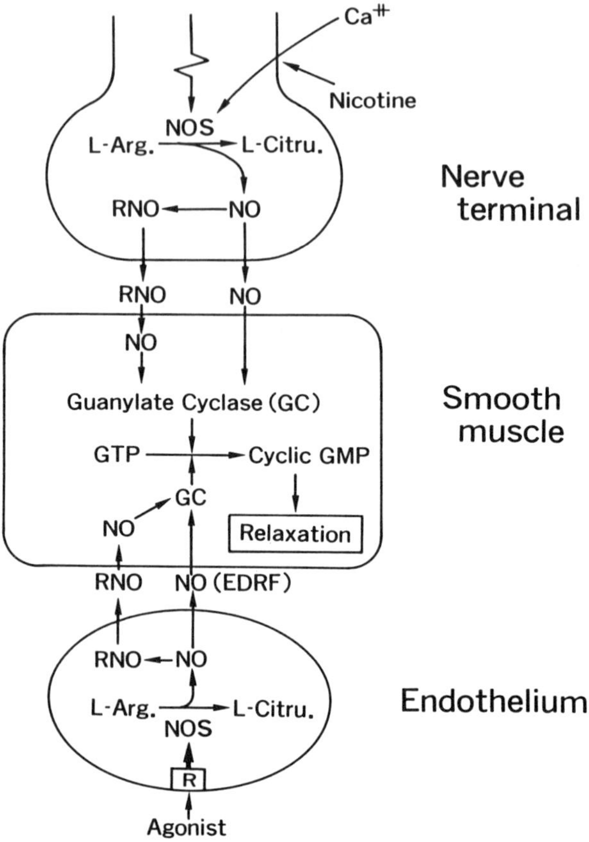

FIGURE 3. Schematic presentation of the possible involvement of NO or S-nitrosothiol (RNO) released from the endothelium (EDRF) and vasodilator nerve in the regulation of cerebroarterial smooth muscle tone. L-Arg. = L-arginine; L-Citru. = L-citrulline; R = receptor for agonists. (From Toda, N. and Okamura, T., *Am. J. Physiol.*, 259, H1511, 1990. With permission.)

REFERENCES

1. **Furchgott, R. F. and Zawadzki, J. V.,** The obligatory role of endothelial cells in the relaxation of arterial smooth muscle by acetylcholine, *Nature,* 288, 373, 1980.
2. **Angus, J. A. and Cocks, T. M.,** Endothelium-derived relaxing factor, *Pharmac. Ther.,* 41, 303, 1989.
3. **Palmer, R. M. J., Ferrige, A. G., and Moncada, S.,** Nitric oxide release accounts for the biological activity of endothelium-derived relaxing factor, *Nature,* 327, 524, 1987.

4. **Furchgott, R. F.,** Studies on relaxation of rabbit aorta by sodium nitrate: the basis for the proposal that the acid-activatable inhibitory factor from bovine retractor penis is inorganic nitrate and the endothelium-derived relaxing factor is nitric oxide, in *Mechanism of Vasodilatation,* Vol. 4, Vanhoutte, P. M., Ed., Raven Press New York, 1988, 401.
5. **Ignarro, L. J., Byrns, R. E., Buga, G. M., and Wood, K. S.,** Endothelium-derived relaxing factor from pulmonary artery and vein possesses pharmacologic and chemical properties identical to those of nitric oxide radical, *Circ. Res.,* 60, 82, 1987.
6. **Palmer, R. M. J., Ashton, D. S., and Moncada, S.,** Vascular endothelial cells synthesize nitric oxide from L-arginine, *Nature,* 333, 664, 1988.
7. **Rees, D. D., Palmer, R. M. J., Hodson, H. F., and Moncada, S.,** A specific inhibitor of nitric oxide formation from L-arginine attenuates endothelium-dependent relaxation, *Br. J. Pharmacol.,* 96, 418, 1989.
8. **Whalley, E. T., Amure, Y. O., and Lye, R. H.,** Analysis of the mechanism of action of bradykinin on human basilar artery in vitro, *Naunyn-Schmiedebergs Arch. Pharmakol.,* 335, 433, 1987.
9. **Kanamaru, K., Waga, S., Fujimoto, K., Itoh, H., and Kubo, Y.,** Endothelium-dependent relaxation of human basilar arteries, *Stroke,* 20, 1208, 1989.
10. **Toda, N.,** Mechanism underlying responses to histamine of isolated monkey and human cerebral arteries, *Am. J. Physiol.,* 258, H311, 1990.
11. **Dauphin, F. and Hamel, E.,** Muscarinic receptor subtype mediating vasodilation in feline middle cerebral artery exhibits M_3 pharmacology, *Eur. J. Pharmacol.,* 178, 203, 1990.
12. **Nakagomi, T., Kassell, N. F., Sasaki, T., Hongo, K., Fujiwara, S., Lehman, R. M., and Vollmer, D. G.,** Effect of hypoxia on endothelium-dependent relaxation of canine and rabbit basilar arteries, *Acta Neurochir.,* 97, 77, 1989.
13. **Lai, F. M., Cobuzzi, A., Shepherd, C., Tanikella, T., Hoffman, A., and Cervoni, P.,** Endothelium-dependent basilar and aortic vascular responses in normotensive and coarctation hypertensive rats, *Life Sci.,* 45, 607, 1989.
14. **Brayden, J. E.,** Membrane hyperpolarization is a mechanism of endothelium-dependent cerebral vasodilation, *Am. J. Physiol.,* 259, H668, 1990.
15. **Toda, N.,** Acetylcholine-induced relaxation in isolated dog cerebral arteries, *J. Pharmacol. Exp. Ther.,* 209, 353, 1979.
16. **Kanamaru, K., Waga, S., Kojima, T., Fujimoto, K., and Itoh, H.,** Endothelium-dependent relaxation of canine basilar arteries, *Stroke,* 18, 932, 1987.
17. **Toda, N., Kawakami, M., Yamazaki, M., and Okamura, T.,** Comparison of endothelium-dependent responses of monkey cerebral and temporal arteries, *Br. J. Pharmacol.,* 102, 805, 1991.
18. **Hatake, K., Kakishita, E., Wakabayashi, I., Sakiyama, N., and Hishida, S.,** Effect of aging on endothelium-dependent vascular relaxation of isolated human basilar artery to thrombin and bradykinin, *Stroke,* 21, 1039, 1990.
19. **Katusic, Z. S., Marshall, J. J., Kontos, H. A., and Vanhoutte, P. M.,** Similar responsiveness of smooth muscle of the canine basilar artery to EDRF and nitric oxide, *Am. J. Physiol.,* 257, H1235, 1989.
20. **Shimokawa, H., Kim, P., and Vanhoutte, P. M.,** Endothelium-dependent relaxation to aggregating platelets in isolated basilar arteries of control and hypercholesterolemic pigs, *Circ. Res.,* 63, 604, 1988.
21. **Katusic, Z. S., Shepherd, J. T., and Vanhoutte, P. M.,** Vasopressin causes endothelium-dependent relaxations of the canine basilar artery, *Circ. Res.,* 55, 575, 1984.
22. **Katusic, Z. S., Shepherd, J. T., and Vanhoutte, P. M.,** Oxytocin causes endothelium-dependent relaxations of canine basilar arteries by activating V_1-vasopressinergic receptors, *J. Pharmacol. Exp. Ther.,* 236, 166, 1986.
23. **Onoue, H., Nakamura, N., and Toda, N.,** Endothelium-dependent and -independent responses to vasodilators of isolated dog cerebral arteries, *Stroke,* 19, 1388, 1988.

24. **Toda, N. and Okamura, T.,** Different susceptibility of vasodilator nerve, endothelium and smooth muscle functions to Ca^{++} antagonists in cerebral arteries, *J. Pharmacol. Exp. Ther.,* 261, 234, 1992.
25. **Toda, N. and Okamura, T.,** Role of nitric oxide in neurally induced cerebroarterial relaxation, *J. Pharmacol. Exp. Ther.,* 258, 1027, 1991.
26. **Kim, P., Lorenz, R. R., Sundt, T. M., Jr., and Vanhoutte, P. M.,** Release of endotheliumderived relaxing factor after subarachnoid hemorrhage, *J. Neurosurg.,* 70, 108, 1989.
27. **Kim, P., Sundt, T. M., Jr., and Vanhoutte, P. M.,** Alterations in endothelium-dependent responsiveness of the canine basilar artery after subarachnoid hemorrhage, *J. Neurosurg.,* 69, 239, 1988.
28. **Nakagomi, T., Kassell, N. F., Sasaki, T., Fujiwara, S., Lehman, R. M., and Torner, J. C.,** Impairment of endothelium-dependent vasodilation induced by acetylcholine and adenosine triphosphate following experimental subarachnoid hemorrhage, *Stroke,* 18, 482, 1987.
29. **Kim, P., Schini, V. B., Sundt, T. M., Jr., and Vanhoutte, P. M.,** Reduced production of cGMP underlies the loss of endothelium-dependent relaxations in the canine basilar artery after subarachnoid hemorrhage, *Circ. Res.,* 70, 248, 1992.
30. **Saito, A., Handa, J., and Toda, N.,** Reactivity to vasoactive agents of canine basilar arteries exposed to experimental subarachnoid hemorrhage, *Surg. Neurol.,* 35, 461, 1991.
31. **Hongo, K., Ogawa, H., Kassell, N. F., Nakagomi, T., Sasaki, T., Tsukahara, T., and Lehman, R. M.,** Comparison of intraluminal and extraluminal inhibitory effects of hemoglobin on endothelium-dependent relaxation of rabbit basilar artery, *Stroke,* 19, 1550, 1988.
32. **Rosenblum, W. I., Nelson, G. H., and Povlishock, J. T.,** Laser-induced endothelial damage inhibits endothelium-dependent relaxation in the cerebral microcirculation of the mouse, *Circ. Res.,* 60, 169, 1987.
33. **Wei, E. P. and Kontos, H. A.,** H_2O_2 and endothelium-dependent cerebral arteriolar dilation, *Hypertension,* 16, 162, 1990.
34. **Rosenblum, W. I.,** Endothelial dependent relaxation demonstrated in vivo in cerebral arterioles, *Stroke,* 17, 494, 1986.
35. **Kontos, H. A., Wei, E. P., and Marshall, J. J.,** In vivo bioassay of endothelium-derived relaxing factor, *Am. J. Physiol.,* 255, H1259, 1988.
36. **Marshall, J. J., Wei, E. P., and Kontos, H. A.,** Independent blockade of cerebral vasodilation from acetylcholine and nitric oxide, *Am. J. Physiol.,* 255, H847, 1988.
37. **Watanabe, M., Rosenblum, W. I., and Nelson, G. H.,** In vivo effect of methylene blue on endothelium-independent dilations of brain microvessels in mice, *Circ. Res.,* 62, 86, 1988.
38. **Rosenblum, W. I., Nishimura, H., and Nelson, G. H.,** Endothelium-dependent L-Arg- and L-NMMA-sensitive mechanisms regulate tone of brain microvessels, *Am. J. Physiol.,* 259, H1396, 1990.
39. **Faraci, F. M., Mayhan, W. G., and Heistad, D. D.,** Responses of rat basilar artery to acetylcholine and platelet products in vivo, *Stroke,* 22, 56, 1991.
40. **Parnavelas, J. G., Kelly, W., and Burnstock, G.,** Ultrastructural localization of choline acetyltransferase in vascular endothelial cells in rat brain, *Nature,* 316, 724, 1985.
41. **Rosenblum, W. I.,** Hydroxyl radical mediates the endothelium-dependent relaxation produced by bradykinin in mouse cerebral arterioles, *Circ. Res.,* 61, 601, 1987.
42. **Kontos, H. A., Wei, E. P., Kukreja, R. C., Ellis, E. F., and Hess, M. L.,** Differences in endothelium-dependent cerebral dilation by bradykinin and acetylcholine, *Am. J. Physiol.,* 258, H1261, 1990.
43. **Yang, S.-T., Mayhan, W. G., Faraci, F. M., and Heistad, D. D.,** Mechanisms of impaired endothelium-dependent cerebral vasodilatation in response to bradykinin in hypertensive rats, *Stroke,* 22, 1177, 1991.

44. **Rosenblum, W. I., McDonald, M., and Wormley, B.,** Calcium ionophore and acetylcholine dilate arterioles on the mouse brain by different mechanisms, *Stroke,* 20, 1391, 1989.
45. **Haberl, R. L., Decker, P. J., and Einhaupl, K. M.,** Angiotensin degradation products mediate endothelium-dependent dilation of rabbit brain arterioles, *Circ. Res.,* 68, 1621, 1991.
46. **Busija, D. W., Leffler, C. W., and Wagerle, L. C.,** Mono-L-arginine-containing compounds dilate piglet pial arterioles via an endothelium-derived relaxing factor-like substance, *Circ. Res.,* 67, 1374, 1990.
47. **Mayhan, W. G.,** Impairment of endothelium-dependent dilatation of basilar artery during chronic hypertension, *Am. J. Physiol.,* 259, H1455, 1990.
48. **Yang, S.-T., Mayhan, W. G., Faraci, F. M., and Heistad, D. D.,** Endothelium-dependent responses of cerebral blood vessels during chronic hypertension, *Hypertension,* 17, 612, 1991.
49. **Ellison, M. D., Erb, D. E., Kontos, H. A., and Povlishock, J. T.,** Recovery of impaired endothelium-dependent relaxation after fluid-percussion brain injury in cats, *Stroke,* 20, 911, 1989.
50. **Mayhan, W. G.,** Impairment of endothelium-dependent dilatation of cerebral arterioles during diabetes mellitus, *Am. J. Physiol.,* 256, H621, 1989.
51. **Toda, N.,** Nicotine-induced relaxation in isolated canine cerebral arteries, *J. Pharmacol. Exp. Ther.,* 193, 376, 1975.
52. **Toda, N.,** Non-adrenergic, non-cholinergic innervation in monkey and human cerebral arteries, *Br. J. Pharmacol.,* 72, 281, 1981.
53. **Toda, N.,** Relaxant responses to transmural stimulation and nicotine of dog and monkey cerebral arteries, *Am. J. Physiol.,* 243, H145, 1982.
54. **Lee, T. J.-F., Su, C., and Bevan, J. A.,** Nonsympathetic dilator innervation of cat cerebral arteries, *Experientia,* 31, 1424, 1975.
55. **Toda, N. and Ayajiki, K.,** Cholinergic prejunctional inhibition of vasodilator nerve function in bovine basilar arteries, *Am. J. Physiol.,* 258, H983, 1990.
56. **Okamura, T., Inoue, S., and Toda, N.,** Action of atrial natriuretic peptide (ANP) on dog cerebral arteries: evidence that neurogenic relaxation is not mediated by release of ANP, *Br. J. Pharmacol.,* 97, 1258, 1989.
57. **Toda, N. and Okamura, T.,** Suppression by N^G-monomethyl-L-arginine of cerebroarterial responses to nonadrenergic, noncholinergic vasodilator nerve stimulation, *J. Cardiovasc. Pharmacol.,* 17(Suppl. 3), S234, 1991.
58. **Toda, N.,** Hemolysate inhibits cerebral artery relaxation, *J. Cereb. Blood Flow Metab.,* 9, 219, 1989.
59. **Toda, N. and Okamura, T.,** Modification by L-N^G-monomethyl arginine (L-NMMA) of the response to nerve stimulation in isolated dog mesenteric and cerebral arteries, *Jpn. J. Pharmacol.,* 52, 170, 1990.
60. **Toda, N. and Okamura, T.,** Possible role of nitric oxide in transmitting information from vasodilator nerve to cerebroarterial muscle, *Biochem. Biophys. Res. Commun.,* 170, 308, 1990.
61. **Toda, N. and Okamura, T.,** Mechanism underlying the response to vasodilator nerve stimulation in isolated dog and monkey cerebral arteries, *Am. J. Physiol.,* 259, H1511, 1990.
62. **Toda, N., Minami, Y., and Okamura, T.,** Inhibitory effects of L-N^G-nitro arginine on the synthesis of EDRF and the cerebroarterial response to vasodilator nerve stimulation, *Life Sci.,* 47, 345, 1990.
63. **Bredt, D. S., Hwang, M., and Snyder, S. H.,** Localization of nitric oxide synthase indicating a neural role for nitric oxide, *Nature,* 347, 768, 1990.
64. **Wood, K. S., Buga, G. M., Byrns, R. E., and Ignarro, L. J.,** Vascular smooth muscle-derived relaxing factor (MDRF) and its close similarity to nitric oxide, *Biochem. Biophys. Res. Commun.,* 170, 80, 1990.

65. **Garthwaite, J., Garthwaite, G., Palmer, R. M. J., and Moncada, S.,** NMDA receptor activation induces nitric oxide synthesis from arginine in rat brain slices, *Eur. J. Pharmacol.,* 172, 413, 1989.
66. **Busse, R. and Mulsch, A.,** Induction of nitric oxide synthase by cytokines in vascular smooth muscle cells, *FEBS Lett.,* 275, 87, 1990.

III. External Factors Influencing Cerebral Blood Flow

Chapter 16

CEREBRAL VASCULAR RESPONSES TO HYPOXIA, HYPER- AND HYPOCAPNIA, AND HYPOTENSION

John W. Phillis

TABLE OF CONTENTS

I. Introduction 250

II. Hypoxia 250
- A. Adenosine 251
- B. Nitric Oxide 253
- C. Prostanoids 254
- D. The ATP-Sensitive K^+ Channel 254

III. Hypercapnia 255
- A. Adenosine 256
- B. Nitric Oxide 256
- C. Prostanoids 257

IV. Hypocapnia 257

V. Hypotension 258
- A. Endothelially Released Factors 259
- B. Adenosine 259

VI. Conclusions 261

References 261

0-8493-5096-0/93/$0.00 + $.50

I. INTRODUCTION

The maintenance of an adequate blood supply to the brain implies a matching of the flow rate in microvessels to the metabolic requirements of the tissues they perfuse. Oxygen and carbon dioxide levels in the tissues are held within narrow physiological limits. This is accomplished by adjustments of microvascular flow to tissue metabolism and, under normal conditions, by the maintenance of relatively constant levels of oxygen and carbon dioxide in the circulating blood. Localized changes in the level of neuronal activity in the brain are closely linked to changes in regional metabolism, which are, in turn, coupled to local cerebral blood flow[1-3] (Chapter 17). Thus, enhanced neuronal activity in an area of the brain leads to a localized increased metabolic rate, as a result of the energy utilization necessary for ion pumping and other activities of the plasma membrane, and to an increased blood supply in that particular region of the brain (Chapter 17).

Maintenance of appropriate levels of oxygen and carbon dioxide in the blood is very important for normal cerebral metabolism. A significant amount of oxygen is utilized for oxidative phosphorylation on a continuing basis by brain tissue and carbon dioxide, the principal end-product of aerobic metabolism, and must be constantly removed from brain tissues. Oxygen and carbon dioxide readily diffuse across the microvessel wall and hence their tensions (partial pressures) in the blood in cerebral microvessels and in surrounding tissues tend to be in equilibrium under normal physiological conditions.

The relationships between the oxygen and carbon dioxide contents of arterial blood and cerebral blood flow have been extensively investigated. Decreases in PaO_2 during hypoxia, or increases in $PaCO_2$ (hypercapnia), reliably increase cerebral perfusion by decreasing cerebrovascular resistance as a result of arterial vasodilation. Conversely, increases in PaO_2 (hyperoxia) or reduction in $PaCO_2$ (hypocapnia) result in decreases in cerebral blood flow. The effects of changes in arterial oxygen or carbon dioxide tensions on cerebral blood flow can occur in the absence of alterations in cerebral metabolic rate of oxygen utilization ($CMRO_2$).[1,2] This establishes that the effects of decreases in PaO_2 or increases in $PaCO_2$ on blood flow are accomplished by a primary influence on cerebral blood vessel diameter rather than as a consequence of changes in cerebral tissue oxidative metabolism. It is on the intrinsic factors responsible for these changes in vascular resistance that the present chapter is focused.

II. HYPOXIA

Decreases in PaO_2 below 40 to 50 mmHg result in arterial dilatation and increased CBF. Following the reduction in PaO_2, detectable increases in pial arterial diameter and CBF occur rapidly (within 30 to 60 s) and steady-state responses are achieved within 5 to 10 min. Blood flow increases to all major areas of the brain, with greater increases in the gray matter in comparison with white matter. Increases in PaO_2 at normal atmospheric pressure have little or no effect on pial arterial tone or CBF when $PaCO_2$ is maintained constant.

The effects of hypoxia on cerebral vessel diameter have been attributed primarily to the release of vasodilator metabolites from the hypoxic brain parenchyma. The identity of the substance(s) involved has, however, been difficult to define. Increases in extracellular K^+ have been implicated in the hypoxia-evoked hyperemia, since extracellular K^+ increases during hypoxia, and elevated K^+ is known to dilate pial arteries. The rise in extracellular K^+ is not, however, pronounced during the early phase of hypoxia and is unlikely to account for the initial rapid increase in CBF. A decrease in pH has also been proposed as the stimulus for the increase in CBF during hypoxia. However, studies on the extracellular pH in the brain have revealed that during the initial phase of hypoxia the brain may be alkalotic.[4]

Potential metabolic regulators of CBF include adenosine, the prostaglandins, endothelium-derived relaxing factors (EDRFs, including nitric oxide), and a role for the ATP-sensitive potassium channel in vascular smooth muscle must also be considered.

A. ADENOSINE

A role for adenosine in hypoxia-evoked cerebral hyperemia is supported by several lines of evidence. Using the freeze-blow technique to prevent its metabolism, Winn et al.[7] were able to demonstrate a rapid increase in brain adenosine levels when PaO_2 was reduced to 30 mmHg. At a PaO_2 of 50 mmHg, adenosine levels underwent a smaller, nonsignificant increase. Using the same technique, these investigators were able to demonstrate an increase in brain adenosine levels within 30 s of the onset of a hypoxia induced by the inhalation of 100% nitrogen. Increases in cerebral interstitial fluid adenosine during hypoxia have been shown by investigators using either microdialysis or cerebral cortical cup techniques[8-13] (Figure 1). Increases in the adenosine content of rat cortical cup superfusates were evident within 2 min of the onset of breathing 100% nitrogen.[10] Hypoxia-evoked adenosine release from the rat cerebral cortex was enhanced when the animals were pretreated with dipyridamole, an adenosine uptake inhibitor; deoxycoformycin, an inhibitor of adenosine deaminase; PD 119,229, an inhibitor of purine nucleoside phosphorylase; or oxypurinol and allopurinol, inhibitors of xanthine oxidase.[14-17]

Further support for a role of adenosine in hypoxia-induced hyperemia has been forthcoming from CBF experiments with adenosine receptor antagonists. Theophylline and caffeine attenuated or blocked hypoxia-evoked hyperemias in several animal models, measured by a variety of experimental techniques.[18-23] Similar results were obtained in humans exposed to hypoxia after aminophylline treatment.[24,25] Moreover, superfusion of cat and rat cerebral

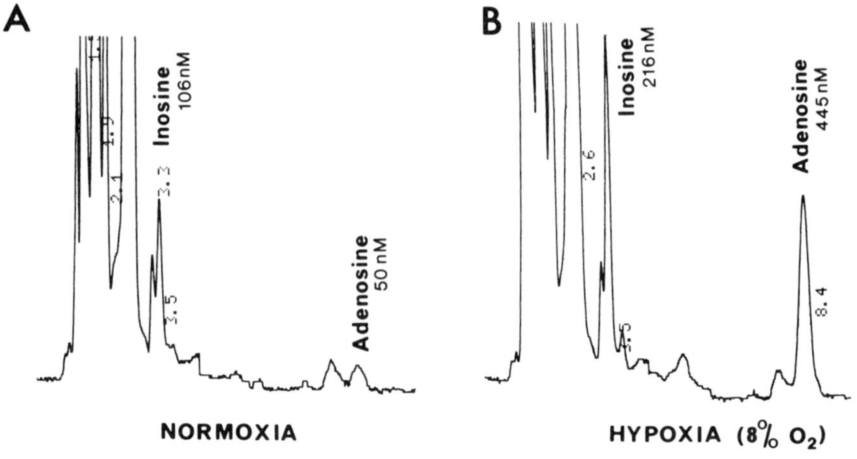

FIGURE 1. HPLC chromatograms of inosine and adenosine in rat cerebral cortical superfusates obtained under (A) normoxic conditions, breathing air, and (B) hypoxic conditions during 10 min of inhalation of 8% oxygen in nitrogen. During hypoxia, the levels of both inosine and adenosine in the superfusate increased.

cortices with adenosine deaminase, to inactivate extracellular adenosine, led to an attenuation of the dilatation of pial vessels during hypoxia[26,27] (Chapter 18).

Potentiation of hypoxia-evoked increases in cerebral blood flow after the administration of inhibitors of adenosine uptake or adenosine deaminase has been reported. A number of agents that inhibit adenosine transport, including dipyridamole, papaverine, lidoflazine, and flunarizine, potentiated the increase in hypoxia-evoked CBF measured by a venous outflow technique in the rat.[20,28] Somewhat unexpectedly, nifedipine, which also potently inhibits adenosine transport,[29] virtually abolished the reactive hyperemia evoked by hypoxia.[30] Further studies demonstrated that nifedipine markedly attenuated the expected increase in adenosine release from the hypoxic rat cerebral cortex.[31] The adenosine deaminase inhibitors deoxycoformycin and erythrohydroxynonyladenine (EHNA) potentiated hypoxia-evoked increases in rat CBF as measured by the venous outflow technique.[32]

Evidence against an involvement of adenosine in hypoxia-evoked cerebral hyperemia has been reported from some laboratories. Topically or systemically administered theophylline has failed to attenuate hypoxic hyperemia in the cat,[33,34] and Dora et al.[35] were unable to detect an effect of topical adenosine deaminase on cerebrocortical vascular volume during hypoxia. The existence of these inconsistencies may reflect differences in the animal species and measurement techniques used, as well as variability in the severity and duration of the hypoxic challenges. Nonpurinergic local mechanisms may predominate, especially when the hypoxia is of long duration.

B. NITRIC OXIDE

A release of endothelium-derived relaxing factor (EDRF), which has been identified as nitric oxide,[36] during hypoxia was observed in isolated segments of basilar and internal carotid arteries.[37] The main action of NO is the stimulation of soluble guanylate cyclase, which causes an increase in cGMP in vascular smooth muscle, leading to relaxation. An involvement of NO in the regulation of cerebral vascular tone during normoxia and its release from dilator nerves has been demonstrated using inhibitors of nitric oxide synthase to block *in vivo* NO formation from L-arginine (Chapter 15).

When pial arterioles on the surface of mouse and rat brains were observed by television microscopy, L-arginine dilated the arterioles, and N^G-monomethyl-L-arginine (L-NMMA) constricted them in a dose-dependent manner.[38,39] Both the dilation and constriction were abolished by endothelial damage,[38] suggesting that there is a continuously acting, endothelium-dependent, L-arginine-dependent, and L-NMMA inhibitable mechanism tending to relax pial arterioles.

Administration of L-NMMA to rats during normoxia resulted in a decrease in CBF of 21% and an increase in cerebral vascular resistance (CVR) of 53%. These effects were reversed by L-arginine, but not by D-arginine.[40] In contrast, the increase in CBF and decrease in CVR during hypoxia in the group of rats which received L-NMMA were similar to that in the control group, indicating that NO is probably not an important factor in the changes in CVR during hypoxia.

In a study on anesthetized, paralyzed, ventilated rats, CBF was measured using a venous outflow technique (retroglenoid sinus) with an extracorporeal return circuit (J. E. Buchanan and J. W. Phillis, unpublished observations). CBF responses to a brief period of hypoxia (8% O_2) were compared prior to and after the administration of the nitric oxide synthase inhibitor N^G-nitro-L-arginine methyl ester (L-NAME; 30 mg/kg). L-NAME did not affect venous outflow from the normoxic brain, even though MABP was increased, demonstrating that cerebrovascular resistance had increased. Nor did L-NAME significantly alter the magnitude of the increase in flow, or the duration of the hyperemia, evoked by the inhalation of 8% O_2. These results support the conclusion that whereas nitric oxide may be involved in the regulation of basal, normoxic, cerebral blood flow, it is not a critical factor in the changes associated with hypoxia.

Nitric oxide may be involved in the increase in cerebral vessel diameter associated with periods of hypoxia plus hypercapnia. Bergfeld and Forrester[41] have shown that a brief exposure to a hypoxic/hypercapnic environment induces a release of ATP from human erythrocytes. Intravascular ATP dilates blood vessel by promoting the release of EDRF from the vascular endothelium,[42] and it is therefore likely that the dilatory action of ATP on cerebral resistance vessels involves nitric oxide release. Elevated levels of ATP have been observed in the circulation for up to 5 min after vigorous body exercise, suggesting that circulating nucleotide could have an influence on the cerebral circulation,[43] involving nitric oxide as a mediator.

C. PROSTANOIDS

Brain tissues have a recognized capacity to synthesize various eicosanoids (see Chapter 19), some of which such as prostacyclin and prostaglandin D_2 have been shown to exert cerebral vasodilatory responses. Evidence supporting a role of vasodilatory prostanoids in the regulation of CBF has come from experiments in which the administration of indomethacin (5 to 10 mg/kg), a potent inhibitor of cyclooxygenase, was observed to decrease blood flow by up to 50%.[44,45] However, other investigators have been unable to observe a reduction in CBF with other nonsteroidal anti-inflammatory agents[46] raising concerns about the actual mechanism of action of indomethacin. When used at lower doses (0.1 mg/kg) indomethacin actually enhanced basal CBF and prolonged the reactive hyperemia following a brief period (24 s) of nitrogen inhalation.[47] The reason for this discrepancy may lie in the inability of indomethacin, in low concentrations, to cross the bloodbrain barrier,[48] although it can effectively inhibit cerebral synthesis of prostanoids when adequate systemic doses (5 to 10 mg/kg) are administered (Chapter 19). The potentiative effects of low doses of indomethacin on hypoxia-evoked cerebral hyperemia may be a consequence of the pronounced ability of this agent to inhibit adenosine uptake.[49] Adenosine uptake into the cerebral capillary endothelium would be reduced after indomethacin administration, thus enhancing extracellular adenosine levels. A similar explanation may account for the ability of indomethacin to potentiate the actions of adenosine on coronary flow in the dog heart.[50] At higher doses (5 to 10 mg/kg), indomethacin is demonstrably able to cross the blood-brain barrier in sufficient amounts to inhibit brain cyclooxygenases and may also reduce adenosine efflux from hypoxic cells, by inhibiting the bidirectional transporter, sufficiently to attenuate hypoxia-elicited increases in CBF.

D. THE ATP-SENSITIVE K^+ CHANNEL

The involvement of ATP-sensitive K^+ channels in cerebrovascular responses to hypoxia must be considered amongst the potential intrinsic mechanisms underlying this phenomenon. An ATP-sensitive K^+ channel has been reported to exist in vascular smooth muscle cells.[51] Blockade of this channel in the isolated guinea pig heart with the sulfonylurea derivative glibenclamide has been shown to reduce hypoxia-induced vasodilation- and adenosine- (but not bradykinin) evoked vasodilation.[52] Glibenclamide reduced the reactive hyperemia in canine hearts elicited by a 30-s coronary occlusion[53] indicating that the ATP-sensitive channel may play a significant role in the coronary vasodilation evoked by the occlusion. Nelson et al.[54] have suggested that this channel may exert its effects on coronary vasomotor tone through its effects on the voltage-dependent Ca^{2+} channel. The open-state probability of this

Ca^{2+} channel depends on the transmembrane potential: at more negative, hyperpolarized levels of transmembrane potential, the channel is more likely to be closed, reducing Ca^{2+} entry into the cell; at less negative, more depolarized levels of potential the channel is more likely to be open, increasing Ca^{2+} entry into the cell, with a resultant vasoconstriction. The ATP-sensitive K^+ channel can influence transmembrane potential depending on whether its open-state probability is high or low. During normoxia, when ATP levels are high within the cell, the channel is usually closed and the cell will be relatively depolarized. When ATP levels fall during hypoxia, the channels will open, hyperpolarizing the cell, reducing Ca^{2+} entry and therefore vasomotor tone.

Masuzawa et al.[55] have demonstrated the presence of ATP-sensitive K^+ channels in the dog middle cerebral artery. Activation of these channels with cromakalim relaxed the endothelium-denuded arterial strips. The relaxant actions of cromakalim were antagonized by glibenclamide. Thus, although the existence of a similar mechanism for hypoxia-evoked cerebrovascular dilation remains to be established, its presence in the coronary vasculature suggests that this must be considered a likely possibility.

III. HYPERCAPNIA

Alterations in $PaCO_2$ have a marked effect on cerebrovascular tone. Hypercapnia causes arterial dilatation and elevated CBF, whereas hypocapnia results in arterial constriction and reduced CBF.[1,2] The cerebrovascular changes are due solely to changes in arterial PCO_2, as alterations in arterial pH, independent of $PaCO_2$, have minimal effects on CBF.[56] Several mechanisms have been proposed to account for the effects of increases in $PaCO_2$ on cerebrovascular tone. These include alterations in the pH of the extracellular fluid of the brain, activation of neural pathways, adenosine, nitric oxide, and prostaglandins.

The hypothesis that $PaCO_2$ affects cerebrovascular tone via changes in the interstitial fluid pH is supported by experimental evidence. CO_2 readily diffuses from the blood to the brain, causing alterations in the pH. Alterations in the pH of CSF perfusing pial arteries had a direct effect on arterial diameter, with acidosis dilating and alkalosis constricting the vessels. Conversely, changes in the CSF PCO_2 and HCO_3^-, independent of changes in pH, had no effect on pial arterial tone. In addition, flushing the cortical surface with CSF at a reduced PCO_2 prevented pial arterial dilation during systemic hypercapnia.[1,2]

The role of peripheral chemoreceptors and neural pathways in the CO_2-induced cerebral vasodilation has been extensively investigated. It is unlikely that neurotransmitters released from the terminals of afferent pathways are involved since destruction of major thalamic and extrathalamic input pathways[57-59] did not alter the cerebrovascular response to hypercapnia. As with the hypoxia-evoked changes in CBF, research on hypercapnia-evoked increases in CBF has been focused on metabolic factors.

A. ADENOSINE

The possibility that endogenously released adenosine is involved in the response to hypercapnia was investigated in an anesthetized, paralyzed, rat cerebral venous outflow model.[60] Animals were mechanically ventilated with a 40% oxygen in nitrogen mixture. At 20 min intervals, at a constant rate of flow, the inspired gas mixture was altered to 10% carbon dioxide, 40% oxygen in nitrogen for periods of between 30 to 90 s. This brief hypercapnic challenge induced a rapid increase in CBF in the absence of any changes in MABP. Caffeine (10 or 20 mg/kg) significantly decreased the peak increase in venous outflow to 44% and 25% of control increases. Dipyridamole (0.1 mg/kg) increased peak flow rates by 92% and deoxycoformycin (0.1 μg/kg) enhanced peak flow rates by 30%. These results suggest that adenosine plays a key role in coupling $PaCO_2$ to cerebral blood flow. Other investigators have reported conflicting findings in that infusion of the adenosine antagonist theophylline produced no significant effect on hypercapnia-induced increases in CBF in rats[61] or arterial diameter (Chapter 18) of cats. Differences in the adenosine antagonist (theophylline), the anesthetics employed, or a longer duration of the CO_2 challenges may account for these disparities.

Further evidence for an involvement of adenosine as a mediator of the hypercapnia-evoked increase in CBF has come from closed cranial window experiments, with videomicroscopy to observe the diameter of rat[27] or cat (Chapter 18) pial arterioles. In both series of experiments, cortical superfusion with an artificial CSF containing adenosine deaminase resulted in a pronounced reduction of arteriolar dilation during the hypercapnic challenge.

Some insights into the potential interactions between hypercapnia and adenosine can be gained from studies on the coronary circulation. A hypercapnic acidosis is associated with an increased potency of adenosine as a coronary vasodilator.[62,63] An increase in adenosine release from the isolated rabbit heart during perfusion with fluids made acidic with CO_2 has been reported[64] and the release of adenosine from vascular endothelial cells is substantially increased upon elevation of the PCO_2 in the perfusion medium.[65] Gerlach et al.[66] have attributed this effect to H^+ activation of a cytosolic 5′-nucleotidase with a resultant enhancement of adenosine formation. Uptake of adenosine into rat brain synaptosomes is highly sensitive to pH,[67] and Mustafa[68] has suggested that increases in adenosine levels during elevation of PCO_2, associated with acidosis, could be a consequence of reductions in adenosine uptake. Since cortical cup release experiments have failed to reveal any increase in adenosine levels during hypercapnia,[5] it appears likely either that elevations in adenosine levels may be localized to the vicinity of the vasculature, or alternatively that the vasodilator potency of extracellular adenosine is enhanced by reductions in pH.

B. NITRIC OXIDE

Topical application of the nitric oxide synthase inhibitors N^G-nitro-L-arginine (L-NA) and L-NMMA inhibited (by up to 93%) the increase in rat sensory cortex blood flow, measured with a laser-Doppler probe, elicited during hypercapnia.[69] The effect of L-NMMA was completely reversed by coapplication of L-arginine. These findings indicate that the powerful effects of CO_2 on the cerebral circulation are mediated by arginine-derived EDRF/nitric oxide.

A similar conclusion was reached in a study of regional cerebral blood flow (cortex, subcortex, brainstem, cerebellum) in the rat brain, with radio-labeled microspheres.[70] L-NAME attenuated by >60% the increases in CBF elicited during hypercapnia in all four regions of the brain. L-NAME also reduced CO_2-elicited increases in rat cerebral blood flow measured by a venous outflow technique (J. E. Buchanan and J. W. Phillis, unpublished observations). In these experiments, L-NAME (10 or 30 mg/kg) reduced the magnitude and duration of hypercapnic hyperemias (Figure 2). The inhibitory effects of L-NAME were reversed by a subsequent application of L-arginine (300 mg/kg), but not by D-arginine.

The cellular source of the EDRF/nitric oxide released during hypercapnia remains uncertain. Potential sources are the vascular endothelium itself, perivascular glia, or the nerve terminals which contain nitric oxide synthase (see Chapter 15).

C. PROSTANOIDS

In several animal species, cyclooxygenase products, probably prostaglandins, contribute to the cerebrovasodilation elicited by hypercapnia (Chapter 19). Studies on adult primates, rats, and gerbils have found inhibition of hypercapnic dilation following administration of indomethacin,[71-73] although other investigators have failed to confirm this result. For a further discussion of the involvement of prostanoids in hypercapnia-evoked increases in CBF, the reader is referred to Chapter 19.

IV. HYPOCAPNIA

Hypocapnia is associated with a powerful vasoconstrictive effect on the cerebral circulation.[1,2] During hypocarbia, CBF decreases in an almost linear fashion until $PaCO_2$ is at 20 to 25 mmHg, at which point further decreases become less pronounced. The mechanisms by which decreased $PaCO_2$ alters cerebrovascular tone is unclear and may relate to decreases in EDRF/nitric oxide formation and release.

Adenosine has been implicated as a factor which limits the extent of the hypocarbia-induced vasoconstriction.[74] Severe hypocarbia (PCO_2 20 mmHg) is associated with an increase in brain adenosine levels,[75] likely resulting from a vasoconstriction-induced hypoxia. The vasoconstriction during hypocarbia was attenuated by dipyridamole and augmented by theophylline, suggesting that adenosine acts to reduce the extent of the vasoconstriction.[74]

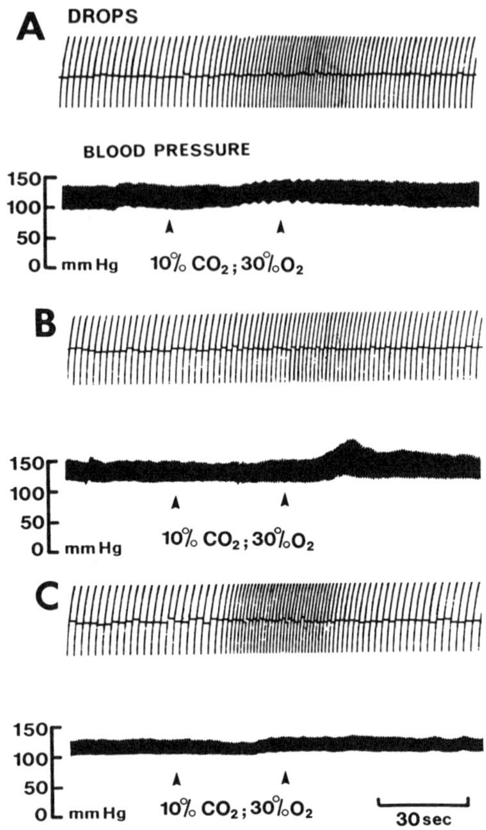

FIGURE 2. Responses of rat cerebral blood flow and arterial blood pressure to hypercapnic episodes. Cerebral blood flow, as represented by outflow from the retroglenoid sinus, is recorded as drops. Hypercapnia was induced by mechanically ventilating the rat with 10% carbon dioxide for 36 s; (A) Control responses, (B) following administration of N^G-nitro-L-arginine methyl ester (30 mg/kg), and (C) after injection of L-arginine (300 mg/kg).

V. HYPOTENSION

Cerebral blood flow is able to respond rapidly to alterations in MABP, so that flow is maintained relatively constant over a wide range of perfusion pressures. The term autoregulation of blood flow is used to describe this phenomenon (see Chapter 3). It implies constriction of the resistance vessels, the arterioles, when blood pressure increases and their dilatation when the pressure decreases. Under steady state conditions, in anesthetized as well as awake animals, autoregulation prevents CBF from changing appreciably over an arterial pressure range of approximately 60 to 150 mmHg.[1,2] Below 60 mmHg pressure, there may be a decrease in cerebral blood flow, even though the cerebral resistance vessels have dilated. Several theories have been proposed to account for the autoregulatory phenomenon, including myogenic, neurogenic, and metabolic theories. Many investigators have favored a myogenic theory, which proposes that the smooth muscle cells of the arterial wall are alone in eliciting the response. These cells would ''sense'' the increased stretch of the vessel wall caused by elevation of blood pressure and respond to increased stretch by a constriction or vice versa. The cellular mechanism involved in this myogenic response may involve changes in the electrical potential across the muscle cell plasma membrane, with depolarization occurring in conjunction with elevated arterial pressures. Membrane depolarization would result in Ca^{2+} entry and an enhanced contractile force[76] (Chapter 2).

A. ENDOTHELIALLY RELEASED FACTORS

Recently, however, evidence has been published indicating a key role of the arterial endothelium in the autoregulation of CBF. The normal increase in vascular tone to stretch is abolished if the endothelium is first removed.[77,78] This finding suggests that vasoconstrictor and vasodilator substances released from the vascular endothelium may be responsible for the autoregulatory response.

Wang et al.[79] used nitro-L-arginine, an inhibitor of nitric oxide synthase, to evaluate the role of nitric oxide in cerebral blood flow autoregulation in rats, when CBF was measured by the ^{133}Xe injection method. Nitro-L-arginine, in doses which suppressed the increases in blood flow during hypercapnia, failed to alter the autoregulation of CBF. Experiments employing the rat venous outflow technique have also failed to detect any significant changes in the CBF autoregulatory response to hypotension after L-NAME administration (Figure 3; J. E. Buchanan and J. W. Phillis, unpublished observations.) Factors other than nitric oxide therefore appear to be responsible for endothelially mediated CBF autoregulation.

B. ADENOSINE

Adenosine has been proposed as a possible metabolic regulator of cerebrovascular resistance. Adenosine is produced in the rat brain during 5 min periods of sustained reduction in arterial blood pressure.[80] With moderate to severe hypotension (MABP = 45 mmHg) brain adenosine levels increased sixfold. Increases in adenosine levels in the brain interstitial fluid, during reductions in MABP below 50 mmHg, have been observed in microdialysis experiments.[81,82] Collectively, these studies demonstrated that although adenosine levels change minimally over a large portion of the autoregulatory range, there is a substantial increase in adenosine levels at blood pressures below 50 mmHg. Adenosine may therefore contribute to the decrease in cerebral vascular resistance at the lower end of the autoregulatory range.

Unfortunately, none of the above studies took into account the likely effect of reductions in cerebral blood flow, which would have occurred at arterial blood pressures below 60 mmHg, on cerebral PO_2 values. Once the

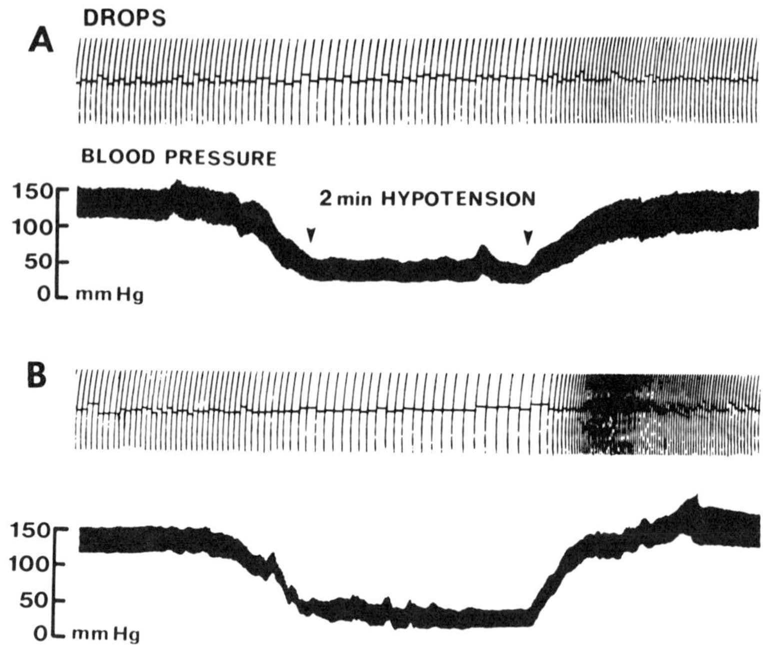

FIGURE 3. Responses of cerebral blood flow and arterial blood pressure to the withdrawal and reinfusion of arterial blood. Blood was withdrawn over a 1 min period; the hypotension was maintained for 2 min; and then blood was reinfused over a 1 min period. After recording the control response (A), L-NAME (10 mg/kg) was administered and 10 min later the hypotensive challenge was repeated (B).

autoregulatory range was exceeded, the decreases in CBF would inevitably have contributed to falls in cerebral PO_2 and increases in PCO_2, both of which may have contributed to elevated interstitial fluid adenosine levels. This point of view is reinforced by the observation[83] that the presence of elevated oxygen in the fluid perfusing the microdialysis probe virtually eliminated the increase in brain interstitial fluid adenosine seen during reduced arterial pressure, clearly demonstrating that the rise in adenosine levels was a consequence of a tissue hypoxia induced by the fall in CBF. Indeed cortical cup estimates of changes in interstitial space adenosine during hypotension (46 mmHg) demonstrated no significant changes in brain adenosine, even though small reductions in PaO_2 (to 80 and 64 mmHg) were associated with increases in adenosine efflux.[10]

To avoid the complications from associated decreases in PO_2 during hypotension, Phillis and DeLong[60] hyperoxygenated ($PaO_2 \cong 140$ mmHg) rats used to study the effects of hypotension on cerebral blood flow and vascular resistance. Under these conditions, the adenosine antagonist, caffeine, failed to alter the CBF response to reductions of MABP to 40 mmHg. The conclusion from these studies is that adenosine is probably not a significant factor in the autoregulation of CBF when secondary tissue oxygen depletion is averted.

VI. CONCLUSIONS

This chapter has explored the possible mechanisms by which cerebral blood flow is adjusted to sustain normal brain function during hypoxia, increases or decreases in arterial PCO_2, and hypotension. Multiple factors, including changes in cerebral interstitial space K^+ and pH levels, are likely to be involved under steady state conditions. The evidence suggests that adenosine is a major factor in initiating hypoxia-evoked vasodilation, and there are also indications for a potential involvement of various eicosanoids. Recent findings emanating from research on the coronary circulation have implicated the ATP-sensitive K^+ channel in hypoxia-evoked vascular dilation, but an involvement of this channel in the cerebrovascular response to hypoxia has, as yet, to be established. Although nitric oxide is demonstrably involved in the regulation of cerebrovascular tone, it currently does not appear to be a key factor in the hypoxia-evoked dilation.

There is positive evidence for an involvement of nitric oxide, adenosine, and the prostanoids in the cerebrovascular dilation elicited during hypercapnia, and all three modulators may share this role. There is less information on the cause of the vasoconstriction associated with hypocapnia, but decreases in nitric oxide and/or adenosine formation, or in their ability to dilate cerebral resistance vessels, may be involved. Although both adenosine and nitric oxide have been proposed as mediators of the cerebral vasodilation associated with hypotension, the current evidence for this appears to be less than convincing. The vasoconstrictor response to hypertension is dependent on the presence of an intact endothelium, suggesting that an endothelially derived constrictor factor may be involved in this response.

REFERENCES

1. **Heistad, D. D. and Kontos, H. A.,** Cerebral circulation, in *Handbook of Physiology, Section 2, The Cardiovascular System,* Vol. 3, Pt. 1, Shepherd, J. T. and Abboud, F. M., Eds., American Physiology Society, Bethesda, MD, 1983, 137.
2. **Busija, D. W. and Heistad, D. D.,** Factors involved in the physiological regulation of the cerebral circulation, *Rev. Physiol. Biochem. Pharmacol.,* 101, 162, 1984.
3. **Kuschinsky, W.,** Coupling of blood flow and metabolism in the brain, *J. Basic Clin. Physiol. Pharmacol.,* 1, 191, 1990.
4. **Astrup, J., Heuser, D., Lassen, N. A., Nilsson, B., Norberg, K., and Siesjo, B. K.,** Evidence against H^+ and K^+ as main factors for the control of cerebral blood flow: a microelectrode study, in *Ciba Foundation Symposium Vol. 56, Cerebral Vascular Smooth Muscle and its Control,* Elsevier, North Holland, 1978, 313.

5. **Phillis, J. W.,** Adenosine in the control of the cerebral circulation, *Cerebrovasc. Brain Metabol. Rev.,* 1, 26, 1989.
6. **Van Wylen, D. G. L., Sciotti, V. M., and Winn, H. R.,** Adenosine and the regulation of cerebral blood flow, in *Adenosine and the Adenine Nucleotides as Regulators of Cellular Function,* Phillis, J. W., Ed., CRC Press, Boca Raton, FL, 1991, 191.
7. **Winn, H. R., Rubio, R., and Berne, R. M.,** Brain adenosine concentration during hypoxia in rats, *Am. J. Physiol.,* 241, H235, 1981.
8. **Zetterstrom, T., Vernet, L., Ungerstedt, U., Tossman, U., Jonzon, B., and Fredholm, B. B.,** Purine levels in the intact rat brain. Studies with an implanted perfused hollow fibre, *Neurosci. Lett.,* 29, 111, 1982.
9. **Van Wylen, D. G. L., Park, T. S., Rubio, R., and Berne, R. M.,** Increases in cerebral interstitial fluid adenosine concentration during hypoxia, local potassium infusion, and ischemia, *J. Cereb. Blood Flow Metab.,* 6, 522, 1986.
10. **Phillis, J. W., Walter, G. A., O'Regan, M. H., and Stair, R. E.,** Increases in cerebral cortical perfusate adenosine and inosine concentrations during hypoxia and ischemia, *J. Cereb. Blood Flow Metab.,* 7, 679, 1987.
11. **Barraco, R. A., Walter, G. A., Polasek, P. M., and Phillis, J. W.,** Purine concentrations in the cerebrospinal fluid of unanesthetized rats during and after hypoxia, *Neurochem. Int.,* 18, 243, 1990.
12. **Meno, J. R., Ngai, A. C., Ibayashi, S., and Winn, H. R.,** Adenosine release and changes in pial arteriolar diameter during transient cerebral ischemia and reperfusion, *J. Cereb. Blood Flow Metab.,* 11, 986, 1991.
13. **Laudignon, N., Farri, E., Beharry, K., and Aranda, J. V.,** Rapid effects of hypoxia on the cerebrospinal fluid levels of adenosine and related metabolites in the newborn and one-month-old piglets, *Biol. Neonate,* 59, 54, 1991.
14. **Phillis, J. W., O'Regan, M. H., and Walter, G. A.,** Effects of two nucleoside transport inhibitors, dipyridamole and soluflazine, on purine release from the rat cerebral cortex, *Brain Res.,* 481, 309, 1989.
15. **Phillis, J. W., O'Regan, M. H., and Walter, G. A.,** Effects of deoxycoformycin on adenosine, inosine, hypoxanthine, xanthine and uric acid release from the hypoxemic rat cerebral cortex, *J. Cereb. Blood Flow Metab.,* 8, 733, 1988.
16. **Phillis, J. W., Walter, G. A., and Simpson, R. E.,** A purine nucleoside phosphorylase inhibitor, 8-amino-9-(2-thienylmethyl)guanine, enhances purine release from the rat cerebral cortex, *Int. J. Purine Pyrimidine Res.,* 1, 17, 1990.
17. **O'Regan, M. H., Phillis, J. W., and Walter, G. A.,** The effects of the xanthine oxidase inhibitors, allopurinol and oxypurinol, on the pattern of purine release from hypoxic rat cerebral cortex, *Neurochem. Int.,* 14, 91, 1989.
18. **Emerson, T. E. and Raymond, R. M.,** Involvement of adenosine in cerebral hypoxic hyperemia in the dog, *Am. J. Physiol.,* 241, H134, 1981.
19. **Hoffman, W. E., Albrecht, R. F., and Miletich, D. J.,** The role of adenosine in CBF increases during hypoxia in young vs. aged rats, *Stroke,* 15, 124, 1984.
20. **Phillis, J. W., Preston, G., and DeLong, R. E.,** Effects of anoxia on cerebral blood flow in the rat brain: evidence for a role of adenosine in autoregulation, *J. Cereb. Blood Flow Metab.,* 4, 586, 1984.
21. **Mori, S., Ngai, A. C., Ko, K. R., and Winn, H. R.,** Role of adenosine in regulation of cerebral blood flow: effects of theophylline during normoxia and hypoxia, *Am. J. Physiol.,* 253, H165, 1987.
22. **Pinard, E., Puiroud, S., and Seylaz, J.,** Role of adenosine in cerebral hypoxic hyperemia in the unanesthetized rabbit, *Brain Res.,* 481, 124, 1989.
23. **Laudignon, N., Farri, E., Beharry, K., Rex, J., and Aranda, J. V.,** Influence of adenosine on cerebral blood flow during hypoxic hypoxia in the newborn piglet, *J. Appl. Physiol.,* 68, 1534, 1990.
24. **McDonnell, M., Ives, N. K., and Hope, P. L.,** Intravenous aminophylline and cerebral blood flow in preterm infants, *Arch. Disease Childhood,* 67, 416, 1992.

25. **Bowton, D. L., Haddon, W. S., Prough, D. S., Adair, N., Alford, P. T., and Stump, D. A.,** Theophylline effect on the cerebral blood flow response to hypoxemia, *Chest,* 94, 371, 1988.
26. **Kontos, H. A. and Wei, E. P.,** Oxygen-dependent mechanisms in cerebral autoregulation, *Ann. Biomed. Eng.,* 13, 329, 1985.
27. **Simpson, R. E. and Phillis, J. W.,** Adenosine deaminase reduces hypoxic and hypercapnic dilatation of rat pial arterioles: evidence for mediation by adenosine, *Brain Res.,* 553, 305, 1991.
28. **Phillis, J. W., DeLong, R. E., and Towner, J. K.,** The effects of lidoflazine and flunarizine on cerebral reactive hyperemia, *Eur. J. Pharmacol.,* 112, 323, 1985.
29. **Phillis, J. W., Swanson, T. H., and Barraco, R. A.,** Interactions between adenosine and nifedipine in the rat cerebral cortex, *Neurochem. Int.,* 6, 693, 1984.
30. **Phillis, J. W., DeLong, R. E., and Towner, J. K.,** The effects of nifedipine and felodipine on cerebral blood flow during anoxic episodes, *Stroke,* 17, 229, 1986.
31. **Phillis, J. W., O'Regan, M. H., and Walter, G. A.,** Effects of nifedipine and felodipine on adenosine and inosine release from the hypoxaemic rat cerebral cortex, *J. Cereb. Blood Flow Metab.,* 8, 179, 1988.
32. **Phillis, J. W., DeLong, R. E., and Towner, J. K.,** Adenosine deaminase inhibitors enhance cerebral anoxic hyperemia in the rat, *J. Cereb. Blood Flow Metab.,* 5, 295, 1985.
33. **Haller, C. and Kuschinsky, W.,** Moderate hypoxia: reactivity of pial arteries and local effect of theophylline, *J. Appl. Physiol.,* 63, 2208, 1987.
34. **Dora, E.,** Effect of theophylline treatment on the functional hyperaemic and hypoxic responses of cerebrocortical microcirculation, *Acta Physiol. Hung.,* 68, 183, 1986.
35. **Dora, E., Koller, A., and Kovach, A. G. B.,** Effect of topical adenosine deaminase treatment on the functional hyperemic and hypoxic responses of the cerebral cortical microcirculation, *J. Cereb. Blood Flow Metab.,* 4, 447, 1984.
36. **Ignarro, L. J., Buga, G. M., Wood, K. S., Byrns, R. E., and Chauduri, G.,** Endothelium-derived relaxing factor produced and released from artery and vein is nitric oxide, *Proc. Natl. Acad. Sci. U.S.A.,* 84, 9265, 1987.
37. **Pearce, W. J., Ashwal, S., and Cuevas, J.,** Direct effects of graded hypoxia on intact and denuded rabbit cranial arteries, *Am. J. Physiol.,* 257, H824, 1989.
38. **Rosenblum, W. I., Nishimura, H., and Nelson, G. H.,** Endothelium-dependent L-Arg- and L-NMMA-sensitive mechanisms regulate tone of brain microvessels, *Am. J. Physiol.,* 259, H1396, 1990.
39. **Faraci, F. M.,** Role of endothelium-derived relaxing factor in cerebral circulation: large arteries vs. microcirculation, *Am. J. Physiol.,* 261, H1038, 1991.
40. **Kozniewska, E., Oseka, M., and Stys, T.,** Effects of endothelium-derived nitric oxide on cerebral circulation during normoxia and hypoxia in the rat, *J. Cereb. Blood Flow Metab.,* 12, 311, 1992.
41. **Bergfeld, G. R. and Forrester, T.,** Release of ATP from human erythrocytes in response to a brief period of hypoxia and hypercapnia, *Cardiovasc. Res.,* 26, 40, 1992.
42. **De Mey, J. G. and Vanhoutte, P. M.,** Role of the intima in cholinergic and purinergic relaxation of isolated canine femoral arteries, *J. Physiol. (London),* 316, 347, 1981.
43. **Forrester, T., Harper, A. M., MacKenzie, E. T., and Thomson, E. M.,** Effect of adenosine triphosphate and some derivatives on cerebral blood flow and metabolism, *J. Physiol. (London),* 296, 343, 1979.
44. **McCulloch, J., Kelly, P. A. T., Grome, J. J., and Pickard, J. D.,** Local cerebral circulatory and metabolic effects of indomethacin, *Am. J. Physiol.,* 243, H416, 1982.
45. **Plotkine, M., El Bouchi, N., Allix, M., Capdeville, C., Bouchon, V., and Boulu, R. G.,** Effect of indomethacin on the coupling of cerebral blood flow to brain metabolism, *J. Pharmacol. (Paris),* 17, 286, 1986.
46. **Houggard, K., Nilsson, B., and Wieloch, T.,** Fatty acid cyclooxygenase inhibitors and the regulation of cerebral blood flow, *Acta Physiol. Scand.,* 117, 585, 1983.

47. **Phillis, J. W., DeLong, R. E., and Towner, J. K.,** Indomethacin and ibuprofen enhance anoxia-induced hyperemia in rat brain, *Eur. J. Pharmacol.*, 124, 85, 1986.
48. **Gamache, D. A. and Ellis, E. F.,** Effect of dexamethasone, indomethacin, ibuprofen, and probenecid on carrageenan-induced brain inflammation, *J. Neurosurg.*, 65, 686, 1986.
49. **Phillis, J. W. and Wu, P. H.,** The effect of various centrally active drugs on adenosine uptake by the central nervous system, *Comp. Biochem. Physiol.*, 72C, 179, 1982.
50. **Glenn, T. M. and Horan, J.,** Modification of adenosine induced changes in coronary flow by methylprednisolone and indomethacin, *Fed. Proc.*, 40, 706, 1981.
51. **Standen, N. B., Quayle, J. M., Davies, N. W., Brayden, J. E., Huang, Y., and Nelson, M. T.,** Hyperpolarizing vasodilators activate ATP-sensitive K^+ channels in arterial smooth muscle, *Science*, 245, 177, 1989.
52. **Daut, J., Maier-Rudolph, W., Von Beckerath, N., Mehrke, G., Gunther, K., and Goedel-Meinen, L.,** Hypoxic dilation of coronary arteries is mediated by ATP-sensitive potassium channels, *Science*, 247, 1341, 1990.
53. **Aversano, T., Ouyang, P., and Silverman, H.,** Blockade of the ATP-sensitive potassium channel modulates reactive hyperemia in the canine coronary circulation, *Circ. Res.*, 69, 618, 1991.
54. **Nelson, M. T., Patlak, J. B., Worley, J. F., and Standen, N. B.,** Calcium channels, potassium channels and voltage dependence of arterial smooth muscle tone, *Am. J. Physiol.*, 259, C3, 1990.
55. **Masuzawa, K., Asano, M., Matsuda, T., Imaizumi, Y., and Watanabe, M.,** Possible involvement of ATP-sensitive K^+ channels in the relaxant response of dog middle cerebral artery to cromakalim, *J. Pharmacol. Exp. Ther.*, 255, 818, 1990.
56. **Harper, A. M. and Bell, R. A.,** The effect of metabolic acidosis and alkalosis on the blood flow through the cerebral cortex, *J. Neurol. Neurosurg. Psychiatry*, 26, 341, 1963.
57. **Iadecola, C., Mraovitch, S., Meeley, M., and Reis, D.,** Lesions of the basal forebrain in rat selectively impair the cortical vasodilation elicited from cerebellar fastigial nucleus, *Brain Res.*, 279, 41, 1983.
58. **Iadecola, C., Arneric, S., Baker, H., Tucker, L., and Reis, D.,** Role of local neurons in cerebrocortical vasodilation elicited from cerebellum, *Am. J. Physiol.*, 252, R1082, 1987.
59. **Harik, S. I., Prado, R., Busto, R., and Ginsberg, M. D.,** Increased cerebral blood flow during hypercapnia is not affected by lesion of the nucleus locus ceruleus, *Stroke*, 17, 1235, 1986.
60. **Phillis, J. W. and DeLong, R. E.,** An involvement of adenosine in cerebral blood flow regulation during hypercapnia, *Gen. Pharmacol.*, 18, 133, 1987.
61. **Morii, S., Ngai, A. C., and Winn, H. R.,** Reactivity of rat pial arterioles and venules to adenosine and carbon dioxide: with detailed description of the closed window technique in rats, *J. Cereb. Blood Flow Metab.*, 6, 34, 1986.
62. **Mustafa, S. J. and Ghai, G.,** Effect of adenosine on the relaxation of coronary arteries at varying pH values, *Basic Res. Cardiol.*, 76, 380, 1981.
63. **Raberger, G., Schutz, W., and Kraupp, O.,** Coronary reactive hyperemia and coronary dilator action of adenosine during normal respiration and hypercapnic acidosis in the dog, *Clin. Exp. Pharmacol. Physiol.*, 2, 373, 1975.
64. **Mustafa, S. J. and Mansour, M. M.,** Effect of perfusate pH on coronary flow and adenosine release in isolated rabbit heart, *Proc. Soc. Exp. Biol. Med.*, 176, 22, 1984.
65. **Nees, S. and Gerlach, E.,** Adenine nucleotide and adenosine metabolism in cultured coronary endothelial cells: formation and release of adenine compounds and possible functional implications, in *Regulatory Function of Adenosine*, Berne, R. M., Rall, T. W., and Rubio, R., Eds., Martinius Nijhoff, The Netherlands, 1983, 347.
66. **Gerlach, E., Becker, B. F., and Nees, S.,** Formation of adenosine by vascular endothelium: a homeostatic and antithrombogenic mechanism, in *Topics and Perspectives in Adenosine*, Gerlach, E. and Becker, B. F., Eds., Springer-Verlag, Berlin, 1987, 309.

67. **Bender, A. S., Wu, P. H., and Phillis, J. W.,** Some biochemical properties of the rapid adenosine uptake system in rat brain synaptosomes, *J. Neurochem.*, 37, 1282, 1981.
68. **Mustafa, S. J.,** Effect of varying pH [H^+] on the metabolism of adenosine in isolated heart cells, *J. Mol. Cell. Cardiol.*, 12, 335, 1980.
69. **Iadecola, C.,** Does nitric oxide mediate the increases in cerebral blood flow elicited by hypercapnia, *Proc. Natl. Acad. Sci. U.S.A.*, 89, 3913, 1992.
70. **Pelligrino, D. A., Koenig, H., and Sharp, A.,** Nitric oxide (NO) synthesis and cerebral vasodilatory responses in the rat, *FASEB J.*, 6, A1462, 1992.
71. **Picard, J. D.,** Role of prostaglandins and archidonic acid derivatives in the coupling of cerebral blood flow to cerebral metabolism, *J. Cereb. Blood Flow Metab.*, 1, 361, 1981.
72. **Sakabe, T. and Siesjo, B. K.,** The effect of indomethacin on the blood flow-metabolism couple in the brain under normal, hypercapnic and hypoxic conditions, *Acta Physiol. Scand.*, 107, 283, 1979.
73. **Crockard, H. A., Iannotti, F., and Ladds, G.,** Cerebrovascular effects of prostaglandin inhibitors in the gerbil, *J. Cereb. Blood Flow Metab.*, 1, 285, 1982.
74. **Ibayashi, S., Ngai, A. C., Meno, J. R., and Winn, H. R.,** The effects of dipyridamole and theophylline on rat pial vessels during hypocarbia, *J. Cereb. Blood Flow Metab.*, 8, 829, 1988.
75. **Winn, H. R., Rubio, R., and Berne, R. M.,** Brain adenosine concentration during hypoxia in rats, *Am. J. Physiol.*, 241, H235, 1981.
76. **Harder, D. R.,** A cellular mechanism for myogenic regulation of cat cerebral arteries, *Ann. Biomed. Eng.*, 13, 335, 1985.
77. **Harder, D. R.,** Pressure-induced myogenic activation of cat cerebral arteries is dependent on intact endothelium, *Circ. Res.*, 60, 102, 1987.
78. **Katusic, Z. S., Shepherd, J. T., and VanHoutte, P. M.,** Endothelium-dependent contraction to stretch in canine basilar arteries, *Am. J. Physiol.*, 252, H671, 1987.
79. **Wang, Q., Paulson, O. B., and Lassen, N. A.,** Is autoregulation of cerebral blood flow in rats influenced by nitro-L-arginine, a blocker of the synthesis of nitric oxide, *Acta Physiol. Scand.*, 145, 297, 1992.
80. **Winn, R. H., Welsh, J. E., Rubio, R., and Berne, R. M.,** Brain adenosine production in rat during sustained alteration in systemic blood pressure, *Am. J. Physiol.*, 239, H636, 1980.
81. **Van Wylen, D. G. L., Park, T. S., Rubio, R., and Berne, R. M.,** Cerebral blood flow and interstitial fluid adenosine during hemorrhagic hypotension, *Am. J. Physiol.*, 255, H1211, 1988.
82. **Park, T. S., Van Wylen, D. G. L., Rubio, R., and Berne, R. M.,** Brain interstitial adenosine and sagittal sinus blood flow during systemic hypotension in piglet, *J. Cereb. Blood Flow Metab.*, 8, 822, 1988.
83. **Park, T. S., Van Wylen, D. G. L., Rubio, R., and Berne, R. M.,** Increased brain interstitial adenosine concentration during hypoxia in the newborn piglet, *J. Cereb. Blood Flow Metab.*, 7, 178, 1987.
84. **Phillis, J. W. and DeLong, R. E.,** The role of adenosine in cerebral vascular regulation during reductions in perfusion pressure, *J. Pharm. Pharmacol.*, 38, 460, 1986.

IV. Metabolic Regulation of Cerebral Blood Flow

Chapter 17

COUPLING OF BLOOD FLOW AND METABOLISM IN THE BRAIN

Wolfgang Kuschinsky

TABLE OF CONTENTS

I. Methodological Approaches 270

II. Metabolic Rate Vs. Functional Activity 270

III. Blood Flow Vs. Metabolic Rate or Functional Activity 271

IV. Static Coupling of Blood Flow with Function and Metabolism .. 271

V. Capillary Perfusion 273

VI. Dynamic Coupling of Blood Flow to Function and Metabolism 275

VII. Does Uncoupling Occur under Physiological Conditions? 277

Acknowledgment 277

References 277

0-8493-5096-0/93/$0.00 + $.50

I. METHODOLOGICAL APPROACHES

It is a matter of dispute, whether or not metabolism and blood flow in the brain are tightly coupled under physiological conditions with the consequence that coupling is disturbed only under extreme conditions such as cerebral ischemia or brain damage.

Recent findings seem to argue against a coupling of blood flow and metabolism in the brain, even under physiological conditions or such moderately altered conditions as anesthesia. This conclusion has been derived from global measurements of cerebral metabolism and blood flow and, more recently, from more local positron emission tomography (PET) studies.[1] The present article presents arguments and findings which do not support such a view.

A close interrelationship between metabolism and blood flow in the brain had first been postulated by Roy and Sherrington in 1890. In recent years, this idea has been extended and verified. Global measurements of whole brain metabolism and blood flow have already demonstrated a direct relationship among functional activity, metabolism, and blood flow.[2] The more recent use of methods that allow determination of blood flow and metabolism in defined regions has disclosed notable differences among the regions. This heterogeneous blood flow, the result of varying local function and metabolic level, exists not only during resting conditions but also with activated brain function, e.g., during the performance of mental tasks.

The coupling of local metabolism and blood flow can be expressed quantitatively by the ratio of metabolism to blood flow. Methods used for such a local analysis include autoradiography, inert gas clearance methods, and PET, with autoradiography and PET being supplementary to one another. Used exclusively in animals, autoradiography has the advantage of high spatial resolution (0.1 to 0.2 mm), whereas PET has a lower resolution (6 to 12 mm), but can be employed in human subjects. There is no question that investigation of local coupling mechanisms requires high spatial resolution methods.

Coupling of function, metabolism, and blood flow in the brain has been analyzed by correlating two of the parameters. The interpretation of correlations between two parameters as an expression of causality leads to three possible conclusions. First, the local metabolic rate for oxygen and glucose may depend on the degree of functional activity. Second, local blood flow may depend on the local metabolic rates for oxygen and glucose. Third, local blood flow may in fact depend on local functional activity.

II. METABOLIC RATE VS. FUNCTIONAL ACTIVITY

Sokoloff's development of the 2-deoxyglucose method has given impetus to studies on the dependency of local metabolic rate on local functional activity.[3] This method allows one to estimate the degree of local functional activity in defined areas of the brain by quantifying local glucose utilization and has disclosed new information regarding the functional patterns of the brain.[4-6] Glucose utilization is turned on and off during various physiological interventions. Visual stimulation in humans increased the local metabolic rate of glucose in the visual cortex, and the metabolic rate depended on the intensity of the visual stimuli. Such positive correlations have been verified for a variety of sensory and motor functions. Although correlations exist during changes in sensory or motor functions, the 2-deoxyglucose method assesses primarily regional glucose utilization and is only assumed to reflect functional activity. Data on the relationship between electrical activity and local glucose utilization are still lacking or are rather indirect.

III. BLOOD FLOW VS. METABOLIC RATE OR FUNCTIONAL ACTIVITY

Because for a long time, local metabolic rates could not be assessed directly, local blood flow was interpreted as to reflect brain activity and metabolic rate. In human subjects, such measurements of local blood flow have greatly extended our knowledge of the dynamics of brain function beyond what was known on the basis of neuroanatomical and clinical studies.

According to this concept of interactions, functional activation of a specific brain area should increase its metabolic rate, as ion fluxes accompanying action potentials lead to an increase in activities of ion pumps in order to restore intra/extracellular ionic homeostasis. The consequence is a higher energy demand of the Na^+, K^+-ATPase as reflected in increased local blood flow. Therefore, the enhanced local blood flow is indicative of increased neuronal activity. For example, a rather high blood flow has been measured in human subjects in the frontal brain areas during rest, which has been interpreted as a ''preparatory simulation of behavior'',[2] given that neurophysiological studies indicate efferent motor functions of the frontal brain area.

Sensory stimulation and voluntary motor activity abolished the pattern and disclosed an activation of the sensory motor cortex as anticipated by the results of neuroanatomical and clinical studies. Further PET studies show that this pattern of high levels of activity in frontal parts of the brain reflects the organism's mental preparation for engaging in future motor activities.

The resting state, therefore, is one of many states which can collectively be described as a continuum of states, with apprehension and relaxation at the opposite poles of the continuum. Accordingly, frontal hyperactivity could not be observed in highly relaxed subjects.[7]

IV. STATIC COUPLING OF BLOOD FLOW WITH FUNCTION AND METABOLISM

In this case of static coupling, a topic that has generated considerable controversy, it now appears that the results of blood flow studies and metabolic

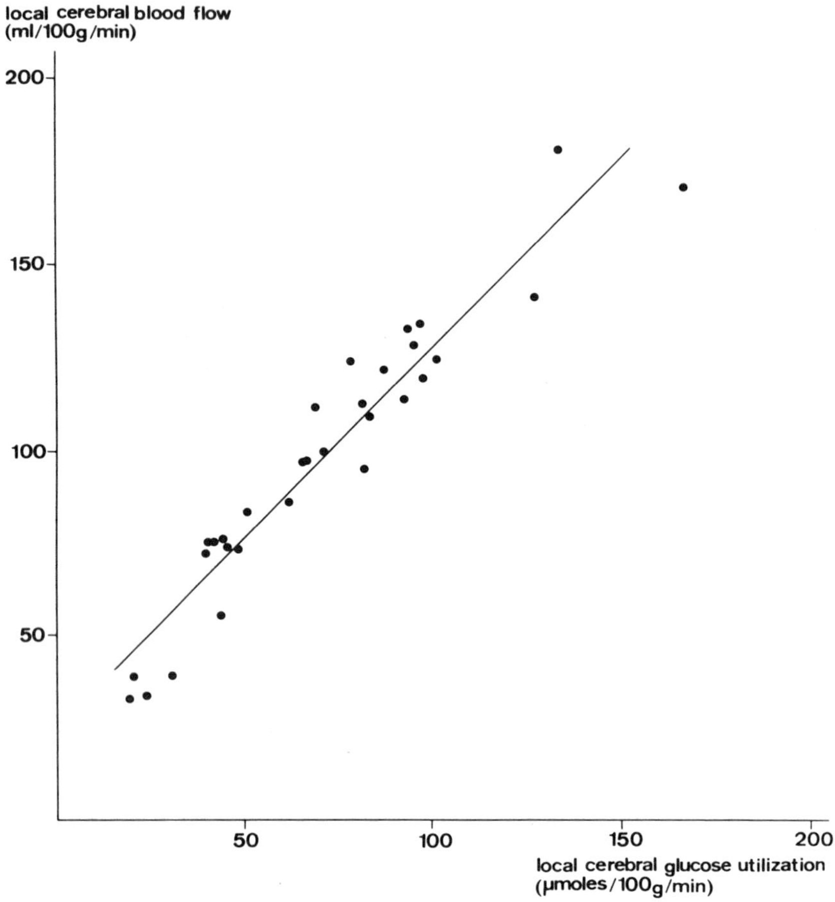

FIGURE 1. Static component of coupling between metabolism and blood flow in the brain. Each point represents the data from one cerebral region. Significant positive correlations exist also for oxygen consumption and blood flow in the brain. The slope of the regression line can be altered by manipulating the experimental conditions.

studies can be matched with some precision. However, blood flow rate and metabolic activity may not under all conditions be interchangeable correlates of brain function, as indicated by analysis of the mechanisms that couple blood flow and cerebral metabolism.

Oxygen consumption, or glucose utilization, correlates directly with blood flow in a given brain area. The results obtained from studies of the rat brain shown in Figure 1 show a correlation that can be observed also in humans by means of PET. This correlation between metabolic rate and blood flow is not, however, invariable. A rather large number of experimental manipulations (e.g., metabolic acidosis,[8] norepinephrine,[9] gamma-hydroxybutyrate,[10] indomethacin,[11] K^+ deficiency[12]) leads to increases or decreases in the slope of the correlation. Thus, the ratio of metabolism over blood flow is being reset, which means that blood flow rate at a given metabolic rate will be either higher or lower.

The hypothesis of resetting, however, depends on the assumption that cerebral glucose utilization is a quantitative measure of metabolic rate. This could well apply to the conditions already mentioned. A change in the nature of the metabolic fuel alone (i.e., the substitution of glucose by other fuels) would not be large enough to explain fully the resetting phenomenon.

The question then is raised: what actually causes resetting? The results point to the weakness of relying exclusively on a global methodological approach for the quantification of metabolic activity and blood flow as, under experimental conditions like those described above, the two parameters actually appear to be dissociated as an apparent sign of uncoupling. The phenomenon formerly described as that of uncoupling is now more clearly defined as a resetting of the coupling characteristics. True uncoupling appears to occur only under extreme pathophysiological conditions, e.g., during ischemia. It should be noted, however, that a true dissociation between blood flow and metabolism still needs to be documented.

V. CAPILLARY PERFUSION

What mechanisms establish coupling at different levels under different experimental conditions? Local differences in capillary density have recently been suggested as one such mechanism.

Local differences in capillary density and a correlation between capillary density and local blood flow have been demonstrated in the brain (Figure 2). Capillary density was also found to correlate with the local glucose utilization.[13] It can be concluded from these data that the local metabolic rate in each brain structure determines its capillary density. The local capillary density is the decisive parameter for the local blood flow. Local blood flow can then be varied by dynamic factors which are released depending on function and metabolism. The local enzymatic pattern may also vary in parallel to the capillary density: a negative correlation was found between capillary density and lactate dehydrogenase, whereas capillary density and cytochrome oxidase were positively correlated.[14]

The question as to what fraction of the brain capillaries is perfused at any given moment under normal condition is highly controversial. Perfusion fractions ranging from half to all of the existing cerebral capillaries have been reported. In numerous studies Weiss[15] has claimed that about half of the capillary bed is perfused at any moment. Capillary cycling has also been claimed by others. A perfusion fraction of 70 to 80% has been observed.[16] Collins et al.[17] have concluded that more than 84% of all capillaries are perfused in the brain structure investigated, which was a part of the superior colliculus. Pawlik et al.[18] found more than 90% of all capillaries being

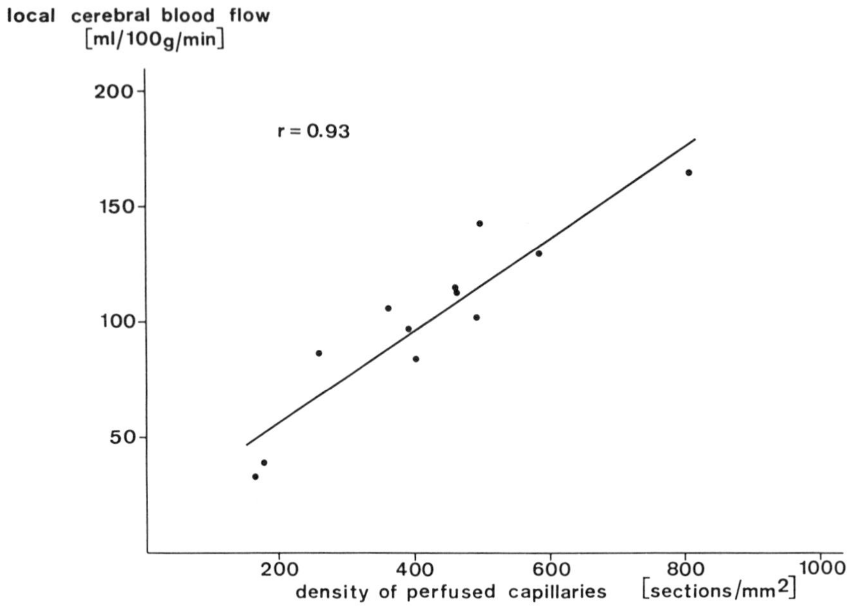

FIGURE 2. Correlation between the density of perfused capillaries in the brain and local blood flow. Each point represents a brain structure in which capillary density or blood flow have been measured. (From Klein, B., et al., *Am. J. Physiol.*, 251, H1333, 1986. With permission.)

perfused. On the other hand, it has been claimed that all capillaries in the brain are perfused at any given moment,[19] which also excludes capillary recruitment during hyperemic conditions.[20] The finding of nonperfused capillaries under normal conditions may be due to methodological flaws of the staining methods employed. The number of perfused and morphologically existing capillaries found by different groups appears to be a function of the sensitivity of the method used. These aspects have been recently summarized.[21]

Three sequential events are of note. First, different levels of functional activity in certain brain structures lead to a heterogeneous distribution of regional metabolic rates. Second, regional metabolism appears to be a determinant for the development of capillaries. Third, capillary density is, then, a critical determinant of regional blood flow rate. Supplementary to the basal rate of blood flow, fluctuations occur, in order to match minute-to-minute changes in metabolic rates. The factors responsible for changes in regional capillary density are still not yet understood. Hypoxia may be one factor, as exposure to hypoxia, which occurs during a certain period of brain development, stimulates capillary growth. The level of coupling, thus, appears to be a function of the extensiveness of capillary development. Hence, this component can be conceptualized as the structural, static, or long-term component of the coupling mechanism.

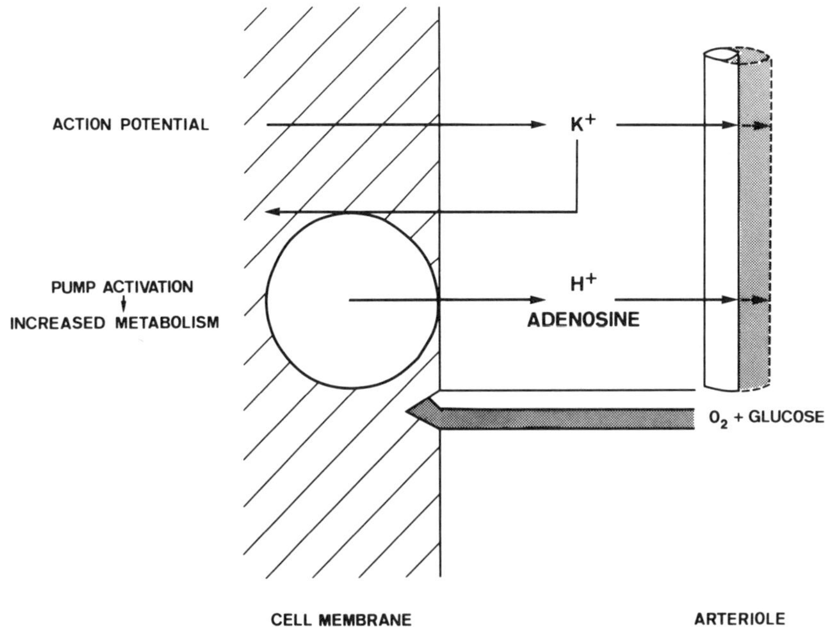

FIGURE 3. Dynamic component of coupling between functional activity, metabolism, and blood flow in the brain. Dynamic coupling consists of two elements: the function dependent element is represented by K^+ and the metabolic element by H^+ and adenosine. Increased concentrations of K^+, H^+, and adenosine dilate the cerebral resistance vessels. The release of K^+ depends on the frequency of action potentials (function dependent element), whereas H^+ and adenosine concentrations increase if there is a mismatch between oxygen/glucose delivery and demand (metabolic element). The impact of both elements on the actual adjustment of vessel diameter may vary from situation to situation.

VI. DYNAMIC COUPLING OF BLOOD FLOW TO FUNCTION AND METABOLISM

In the brain, as in other organs, local blood flow is adjusted to the minute-by-minute functional activity and metabolic demands. This is achieved by the vasomotor action of the cerebral arteries and arterioles.

The vasomotor response occurs within seconds and allows for rapid changes in regional blood flow.[22,23] It is referred to as the acute, or dynamic, component of coupling. Its essentials are given in Figure 3. Increased neuronal activity, as seen in a higher frequency of action potentials, leads to the release of intracellular K^+ into the extracellular space. Since the extracellular space in the brain is small (about 15%) and the intra/extracellular K^+ concentration gradient high, a considerable increase results in the extracellular K^+ concentration, which in turn dilates the cerebral resistance vessels. This, together with the information forwarded by the action potential, results in the quick adjustment of blood flow to the increased functional activity.

The original extra/intracellular distribution of ions then has to be reestablished on a long-term basis. Pumps are activated to carry K^+ back into and Na^+ out of the cells. Increased pump activity is accompanied by increased metabolic activity. This is the very basis for neuroimaging which makes use of the metabolic activity as an indicator of function. The signals for metabolically induced vasodilatation, of which H^+ and adenosine have been identified, continue to be released as long as a mismatch occurs between the oxygen/glucose demand and supply.

Vasodilation induced by these factors counteracts this mismatch and thus permits a fine tuning of adequate blood supply to the tissue. Hence, acute, dynamic coupling occurs by two mechanisms, the feedforward mechanism utilized by K^+ and the feedback mechanism used by H^+ and adenosine, which are key mechanisms in both circulatory and respiratory physiology.

For over a decade, controversies have persisted regarding the quantitative contributions of these regional factors to dynamic coupling. While K^+ is now accepted as an initial mediator of coupling, controversy persists regarding the quantitative contributions made by H^+ and adenosine to dynamic coupling. Some studies show that extracellular pH decreases immediately as neuronal activity increases, whereas others report a decrease in pH that lags behind the onset of neuronal activity by some seconds (for references see 24). With regard to adenosine, the situation may become more clear in the near future. Previous experiments have indicated an increase in brain tissue adenosine concentration during the starting phase of bicuculline-induced seizures.[25,26] With regard to the interstitial adenosine concentration which may be more relevant with regard to the action on vascular diameter, studies using the brain dialysis technique confirm an increase in adenosine release although its extent is not overwhelming.[27] However, a precise time characteristic has not yet been obtained for the first seconds of functional hyperemia.

These inconsistencies can be reconciled if one considers the conditions under which K^+, H^+, and adenosine leave the cell. While the release of K^+ is dependent on the neuronal firing rate, H^+ and adenosine accumulate in the tissues when a mismatch occurs between oxygen demand and delivery. Therefore, fine tuning by the H^+-adenosine metabolic mechanism is likely to become effective after a time lag and to have a greater effect in those cases in which the K^+ mechanism alone is not sufficient to yield an adequate O_2 supply.

The effect of the H^+-adenosine mechanism, therefore, depends on the regional conditions. Its impact is expected to be small where neural activation is accompanied by increased pO_2. In contrast, it can be expected to play a major role in oxygen deficiency, e.g., hypoxia and ischemia. Hence, the extent to which vascular resistance is controlled by metabolic mechanisms determines the ratio metabolic activity: blood flow.

In a region with weak metabolic control of vascular resistance, blood flow will be dependent less on the metabolic factors and more on the K^+

concentration in the interstitium. In such a region, the conditions result in a slope of the ratio metabolic activity: blood flow that will be different from that of other brain areas, although an uncoupling is not implied.

VII. DOES UNCOUPLING OCCUR UNDER PHYSIOLOGICAL CONDITIONS?

Local uncoupling has been postulated for somatosensory stimulation in humans.[1] This postulate, derived from PET studies, appears to be a contradiction in terms, however. It is based on a greater percentage increase in local blood flow (+29%), than in local oxygen consumption (+5%), and maximal increase of these parameters as measured in the contralateral brain hemisphere during cutaneous vibration of the finger pads of one hand. This notion of uncoupling, at first, seems plausible. However, the coupling sequence (i.e., neuronal activity — metabolism — blood flow) may not fully describe all aspects of the coupling procedure. The procedure may be cut short by the influence of neuronal activity on the cerebral vessels. The neuronal activity may be related directly to the interstitial K^+ concentration or to the cotransmission of vasoactive peptides, thereby modifying the metabolic link between neuronal activity and local hemodynamics. Dissociation, or partial dissociation, between regional oxygen consumption and blood flow would then be expected to result in a greater increase in blood flow than in metabolic rate. This, however, does not indicate uncoupling but rather a specific type of coupling. The greater increase in blood flow than in metabolism leads to regional hyperperfusion, the result being a smaller arteriovenous difference of substrates, e.g., glucose and oxygen. In conclusion, the coupling phenomenon is not fully described by relating blood flow rate to metabolic rate only, a scheme that is too simplistic (Figure 1). The events outlined in Figure 3 cannot be neglected in such an analysis.

ACKNOWLEDGMENT

Supported by the Deutsche Forschungsgemeinschaft.

REFERENCES

1. **Fox, P. T. and Raichle, M. E.,** Focal physiological uncoupling of cerebral blood flow and oxidative metabolism during somatosensory stimulation in human subjects, *Proc. Natl. Acad. Sci. U.S.A.*, 83, 1140, 1986.
2. **Ingvar, D. H.,** Mental illness and regional brain metabolism, *Trends in Neurosci.*, 5, 199, 1982.

3. **Sokoloff, L., Reivich, M., Kennedy, C., DesRosiers, M. H., Patlak, C. S., Pettigrew, K. D., Sakurada, O., and Shinohara, M.,** The (^{14}C)deoxyglucose method for the measurement of local cerebral glucose utilization: theory, procedure, and normal values in the conscious and anesthetized albino rat, *J. Neurochem.*, 28, 897, 1977.
4. **Heiss, W. D., Pawlik, G., Herholz, K., Wagner, R., and Wienhard, K.,** Regional cerebral glucose metabolism in man during wakefulness, sleep, and dreaming, *Brain Res.*, 327, 362, 1985.
5. **McCulloch, J.,** Mapping functional alterations in the CNS with (^{14}C)deoxyglucose, in *Handbook of Psychopharmacology,* Iversen, L. L., Iversen, S. D., and Snyder, S. H., Eds., Vol. 15, Plenum Press, New York, 1982, 321.
6. **Sokoloff, L., Ed.,** Brain imaging and brain function, Vol. 63, Raven Press, New York, 1985.
7. **Mazziotta, J. C., Phelps, M. E., Miller, J., and Kuhl, D. E.,** Tomographic mapping of human cerebral metabolism: normal unstimulated state, *Neurology,* 31, 503, 1981.
8. **Kuschinsky, W., Suda, S., and Sokoloff, L.,** Local cerebral glucose utilization and blood flow during metabolic acidosis, *Am. J. Physiol.*, 241, H772, 1981.
9. **Kuschinsky, W., Suda, S., Bünger, R., Yaffe, S., and Sokoloff, L.,** The effects of intravenous norepinephrine on the local coupling between glucose utilization and blood flow in the rat brain, *Pfluegers Arch.*, 398, 134, 1981.
10. **Kuschinsky, W., Suda, S., and Sokoloff, L.,** Influence of gamma-hydroxybutyrate on the relationship between local cerebral glucose utilization and local cerebral blood flow in the rat brain, *J. Cereb. Blood Flow Metab.*, 5, 58, 1985.
11. **McCulloch, J., Kelly, P. A. T., Grome, J. J., and Pickard, J. D.,** Local cerebral circulatory and metabolic effects of indomethacin, *Am. J. Physiol.*, 243, H416, 1982.
12. **Schröck, H. and Kuschinsky, W.,** Cerebral blood flow, glucose use, and CSF ionic regulation in potassium-depleted rats, *Am. J. Physiol.*, 254, H250, 1988.
13. **Klein, B., Kuschinsky, W., Schröck, H., and Vetterlein, F.,** Interdependency of local capillary density, blood flow and metabolism in the rat brain, *Am. J. Physiol.*, 251, H1333, 1986.
14. **Borowsky, I. W. and Collins, R. C.,** Metabolic anatomy of brain: a comparison of regional capillary density, glucose metabolism, and enzyme activities, *J. Comp. Neurol.*, 288, 401, 1989.
15. **Weiss, H. R.,** Measurement of cerebral capillary perfusion with a fluorescent label, *Microvasc. Res.*, 36, 172, 1988.
16. **Kikano, G. E., LaManna, J. C., and Harik, S. I.,** Brain perfusion in acute and chronic hyperglycemia in rats, *Stroke,* 20, 1027, 1989.
17. **Collins, R. C., Wagmann, I. L., Lymer, L., and Matter, J. M.,** Distribution and recruitment of capillaries in rat brain (abstract), *J. Cereb. Blood Flow Metab.*, 7(Suppl. 1), 336, 1987.
18. **Pawlik, G., Rackl, A., and Bing, R. J.,** Quantitative capillary topography and blood flow in the cerebral cortex of cats: an in vivo microscopic study, *Brain Res.*, 208, 35, 1989.
19. **Göbel, U., Theilen, H., and Kuschinsky, W.,** Congruence of total and perfused capillary network in rat brains, *Circ. Res.*, 6, 271, 1990.
20. **Göbel, U., Klein, B., Schröck, H., and Kuschinsky, W.,** Lack of capillary recruitment in the brain of awake rats during hypercapnia, *J. Cereb. Blood Flow Metab.*, 9, 491, 1989.
21. **Kuschinsky, W. and Paulson, O. B.,** Capillary circulation in the brain, *Cerebrovasc. Brain Metab. Rev.*, 4, 261, 1992.
22. **Kuschinsky, W. and Wahl, M.,** Local chemical and neurogenic regulation of cerebral vascular resistance, *Physiol. Rev.*, 58, 656, 1978.
23. **Leniger-Follert, E.,** Mechanisms of regulation of cerebral microflow during bicuculline-induced seizures in anaesthetized cats, *J. Cereb. Blood Flow Metab.*, 4, 150, 1984.

24. **Kuschinsky, W.,** Role of hydrogen ions in regulation of cerebral blood flow and other regional flows, in *Advances in Microcirculation,* Vol. 11, Altura, B. M., Davis, E., and Harders, H., Eds., S. Karger, Basel, 1982, 1.
25. **Schrader, J., Wahl, M., Kuschinsky, W., and Kreutzberg, G. W.,** Increase of adenosine content in cerebral cortex of the cat during bicuculline-induced seizure, *Pfluegers Arch.,* 387, 245, 1980.
26. **Winn, H. R., Welsh, J. E., Rubio, R., and Berne, R. M.,** Changes in brain adenosine during bicuculline induced seizures in rats. Effects of hypoxia and altered systemic blood pressure, *Circ. Res.,* 47, 568, 1980.
27. **Park, T. S., van Wylen, D. G. L., Rubio, R., and Berne, R. M.,** Interstitial fluid adenosine and sagittal sinus blood flow during bicuculline-seizures in newborn piglets, *J. Cereb. Blood Flow Metab.,* 7, 633, 1987.

Chapter 18

CEREBROVASCULAR FLOW REGULATION BY ADENOSINE

Enoch P. Wei and Hermes A. Kontos

TABLE OF CONTENTS

I. Introduction 282

II. Cerebrovascular Effects of Adenosine 282

III. Role of Adenosine in Cerebral Circulation 283
- A. Normoxia 283
- B. Hypoxia 283
- C. Seizures 285
- D. Hypotension 286
- E. Autoregulation 286
- F. Hypercapnia 288
- G. Hypocapnia 291
- H. Ischemia/Reperfusion 292

IV. Summary 292

Acknowledgment 293

References 293

0-8493-5096-0/93/$0.00 + $.50

I. INTRODUCTION

The brain is well known for its high resting metabolic rate and its heavy dependence on oxygen supply. Normally cerebral blood flow (CBF) remains relatively constant over a wide range of blood pressures; however, CBF will change in order to meet the metabolic demands of the brain. This close relationship between CBF and metabolism is believed to be dependent upon the production of vasodilator metabolites from brain cells and the abundance of these metabolites to be dependent upon the blood flow. A number of candidates have been proposed to be the metabolic mediator on CBF and all seem to have received some evidence of support. But, the accumulated evidence showed that none of these proposed candidates alone can account for all the changes in CBF during associated alterations in oxygen supply and demand. It has, therefore, been suggested that possibly several mediators are involved in the metabolic adjustments of CBF.

In the light of the ubiquity of adenosine receptors and of the fact that all cells under stress can release adenosine into the surrounding interstitial fluid, adenosine is understandably the most widely studied among the candidates in recent years. Based on the available evidence adenosine also emerges as the most promising vasodilator metabolite so far, since a rapid rise of adenosine levels has been found in brain in a number of situations such as cerebral hypoxia,[1] hypotension,[2] ischemia,[3] electrical stimulation,[4] and drug-induced seizures.[5,6]

The production and metabolism of adenosine and its role on CBF were recently reviewed in detail.[7,8] Therefore, for the remainder of this chapter we will examine additional evidence on the role of adenosine as a vasodilator metabolite obtained by using the cranial window technique in cats.

II. CEREBROVASCULAR EFFECTS OF ADENOSINE

In comparison with other vascular beds, blood flow in the brain is regulated primarily by intrinsic mechanisms. As explained by Winn et al.,[9] increased production of adenosine in brain reflects cerebral, not systemic, events. The vasodilator effect of adenosine can be easily demonstrated on the pial vessels, whether it is applied topically by superfusion,[10] by microinjection in the immediate vicinity of these arterioles,[11] or by topical application in the space under a cranial window.[12-14] As shown in Figure 1, the dilator action of adenosine on pial vessels can be blocked with adenosine deaminase. Adenosine deaminase is a specific enzyme catalyzing the breakdown of adenosine to inosine and in itself does not have any significant action on pial vessels during normoxia. Furthermore, adenosine deaminase exerts no effect on vasodilation induced by topical application of 2-chloroadenosine (Figure 1)[12,15] or histamine (data not shown). Its effect on adenosine, therefore, appears to be specific. Hence it can be used as a tool to investigate the role of adenosine in various responses.

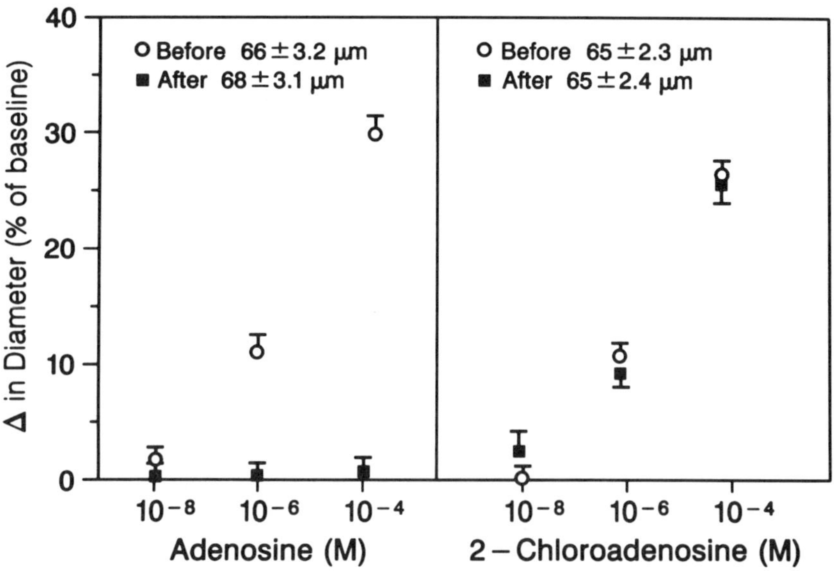

FIGURE 1. Changes of pial arteriolar diameter (mean ± SE) to adenosine, and 2-chloroadenosine before and after 10-min exposure of the brain cortex to adenosine deaminase (5 U/ml CSF). Adenosine deaminase inhibits the dilation of pial arterioles (18 vessels, 6 animals) to adenosine, but it does not affect the response to 2-chloroadenosine (21 vessels, 5 animals). Baseline diameters from which the percent changes were derived are shown in the insert.

III. ROLE OF ADENOSINE IN CEREBRAL CIRCULATION

A. NORMOXIA

The role of adenosine during normoxia has been discussed at length by Van Wylen et al.[7] Presumably, should adenosine contribute to the resting tone in the cerebral circulation, then the inhibition of adenosine action would result in vasoconstriction. However, there has been considerable heterogeneity in the reports of responses in resting CBF or pial vessel caliber, with some increasing, others decreasing, and still others remaining unchanged, following administration of adenosine receptor antagonists. Some of the discrepancies can be attributed to indirect effects following the systemic administration of adenosine blockers. Studies with topical application of theophylline or adenosine deaminase appear to be less controversial. Generally there was little or no change in resting pial vessel diameter,[11,13,14,16,17] suggesting that no accumulation of vasodilator metabolites takes place during normoxia.

B. HYPOXIA

An increased brain adenosine concentration has been demonstrated in arterial hypoxia induced by inhalation of gas mixtures containing low

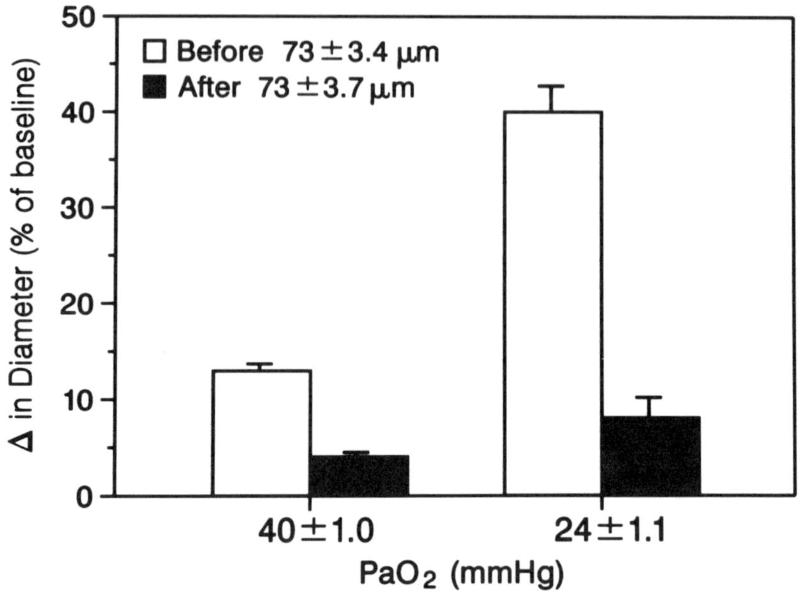

FIGURE 2. Responses of pial arterioles (15 vessels, 5 animals) to 2 levels of arterial hypoxia before and after topical application of adenosine deaminase (5 U/ml CSF). Hypoxic vasodilation was significantly inhibited following adenosine deaminase.

concentrations of oxygen. The elevated production of adenosine under these conditions may be the result of hypoxia of the neural cells, which leads to increased production of adenosine and subsequent dilation of blood vessels supplying that region, thus increasing oxygen delivery.

As shown in our previous studies,[18] the dilator action of arterial hypoxia on cerebral arterioles is mediated by local mechanisms, since it can be counteracted almost completely by supplying sufficient oxygen via topical application of oxygenated fluorocarbons which have a high carrying capacity for oxygen. In these experiments, after a steady state was established following induction of arterial hypoxia, the space under the cranial window was superfused with oxygenated CSF and fluorocarbons equilibrated with either 100% N_2 or 100% O_2. Oxygenated CSF caused a moderate reduction of vasodilation, whereas oxygenated fluorocarbons almost abolished the vasodilation. Deoxygenated fluorocarbons, on the other hand, had no effect on hypoxic vasodilation. Reduction of hypoxic vasodilation can also be achieved by superfusing the space under the cranial window with synthetic allosteric modifiers of hemoglobin (Hb) which decrease the oxygen affinity of Hb, thus increasing the amount of oxygen released by Hb to tissues.[19] If the surface of the brain is treated with adenosine deaminase, the hypoxia-induced dilation is greatly diminished, as shown in Figure 2.

Using the cranial window technique in rats, Morii et al.[13] observed a similar attenuation of hypoxic hyperemia and pial vasodilation after intraperitoneal administration of theophylline. Theophylline, in the doses used, blocked adenosine receptors and prevented the vasodilator action of adenosine. Moreover, they found that during hypoxia induced by 7% O_2 inhalation adenosine concentrations increased by more than threefold in the interstitial fluid.

Despite ample evidence supporting the involvement of adenosine in hypoxia-induced cerebral vasodilation as reviewed by Van Wylen et al.,[7] conflicting results with topical treatment of adenosine deaminase or theophylline did arise from other laboratories.[12,17] Although the reasons for the discrepancies are not obvious, there were differences in the approach of cerebrocortical observation from these laboratories. For instance, Dora et al. used the detection method of surface fluororeflectometry and a more potent hypoxic stimulus in 6% O_2 for 3 to 4 min. It should be noted that fluorescein administration generally causes substantial dilation in the resting pial vessel diameter. In addition, they measured vascular volume which includes both the surface and the underlying vessels. It has been shown that topically applied adenosine easily penetrates the brain tissues, but a residual dilator effect on the underlying vessels persists despite repeated wash-out in the space under the cranial window.[20] On the other hand, brain tissue is not readily accessible to topically applied adenosine deaminase due to its large molecular weight. It is even more difficult to assess the negative findings from Haller and Kuschinsky, who used microapplication in an open preparation with the exposed brain surface covered with mineral oil.[17] It is uncertain whether the lipid soluble theophylline could be diluted by the surrounding mineral oil. Based on their negative findings with adenosine as a possible vasodilator mediator, Haller and Kuschinsky went on to conclude that adenosine may not be the main causative factor for the hypoxic hyperemia. Instead, they suggested that other chemical factors such as K^+ and H^+ could contribute to the dilation during mild to moderate hypoxia. Of course, the roles of these candidates as vasodilator metabolites on the regulation of CBF are much less well defined.

C. SEIZURES

Generalized seizures are usually linked to an increase in cerebral metabolism, CBF, and dilation of pial arterioles.[21-23] Rapid increases in adenosine concentration have been found in bicuculline-induced seizures in cats and rats.[24,25] In terms of cranial window studies, the vasodilation that follows metrazol-induced seizures could be partially reversed by superfusion of oxygenated fluorocarbons in the space under the cranial window, suggesting that seizure-induced vasodilation is mediated at least in part by a local oxygen-dependent mechanism.[18,26] Dora et al.[12] detected no evidence favoring the involvement of adenosine in the vasodilation of arterial hypoxia, topical cyanide poisoning, or direct electrical stimulation; nevertheless, they found some evidence of adenosine participating in seizure-induced hyperemia.

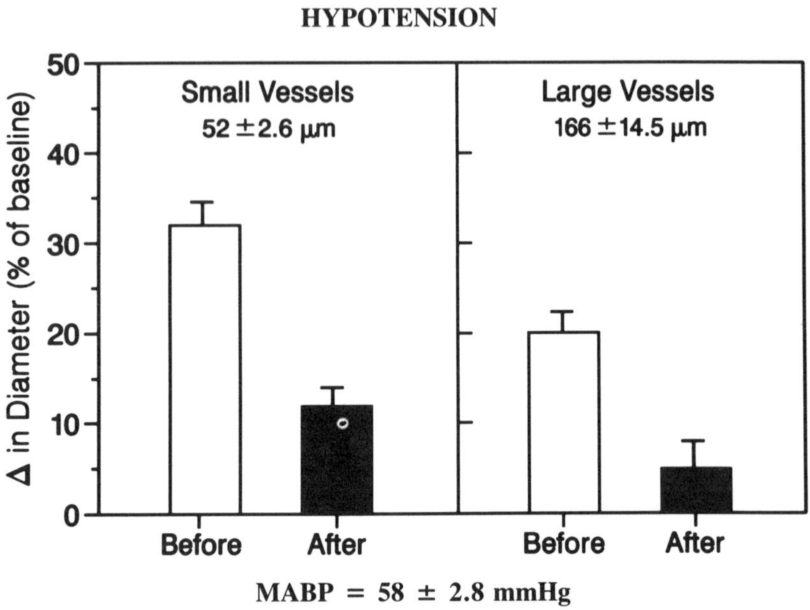

FIGURE 3. Responses of pial arterioles (21 small and 15 large, 5 animals) to hypotension before and after treatment of adenosine deaminase (5 U/ml CSF). Vasodilation to hypotension was significantly reduced following adenosine deaminase.

Pretreatment with either theophylline or adenosine deaminase in their studies slightly decreased the vasodilator effect of metrazol-induced seizures.

D. HYPOTENSION

Cerebral arterioles dilate readily to reductions in blood pressure.[27] Tissue hypoxia is believed to be the dominant mechanism involved in the vasodilation associated with hypotension.[18] As is in the case with arterial hypoxia, this hypotension-induced vasodilation could be abolished with increased local delivery of oxygen by superfusion of oxygenated fluorocarbon over the brain surface. Superfusion of deoxygenated fluorocarbon had no effect.[18] The local oxygen-dependent mechanisms responding to arterial hypotension can also be demonstrated by superfusing over the brain surface certain allosteric modifiers of Hb, which increase the amount of O_2 delivery to the tissues by decreasing the O_2 affinity of Hb.[19] When adenosine deaminase was topically applied during a steady state hypotensive hyperemia, the induced vasodilation was greatly diminished in both small (resting diameter < 100 µm) and large (resting diameter ≥ 100 µm) pial precapillary vessels (Figure 3).

E. AUTOREGULATION

The consensus is that cerebral autoregulation is the result of local regulatory mechanisms. However, as in other vascular beds, both myogenic and

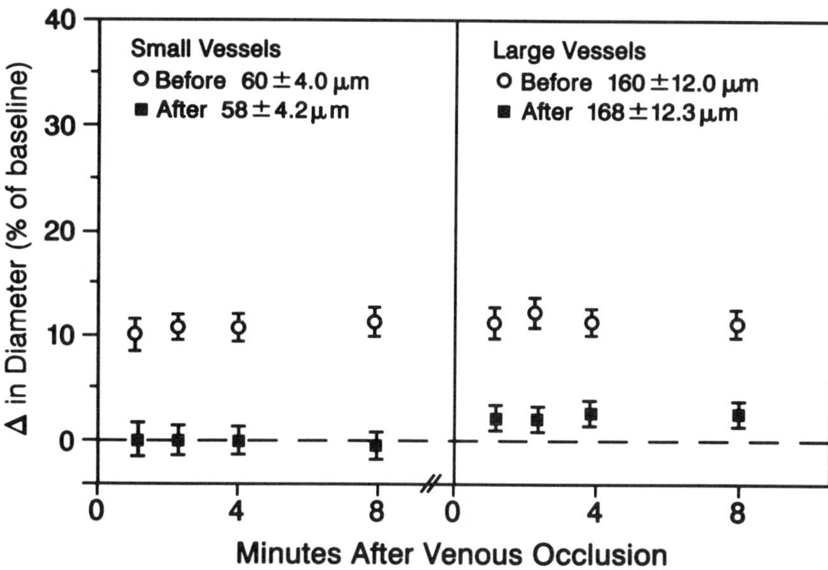

FIGURE 4. Responses of pial arterioles (15 small and 16 large, 5 animals) to occlusion of superior vena cava before and after treatment with adenosine deaminase (5 U/ml CSF). Vasodilation to venous occlusion was virtually abolished following adenosine deaminase.

metabolic mechanisms have been proposed to explain the phenomenon. It was suggested that the responses of arterioles to elevated venous pressure could distinguish the dominant mechanism of autoregulation.[28] Increased venous pressure causes an increased intravascular pressure and, hence, increased transmural pressure which is transmitted upstream to the capillaries and arterioles. On the other hand, increased venous pressure also causes decreased flow. Therefore, if the dominant mechanism of autoregulation is metabolic, one would expect to see vasodilation in response to the accumulation of vasodilator metabolites. We demonstrated earlier that an elevated venous pressure, caused by occlusion of the superior vena cava in anesthetized cats, resulted in cerebral arteriolar dilation.[29] However, when the space under the cranial window was perfused with fluorocarbons equilibrated with 100% O_2, thus eliminating the release of vasodilator metabolites, the response to increased venous pressure was a small vasoconstriction, consistent with the expected outcome of the operation of myogenic mechanisms.[30] Based on these experiments in anesthetized cats, the dominant mechanism of autoregulation in cerebral arterioles, at least in the face of decreasing pressure, is a metabolic mechanism which depends on changes of oxygen tension in the parenchymal tissues. When adenosine deaminase was applied in the space under the cranial window, vasodilation to venous occlusion was virtually abolished as shown in Figure 4.

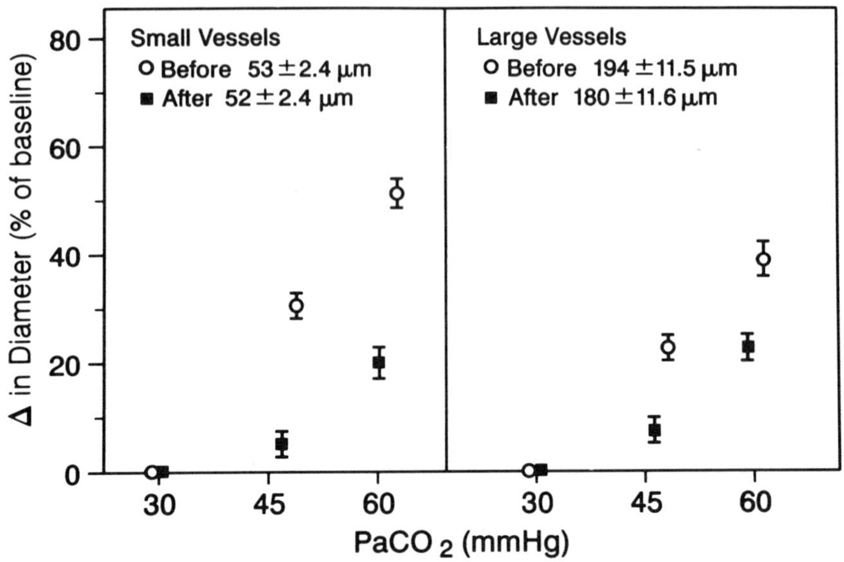

FIGURE 5. Responses of pial arterioles (27 small and 15 large, 5 animals) to hypercapnia before and after treatment with adenosine deaminase (5 U/ml CSF). Hypercapnic vasodilation was significantly reduced following adenosine deaminase.

F. HYPERCAPNIA

Hypercapnia relaxes cerebral arterioles and increases CBF.[31] Since decreased extracellular O_2 and increased CO_2 levels are invariably linked to increased cerebral metabolism, adenosine has been considered as a possible mediator in hypercapnia. This possibility that endogenously released adenosine could play a role in response to hypercapnia was investigated in the anesthetized rat by Phillis and DeLong.[32] Arterial hypercapnia was induced by inhalation of 10% CO_2 for 30 to 90 s. Caffeine, an adenosine antagonist, decreased the peak increases in CBF. On the other hand, dipyridamole, an uptake inhibitor, and deoxycoformycin, an adenosine deaminase inhibitor, elevated CBF. These results suggested that adenosine played an important role in coupling increased $PaCO_2$ to CBF.

In terms of cranial window studies in cats, Figure 5 shows the responses of pial arterioles to 5 and 7.5% CO_2 inhalation before and after local application of adenosine deaminase. Adenosine deaminase greatly diminishes the hypercapnic hyperemia. Since deamination of adenosine with adenosine deaminase is expected to generate ammonia, the local pH is likely to rise as a result of the generation of ammonia. Local alkalosis, therefore, may explain the diminished response of pial arterioles to CO_2 following adenosine deaminase.[33,34] However, as shown in Figure 6, the presence of ammonia per se does not inhibit the vasodilation of pial vessels in reaction to hypercapnia.

Negative findings have been reported by other investigators. Emerson and Raymond[35] and Morii et al.[13] found that theophylline had no effect on

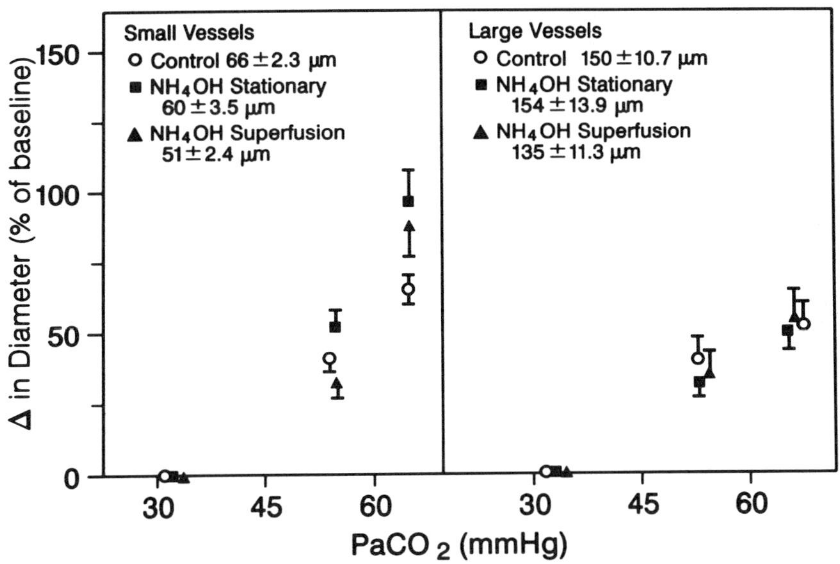

FIGURE 6. Responses of pial arterioles (27 small and 16 large, 5 animals) to hypercapnia with the space under the cranial window exposed to stationary or superfusing solution of NH_4OH. Responsiveness of pial arterioles to hypercapnia was not altered by NH_4OH.

the cerebral hyperemia induced by hypercapnia. However, most of the discrepancies could be attributed to the differences in the experimental design. Both above-mentioned groups happened to use 15% CO_2 inhalation to induce vasodilation for a duration of 2 to 5 min and 2 to 3 min, respectively. It should be noted that inhalation of a 7.5% CO_2 gas mixture could have conceivably induced maximal pial dilation. Moreover, vasodilation generally would not have reached a steady state in response to arterial hypercapnia within 2 to 5 min. In other words, cerebral vessels were still on their way to reach their maximal dilation during the initial minutes of hypercapnia; there fore, the effect of theophylline may not have been realized in the face of increasing hypercapnic vasodilation, or possibly the inhibitory effect of theophylline was minimal in overcoming the hypercapnic hyperemia induced by an extremely potent stimulus in 15% CO_2. Hoffman et al.[36] also reported negative findings on the role of adenosine in response to arterial hypercapnia. Therefore, they suggested that theophylline treatment was specific for hypoxic hyperemia and adenosine release. The concentration of hypercapnic gases used in their experiments was not specified. If, like the two previously mentioned groups, they used extremely high concentration of CO_2, the absence of a reduction of CBF after treatment with theophylline may be explained.

Increased adenosine concentration in the brain during hypercapnia has not been documented. However, some insights on potential mechanisms can be gained from studies on the coronary circulation which also responds with increased blood flow to arterial hypercapnia. Some studies on the coronary

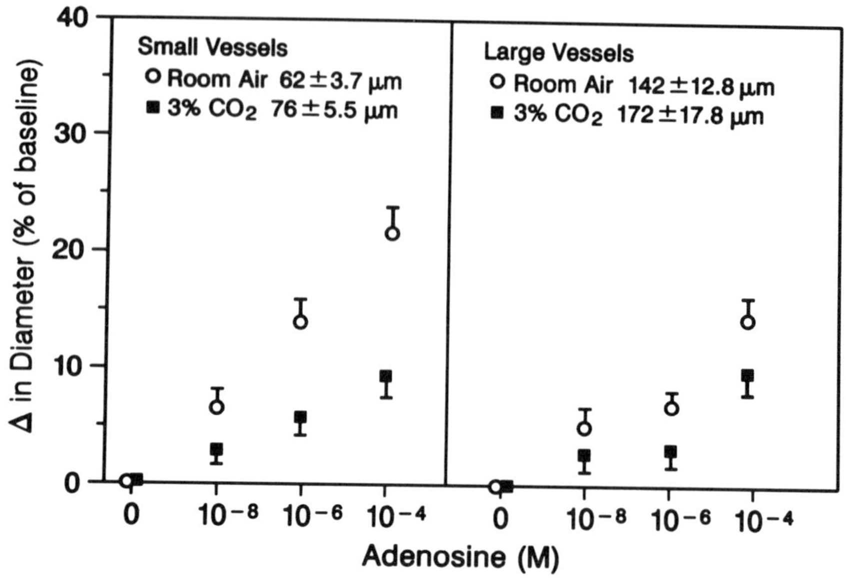

FIGURE 7. Responses of pial arterioles (11 small and 10 large, 3 animals) to adenosine before and after 3% CO_2 inhalation. Vasodilation to adenosine was not affected in the presence of hypercapnia.

circulation showed an association of hypercapnic acidosis with increased potency of exogenous adenosine, suggesting that acidosis sensitizes the coronary vessels to adenosine.[37-39] However, evidence that would show hypercapnic acidosis potentiating the action of adenosine is lacking in the brain. In the presence of mild hypercapnia, induced by inhalation of 3% CO_2, pial arterioles continued to dilate further in response to topical application of adenosine as shown in Figure 7. But, the degree of dilation to adenosine was not accentuated.

In additional experiments we found that the presence of an intact adenosine receptor is essential for the depressant effect of adenosine deaminase on the vasodilation from hypercapnia to be expressed. In these experiments we examined the effect of adenosine deaminase on the steady state vasodilation from hypercapnia, due to inhalation of 5% CO_2, after topical administration of theophylline. As seen in Figure 8, the response to hypercapnia was unaffected by theophylline. Subsequent administration of adenosine deaminase did not influence the response to hypercapnia. It is clear, therefore, that the presence of an intact adenosine receptor is necessary for the depressant effect of adenosine deaminase on the response to CO_2 to be expressed. Blockade of the adenosine receptor by theophylline in itself does not depress the response to CO_2 but prevents the depressant effect of adenosine deaminase.

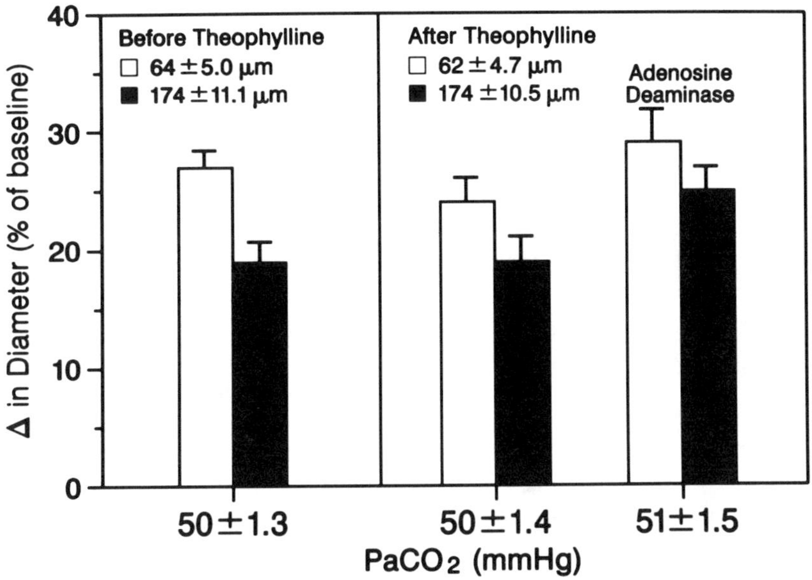

FIGURE 8. Responses of 17 small (open columns) and 12 large (solid columns) pial arterioles to 5% CO_2 inhalation before and after theophylline (2.5 μg/ml CSF) in 5 animals. Theophylline has no effect on pial dilation to hypercapnia, as shown in the middle columns, but it prevents the inhibitory effect of adenosine deaminase (5 U/ml CSF), as shown in the right-hand columns.

G. HYPOCAPNIA

Arterial hypocapnia exerts a powerful vasoconstrictor effect on cerebral blood vessels. While the responses of pial arterioles to hypercapnia are strongly size dependent, with smaller vessels responding more vigorously than the larger ones,[40,41] the responses of the same vessels to hypocapnia are size independent.[40] An increased concentration of adenosine in brain tissue was found during hypocapnia ($PaCO_2 < 20$ mmHg), presumably due to tissue hypoxia created by hypocapnic vasoconstriction at these low levels of $PaCO_2$.[1] The released adenosine was believed to represent a protective mechanism which limits the degree of vasoconstriction during hypocapnia. Ibayashi et al.[42] were able to demonstrate that the vasoconstriction during hypocapnia was attenuated by dipyridamole and augmented by theophylline. But similar findings were not observed in our cat cranial window model. Whether the surface of the brain was pre- or post-treated with adenosine deaminase, steady-state diameter readings showed that hypocapnia produced the same degree of vasoconstriction in pial arterioles (data not shown).

Evidence from patient studies, however, seems to favor the findings of Ibayashi et al. Sollevi et al.[43] examined the effects of intravenous administration of adenosine on CBF in seven patients with cerebral arteriovenous malformations. Six of their patients were normally ventilated and the seventh hyperventilated. In comparison with normally ventilated patients, their findings of CBF, CVR, and MABP on the hyperventilated patient implied that hyperventilation was able to counteract the cerebral vasodilator effect of adenosine.

H. ISCHEMIA/REPERFUSION

Elevated adenosine levels due to cerebral ischemia have been documented in a number of studies. More recently, an increased concentration in the brain during reperfusion following cerebral ischemia has been reported. Sciotti et al.[44] found that interstitial adenosine concentration peaked during initial minutes (5 to 10 min) of reperfusion following 10-min cerebral ischemia (forebrain) by bilateral carotid occlusion. Similar findings were reported by Meno et al.[45] who examined the changes of CSF concentrations of adenosine, inosine, and hypoxanthine as well as pial arteriolar diameter following transient fore-brain ischemia. They found that the concentration of adenosine in CSF increased 13.8-fold during the first 5 min of reperfusion. Concomitantly arteriolar diameter increased significantly. Their next measurements at 30 min after reperfusion showed diminished values for both adenosine concentration and vessel caliber. Therefore, they hypothesized that the increase in adenosine concentration during the initial minutes of reperfusion could account for the changes in CBF.

In our cat model there was a marked hyperemia and pial arteriolar dilation immediately following ischemia/reperfusion. The elevated CBF lasted for 30 to 45 min whereas pial arteriolar dilation persisted up to a period of 2 h after the onset of reperfusion.[46] With respect to the possible role of adenosine, we obtained negative results in cerebral ischemia/reperfusion experiments conducted in cats equipped with double cranial windows. The brain surface under one window was pretreated with adenosine deaminase prior to a 10-min period of global cerebral ischemia, and changes in vessel caliber from both cranial windows during reperfusion were compared for the duration of 1 h. Although vessels from the treated side failed to respond to a local application of adenosine, their dilation during the reperfusion period was not significantly different from what was found in the untreated window.

Therefore, while it is still uncertain whether adenosine plays an important role in the vasodilation seen during the initial minutes of ischemia/reperfusion, its contribution appears to be insignificant during the sustained dilation which prevails 30 to 60 min following reperfusion.

IV. SUMMARY

Evidence from cranial window studies supports the suggestions that adenosine closely meets the criteria for a metabolic mediator of CBF regulation. As outlined in Figure 9, when oxygen supply and demand are unbalanced as a result of decreased oxygen supply, reduced arterial oxygen tension, or

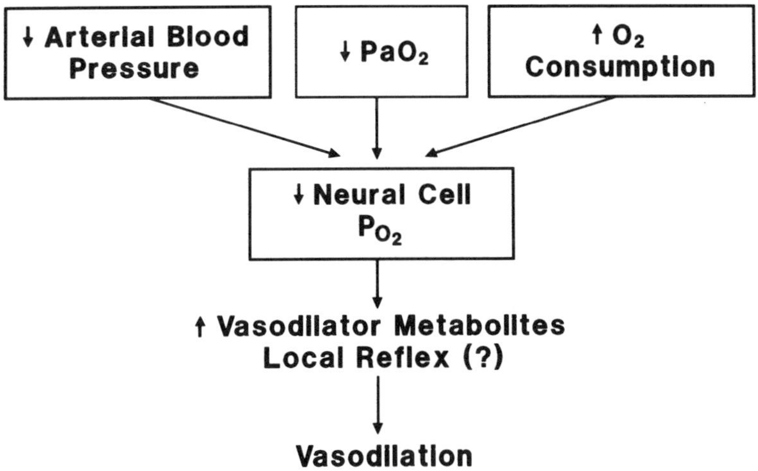

FIGURE 9. Diagrammatic representation of proposed action of adenosine as a metabolic mediator on CBF regulation.

increased metabolic activity, brain adenosine production is elevated in response to hypoxia of the neural cells. Subsequently blood vessels supplying that region are dilated, thus increasing the oxygen supply.

ACKNOWLEDGMENT

Supported by Grant HL 21851 from the National Institutes of Health.

REFERENCES

1. **Winn, H. R., Rubio, R., and Berne, R. M.,** Brain adenosine concentration during hypoxia in rats, *Am. J. Physiol.*, 241, H235, 1981.
2. **Winn, H. R., Welsh, J. E., Rubio, R., and Berne, R. M.,** Brain adenosine production in rat during sustained alteration in systemic blood pressure, *Am. J. Physiol.*, 239, H636, 1980.
3. **Winn, J. R., Rubio, R., and Berne, R. M.,** Brain adenosine production in the rat during 60 seconds of ischemia, *Circ. Res.*, 45, 486, 1979.
4. **Rubio, R., Berne, R. M., Bockman, E. L., and Curnish, R. R.,** Relationship between adenosine concentration and oxygen supply in rat brain, *Am. J. Physiol.*, 228, 1896, 1975.
5. **Park, R. S., Van Wylen, D. G. L., Rubio, R., and Berne, R. M.,** Interstitial fluid adenosine and cerebral blood flow during bicuculline-seizures in newborn piglet, *J. Cereb. Blood Flow Metab.*, 7, 633, 1987.
6. **Winn, J. R., Welsh, J. E., Rubio, R., and Berne, R. M.,** Changes in brain adenosine during bicuculline-induced seizures in rats, *Circ. Res.*, 47, 568, 1980.

7. **Van Wylen, D. G. L., Sciotti, V. M., and Winn, H. R.,** Adenosine and the regulation of cerebral blood flow, in *Adenosine and Adenine Nucleotides as Regulators of Cellular Function,* Phillis, J. W., Ed., CRC Press, Boca Raton, FL 1991, Chapt. 15.
8. **Phillis, J. W.,** Adenosine in the control of the cerebral circulation, *Cerebrovasc. Brain Metab. Rev.,* 1, 26, 1989.
9. **Winn, J. R., Rubio, R., and Berne, R. M.,** The role of adenosine in the regulation of cerebral blood flow, *J. Cereb. Blood Flow Metab.,* 1, 239, 1981.
10. **Berne, R. M., Rubio, R., and Curnish, R. R.,** Release of adenosine from ischemic brain. Effect on cerebral vascular resistance and incorporation into cerebral adenine nucleotides, *Circ. Res.,* 35, 262, 1974.
11. **Wahl, M. and Kuschinsky, W.,** The dilatory action of adenosine on pial arteries of cat and its inhibition by theophylline, *Pfluegers Arch.,* 362, 55, 1976.
12. **Dora, E., Koller, A., and Kovach, A. G. B.,** Effect of topical adenosine deaminase treatment on the functional hyperemic and hypoxic responses of cerebrocortical microcirculation, *J. Cereb. Blood Flow Metab.,* 4, 447, 1984.
13. **Morii, S., Ngai, A. C., Ko, K. R., and Winn, H. R.,** Role of adenosine in regulation of cerebral blood flow: effects of theophylline during normoxia and hypoxia, *Am. J. Physiol.,* 253, 165, 1987.
14. **Wei, E. P. and Kontos, H. A.,** Role of adenosine in cerebral arteriolar dilation from arterial hypoxia, *J. Cereb. Blood Flow Metab.,* 1(Suppl. 1), S395, 1981.
15. **Winn, H. R., Rubio, R., Curnish, R. R., and Berne, R. M.,** Changes in regional cerebral blood flow (rCBF) caused by increases in CSF concentrations of adenosine and 2-chloroadenosine (CHL-ADO), *J. Cereb. Blood Flow Metab.,* 1(Suppl. 1), S401, 1981.
16. **Dora, E.,** Effect of theophylline treatment on the functional hyperemic and hypoxic responses of cerebrocortical microcirculation, *Acta Physiol. Hung.,* 68, 183, 1986.
17. **Haller, C. and Kuschinsky, W.,** Moderate hypoxia: reactivity of pial arteries and local effects of theophylline, *J. Appl. Physiol.,* 63, 2208, 1987.
18. **Kontos, H. A., Wei, E. P., Raper, A. J., Rosenblum, W. I., Navari, R. M., and Patterson, J. L., Jr.,** Role of tissue hypoxia in local regulation of cerebral microcirculation, *Am. J. Physiol.,* 234, H582, 1978.
19. **Wei, E. P. and Kontos, H. A.,** Effect of local change in oxygen saturation of hemoglobin on cerebral vasodilation from hypoxia and hypotension, *FASEB J.,* 6, A1262, 1992.
20. **Haberl, R. L., Heizer, M. L., and Ellis, E. F.,** Laser-Doppler assessment of brain microcirculation: effect of local alterations, *Am. J. Physiol.,* 256, H1255, 1989.
21. **Chapman, A. G., Meldrum, B. S., and Siesjo, B. K.,** Cerebral metabolic changes during prolonged epileptic seizures in rats, *J. Neurochem.,* 28, 1025, 1977.
22. **Meldrum, B. S. and Nilsson, B.,** Cerebral blood flow and metabolic rate early and late in prolonged epileptic seizures induced in rats by bicuculline, *Brain,* 99, 523, 1976.
23. **Kuschinsky, W. and Wahl, M.,** Perivascular pH and pial arterial diameter during bicuculline induced seizures in cats, *Pfluegers Arch.,* 382, 81, 1979.
24. **Schrader, J., Wahl, M., Kuschinsky, W., and Kreutzberg, G. W.,** Increase of adenosine content in cerebral cortex of the cat during bicuculline-induced seizure, *Pfluegers Arch.,* 387, 245, 1980.
25. **Winn, H. R., Rubio, R., and Berne, R. M.,** Brain adenosine production during the initial 60 seconds of bicuculline seizures in rats, *Acta Neurol. Scand.,* 72(Suppl.), 536, 1979.
26. **Wei, E. P., Kontos, H. A., Rosenblum, W. I., and Patterson, J. L., Jr.,** Reduction of seizure-induced cerebral vasodilation by increased local delivery of oxygen, *Acta Neurol. Scand.,* 64(Suppl.), 228, 1977.
27. **Kontos, H. A., Wei, E. P., Navari, R. M., Levasseur, J. E., Rosenblum, W. I., and Patterson, J. L., Jr.,** Responses of cerebral arteries and arterioles to acute hypotension and hypertension, *Am. J. Physiol.,* 234, H371, 1978.
28. **Johnson, P. C.,** Review of previous studies and current theories of autoregulation, *Circ. Res.,* 14–15(Suppl. 1), 2, 1964.

29. **Wei, E. P. and Kontos, H. A.,** Responses of cerebral arterioles to increased venous pressure, *Am. J. Physiol.,* 243, 442, 1982.
30. **Kontos, H. A. and Wei, E. P.,** Oxygen-dependent mechanisms in cerebral autoregulation, *Ann. Biomed. Eng.,* 13, 329, 1985.
31. **Heistad, D. D. and Kontos, H. A.,** Cerebral circulation, in *The Cardiovascular System,* Vol. 3, *Peripheral Circulation and Organ Blood Flow,* Part 1, Shepherd, J. T. and Abboud, F. M., Eds., American Physiology Society, Washington, D.C., 1983, Chap. 5.
32. **Phillis, J. W. and DeLong, R. E.,** An involvement of adenosine in cerebral blood flow regulation during hypercapnia, *Gen. Pharmacol.,* 18, 133, 1987.
33. **Kontos, H. A., Raper, A. J., and Patterson, J. L., Jr.,** Analysis of vasoactivity of local pH, PCO_2 and bicarbonate on pial vessels, *Stroke,* 8, 358, 1977.
34. **Kontos, H. A., Wei, E. P., Raper, A. J., and Patterson, J. L., Jr.,** Local mechanism of CO_2 action on cat pial arterioles, *Stroke,* 8, 226, 1977.
35. **Emerson, T. E., Jr. and Raymond, R. M.,** Involvement of adenosine in cerebral hypoxic hyperemia in the dog, *Am. J. Physiol.,* 241, H134, 1981.
36. **Hoffman, W. E., Albrecht, R. F., and Miletich, D. J.,** The role of adenosine in CBF increases during hypoxia in young vs aged rats, *Stroke,* 15, 124, 1984.
37. **Mustafa, S. J. and Ghai, G.,** Effect of adenosine on the relaxation of coronary arteries at varying pH values, *Basic Res. Cardiol.,* 76, 380, 1981.
38. **Raberger, G., Schutz, W., and Kraupp, O.,** Coronary reactive hyperemia and coronary dilator action of adenosine during normal respiration and hypercapnia acidosis in the dog, *Clin. Exp. Pharmacol. Physiol.,* 2, 373, 1975.
39. **Wexels, J. C.,** Adenosine modifies canine myocardial blood flow response to hypocapnia and hypercapnia, while aminophylline and verapamil do not, *Scand. J. Clin. Lab. Invest.,* 47, 691, 1987.
40. **Wei, E. P., Kontos, H. A., and Patterson, J. L., Jr.,** Dependence of pial arteriolar response to hypercapnia on vessel size, *Am. J. Physiol.,* 238, H697, 1980.
41. **Morii, S., Ngai, A. C., and Winn, H. R.,** Reactivity of rat pial arterioles and venules to adenosine and carbon dioxide: with detailed description of the closed cranial window technique in rats, *J. Cereb. Blood Flow Metab.,* 6, 34, 1986.
42. **Ibayashi, S., Ngai, A. C., Meno, J. R., and Winn, R.,** The effects of dipyridamole and theophylline on rat pial vessels during hypocarbia, *J. Cereb. Blood Flow Metab.,* 8, 829, 1988.
43. **Sollevi, A., Ericson, K., Eriksson, L., Lindqvist, C., Largerkranser, M., and StoneElander, S.,** Effect of adenosine on human cerebral blood flow as determined by positron emission tomography, *J. Cereb. Blood Flow and Metab.,* 7, 673, 1987.
44. **Sciotti, V., Litchomore, T., and Van Wylen, D. G. L.,** Interstitial fluid (ISF) purine metabolite levels during and after cerebral ischemia (ISC), *FASEB J.,* 4, A1095, 1990.
45. **Meno, J. R., Ngai, A. C., Ibayashi, S., and Winn, H. R.,** Adenosine release and changes in pial arteriolar diameter during transient cerebral ischemia and reperfusion, *J. Cereb. Blood Flow and Metab.,* 11, 986, 1991.
46. **Tasdemiroglu, E., Macfarlane, R., Wei, E. P., Kontos, H. A., and Moskowitz, M. A.,** Pial vessel caliber and cerebral blood flow become dissociated during ischemia/reperfusion in cats, *Am. J. Physiol.,* 263, H533, 1992.

Chapter 19

ROLE OF THE EICOSANOIDS IN CEREBRAL HEMODYNAMICS

Charles W. Leffler, William M. Armstead, and Masaaki Shibata

TABLE OF CONTENTS

I. Vascular Activity 298

II. Synthesis 299

III. Functional Significance 300

IV. Injury 305

References 306

0-8493-5096-0/93/$0.00 + $.50

I. VASCULAR ACTIVITY

Eicosanoids can affect cerebral vascular smooth muscle tone. The eicosanoids most studied, both *in vitro* and *in vivo,* are the prostanoids (earlier work reviewed by White and Hagen[1]). Products of arachidonic acid metabolism via prostaglandin (PG) H synthase include dilators and constrictors. *In vitro,* most efforts have centered around the larger cerebral arteries. Not only do $PGF_{2\alpha}$ and thromboxane (TX) A_2[2,3] constrict large cerebral arteries, but, also PGE_2 has been reported to cause constriction of large cerebral arteries,[3-6] although dilation is seen at lower doses.[6] PGI_2, on the other hand, dilates even large cerebral arteries,[3,7-10] but the dilation appears to be greater in small arteries.[11]

The prostanoid family contains dilators and constrictors of pial arteries and arterioles, important resistance vessels in the cerebral circulation.[12] Topical arachidonic acid universally causes dilation of pial arterioles.[5,13-16] In adults much of this dilation may result from activated oxygen,[16,17] while in newborns the dilation appears to be from prostanoids. Among the dilator prostanoids are PGI_2 and PGE_2.[18,19] In newborn pigs,[20] but not adult cats,[18,19] PGI_2 causes dilation at lower concentrations than PGE_2. Constrictor prostanoids include TXA_2 and $PGF_{2\alpha}$. Data are not available *in vivo* on effects of TXA_2 due to its rapid hydrolysis, but U46619, a TXA_2/PGH_2 receptor agonist, causes constriction of pial arterioles.[19,21,22] Topical PGH_2 produces vasodilation, after initial constriction, due to conversion to dilator prostanoids.[7,22] $PGF_{2\alpha}$ constricts pial arterioles of rats,[23] piglets,[22] or humans (*in vitro*).[24] However, cat pial arterioles *in vivo* do not constrict in response to $PGF_{2\alpha}$[23] while $PGF_{2\alpha}$ constricts the feline basilar artery nicely.[25] The primary prostanoid produced by rodent brain,[26] PGD_2 appears to be a vasodilator that is less potent than PGE_2 or PGI_2.[18]

Products of 5-lipoxygenase can also alter cerebral vascular tone. Leukotrienes constrict cerebral vessels of various sizes from numerous species,[3,27-29] but these effects may be less than on peripheral vessels.[30,31] These compounds, in addition to their ability to constrict the cerebral vasculature, can alter blood-brain barrier properties, but effects of leukotrienes on cerebral arterioles, in terms of production of leaky sites, may also be less than on peripheral arterioles.[30]

Similarly to prostanoids, metabolites of arachidonic acid via 15-lipoxygenase include both constrictors and dilators. 15-HETE constricts pial arterioles when topically applied in newborn pigs[32] while alternative products of 15-lipoxygenase, the lipoxins, cause dilation.[33] Little is known of the functional significance of the 15-lipoxygenase products in control of the cerebral circulation, but the potential to produce both vasodilation and vasoconstriction by alternative products of this pathway and the ability of brain to produce these compounds (see below) make them of particular interest.

Products of cytochrome P_{450} metabolism of arachidonic acid[34-37] can affect cerebral vascular tone. The epoxide derivatives (EETs) dilate pial arterioles while in the hydrolysis products, the diols, have little activity[38] (and unpublished observations). The PGH synthase derivatives of cytochrome P_{450} metabolized arachidonic acid[39] are dilators in the cerebral circulation, and activated oxygen is produced during the metabolism by PGH synthase of cytochrome P_{450} products.

Therefore, eicosanoids include many potentially important compounds for control of cerebral hemodynamics.

II. SYNTHESIS

Eicosanoids are synthesized by brain, further suggesting that they can contribute to control of cerebral circulation. Prostanoids can be found in whole brain and fluids surrounding the brain.[40-43] The prostanoid profile depends upon species and age. In rodents the predominant prostanoid in brain is PGD_2.[26] However, in dog brain, PGD_2 levels are low and 6-keto-$PGF_{1\alpha}$ levels are high.[44] In human brain, $PGF_{2\alpha}$ is the most abundant prostanoid, followed by PGE_2, but prostacyclin is the principal prostanoid in human CSF.[45] In newborn pigs, 6-keto-$PGF_{1\alpha}$ and PGE_2 are dominant components of the prostanoid profile in cortical periarachnoid fluid while $PGF_{2\alpha}$ is much more prominent in adult rabbits.[13,41,46-48] Prostanoids vary among cerebral fluid compartments. In piglets, prostanoids have been measured in plasma, cisterna magna subarachnoid fluid, cortical periarachnoid fluid collected by placing a closed cranial window over the parietal cortex, and in extracts of whole brain.[46,49] Whole brain and cortical periarachnoid CSF have similar profiles and relatively high concentrations. In contrast, CSF from the cisterna magna has levels of prostanoids similar to those in plasma suggesting these prostanoids originated in the CSF as it was formed and do not represent to a large extent production of prostanoids by brain tissue.[46] Cellular sources of prostanoids found in brain and cortical periarachnoid CSF are not known. Endothelia, smooth muscle, glia, and neurons can all produce prostanoids.[50-52] Thromboxane and prostacyclin in cortical CSF are likely to include vascular origin,[40] with much of the 6-keto-$PGF_{1\alpha}$ originating with endothelial cells.[47,52] Vascular smooth muscle, in culture, does not appear to produce TXA_2 suggesting that the TXB_2 originates with alternative cell types.[52] PGE_2 may include neural origin while glia can produce a variety of prostanoids.[51]

Brain also produces leukotrienes.[53-55] Some have reported increases in leukotrienes following cerebral ischemia while others have been unable to detect elevations following ischemia in alternative animal models.[49,56,57] Cellular sources of leukotrienes are not known, although *in vitro* and *in vivo* data suggest neurons and glia as possibilities.[55,58,59]

5-, 12-, and 15-HETE[60] have been reported to occur in brain tissues. Since brain can produce both 15-HETE and lipoxins,[61,62] the lipoxygenase pathways can provide both dilator and constrictor influences to the cerebral circulation (see above) similarly to the PGH synthase pathway.

III. FUNCTIONAL SIGNIFICANCE

Eicosanoids can affect vascular tone, brain produces eicosanoids, and production of these compounds can be affected by physiological and pathological conditions. Nevertheless, the functional significance of these eicosanoids in regulation of cerebral vascular tone remains somewhat controversial, although the reasons for some apparently conflicting findings in similar experiments are becoming increasingly clear. The role of prostanoids in the cerebral circulation is species specific. Further, contributions of prostanoids to control of cerebral circulation may be more prominent in newborns than in adults, but, due to the use of different species for study of cerebral circulation of newborns and adults, the greater role of prostanoids in newborn than in adult cerebral circulation has not been established with certainty.

Demonstration of the functional significance of a relationship between a purported mediator and a response must include either inhibition of the synthesis of the mediator, scavenging of the mediator, or receptor blockade. Many hypothesized physiological roles for prostanoids in control of cerebral circulation involve dilator effects, but effective receptor blockers for dilator prostanoids do not exist and effective removal is not possible. Therefore, much information related to the functional significance of eicosanoids is from experiments using inhibitors of PGH synthase. The most frequently used inhibitor is indomethacin, a compound that does not readily cross the blood-brain barrier but can effectively inhibit cerebral synthesis of prostanoids when adequate systemic doses (e.g., 5 mg/kg) are employed.[13,46]

Two groups of dilators are produced from PGH synthase metabolism of arachidonic acid, prostanoids and activated oxygen species. Thus, effects upon cerebral circulation caused by inhibition of PGH synthase could be caused by inhibition of production of activated oxygen, by inhibition of production of prostanoids, or by both. Experiments addressing the question of relative contributions of activated oxygen and prostanoids to responses depending upon activity of PGH synthase yielded opposite results in adult cats and rabbits compared to newborn pigs. In adult cats and rabbits, PGH synthase does not appear to be involved in hypercapnic vasodilation (see below), but dilation to topical arachidonic acid and bradykinin does involve PGH synthase. In these experiments dilation, as the result of PGH synthase metabolism of arachidonic acid, was found to result from superoxide anion, hydrogen peroxide, and/or hydroxyl radical; dilation, in response to topical arachidonic acid or bradykinin, is blocked by superoxide dismutase, catalase, and free radical scavengers.[17,39] Also, in adult mice, superoxide dismutase, catalase, or deferoxamine inhibited pial arteriolar dilation in response to bradykinin suggesting hydroxyl radical involvement.[63] By contrast, in piglets, where PGH synthase metabolism of arachidonic acid is involved in vasodilation in response to hypercapnia, very aggressive treatment with scavengers of superoxide anion, hydrogen peroxide, and hydroxyl radical did not affect vasodilation in response to hypercapnia.[64] Dilation to hypercapnia was totally abolished by indomethacin treatment (see below). These data suggest that, in contrast to adult rabbits and cats, in newborn pigs prostanoids rather than activated oxygen are the functional dilator products of arachidonic acid metabolism by PGH synthase.

Further complicating the question of the functional significance of prostanoids in control of cerebral circulation is the question of whether prostanoids contribute to the maintenance of resting blood flow. Once again, the answer to this question appears to depend upon species and age. In adult rabbits, cats, and dogs indomethacin does not affect cerebral blood flow in chronically instrumented or acutely prepared anesthetized animals.[14,65,66] Conversely, in baboons, gerbils, and goats, cerebral blood flow is reduced by indomethacin pretreatment.[67-70] Most of the available data on newborns derives from piglets, puppies, and human infants. In all these, there is a decrease in cerebral blood flow following treatment with indomethacin,[71-76] although the human data cannot be treated as necessarily the response of a healthy, full-term infant. In human newborns, compared to newborn pigs,[77] apparent decreases in cerebral blood flow are surprisingly great considering the very low doses (typically 0.2 mg/kg) used, suggesting indomethacin may cross the blood-brain barrier of the premature human infant more readily than of the term piglet or that endothelially derived prostanoids are very important in maintenance of cerebral blood flow in premature babies. In piglets the effect of indomethacin is quite uniform throughout the brain producing a consistent decrease of about 20 to 25% cerebral blood flow when a dose of 5 mg/kg i.v. is used.[71] In fetal lambs *in utero,* aspirin and indomethacin also decrease resting cerebral blood flow.[78,79] Therefore, it appears that prostanoids are involved in maintenance of resting cerebral blood flow in the perinatal period.

The subject of effects of PGH synthase inhibition on hypercapnic cerebral vasodilation has been controversial even though differing results obtained by different investigators appear to be explained in some cases by species variation and the difference in responses related to age. Studies in adult primates, rats, and gerbils found inhibition of hypercapnic vasodilation following indomethacin.[67-69] On the other hand, some investigators using rabbits, dogs, and cats were unable to detect any effect of indomethacin on hypercapnic cerebral vasodilation.[14,15,65,66,80] Conversely, others reported inhibition of hypercapnic cerebral vasodilation following indomethacin in these same three species.[8185] Reasons for these disparities in the same species do remain unclear. In newborn pigs, and apparently newborn humans, hypercapnic cerebral vasodilation is reduced or abolished when PGH synthase is inhibited (Figure 1).[73-75,86,87] This finding coupled with measurements of increased cerebral synthesis of prostanoids induced by hypercapnia (Figure 2)[46,87] and the inability of radical scavengers to alter the response (see above) strongly suggest that prostanoids play a role in hypercapnic cerebral vasodilation in newborn pigs and human infants. Cerebral vasoconstriction in response to hypocapnia is not altered by PGH synthase inhibition;[88] so it appears that cerebral vascular responses to CO_2 involve multiple mechanisms depending upon either:

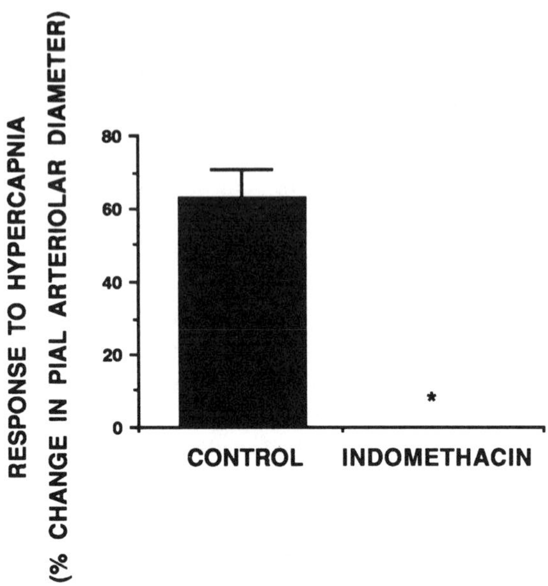

FIGURE 1. Effects of indomethacin (5 mg/kg, i.v.) on dilation of newborn pig pial arterioles to hypercapnia ($PaCO_2$ @ 70 mmHg); n = 7. $*p < 0.05$ compared to control (no indomethacin).

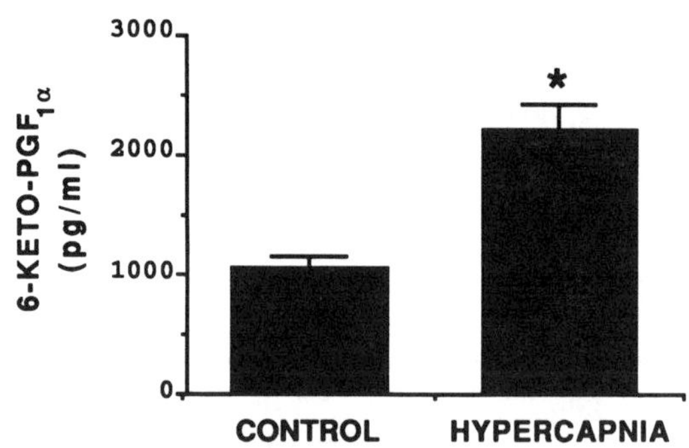

FIGURE 2. Effects of hypercapnia ($PaCO_2$ @ 70 mmHg) on cortical periarachnoid CSF concentration of 6-keto-$PGF_{1\alpha}$ in newborn pigs; n = 23. $*p < 0.05$ compared to control (normocapnia).

(1) whether the change is an increase or a decrease from the physiological baseline or (2) the direction of change per se.

Data on prostanoid contributions to autoregulatory cerebral vasodilation appear largely consistent and suggest that dilator prostanoids can contribute to autoregulatory cerebral vasodilation. In newborn pigs and adult rats, hypotension increases cerebral prostanoid synthesis.[20,89,90] In piglets, autoregulatory vasodilation is reversed by treatment with indomethacin.[20,91] In dogs in hemorrhagic shock, indomethacin decreases cerebral blood flow.[92] In anesthetized baboons, indomethacin decreased resting cerebral blood flow, but the relative vascular response to hemorrhage was not changed.[93] However, the absolute cerebral blood flow was reduced about 30% at all pressures between 60 and 30 mmHg so that cerebral oxygen consumption decreased at higher arterial pressures in indomethacin-treated baboons than in controls. In newborn pigs, vasoconstriction in response to hypertension does not appear to be affected greatly by inhibition of prostanoid synthesis (unpublished data). Thus, similarly to CO_2, the mechanisms involved in cerebral autoregulatory responses, at least in newborn pigs, do not appear to be uniform throughout the pressure range.

Constrictor prostanoids may be involved in control of cerebral circulation. For example, cortical spreading depression in rabbits is accompanied by cerebral vasodilation that follows the depolarization across the cerebral surface.[94] Depolarization and vasodilation are accompanied by increased cerebral prostanoids, particularly $PGF_{2\alpha}$.[48] Indomethacin augments the vasodilation suggesting constrictor prostanoids reduce the vasodilation.[48,94] Endothelium-dependent contraction of dog basilar arteries in response to stretch or nicotine can be inhibited by blockers of PGH synthase and may involve TXA_2,[95,96] although superoxide anion has also been found to constrict canine basilar artery.[97]

Prostanoids interact with numerous nonprostanoid mediators. These interactions can be categorized as participation, attenuation, or permission. Data include measurements of cortical periarachnoid fluid prostanoids as indices of cerebral prostanoid synthesis and effects of inhibition of PGH synthase. In piglets, with the exception of phorbol 12,13-dibutyrate,[9] if the treatment causes an increase in cortical periarachnoid prostanoids, indomethacin can alter the pial arteriolar response to that treatment, and if the treatment does not effect cortical periarachnoid prostanoids, indomethacin does not alter the response to the treatment (Table 1). Such a combination strongly suggests that effects of indomethacin involve prostanoids. In the participation category, for example, in newborn pigs, topical histamine causes an increase in cerebral prostanoid synthesis, and vasodilation to histamine is blocked by pretreatment with indomethacin[99] suggesting that prostanoid synthesis is necessary for histamine-induced cerebral vasodilation. In adult mice and cats, vasodilation in response to bradykinin is similarly reduced by inhibition of PGH synthase.[17,63] However, in mice and cats the PGH synthase products causing vasodilation are activated oxygen species rather than prostanoids. Dilator prostanoids can attenuate constrictor responses. For example, sympathetic nerve stimulation or topical norepinephrine constricts pial arterioles.[117] In newborn pigs, such stimulation is accompanied by increased cerebral prostanoid synthesis.[111] Inhibition of this synthesis can augment constriction in response to the catecholamine.[111] A permissive association between prostanoids and another agonist is seen in the response of piglet pial arterioles to acetylcholine. Acetylcholine produces dose-dependent vasoconstriction[114] that

TABLE 1
Effects of Treatments on Cortical Periarachnoid CSF Prostanoids and the Effects of Indomethacin (Indo) (5 mg/kg) on Pial Arteriolar Responses to Those Treatments in Newborn Pigs

Dilators	Increase prostanoids?	Effect of indo. of dilation	Reference
Hypercapnia	Yes	Blocks	13, 46, 86, Fig. 1
Hypotension	Yes	Blocks	20
Histamine	Yes	Blocks	99
KC-404	Yes	Blocks	100
Arachidonate	Yes	Blocks	13
Interleukin 1α	Yes	Blocks	101
Seizures (bicuculline)	Yes	Attenuates	102
Pressure ventilation	Yes	Blocks	103–105
Methionine enkephalin	Yes	Blocks	106
Leucine enkephalin	Yes	Blocks	106
Dynorphin (normotension)	Yes	Blocks	106
Bradykinin	Yes	Attenuates	107 and unpublished data
Isoproterenol	No	No effect	108
Lipoxins (A_4 and B_4)	No	No effect	33
NMDA	No	No effect	109
Constrictors		**Effect of indo. on constriction**	
15-HETE	Yes	Potentiates	32
β-Endorphin	Yes	Potentiates	106
Dynorphin (hypotension)	Yes	Potentiates	106
Vasopressin (hypotension)	Yes	Potentiates	110
Norepinephrine	Yes	Potentiates	111
Platelet activating factor	No	No effect	112
Dopamine	No	No effect	113
Phorbol 12,13 dibutyrate	Yes	No effect[a]	98
Acetylcholine	Yes	Blocks (see text)	22, 114–116

[a] The effect of indomethacin on pial arteriolar constriction to PDB was only examined at one high dose of PDB. Whether indomethacin can potentiate constriction in response to lower doses is unknown.

is blocked by indomethacin[115] suggesting prostanoids are involved and acetylcholine does not produce endothelial-dependent dilation. Accompanying acetylcholine-induced constriction is a large increase in cerebral prostanoid synthesis, but the predominant prostanoids produced are dilators.[116] The constrictor response to acetylcholine appears to involve an interaction between muscarinic-1 and TXA_2/PGH_2 receptors.[22] Thus, following indomethacin, acetylcholine applied to piglet pial arterioles produces no response. However, if subthreshold concentrations of agonists for the TXA_2/PGH_2 receptor (U46619, PGH_2, or $PGF_{2\alpha}$) are maintained under the cranial window of a piglet pretreated with indomethacin, acetylcholine produces dose-dependent vasoconstriction that is greater than that produced in response to acetylcholine without indomethacin. Thus, it seems that activation of the TXA_2/PGH_2 receptor permits muscarinic vasoconstriction to occur, and vasodilator prostanoids produced simultaneously attenuate this vasoconstriction.

IV. INJURY

Cerebral injury can increase eicosanoid synthesis and modify the cerebral eicosanoid profile. The significance of these eicosanoids to the cerebral circulation following cerebral injury is not thoroughly understood.

During cerebral ischemia, free arachidonic acid accumulates in brain,[118-120] is converted to eicosanoids, and activated oxygen upon reperfusion.[121-124] Activated oxygen can produce endothelial injury and selective loss of responses.[17,125,126] The major source of activated oxygen during cerebral reperfusion appears to be PGH synthase rather than xanthine oxidase.[124] Cerebral ischemia causes loss of endothelial-dependent responses in cats[127] and of prostanoid-associated responses in piglets.[128,129] The loss of prostanoid-associated responses in piglets appears to relate to a failure to release arachidonic acid in response to appropriate stimuli. Such failure could be caused by depletion of specific arachidonic acid pools during ischemia.[130] Following cerebral ischemia, in some animal models, leukotrienes are produced by brain.[57,131-133] These leukotrienes could cause vasoconstriction[29] and alter blood-brain barrier properties.[134] Following cerebral ischemia in another animal model, no increase in leukotriene synthesis was detected[49] suggesting the cerebral eicosanoid system's response to cerebral ischemia may be species and age dependent.

Following intracranial hemorrhage, activated oxygen and eicosanoids are produced.[56,135,136] Superoxide and thromboxane are generated by platelets[136-138] and high levels of leukotrienes tend to be produced.[56] Hemolysate can inhibit PGI_2 synthesis by cerebral vessels *in vitro*.[139] Following prolonged exposure to extravascular intracranial blood, responses that require dilator prostanoids can be lost.[140] Constrictor prostanoids and leukotrienes have been implicated in cerebral vasospasm, a severe complication of intracranial hemorrhage.[56,137,138,141]

Following percussive brain injury, generation of activated oxygen results from metabolism of arachidonic acid by PGH synthase.[142,143] Other possible sources of activated oxygen species involve oxidation of catecholamines[144,145] from enhanced sympathetic outflow following percussive brain injury.[146,147] Increased eicosanoids and free radicals could alter cerebral vascular tone and responsiveness following traumatic brain injury.[143,148] Morphological lesions of vascular endothelium observed following percussive brain injury are reduced by free radical scavengers,[148] but contributions of eicosanoids to alterations in cerebral hemodynamics subsequent to traumatic brain injury are not clearly understood.

REFERENCES

1. **White, R. P. and Hagen, A. A.,** Cerebrovascular actions of prostaglandins, *Pharmacol. Ther.,* 18, 313, 1982.
2. **Ellis, E. F., Nies, A. S., and Oates, J. A.,** Cerebral arterial smooth muscle constriction by thromboxane A_2, *Stroke,* 8, 480, 1977.
3. **Holst, H., Granstrom, E., Hamarsträm, S., Samuelsson, B., and Steiner, L.,** Effects of leukotrienes C_4, D_4, prostacyclin, and thromboxane A_2 on isolated human cerebral arteries, *Acta Neurochir.,* 62, 177, 1982.
4. **White, R. P.,** Multiplex origins of cerebral vasopressin, in *Cerebrovascular Diseases,* Eleventh Princeton Conference, Price, T. R. and Nelson, E. D., Eds., Raven Press, New York, 1979, 307.
5. **Hayashi, S., Park, M. K., and Kuehl, T. J.,** Effects of prostaglandins and arachidonic acid on baboon cerebral and mesenteric arteries, *Prostaglandins,* 32, 587, 1986.
6. **Whalley, E. T., Schilling, L., and Wahl, M.,** Cerebrovascular effects of prostanoids: *in vitro* studies in feline middle cerebral and basilar artery, *Prostaglandins,* 38, 625, 1989.
7. **Chapleau, C. E. and White, R. P.,** Effects of prostacyclin on the canine isolated basilar artery, *Prostaglandins,* 17, 573, 1979.
8. **Chapleau, C. E., White, R. P., and Robertson, J. T.,** Cerebral vasodilation and prostacyclin. The effects of aspirin and meclofenamate *in vitro, J. Neurosurg.,* 53, 188, 1980.
9. **Toda, N.,** Responses to prostaglandins H_2 and I_2 of isolated dog cerebral and peripheral arteries, *Am. J. Physiol.,* 238, H111, 1980.
10. **Shirahase, H., Usi, H., Manabe, K., Kurachashi, K., and Fujiwara, M.,** Vasorelaxing effects of prostaglandin I_2 on the canine basilar and coronary arteries, *J. Pharmacol. Exp. Ther.,* 248, 769, 1989.
11. **Toda, N. and Miyazaki, M.,** Heterogenous responses to vasodilators of dog proximal and distal middle cerebral arteries, *J. Cardiovasc. Pharmacol.,* 6, 1230, 1984.
12. **Busija, D. W. and Heistad, D. D.,** Factors involved in physiological regulation of cerebral blood flow, *Rev. Physiol. Pharmacol. Biochem.,* 101, 161, 1984.
13. **Leffler, C. W. and Busija, D. W.,** Arachidonate metabolism on the cerebral surface of newborn pigs, *Prostaglandins,* 30, 811, 1985.
14. **Busija, D. W.,** Role of prostanoids in the response of the cerebral circulation to carbon dioxide in awake rabbits, *J. Cereb. Blood Flow Metab.,* 3, 376, 1983.
15. **Wei, E. P., Ellis, E. F., and Kontos, H. A.,** Role of prostaglandins in pial arteriolar responses to CO_2 and hypoxia, *Am. J. Physiol.,* 238, H226, 1980.
16. **Kontos, H. A. and Wei, E. P.,** Cerebral arteriolar damage by arachidonic acid and prostaglandin G_2, *Science,* 209, 1242, 1980.
17. **Kontos, H. A., Wei, E. P., Povlishock, J. T., and Christman, C. W.,** Oxygen radicals mediate the cerebral arteriolar dilation from arachidonate and bradykinin in cats, *Circ. Res.,* 55, 295, 1984.
18. **Ellis, E. F., Wei, E. P., and Kontos, H. A.,** Vasodilation of cat cerebral arterioles by prostaglandins D_2, E_2, G_2, and I_2, *Am. J. Physiol.,* 237, H381, 1979.
19. **Wahl, M., Schilling, L., and Whalley, E. T.,** Cerebrovascular effects of prostanoids. *In situ* studies in pial arteries of the cat, *Arch. Pharmacol.,* 340, 314, 1989.
20. **Leffler, C. W. and Busija, D. W.,** Prostanoids and pial arteriolar diameter in hypotensive newborn pigs, *Am. J. Physiol.,* 252, H687, 1987.
21. **Haberl, R. L., Heizer, M. L., and Ellis, E. F.,** Effects of the thromboxane A_2 mimetic U46619 on pial arterioles of rabbits and rats, *Stroke,* 18, 796, 1987.
22. **Armstead, W. M., Mirro, R., Busija, D. W., and Leffler, C. W.,** Permissive role of prostanoids in acetylcholine-induced cerebral vasoconstriction, *J. Pharmacol. Exp. Ther.,* 251, 1012, 1989.

23. **Ellis, E. F., Wei, E. P., Cockerall, C. S., Choi, S., and Kontos, H. A.,** The effects of $PGF_{2\alpha}$ on *in vivo* cerebral arteriolar diameters in cats and rats, *Prostaglandins,* 26, 917, 1983.
24. **Uski, T. K., Andersson, K.-E., Brandt, L., and Ljunggren, B.,** Characterization of the prostanoid receptors and of the contractile effects of prostaglandin $F_{2\alpha}$ in human pial arteries, *Acta Physiol. Scand.,* 121, 369, 1984.
25. **Uski, T. K. and Andersson, K.-E.,** Effects of prostanoids on isolated feline cerebral arteries. II. Roles of extra- and intracellular calcium for the prostaglandin $F_{2\alpha}$-induced constriction, *Acta Physiol. Scand.,* 120, 197, 1984.
26. **Abdel-Halim, M. S., Hamberg, M., Sjoquist, B., and Anggard, E.,** Identification of prostaglandin D_2 as a major prostaglandin in homogenates of rat brain, *Prostaglandins,* 14, 633, 1977.
27. **Rosenblum, W. I.,** Constricting effect of leukotrienes on cerebral arterioles of mice, *Stroke,* 16, 262, 1985.
28. **Jancar, S., Schulz, R., Krueger, C., and Cook, D. A.,** Mechanisms of arachidonic acid-induced constrictions of canine cerebral arteries, *Eur. J. Pharmacol.,* 136, 345, 1987.
29. **Busija, D. W., Leffler, C. W., and Beasley, D. G.,** Effects of leukotrienes C_4, D_4, and E_4 on cerebral arteries of newborn pigs, *Pediatr. Res.,* 20, 973, 1986.
30. **Mayhan, W. G., Sahagun, G., Spector, R., and Heistad, D. D.,** Effects of leukotriene C_4 on the cerebral microvasculature, *Am. J. Physiol.,* 251, H471, 1986.
31. **Tostiharu, K., Little, M. H., and Ellis, E. F.,** Effect of leukotrienes, 12-HETE, histamine, bradykinin, and 5-hydroxytryptamine on *in vivo* rabbit cerebral arteriolar diameter, *J. Cereb. Blood Flow Metab.,* 5, 554, 1985.
32. **Lovelady, G. K., Mirro, R., Armstead, W. M., Busija, D. W., and Leffler, C. W.,** Effect of 15-HETE on cerebral arterioles of newborn pigs, *Prostaglandins,* 36, 507, 1988.
33. **Busija, D. W., Armstead, W., Leffler, C. W., and Mirro, R.,** Lipoxins A_4 and B_4 dilate cerebral arterioles of newborn pigs, *Am. J. Physiol.,* 256, H468, 1989.
34. **Chalos, N., Falck, J. R., Wixtrom, C., and Capdevila, J.,** Novel epoxides formed during the liver cytochrome P-450 oxidation of arachidonic acid, *Biochem. Biophys. Res. Comm.,* 104, 916, 1982.
35. **Capdevila, J., Marnett, L. J., Chacon, N., Prough, R. A., and Estabrook, R. W.,** Cytochrome P-450-dependent oxygenation of arachidonic acid to hydroxyeicosatetraenoic acids, *Proc. Natl. Acad. Sci. U.S.A.,* 79, 767, 1982.
36. **Capdevila, J., Chacos, N., Werringloer, J., Prouch, R. A., and Estabrook, R. W.,** Liver microsonal cytochrome P-450 and the oxidative metabolism of arachidonic acid, *Proc. Natl. Acad. Sci. U.S.A.,* 78, 5362, 1981.
37. **Carroll, M. A., Garcia, M. P., Falck, J. R., and McGiff, J. C.,** 5,6-epoxyeicosatrienoic acid, a novel arachidonate metabolite. Mechanisms of vasoactivity in the rat, *Circ. Res.,* 67, 1082, 1990.
38. **Amruthesh, S. C., Falck, J. R., and Ellis, E. F.,** Brain synthesis and cerebrovascular action of epoxygenase metabolites of arachidonic acid, *J. Neurochem.,* 58, 503, 1992.
39. **Ellis, E. F., Police, R. F., Yancey, L., McKinney, J. S., and Amruthesh, S. C.,** Dilation of cerebral arterioles by cytochrome P-450 metabolites of arachidonic acid, *Am. J. Physiol.,* 259, H1171, 1990.
40. **Hagen, A. A., White, R. P., and Robertson, J. T.,** Synthesis of prostaglandins and thromboxane B_2 by cerebral arteries, *Stroke,* 10, 306, 1979.
41. **Abdel-Halim, M. S., Lunden, I., Cseh, G., and Anggard, E.,** Prostaglandin profiles in nervous tissue and blood vessels of the brain of various animals, *Prostaglandins,* 19, 249, 1980.
42. **Wolfe, L. S.,** Eicosanoids: prostaglandins, thromboxanes, leukotrienes, and other derivatives of carbon-20 unsaturated fatty acids, *J. Neurochem.,* 38, 1, 1982.

43. **Romero, S. D., Chyatte, D., Byer, D. E., Romero, J. C., and Yaksh, T. Y.,** Measurement of prostaglandins in the cerebrospinal fluid in cat, dog, and man, *J. Neurochem.*, 43, 1642, 1984.
44. **Walker, V., Pickard, J. D., Smythe, P., Eastwood, S., and Perry, A.,** Effects of subarachnoid hemorrhage on intracranial prostaglandins, *J. Neurol. Neurosurg. Psychiatry,* 46, 119, 1983.
45. **Abdel-Halim, M. S., Van Holst, H., Meyerson, B., Sachs, C., and Anggard, E.,** Prostaglandin profiles in tissues and blood vessels from human brain, *J. Neurochem.*, 34, 1331, 1980.
46. **Leffler, C. W. and Busija, D. W.,** Prostanoids in cortical subarachnoid cerebrospinal fluid and pial arterial diameter in newborn pigs, *Circ. Res.*, 57, 689, 1985.
47. **Katz, B., Sofonio, M., Lyden, P. O., and Mitchell, M. D.,** Prostaglandin concentrations in cerebrospinal fluid of rabbits under normal and ischemic conditions, *Stroke,* 19, 349, 1988.
48. **Shibata, M., Leffler, C. W., and Busija, D. W.,** Prostanoids attenuate pial arteriole dilation induced by cortical spreading depression in rabbits, *Am. J. Physiol.*, 261, R828, 1991.
49. **Hsu, P., Zuckerman, S., Mirro, R., Armstead, W. M., and Leffler, C. W.,** Effects of ischemia/reperfusion on brain tissue prostanoids and leukotrienes in newborn pigs, *Prostaglandins,* 42, 557, 1991.
50. **Goehlert, U. G., Ng-Ying-Kin, N. M. K., and Wolfe, L. S.,** Biosynthesis of prostacyclin in cat cerebral microvenule and the choroid plexus, *J. Neurochem.*, 36, 1192, 1981.
51. **Seregi, A., Keller, M., Jackish, R., and Hartting, G.,** Comparison of the prostanoid synthesizing capacity in homogenates from primary neuronal and astroglial cell cultures, *Biochem. Pharmacol.*, 33, 3315, 1984.
52. **Moore, S. A., Spector, A. A., and Hart, M. N.,** Eicosanoid metabolism in cerebromicrovascular endothelium, *Am. J. Physiol.*, 254, C37, 1988.
53. **Dembinska-Kiec, Simmet, T., and Peskar B.,** Formation of leukotriene C_4-like material by rat brain tissue, *Eur. J. Pharmacol.*, 99, 57, 1984.
54. **Simmet, T., Luck, W., Delank, W. K., and Peskar, B. A.,** Formation of cysteinyl leukotrienes by human brain tissues, *Brain Res.*, 456, 344, 1988.
55. **Hynes, N., Bishai, I., Lees, J., and Coceani, F.,** Leukotrienes in brain: natural occurrence and induced changes, *Brain Res.*, 553, 4, 1991.
56. **Kiwak, K. J., Moskowitz, M. A., and Levine, L.,** Leukotriene production in gerbil brain after ischemic insults, subarachnoid hemorrhage, and concussive injury, *J. Neurosurg.*, 62, 865, 1985.
57. **Moskowitz, M. A., Kiwak, K. J., Hekimian, K., and Levine, L.,** Synthesis of compounds with properties of leukotrienes C_4 and D_4 in gerbil brains after ischemia and reperfusion, *Science,* 224, 886, 1984.
58. **Hartang, H. P., Heininger, K., and Toyko, K. V.,** Primary rat astroglial cultures can generate leukotriene B_4, *J. Neuroimmunol.*, 19, 237, 1988.
59. **Simmett, T., Seregi, A., and Hertting, G.,** Characterization of seizure-induced cysteinyl-leukotriene formation in brain tissue of convulsion-prone gerbils, *J. Neurochem.*, 50, 1738, 1988.
60. **Moore, S. A., Figard, P. H., Spector, A. A., and Hart, M. N.,** Brain microvessels produce 12-Hydroxyeicosatetraenoic acid, *J. Neurochem.*, 53, 376, 1989.
61. **Adesuyi, S. A., Cockrell, C. S., Gamache, D. A., and Ellis, E. F.,** Lipoxygenase metabolism of arachidonic acid in brain, *J. Neurochem.*, 45, 770, 1985.
62. **Samuelsson, B., Dahlen, B. S. E., Lindgren, J. A., Roazer, C. A., and Serhan, C. N.,** Leukotrienes and lipoxins: structures, biosynthesis, and biological effects, *Science,* (Washington, D.C.) 237, 1171, 1987.

63. **Rosenblum, W. I.,** Hydroxyl radical mediates the endothelium-dependent dilation produced by bradykinin in mouse cerebral arterioles, *Circ. Res.,* 61, 601, 1987.
64. **Leffler, C. W., Mirro, R., Thompson, C., Shibata, M., Armstead, W. M., Pourcyrous, M., and Thelin, O.,** Activated oxygen species do not mediate hypercapnia-induced cerebral vasodilation in newborn pigs, *Am. J. Physiol.,* 261, H335, 1991.
65. **Busija, D. W. and Heistad, D. D.,** Effects of indomethacin on cerebral blood flow during hypercapnia in cats, *Am. J. Physiol.,* 244, H519, 1983.
66. **Jackson, E. K., Gerkins, J. F., Zimmerman, J. B., Lederman, H. D., Oates, J. A., Workman, R. J., and Branch, R. A.,** Prostaglandin biosynthesis does not participate in hypercapnia-induced cerebral vasodilation in the dog, *J. Pharmacol. Exp. Ther.,* 226, 486, 1983.
67. **Crockard, H. A., Iannotti, F., and Lads, G.,** Cerebrovascular effects of prostaglandin inhibitors in the gerbil, *J. Cereb. Blood Flow Metab.,* 2, 67, 1982.
68. **Pickard, J. D. and Mackenzie, E. T.,** Inhibition of prostaglandin synthesis and the response of the baboon cerebral circulation to carbon dioxide, *Nature New Biol.,* 245, 187, 1973.
69. **Sakabe, T. and Siesjö, B. K.,** The effect of indomethacin on the blood flow metabolism couple in the brain under normal, hypercapnic and hypoxic conditions, *Acta Physiol. Scand.,* 107, 283, 1979.
70. **Hoffman, W. E., Albrecht, R. F., Pelligrino, D., and Miletich, D. J.,** Effects of prostaglandins on the cerebral circulation in the goat, *Prostaglandins,* 23, 897, 1982.
71. **Leffler, C. W., Busija, D. W., Fletcher, A. M., Beasley, D. G., Hessler, J. R., and Green, R. S.,** Effects of indomethacin upon cerebral hemodynamics of newborn pigs, *Pediatr. Res.,* 19, 1160, 1985.
72. **Lundell, B. P., Sonesson, S. E., and Cotton, R. B.,** Ductus closure in preterm infants. Effects on hemodynamics, *Acta Pediatr. Scand. Suppl.,* 329, 140, 1986.
73. **Cowan, F.,** Indomethacin, patent ductus arteriosus, and cerebral blood flow, *J. Pediatr.,* 109, 314, 1986.
74. **Laudignon, N., Chemtob, S., Bard, H., and Aranda, J. V.,** Effect of indomethacin on cerebral blood flow velocity of premature newborns, *Biol. Neonate,* 54, 254, 1988.
75. **Edwards, A. D., Wyatt, J. S., Richardson, C. E., Potter, A., Cope, M., Delpy, D. T., and Reynolds, E. O. R.,** Effects of indomethacin on cerebral hemodynamics in very preterm infants, *Lancet,* 335, 1491, 1990.
76. **Ment, L. R., Stewart, W. B., Duncan, C. D., Scott, D. T., and Lambrecht, R.,** Beagle puppy model of intraventricular hemorrhage. Effect of indomethacin on cerebral blood flow, *J. Neurosurgery,* 58, 857, 1983.
77. **Leffler, C. W., Busija, D. W., and Beasley, D. G.,** Effect of therapeutic dose of indomethacin on the cerebral circulation of newborn pigs, *Pediatr. Res.,* 21, 188, 1987.
78. **Heymann, M. A. and Rudolph, A. M.,** The effect of acetylsalicylic acid on the ductus arteriosis and circulation in fetal lambs *in utero, Circ. Res.,* 38, 418, 1976.
79. **Hohimer, A. R., Richardson, B. S., Bissonnette, J. M., and Machida, C. M.,** The effect of indomethacin on breathing movements and cerebral blood flow and metabolism in the fetal sheep, *J. Dev. Physiol.,* 7, 217, 1985.
80. **Cuypers, J., Cuevas, A., and Duisberg, R.,** Effect of indomethacin on CO_2-induced hyperemia (CO_2-response) in the rabbit brain, *Neurochirurgia,* 21, 62, 1978.
81. **Ruszczewsi, P. and Herbacynska-Cedro, K.,** Release of prostaglandin-like substance into cerebral venous blood in conditions injurious to brain in the dog, *Acta Physiol. Pol.,* 29, 498, 1978.
82. **Vlahov, V.,** The role of prostaglandins in the regulation of cerebral vessel wall reactivity, in *The Cerebral Vessel Wall,* CervosNavarro, J., Betz, E., Matakas, F., and Wullenweber, R., Raven Press, New York, 1976, 143.

83. **Shigeno, S., Fritschka, E., Shigeno, T., and Brock, M.,** Effect of indomethacin on CBF during and after focal erebral ischemia in the cat, *J. Cereb. Blood Flow Metab.*, 3(Suppl. 1), S309, 1983.
84. **Bill, A.,** Effects of indomethacin on regional blood flow in conscious rabbits: a microsphere study, *Acta Physiol. Scand.*, 105, 437, 1979.
85. **Pinard, E., Rougier, P., and Seylaz, J.,** Effects of inhibition of prostaglandin synthesis on cerebral blood flow and its regulation, *J. Cereb. Blood Flow Metab.*, 3(Suppl 1), S305, 1983.
86. **Wagerle, L. C. and Mishra, O. P.,** Mechanisms of CO_2 responses in cerebral arteries of the newborn pig: role of phospholipase, cyclooxygenase, and lipoxygenase pathways, *Circ. Res.*, 62, 1019, 1988.
87. **Wagerle, L. C., DeGuilio, P. A., Mishra, O. P., and DelivoriaPapadopoulos., M.,** Effect of dexamethasone on cerebral prostanoid formation and pial arteriolar reactivity to CO_2 in newborn pigs, *Am. J. Physiol.*, 260, H1313, 1991.
88. **Mirro, R., Pharris, L. J., Armstead, W. M., Shibata, M., and Leffler, C. W.,** Cerebral vasoconstriction during hyperventilation is not prostanoid dependent, *Pediatr. Res.*, 31, 213A, 1992.
89. **Chemtob, S., Beharry, K., Rex, J., Varma, D. R., and Aranda, J. V.,** Prostanoids determine the range of cerebral blood flow autoregulation on newborn piglets, *Stroke*, 21, 777, 1990.
90. **Shohami, E. and Sidi, A.,** Accumulation of prostacyclin in rat brain during hemorrhagic hypotension-possible role of PGI_2 in autoregulation, *J. Cereb. Blood Flow Metab.*, 4, 107, 1984.
91. **Leffler, C. W., Busija, D. W., Beasley, D. G., and Fletcher, A. M.,** Maintenance of cerebral circulation during hemorrhagic hypotension in newborn pigs: role of prostanoids, *Circ. Res.*, 59, 562, 1986.
92. **Leffler, C. W. and Passmore, J. C.,** Effects of indomethacin on hemodynamics of dogs in refractory hemorrhagic shock, *J. Surg. Res.*, 23, 392, 1977.
93. **Pickard, J. D., MacDonell, L. A., Mackenzie, E. T., and Harper, A. M.,** Response of the cerebral circulation in baboons to changing perfusion pressure after indomethacin, *Circ. Res.*, 40, 198, 1977.
94. **Shibata, M., Leffler, C. W., and Busija, D. W.,** Cerebral hemodynamics during cortical spreading depression in rabbits, *Brain Res.*, 530, 267, 1990.
95. **Katusic, Z. S., Shepherd, J. T., and Vanhoutte, P. M.,** Endothelium-dependent contraction to stretch in canine basilar arteries, *Am. J. Physiol.*, 252, H671, 1987.
96. **Shirahase, H., Usui, H., Kurahashi, K., Fujiwara, M., and Fukini, K.,** Endothelium-dependent contraction induced by nicotine in isolated canine basilar artery: possible involvement of a thromboxane $A_2(TXA_2)$ like substance, *Life Sci.*, 42, 437, 1988.
97. **Katusic, Z. S. and Vanhoutte, P. M.,** Superoxide anion is an endothelium-dependent contracting factor, *Am. J. Physiol.*, 257, H33, 1989.
98. **Busija, D. W. and Leffler, C. W.,** Effects of phorbol esters on pial arteriolar diameter and brain production of prostanoids in piglets, *Circ. Res.*, 69, 1253, 1991.
99. **Mirro, R., Busija, D. W., Armstead, W. M., and Leffler, C. W.,** Histamine dilates pial arterioles of newborn pigs through prostanoid production, *Am. J. Physiol.*, 254, H1023, 1988.
100. **Armstead, W. M., Mirro, R., Leffler, C. W., and Busija, D. W.,** The role of prostanoids in the mediation of responses to KC-404, a novel cerebrovasodilator, *J. Pharmacol. Exp. Ther.*, 244, 138, 1988.
101. **Shibata, M., Leffler, C. W., and Busija, D. W.,** Recombinant human interleukin-1α dilates pial arterioles and increases cerebrospinal fluid prostanoids in piglets, *Am. J. Physiol.*, 259, H1486, 1990.
102. **Busija, D. W. and Leffler, C. W.,** Role of prostanoids in cerebrovascular responses during seizures in piglets, *Am. J. Physiol.*, 256, H120, 1989.

103. **Mirro, R., Armstead, W. M., Busija, D. W., Green, R. S., and Leffler, C. W.,** Increasing ventilation pressure increases cortical subarachnoid cerebrospinal fluid prostanoids in newborn pigs, *Pediatr. Res.*, 22, 647, 1987.
104. **Mirro, R., Leffler, C. W., Armstead, W. M., Beasley, D. G., and Busija, D. W.,** Indomethacin restricts cerebral blood flow during pressure ventilation of newborn pigs, *Pediatr. Res.*, 24, 59, 1988.
105. **Mirro, R., Leffler, C. W., Armstead, W. M., and Busija, D. W.,** Pressure ventilation increases brain vascular prostacyclin production in newborn pigs, *Pediatr. Res.*, 28, 609, 1990.
106. **Armstead, W. M., Mirro, R., Busija, D. W., and Leffler, C. W.,** Prostanoids modulate opioid cerebrovascular responses in newborn pigs, *J. Pharmacol. Exp. Ther.*, 255, 1083, 1990.
107. **Lowery-Smith, L., Mirro, R., Hsu, P., and Leffler, C. W.,** Bradykinin increases cerebral vascular endothelial inositol phosphate turnover and prostacyclin synthesis in newborn pigs, *Pediatr. Res.*, 31, 210A, 1992.
108. **Leffler, C. W. and Busija, D. W.,** Arachidonic acid metabolites and perinatal cerebral hemodynamics, *Sem. Perinatol.*, 11, 31, 1987.
109. **Busija, D. W. and Leffler, C. W.,** Dilator effects of amino acid neurotransmitters on piglet pial arterioles, *Am. J. Physiol.*, 257, H1200, 1989.
110. **Armstead, W. M., Mirro, R., Busija, D. W., and Leffler, C. W.,** Vascular responses to vasopressin are tone-dependent in the cerebral circulation of the newborn pig, *Circ. Res.*, 64, 136, 1989.
111. **Busija, D. W. and Leffler, C. W.,** Eicosanoid synthesis elicited by norepinephrine in piglet parietal cortex, *Brain Res.*, 403, 243, 1987.
112. **Armstead, W. M., Pourcyrous, M., Mirro, R., Leffler, C. W., and Busija, D. W.,** Platelet activating factor: a potent constrictor of cerebral arterioles in newborn pigs, *Circ. Res.*, 62, 1, 1988.
113. **Busija, D. W. and Leffler, C. W.,** Effects of dopamine on pial arteriolar diameter and CSF prostanoid levels in piglets, *J. Cereb. Blood Flow Metab.*, 9, 264, 1989.
114. **Armstead, W. M., Mirro, R., Leffler, C. W., and Busija, D. W.,** Acetylcholine produces cerebrovascular constriction through activation of muscarinic-1 receptors in the newborn pig, *J. Pharmacol. Exp. Ther.*, 247, 926, 1988.
115. **Wagerle, L. C. and Busija, D. W.,** Cholinergic mechanisms in the cerebral circulation of the newborn piglet: effect of inhibitors of arachidonic acid metabolism, *Circ. Res.*, 64, 1030, 1989.
116. **Busija, D. W., Wagerle, L. C., Pourcyrous, M., and Leffler, C. W.,** Acetylcholine dramatically increases prostanoid synthesis in piglet parietal cortex, *Brain Res.*, 439, 122, 1988.
117. **Busija, D. W., Leffler, C. W., and Wagerle, L. C.,** Responses of newborn pig pial arteries to sympathetic nervous stimulation and exogenous norepinephrine, *Pediatr. Res.*, 19, 1210, 1985.
118. **Westerberg, E., Deshpande, K. J. K., and Wieloch, T.,** Regional differences in arachidonic acid release in rat hippocampal CA_1 and CA_3 regions during cerebral ischemia, *J. Cereb. Blood Flow Metabol.*, 7, 189, 1987.
119. **Kishore, K., Bhakoo, H., Crockard, A., and Lascelles, P. T.,** Regional studies of changes in brain fatty acids following experimental ischemia and reperfusion in the gerbil, *J. Neurochem.*, 43, 1025, 1984.
120. **Abe, K., Kogure, K., Yamamoto, H., Imazawa, M., and Miyamoto, K.,** Mechanisms of arachidonic acid liberation during ischemia in gerbil cerebral cortex, *J. Neurochem.*, 48, 503, 1987.
121. **Stevens, M. K. and Yaksh, T. L.,** Time course of release *in vivo* of PGE_2, $PGF_{2\alpha}$, 6keto-$PGF_{1\alpha}$, and TXB_2 into the brain extracellular space after 15 min of complete global ischemia in the presence and absence of cyclooxygenase inhibition, *J. Cereb. Blood Flow Metabol.*, 8, 790, 1988.

122. **Dorman, R. V.,** Effects of cerebral ischemia and reperfusion on prostanoid accumulation in unanesthetized and pentobarbital-treated gerbils, *J. Cereb. Blood Flow Metab.,* 8, 609, 1988.
123. **Johshita, H., Asano, T., Hanamura, T., and Takakura, K.,** Effects of indomethacin and a free radical scavenger on cerebral blood flow and edema after cerebral artery occlusion in cats, *Stroke,* 20, 788, 1983.
124. **Armstead, W. M., Mirro, R., Busija, D. W., and Leffler, C. W.,** Postischemic generation of superoxide anion by newborn pig brain, *Am. J. Physiol.,* 255, H401, 1988.
125. **Wei, E. P., Christman, C. W., Kontos, H. A., and Povlishock, J. T.,** Effects of oxygen radicals on cerebral arterioles, *Am. J. Physiol.,* 248, H157, 1985.
126. **Leffler, C. W., Busija, D. W., Armstead, W. M., Shanklin, D. R., Mirro, R., and Thelin, O.,** Activated oxygen and arachidonate effects on newborn cerebral arterioles, *Am. J. Physiol.,* 259, H1230, 1990.
127. **Mayhan, W. G., Amundsen, S. M., Faraci, F. M., and Heistad, D. D.,** Responses of cerebral arteries after ischemia and reperfusion in cats, *Am. J. Physiol.,* 255, H879, 1988.
128. **Leffler, C. W., Busija, D. W., Armstead, W. M., and Mirro, R.,** Postischemic cerebral microvascular responses to norepinephrine and hypotension in newborn pigs, *Stroke,* 20, 541, 1989.
129. **Leffler, C. W., Busija, D. W., Armstead, W. M., Mirro, R., and Beasley, D. G.,** Ischemia alters cerebral vascular responses to hypercapnia and acetylcholine in piglets, *Pediatr. Res.,* 28, 1989.
130. **Leffler, C. W., Mirro, R., Armstead, W. M., and Shibata, M.,** Topical arachidonic acid restores pial arteriolar dilation to hypercapnia of postischemic newborn pig brain, *Am. J. Physiol.,* 263, H746, 1992.
131. **Saito, K., Levine, L., and Moskowitz, M.,** Blood components contribute to rise in gerbil brain levels of leukotriene-like immunoreactivity after ischemia and reperfusion, *Stroke,* 19, 1395, 1988.
132. **Aktan, S., Aykut, C., Oktay, S., Yegen, B., Keles, E., Aykac, I., and Ercan, S.,** The alterations of leukotriene C_4 and prostaglandin E_2 levels following different ischemic periods in the rat brain tissue, *Prostaglandins, Leukotrienes, and Essential Fatty Acids,* 42, 67, 1991.
133. **Aktan, S., Aykut, C., and Ercan, S.,** Leukotriene C_4 and prostaglandin E_2 activities in the serum and cerebrospinal fluid during acute cerebral ischemia, *Prostaglandins, Leukotrienes, and Essential Fatty Acids,* 43, 247, 1991.
134. **Dahlen, S.-E., Bjork, J., Hedovist, P., Arfors, K.-E., Hammarstrom, A., Lingren, J.-A., and Sammuelsson, B.,** Leukotrienes promote plasma leakage and leukocytes adhesion in postcapillary venous: *in vivo* effects with relevance to the acute inflammatory response, *Proc. Natl. Acad. Sci. U.S.A.,* 78, 3887, 1981.
135. **Sano, K., Asano, T., Tanishima, T., and Sasaki, T.,** Lipid peroxidation as a cause of cerebral vasospasm, *Neurol. Res.,* 2, 253, 1980.
136. **Mirro, R., Armstead, W. M., Busija, D. W., and Leffler, C. W.,** Blood induced superoxide anion generation by newborn pig cerebral cortex, *Am. J. Physiol.,* 257, H1560, 1989.
137. **Sasaki, T., Wakai, S., Asano, T., Takakura, K., and Sano, K.,** Prevention of cerebral vasospasm after SAH with a thromboxane synthesis inhibitor, OKY-1581, *J. Neurosurg.,* 57, 74, 1982.
138. **Schumacher, M. A. and Alksne, J. F.,** Mechanisms of whole blood-induced cerebral arterial contraction, *Neurosurgery,* 9, 275, 1981.
139. **Noboru, T.,** Hemolysate inhibits cerebral artery relaxation, *J. Cereb. Blood Flow Metab.,* 8, 46, 1988.
140. **Busija, D. W. and Leffler, C. W.,** Selective attenuation by perivascular blood of prostanoid-dependent cerebrovascular dilation in piglets, *Stroke,* 22, 484, 1991.

141. **Lang, S. A. and Maron, M. B.,** Role of prostaglandins in blood-induced vasoconstriction of canine cerebral arteries, *J. Cereb. Blood Flow Metab.*, 8, 109, 1988.
142. **Ellis, E. F., Wright, K. F., Wei, E. P., and Kontos, H. A.,** Cyclooxygenase products of arachidonic acid metabolism in cat cerebral cortex after experimental concussive brain injury, *J. Neurochem.*, 37, 892, 1981.
143. **Kontos, H. A. and Wei, E. P.,** Superoxide production in experimental brain injury, *J. Neurosurg.*, 64, 803, 1986.
144. **Cadet, J. L.,** Free radical mechanisms in the central nervous system: an overview, *Int. J. Neurosci.*, 40, 13, 1988.
145. **Cohen, G.,** Oxy-radical toxicity in catecholamine neurons, *Neurotoxicology,* 5, 77, 1984.
146. **Clifton, G. L., Ziegler, M. G., and Grossman, R. G.,** Circulating catecholamines and sympathetic activity after head injury, *Neurosurgery,* 8, 10, 1981.
147. **Clifton, G. L., Robertson, C. S., Kyper, K., Taylor, A. A., Dhekne, R. D., and Grossman, R. G.,** Cardiovascular response to severe head injury, *J. Neurosurg.*, 59, 447, 1983.
148. **Wei, E. P., Kontos, H. A., Dietrich, W. D., Povlishock, J. T., and Ellis, E. F.,** Inhibition by free radical scavengers and cyclooxygenase inhibitors of pial arteriolar abnormalities from concussive brain injury in cats, *Circ. Res.*, 4895, 1981.

Chapter 20

EFFECTS OF BRADYKININ IN THE CEREBRAL MICROCIRCULATION

M. Wahl and L. Schilling

TABLE OF CONTENTS

I. Introduction 316

II. Vasomotor Effects of BK in Cerebral Arteries and Veins 316

III. Effects of Kininase II Inhibitors on the Vasomotor Action of BK 317

IV. Effects of BK on Blood-Brain Barrier (BBB) Permeability 318

V. Kinin Receptors in Cerebral Arteries 319

VI. Mechanisms Mediating the BK Induced Effects 320

VII. BK as a Mediator of Brain Edema 322

References 323

0-8493-5096-0/93/$0.00 + $.50

I. INTRODUCTION

Bradykinin (BK), which has been reported to elicit vasomotor responses and to change the permeability of the vessel wall in many vascular beds,[1] can be formed in blood and brain. All components of an intracerebral kallikrein-kinin system have been described. Kininogen- and kininogenase-like activity have been found in various cerebral areas of different species.[2-8] BK is present in fibers and cell bodies of the brain, especially in hypothalamus and cerebral cortex.[3,9-11] Several enzymes with kininase-like activity have been detected in various regions of the brain.[12-24] Part of the kininase-like activity is due to kininase II which can be blocked by angiotensin converting enzyme inhibitors.

BK appears to be involved in the mediation of secondary brain damage[25] following cold lesion,[26] fluid percussion injury,[27] or ischemia.[28] Thus, BK is favored to be a mediator of vasogenic brain edema besides arachidonic acid and histamine.[29]

The kinin receptors mediating the vasomotor effects have been identified by the rank order of potency of different agonists and antagonists and by ligand binding.[1,30,31] Whereas the expression of the B_1-kinin receptor can only be induced under distinct conditions,[32] the vasomotor effect of BK appears to be mainly mediated by B_2-kinin receptors. Whether B_3-kinin receptors, which have been detected recently in the airways,[33] are also present in vascular smooth muscle is still unclear.

The present chapter, which is an updated review of items published previously,[29,34] will deal with the vasomotor and permeability effects of BK and the underlying mechanisms in the cerebral circulation.

II. VASOMOTOR EFFECTS OF BK IN CEREBRAL ARTERIES AND VEINS

The vasomotor action of BK has been studied *in vitro* by measuring the isometric contraction in segments of cerebral vessels. The results obtained were dependent in part on the species, the cerebral region, and the experimental design. This became obvious especially from the results obtained in cerebral arteries with stretch-induced tone but without precontraction. BK induced contraction in canine arteries,[35] but no response or dilatation in human or feline arteries in the absence and presence of antagonists or other autacoids or transmitters, respectively.[36-41] After pharmacological precontraction, relaxing effects of BK were recorded in all isolated extraparenchymal arteries tested[35-37,41-47] with the exception of the nonresponding feline basilar artery.[35,38,39] Concentration-dependent relaxations were found in the range of 10^{-9} to 10^{-5} *M* BK. Intraparenchymal arteries also dilated to BK,[48] whereas the relaxation of rabbit basilar artery was reversed to contraction during repeated intermittent application of BK over 10 h.[32,47] In precontracted human pial veins, BK induced moderate relaxation and contraction below and above 10^{-6} *M*, respectively.[49]

In situ, bradykinin is a potent dilator of extraparenchymal cerebral arteries. Employing perivascular microapplication BK was found to induce concentration-dependent dilatations of feline pial arteries with an EC_{50} of 4.4×10^{-7} *M* and a maximal response of 45%.[37,38,50] These results demonstrate that BK has a similar potency and efficacy as adenosine[51] and histamine.[52] Thus, BK appears to be an important autacoid for the local adjustment of cerebral microcirculation.[53] Similar responses were found during cortical superfusion of BK in an open or closed cranial window in several species.[54-65] After 30 min of cortical superfusion, the dilating effect of BK was diminished, which may be due to tachyphylaxis.[62,63] A reduced dilating action of BK has been found due to aging,[60] chronic hypertension,[59] and cortical spreading depression.[66]

Endogenous BK could be released from brain kininogen by cortical superfusion of kallikrein. The concomitant dilatation was inhibited by the kallikrein-inhibitor aprotinin.[55] According to the arterial dilatation induced by BK acting from the extravascular side, an increase of cerebral blood flow (CBF) was measured during ventriculo-cisternal perfusion with bradykinin.[67] The diameter of feline pial veins was reduced concentration dependently above 4×10^{-7} *M* BK during cortical superfusion.[62,63] This might be explained by an active constriction of pial veins as found in isolated human pial veins above 10^{-6} *M* BK.[49]

In contrast to the results obtained during extravascular application, intracarotid infusion of BK in cats inducing concentrations of 10^{-6} to 10^{-5} *M* in the sagittal sinus blood, did not alter the diameter of pial arteries and veins[63] or CBF.[68] These findings clearly indicate that the kinin receptors inducing vasomotor responses can only be reached by BK from the extravascular side.

III. EFFECTS OF KININASE II INHIBITORS ON THE VASOMOTOR ACTION OF BK

Several enzymes with kininase-like activity have been found in the brain (see Introduction). Part of the total cerebral kininase activity is due to kininase II (K II). Two peptidylpeptidases are considered to belong to the family of kininase II, one (K II-ACE) appears to be identical with the angiotensin-converting enzyme (ACE)[69] and one (K II-NEP) with the neutral endopeptidase (NEP).[70] However, several isoenzymes of ACE with varying molecular weight and localization have been detected in the brain.[71] Kininase II (KII-ACE) can be inhibited by several compounds such as BK-potentiating peptides 5a (BPP_{5a}) and 9a (BPP_{9a}), BK potentiator C, and captopril which can be employed *in vitro* and *in situ*. These compounds were used to test whether kininase II is present in the vessel wall, the perivascular fluid, the surrounding tissue of extraparenchymal arteries, or the cerebrospinal fluid (CSF) and whether it is involved in the degradation of BK.

Studies employing isolated cerebral arteries of different species (cat, rabbit, man) failed to detect an influence of the inhibitors on the dilating effect of BK.[37,39,41] That these findings do not indicate the absence of KII-ACE in the vessel wall of the arteries tested was confirmed by testing the vasomotor effect of angiotensin I (AI). To induce contraction, AI has to be converted to AII by KII-ACE. This could be inhibited by the blocking agents demonstrating that KII-ACE is present in the vessel wall and important for the conversion of AI to AII but not for the degradation of BK.[39,41]

In situ studies employing perivascular microapplication revealed data corresponding to those obtained in the isolated arteries. Again, the dilating effect of BK was not potentiated by the KII-ACE inhibitors.[37] However, captopril reduced the constrictor response of feline pial arteries to AI, thus confirming the presence of KII-ACE in the perivascular fluid and/or the vessel wall.[72] KII-ACE activity was also determined in cisternal CSF using a bioassay which showed that the conversion of AI to AII and the breakdown of BK could be inhibited by captopril.[72]

The data obtained *in vitro* and *in situ* demonstrate that kininase II (KII-ACE) is present in the vessel wall, the perivascular space or the adjacent tissue, and in the CSF. Kininase II is necessary for the conversion of AI to AII but unimportant for the degradation of BK. Thus, other enzymes with kininase-like activity such as carboxypeptidase, which has been localized in the wall of cerebral vessels,[73] may be involved in the degradation of BK.

IV. EFFECTS OF BK ON BLOOD-BRAIN BARRIER (BBB) PERMEABILITY

The influence of extravascular BK on feline BBB permeability was studied by intravital fluorescence microscopy.[62-64] Under control conditions, all tracers tested were restricted to the intravascular space in the period of observation lasting 3 h. Cortical superfusion with BK dissolved in inert artificial CSF-induced extravasation of Na^+ fluorescein (mol wt, 367) at 4×10^{-7} to 4×10^{-6} *M*. Leakage started as single fluorescent spots around small veins which are known to have a lower transmural electrical resistance than arteries.[74] It became diffuse with duration of exposure and with higher concentrations. Extravasation of fluorescein isothiocyanate (FITC) labeled albumin (mol wt, 67,000) or FITC dextran (mol wt, 19,400–62,000) could not be induced in the cat even at BK concentrations up to 4×10^{-3} M.[63] These data demonstrate that BK selectively opens BBB only for small compounds. In contrast, cortical superfusion with Na^+ arachidonate[75] or histamine[76] showed that these compounds also increased BBB permeability for tracers with a mol wt of 62,000 and 145,000, respectively. From the hydrodynamic radius of Na^+ fluorescein one can estimate that BK increased BBB permeability by opening functional pores with a diameter of at least 11 Å. The upper limit of the pore size was not determined exactly, but FITC dextran (mol wt, 19,000) with a Stokes' radius of 30 Å could definitely not penetrate BBB during superfusion with BK.[63] Since vesicular transport was not increased in the cat,[77] widening of tight junctions due to BK-induced contraction of endothelial cells may be a mechanism.[63] Correspondingly, Unterberg et al.[63] found that the BK-induced opening of BBB could be inhibited by isoproterenol which may be explained by a relaxation of endothelial cells.[78] Further support to the hypothesis that BK opens tight junctions has been given recently. Revest et al.[79] found that BK increased the intracellular Ca^{2+} concentration in cultured rat brain capillary endothelial cells. In addition, BK or a rise in cytosolic Ca^{2+} concentration increased ion permeability of frog cerebral venules[80,81] which might be explained by a shortening of contractile proteins within the endothelial cells.[82] However, divergent results were obtained during intravascular administration of BK. Increased pinocytosis and leakage of horseradish peroxidase (mol wt, 40,000) have been found in the rat after intracarotid infusion of 10^{-5} *M* BK.[83] In contrast, others[84,85] were unable to detect extravasation of the tracers ink or Evans Blue into the brain after intravenous injection of 10^{-6} to 10^{-5} *M* BK per kg body weight. However, an increased ionic conductance was detected in frog pial venules during intravascular administration of BK.[80] Similarly, intracarotid infusion of BK leading to concentrations of 10^{-6} to 10^{-5} *M* in sagittal sinus blood evoked leakage of Na^{+} fluorescein but not of FITC dextran (mol wt, 62,000) from cat pial vessels.[63] From these results it is evident that very similar concentrations reaching the kinin receptors from both intra- and extravascular side can open the BBB.

The bradykinin-induced leakage of Na^{+} fluorescein is primarily caused by an increased permeability of the vessel wall because intra- and extravascular BK caused a comparable extravasation without and with concomitant arterial dilatation, respectively.[63] Arterial vasodilatation that increases the transmural driving force and the vascular surface area is per se not sufficient to induce penetration of the tracers. However, there is no doubt that arterial dilatation augments leakage if permeability is increased at all.[64]

V. KININ RECEPTORS IN CEREBRAL ARTERIES

Kinin receptors of cerebral arteries were characterized by studying the vasomotor effects of agonists and antagonists of various affinity. According to Regoli and Barabé[1] the rank order of apparent affinities for the agonist were methionyl-lysyl-BK (M-L-BK) > des-Arg^9-BK > BK for B_1-kinin receptors and BK > M-L-BK > des-Arg^9-BK for B_2-kinin receptors.

In vitro studies employing these agonists demonstrated that the relaxation of large arteries of the circle of Willis of several species including man was mediated by B_2-kinin receptors.[32,38,86] Correspondingly, the dilating effects of kinin agonists could be inhibited by the B_2-kinin receptor antagonist Thi^{5,8} D-Phe^7-BK[41] but not by the B_1-kinin receptor antagonist des-Arg^9-Leu^8-BK.[38] The contraction of rabbit isolated basilar artery which could be elicited by repeated intermittent application of BK over several hours is mediated by B_1-kinin receptors. Since this could be prevented by preincubation with cycloheximide, an inhibitor of protein synthesis, a *de novo* expression of B_1 receptors was suggested.[32]

In situ investigations of the feline extraparenchymal (pial) small arteries confirmed the results obtained in the isolated large arteries. Again, the rank order of potency of the agonists showed that the dilatation was mediated by B_2-kinin receptors.[38,63] Correspondingly, a B_1-kinin receptor antagonist did not change the BK-induced dilatation.[38,63] Employing the B_2-kinin receptor antagonist Thi,[5,8] D-Phe[7]-BK, the dilating effect of exogenous and endogenous BK could be inhibited in the rabbit.[54] Since the first generation of B_2-kinin receptor antagonists was converted to B_1-kinin receptor antagonists,[87] a reinvestigation with a new more specific B_2-kinin receptor antagonist would be worthwhile. Since the vasomotor response is endothelium dependent (see Section VI) and could only be elicited by extravascular but not by intravascular BK[63] this B_2 receptor has to be localized to the antiluminal side of the endothelial cell.

The effect of BK on BBB permeability was not inhibited by a B_1-kinin receptor antagonist. Furthermore, since the extravasation of Na^+ fluorescein could not be induced by a B_1-kinin receptor agonist and was not inhibited by a B_1-kinin receptor antagonist,[63] the effect of BK on cerebrovascular permeability was obviously mediated by B_2-kinin receptors, similar as in most parts of the peripheral circulation.[86] Since intra- and extravascular BK open the BBB, these B_2-kinin receptors have to be localized to the luminal and antiluminal side of the endothelium.

VI. MECHANISMS MEDIATING THE BK INDUCED EFFECTS

The opening of the BBB is mediated by B_2-kinin receptors[63] which stimulate phosphoinositide turnover in cerebral microvessels.[88] This may induce an activation of protein kinase C which is involved in the permeability increasing effect of BK in microvessels of the hamster cheek pouch.[89] In accordance with such a mechanism were findings obtained in cultured cerebral endothelial cells in which BK or phorbol ester stimulated the fluid-phase endocytosis of a fluorescent tracer.[90] That activation of protein kinase C appears not to open the interendothelial tight junction might be concluded from the finding that phorbol myristate acetate did not reduce the transmural electrical resistance in frog cerebral venules.[81] On the other hand, BK reduced the transmural electrical resistance of frog cerebral venules[80] which would be compatible with an opening of interendothelial tight junctions or transendothelial channels. These findings indicate that further *in situ* investigations are necessary to elucidate the role of protein kinase C in opening of BBB.

Since opening of BBB by BK was prevented in the rat by pretreatment with indomethacin or trifluoperazine, which can suppress prostanoid formation, a coupling between the kallikrein-kinin and prostanoid systems was suggested.[83] If this were the case, pretreatment with dexamethasone, thus inhibiting phospholipase A_2, should reduce the permeability increasing effect of BK. However, such an effect of dexamethasone could not be proven in the cat.[91] An interaction between the kallikrein-kinin system, arachidonic acid, and free radicals has been suggested by Ellis et al.[92] These authors believe that brain injury induces, either directly or by activation of the kallikrein-kinin system, a release of arachidonic acid. Free radicals are generated when arachidonic acid is further metabolized via the cyclooxygenase pathway. Thus, the authors concluded that the arterial dilatation and endothelial lesions after concussive brain injury were finally mediated by free radicals. However, investigations of Unterberg et al.[63,75,93] and Wahl et al.[64] do not support this hypothesis. These authors found divergent vasomotor and permeability effects of BK, arachidonic acid, and free radicals in their experimental model, which were not compatible with the concept of Ellis et al.[92] Considering these and the below mentioned findings, it appears likely that several processes varying with animal species, vascular region, and other unidentified factors are involved in the mediation of BK-induced effects.

The vasomotor effect of BK is endothelium dependent as has been shown *in vitro* and *in situ*.[41,42,44,46,94,95] Since the dilating effect could only be elicited by extravascular BK, the B_2-kinin receptors have to be localized at the antiluminal endothelial membrane. Evidence is now accumulating that the dilating effect of BK can be mediated by several mechanisms, such as a release of endothelium-derived relaxing factor (EDRF), prostanoids, free radicals, H_2O_2, or leukotrienes.

EDRF, which is identified as nitric oxide (NO)[96,97] or a NO-containing moiety like nitrosothiol,[94] is derived from the terminal guanido group of L-arginine by the NO synthase.[98] The relaxing effect of NO is due to activation of the soluble guanylate cyclase and formation of cGMP in the smooth muscle cell.[99] cGMP may act by a reduction of either the cytosolic Ca^{2+} concentration or the Ca^{2+} sensitivity of the contractile proteins.[100,101] BK which has been found to be released also from endothelial cells of the peripheral circulation[102] may thus also have autocrine functions. BK has been shown to increase arginine uptake and intracellular Ca^{2+} concentration in peripheral endothelial cells thus activating NO synthase and releasing NO.[102,103] By such a mechanism the dilating effect of BK appears to be mediated in some cerebral arteries like the basilar artery of dog and rat, which were tested *in vitro* and *in situ*, respectively.[45,59] However, *in situ* NO appears not to mediate the dilating effect of BK in pial arteries of rat[61] and cat.[58] *In situ* studies employing several scavengers of free radicals have suggested that the dilating effect of BK is mediated via release of hydroxyl radicals in pial arteries of mouse[104] and cat[57,58,94] and of H_2O_2 in the rat.[65] Since the dilating action of BK can be reduced or blocked by inhibitors of cyclooxygenase, prostacyclin (PGI_2) has been suggested as a mediator in peripheral vessels.[105,106] That such a mechanism may also act in cerebral arteries was supported by results in rabbit pial arteries *in situ*.[55] However, the involvement of dilating prostanoids in the response to BK could not be demonstrated in isolated middle cerebral or basilar arteries of cats and humans.[36-39,41,43] Since in one of these studies[41] the dilating effect of BK could be reduced by BW755C, an inhibitor of cyclo- and lipoxygenase, the involvement of lipoxygenase products was suggested for human basilar artery.

In vessels of the peripheral circulation, the constrictor effect of BK was independent of endothelium or prostanoids.[107] Accordingly, one might assume that the B_1-kinin receptors mediating contraction of the rabbit isolated basilar artery[32] are localized on smooth muscle cells.

VII. BK AS A MEDIATOR OF BRAIN EDEMA

Evidence has been accumulated that kinins are involved in the formation of vasogenic brain edema. It has been reported that ventriculo-cisternal perfusion with artificial CSF containing 2.5×10^{-6} *M* BK significantly raised brain tissue water content.[108] After a cryogenic lesion of the exposed feline cortex, plasma kininogen was taken up into the focal necrotic and perifocal tissue. Generation of kinins, in particular in perifocal oedematous tissue, was increased by additional cerebral ischemia due to marked rise of intracranial pressure.[26] For these conditions, BK concentrations of 10^{-7} to 10^{-6} *M* can be calculated for the interstitial fluid, which is effective to open BBB permeability and to induce vasodilatation. Similarly, a significant increase of brain kininogen content starting 10 min and reaching an approximately fourfold increase 15 h after fluid percussion injury was detected in the rat. It was accompanied by protein leakage and increase of cerebral tissue water content.[27] Furthermore, tissue kininogen and kinin content were increased after traumatic spinal cord injury.[109]

Further evidence for a mediator role of BK in brain edema was provided by therapeutic studies in rabbits with cold-induced brain swelling.[110] Inhibition of kinin formation by aprotinin reduced significantly the hemisphere swelling. Similarly, activation of the cerebral kallikrein-kinin system and formation of brain edema due to ischemia induced by bilateral carotid occlusion could be reduced by treatment with aprotinin.[28] Furthermore, the arterial dilatation following fluid percussion neural trauma could be reduced by pretreatment with a B_2-kinin receptor antagonist.[92]

Thus, five criteria which have been designated as characteristics for a mediator role of vasogenic brain edema[29] favor the role of BK: (1) it has been found to increase BBB permeability, (2) to dilate arteries thus increasing the driving force for bulk flow into the brain, (3) it induces brain edema, (4) its tissue concentration is increased under pathological conditions which are accompanied by edema and (5) positive therapeutic results were obtained with inhibition of the kinin formation or B_2-kinin receptor antagonist.

REFERENCES

1. **Regoli, D. and Barabé, J.,** Pharmacology of bradykinin and related kinins, *Pharmacol. Rev.*, 32, 1, 1980.
2. **Chao, J., Woodley, C., Chao, L., and Margolius, H. S.,** Identification of tissue kallikrein in brain and in the cell-free translation product encoded by brain mRNA, *J. Biol. Chem.*, 258, 15173, 1983.
3. **Hori, S.,** The presence of bradykinin-like polypeptides, kinin-releasing and destroying activity in brain, *Jpn. J. Physiol.*, 18, 772, 1968.
4. **Kariya, K., Okamoto, H., and Kira, K.,** Kinin-forming enzyme in rat brain mitochondria fraction and biological activity of a kinin released from rat plasma kininogen by this enzyme, *Jpn. J. Pharmacol.*, 34, 203, 1984.
5. **Powers, C. A. and Nasjletti, A.,** A novel kinin-generating protease (kininogenase) in the porcine anterior pituitary, *J. Biol. Chem.*, 257, 5594, 1982.
6. **Powers, C. A. and Nasjletti, A.,** A kininogenase resembling glandular kallikrein in the rat pituitary pars intermedia, *Endocrinology*, 112, 1194, 1983.
7. **Shikimi, T., Kema, R., Matsumoto, M., Yamahata, Y., and Miyata, S.,** Studies on kinin-like substances in brain, *Biochem. Pharmacol.*, 22, 567, 1973.
8. **Shisheva, A., Printz, M. P., Paul, M., and Ganten, D.,** Evidence for kinin forming activity in rat brain, *Fed. Proc.*, 43, 1021, 1983.
9. **Correa, F. M. A., Innis, R. B., Uhl, G. R., and Snyder, S. H.,** Bradykinin-like immunoreactive neuronal systems localized histochemically in rat brain, *Proc. Natl. Acad. Sci. U.S.A.*, 76, 1489, 1979.
10. **Pela, I. R., Gardey-Levassort, C., Lechat, P., and Rocha e Silva, M.,** Brain kinins and fever induced by bacterial pyrogens in rabbits, *J. Pharm. Pharmacol.*, 27, 793, 1975.
11. **Perry, D. C. and Snyder, S. H.,** Identification of bradykinin in mammalian brain, *J. Neurochem.*, 43, 1072, 1984.
12. **Almenoff, J., Wilk, S., and Orlowski, M.,** Membrane bound pituitary metalloendopeptidease: apparent identity to enkephalinase, *Biochem. Biophys. Res. Commun.*, 102, 206, 1981.
13. **Arregui, A., Emson, P. C., and Spokes, E. G.,** Angiotensin-converting enzyme in substantia nigra: reduction of activity in Huntington's disease and after intrastriatal kainic acid in rats, *Eur. J. Pharmacol.*, 52, 121, 1978.
14. **Camargo, A. C. M., Caldo, H., and Reis, M. L.,** Susceptibility of a peptide derived from bradykinin to hydrolysis by brain endooligopeptidases and pancreatic proteinases, *J. Biol. Chem.*, 254, 5304, 1979.
15. **Correa, F. M. A., Plunkett, L. M., Saavedra, J. M., and Hichens, M.,** Quantitative autoradiographic determination of angiotensin converting enzyme (kininase II) binding in individual rat brain nuclei with ^{125}I-^{351}A, a specific enzyme inhibitor, *Brain Res.*, 347, 192, 1985.
16. **Correa, F. M. A., Plunkett, L. M., and Saavedra, J. M.,** Quantitative distribution of angiotensin-converting enzyme (kininase II) in discrete areas of the rat brain by autoradiography with computerized microdensitometry, *Brain Res.*, 375, 259, 1986.
17. **Fuxe, K., Ganten, D., Köhler, C., Schüll, B., and Speck, G.,** Evidence for differential localization of angiotensin-I converting enzyme and renin in the corpus striatum of rat, *Acta Physiol. Scand.*, 110, 321, 1980.
18. **Gimbrone, M. A., Majeau, G. R., Atkinson, W. J., Sadler, W., and Cruise, S. A.,** Angiotensin-converting enzyme activity in isolated brain microvessels, *Life Sci.*, 25, 1075, 1979.
19. **Kariya, K., Kawauchi, R., and Okamoto, H.,** Regional distribution of kininase in rat brain, *J. Neurochem.*, 36, 2086, 1981.

20. **Oliveira, E. B., Martins, A. R., and Camargo, C. M.,** Isolation of brain endopeptidases: influences of size and sequence of substrates structurally related to bradykinin, *Biochemistry,* 15, 1967, 1976.
21. **Poth, M. M., Heath, R. G., and Ward, M.,** Angiotensin-converting enzyme in human brain, *J. Neurochem.,* 25, 83, 1975.
22. **Walter, R., Simmons, W. H., and Yoshimoto, T.,** Proline specific endo- and exopeptidase, *Mol. Cell. Biochem.,* 30, 111, 1980.
23. **Wilk, S. and Orlowski, M.,** Degradation of bradykinin by isolated neutral endopeptidases of brain and pituitary, *Biochem. Biophys. Res. Commun.,* 90, 1, 1979.
24. **Yang, H. Y. T. and Neff, N. H.,** Distribution and properties of angiotensin converting enzyme of rat brain, *J. Neurochem.,* 19, 2443, 1972.
25. **Baethmann, A., Oettinger, W., Rothenfußer, W., Kempski, O., Unterberg, A., and Geiger, R.,** Brain edema factors: current state with particular reference to plasma constituents and glutamate, in *Advances in Neurology,* Vol. 28, *Brain Edema,* CervosNavarro, J. and Ferszt, R., Eds., Raven Press, New York, 1980, 171.
26. **Maier-Hauff, K., Baethmann, A., Lange, M., Schürer, L., and Unterberg, A.,** The kallikrein-kinin system as mediator in vasogenic brain edema. II. Studies on kinin formation in focal and perifocal brain tissue, *J. Neurosurg.,* 61, 97, 1984.
27. **Ellis, E. F., Chao, J., and Heizer, M. L.,** Brain kininogen following experimental brain injury: evidence for a secondary event, *J. Neurosurg.,* 71, 437, 1989.
28. **Kamiya, T., Katayama, Y., Inamura, K., Shimizu, J., Obo, R., Iida, S., Kashiwagi, F., and Terashi, A.,** Activation of bradykinin augments ischemic brain edema, *J. Cereb. Blood Flow Metab.,* 9(Suppl. 1), S73, 1989.
29. **Wahl, M., Unterberg, A., Baethmann, A., and Schilling, L.,** Mediators of blood brain barrier dysfunction and formation of vasogenic brain edema, *J. Cereb. Blood Flow Metab.,* 8, 621, 1988.
30. **Regoli, D., Dion, S., Rhaleb, N.-E., Drapeau, G., and D'Orleans-Juste, P.,** Vasoactive peptides and their receptors, *Blood Vessels,* 27, 137, 1990.
31. **Regoli, D., Rhaleb, N.-E., Dion, S., and Drapeau, G.,** New selective bradykinin receptor antagonists and bradykinin B_2 receptor characterization, *Trends Pharmacol. Sci.,* 11, 156, 1990.
32. **Whalley, E. T., Fritz, H., and Geiger, R.,** Kinin receptors and angiotensin converting enzyme in rabbits basilar arteries, *Naunyn-Schmiedebergs Arch. Pharmakol.,* 324, 296, 1983.
33. **Farmer, S. G., Burch, R. M., Meeker, S. A., and Wilkins, D. E.,** Evidence for a pulmonary B_3 bradykinin receptor, *Mol. Pharmacol.,* 36, 1, 1989.
34. **Wahl, M., Unterberg, A., Whalley, E. T., Baethmann, A., Young, A. R., Edvinsson, L., and Wagner, F. F. W.,** Effects of bradykinin on cerebral haemodynamics and blood brain barrier function, in *Peptidergic Mechanisms in the Cerebral Circulation,* Edvinsson, L. and McCulloch, J., Eds., Horwood, Chichester, 1987, 166.
35. **Toda, N.,** Actions of bradykinin on isolated cerebral and peripheral arteries, *Am. J. Physiol.,* 232, H267, 1977.
36. **Wahl, M., Young, A. R., Edvinsson, L., and Wagner, F.,** Effects of bradykinin on pial arteries and arterioles in vitro and in situ, *J. Cereb. Blood Flow Metab.,* 3, 231, 1983.
37. **Wahl, M., Young, A. R., Edvinsson, L., and Wagner, F.,** Effects of kininase II inhibitors on the vasomotor response to bradykinin of feline intracranial and extracranial arteries in vitro and in situ, *J. Cereb. Blood Flow Metab.,* 3, 339, 1983.
38. **Whalley, E. T. and Wahl, M.,** Analysis of bradykinin receptor mediating relaxation of cat cerebral arteries in vivo and in vitro, *Naunyn-Schmiedebergs Arch. Pharmakol.,* 323, 66, 1983.
39. **Whalley, E. T. and Wahl, M.,** The effect of kininase II inhibitors on the response of feline cerebral arteries to bradykinin and angiotensin, *Pfluegers Arch.,* 398, 175, 1983.

40. **Whalley, E. T.,** Metabolism of bradykinin and angiotensin I by human basilar artery and rabbit aorta, *Naunyn-Schmiedebergs Arch. Pharmakol.*, 335, 551, 1987.
41. **Whalley, E. T., Amure, Y. O., and Lye, R. H.,** Analysis of the mechanism of action of bradykinin on human basilar artery in vitro, *Naunyn-Schmiedebergs Arch. Pharmakol.*, 335, 433, 1987.
42. **Hardebo, J. E., Hanko, J., Kährström, J., and Owman, C.,** Endothelium-dependent relaxation in cerebral arteries, *J. Cereb. Blood Flow Metab.*, 5(Suppl. 1), S533, 1985.
43. **Hatake, K., Kakishita, E., Wakabayashi, I., Sakiyama, N., and Hishida, S.,** Effect of aging on endothelium-dependent vascular relaxation of isolated human basilar artery to thrombin and bradykinin, *Stroke*, 21, 1039, 1990.
44. **Katusic, Z. S., Shepherd, J. T., and Vanhoutte, P. M.,** Oxytocin causes endothelium-dependent relaxations of canine basilar arteries by activating V1-vasopressinergic receptors, *J. Pharmacol. Exp. Ther.*, 236, 166, 1986.
45. **Katusic, Z. S., Marshall, J. J., Kontos, H. A., and Vanhoutte, P. M.,** Similar responsiveness of smooth muscle of the canine basilar artery to EDRF and nitric oxide, *Am. J. Physiol.*, 257, H1235, 1989.
46. **Verrecchia, C., Hamel, E., Edvinsson, L., MacKanzie, E. T., and Seylaz, J.,** Role of the endothelium in the pial artery responses to several vasoactive peptides, *Acta Physiol. Scand.*, 127(Suppl. 552), 33, 1986.
47. **Whalley, E. T., Wahl, M., and Sampaio, C. A. M.,** Angiotensin-converting enzyme, bradykinin, angiotensin and cerebral vessel reactivity, *Hypertension*, 5(Suppl. V), V34, 1983.
48. **Dacey, R. G., Jr. Bassett, J. E., and Takayasu, M.,** Vasomotor responses of rat intracerebral arterioles to vasoactive intestinal peptide, substance P, neuropeptide Y, and bradykinin, *J. Cereb. Blood Flow Metab.*, 8, 254, 1988.
49. **Hardebo, J. E., Kährström, J., Sercombe, R., Owman, C., Salford, L. G., and Verrecchia, C.,** Vasomotor responses of cerebral veins in animals and man, in *Neural Regulation of Brain Circulation*, Owman, C. and Hardebo, J. E., Eds., Elsevier, New York, 1986, 481.
50. **Wahl, M.,** The effect of opiate-like substances and bradykinin on cerebrovascular resistance in cats, in *Cerebral Blood Flow: Effects of Nerves and Neurotransmitters*, Heistad, D. D. and Marcus, M. L., Eds., Elsevier, New York, 1982, 235.
51. **Wahl, M. and Kuschinsky, W.,** The dilatatory action of adenosine on pial arteries of cats and its inhibition by theophylline, *Pfluegers Arch.*, 362, 55, 1976.
52. **Wahl, M. and Kuschinsky, W.,** The dilating effect of histamine on pial arteries of cats and its mediation by H_2 receptors, *Circ. Res.*, 44, 161, 1979.
53. **Wahl, M.,** Local chemical, neural, and humoral regulation of cerebrovascular resistance vessels, *J. Cardiovasc. Pharmacol.*, 7, S36, 1985.
54. **Ellis, E. F., Heizer, M. L., Hambrecht, G. S., Holt, S. A., Stewart, J. M., and Vavrek, R. J.,** Inhibition of bradykinin-induced and kallikrein-induced cerebral arteriolar dilation by a specific bradykinin antagonist, *Stroke*, 18, 792, 1987.
55. **Kamitani, T., Little, M., and Ellis, E. F.,** Evidence for a possible role of the brain kallikrein-kinin system in the modulation of the cerebral circulation, *Circ. Res.*, 57, 545, 1985.
56. **Kamitani, T., Little, M. H., and Ellis, E. F.,** Effect of leukotrienes, 12-HETE, histamine, bradykinin, and 5-hydroxytryptamine on in vivo rabbit cerebral arteriolar diameter, *J. Cereb. Blood Flow Metab.*, 5, 554, 1985.
57. **Kontos, H. A., Wei, E. P., Povlishock, J. T., and Christman, C. W.,** Oxygen radicals mediate the cerebral arteriolar dilatation from arachidonate and bradykinin in cats, *Circ. Res.*, 55, 295, 1984.
58. **Kontos, H. A., Wei, E. P., Kukreja, R. C., Ellis, E. F., and Hess, M. L.,** Differences in endothelium-dependent cerebral dilation by bradykinin and acetylcholin, *Am. J. Physiol.*, 258, H1261, 1990.

59. **Mayhan, W. G.,** Impairment of endothelium-dependent dilatation of basilar artery during chronic hypertension, *Am. J. Physiol.*, 259, H1455, 1990.
60. **Mayhan, W. G., Faraci, F. M., Baumbach, G. L., and Heistad, D. D.,** Effects of aging on response of cerebral arterioles, *Am. J. Physiol.*, 258, H1138, 1990.
61. **Parsons, A. A., Wang, Q., Schilling, L., Lassen, N. A., and Wahl, M.,** Effects of N^G-nitro-L-arginine (NOLAG) on rat pial arterioles in situ, *Pfluegers Arch. Eur. J. Physiol.*, 419(Suppl. 1), R112, 1991.
62. **Unterberg, A., Wahl, M., and Baethmann, A.,** Effects of bradykinin on cerebrovascular permeability and resistance, *J. Cereb. Blood Flow Metab.*, 3(Suppl. 1), S234, 1983.
63. **Unterberg, A., Wahl, M., and Baethmann, A.,** Effects of bradykinin on permeability and diameter of pial vessels in vivo, *J. Cereb. Blood Flow Metab.*, 4, 574, 1984.
64. **Wahl, M., Unterberg, A., and Baethmann, A.,** Intravital fluorescence microscopy for the study of blood-brain-barrier function, *Int. J. Microcirc. Clin. Exp.*, 4, 3, 1985.
65. **Yang, S.T., Mayhan, W. G., Faraci, F. M., and Heistad, D. D.,** Mechanism of impaired endothelium-dependent cerebral vasodilatation in response to bradykinin in hypertensive rats, *Stroke,* 22, 1177, 1991.
66. **Wahl, M., Lauritzen, M., and Schilling, L.,** Change of cerebrovascular reactivity after cortical spreading depression in cats and rats, *Brain Res.*, 411, 72, 1987.
67. **Unterberg, A., Baethmann, A., and Hack, U.,** Cerebral blood flow and metabolism during bradykinin exposure, in *Cerebral Blood Flow, Metabolism and Epilepsy,* Baldy-Moulinier, M., Ingvar, D. H., and Meldrum, B. S., Eds., John Libbey, London, 1983, 174.
68. **Unterberg, A., Hack, U., and Baethmann, A.,** Blood flow, metabolism, and function of the brain during cerebral administration of bradykinin, in *Advances in Neurosurgery,* Vol. 13, Dietz, H., Brock, M., and Klinger, M., Eds., Springer, Berlin, 1985, 326.
69. **Erdös, E. G.,** Kininases, in *Handbook of Experimental Pharmacology,* Suppl. to Vol. 25, Erdös, E. G., Ed., Springer, Heidelberg, 1979, 427.
70. **Bhoola, K. D., Figueroa, C. D., and Worthy, K.,** Bioregulation of kinins, kallikreins, kininogens, and kininase, *Pharmacol. Rev.*, 44, 1, 1992.
71. **Strittmatter, S. M. and Snyder, S. H.,** Angiotensin converting enzyme immunohistochemistry in rat brain and pituitary gland: correlation of isozyme type with cellular localization, *Neuroscience,* 21, 407, 1987.
72. **Whalley, E. T. and Wahl, M.,** Cerebrovascular reactivity to angiotensin and angiotensin converting enzyme activity in cerebrospinal fluid, *Brain Res.*, 438, 1, 1988.
73. **Ward, P. E. and Bausback, H. H.,** Kinin degradation by purified cerebral microvessels, *FASEB J.*, 2, A1381, 1988.
74. **Butt, A. M., Jones, H. C., and Abbott, N. J.,** Electrical resistance across the blood-brain barrier in anaesthetized rats: a developmental study, *J. Physiol.*, 429, 47, 1990.
75. **Unterberg, A., Wahl, M., Hammersen, F., and Baethmann, A.,** Permeability and vasomotor response of cerebral vessels during exposure to arachidonic acid, *Acta Neuropathol.*, 73, 209, 1987.
76. **Schilling, L., Ksoll, E., and Wahl, M.,** Effects of histamine on vasomotor response and permeability of extraparenchymal cerebral vessels, *J. Cereb. Blood Flow Metab.*, 7(Suppl. 1), S506, 1987.
77. **Unterberg, A.,** Veränderungen der Blut-Hirn-Schrankenfunktion und der zerebralen Vasomotorik durch Mediatoren des sekundären Hirnschadens, *Habilitationsschrift,* München, Germany, 1987.
78. **Svensjö, E., Arfors, K.-E., Raymond, R. M., and Grega, G. J.,** Morphological and physiological correlation of bradykinin-induced macromolecular efflux, *Am. J. Physiol.*, 236, H600, 1979.
79. **Revest, P. A., Abbott, N. J., and Gillespie, J. I.,** Receptor-mediated changes in intracellular (Ca^{2+}) in cultured rat brain capillary endothelial cells, *Brain Res.*, 549, 159, 1991.

80. **Olesen, S.-P. and Crone, C.,** Substances that rapidly augment ionic conductance of endothelium in cerebral venules, *Acta Physiol. Scand.*, 127, 233, 1986.
81. **Olesen, S.-P.,** Regulation of ion permeability in frog brain venules. Significance of calcium, cyclic nucleotides and protein kinase C, *J. Physiol.*, 387, 59, 1987.
82. **Owman, C., Edvinsson, L., Hardebo, J. E., Gröschel, Stewart, U., Unsicker, K., and Walles, B.,** Immunohistochemical demonstration of actin and myosin in brain capillaries, in Cerebral Function, Metabolism, and Circulation, Ingvar, D. H. and Lassen, N. A. Eds., Munksgaard, Copenhagen, 1977, 384.
83. **Raymond, J. J., Robertson, D. M., and Dinsdale, H. B.,** Pharmacological modification of bradykinin induced breakdown of the blood-brain barrier, *Can. J. Neurol. Sci.*, 13, 214, 1986.
84. **Gabbiani, G., Basonnel, M. L., and Majno, G.,** Intraarterial injections of histamine, serotonin, or bradykinin: a topographic study of vascular leakage, *Proc. Soc. Exp. Biol. Med.*, 135, 447, 1970.
85. **Saria, A., Lindberg, J. M., Skofitsch, G., and Lembeck, F.,** Vascular protein leakage in various tissues induced by substance P, capsaicin, bradykinin, serotonin, histamine and by antigen challenge, *Naunyn-Schmiedebergs Arch. Pharmakol.*, 324, 212, 1983.
86. **Whalley, E. T., Nwator, I. A., Stewart, J. M., and Vavrek, R. J.,** Analysis of the receptor mediating vascular actions of bradykinin, *Naunyn-Schmiedebergs Arch. Pharmakol.*, 336, 430, 1987.
87. **Regoli, D., Drapeau, G., Rovero, P., Dion, S., Rhaleb, N. E., Barabé, J., D'Orlans-Juste, P., and Ward, P.,** Conversion of kinins and their antagonists into B_1 receptor activators and blockers in isolated vessels, *Eur. J. Pharmacol.*, 127, 219, 1986.
88. **Homayoun, P. and Harik, S. I.,** Bradykinin receptors of cerebral microvessels stimulate phosphoinositide turnover, *J. Cereb. Blood Flow Metab.*, 11, 557, 1991.
89. **Murray, M. A., Heistad, D. D., and Mayhan, W. G.,** Role of protein kinase C in bradykinin-induced increase in microvascular permeability, *Circ. Res.*, 68, 1340, 1991.
90. **Guillot, F. L. and Audus, K. L.,** Angiotensin peptide regulation of fluid-phase endocytosis in brain microvessel endothelial cell monolayers, *J. Cereb. Blood Flow Metab.*, 10, 827, 1990.
91. **Schürer, L., Temesvari, P., Wahl, M., Unterberg, A., and Baethmann, A.,** Blood-brain barrier permeability and vascular reactivity to bradykinin after pretreatment with dexamethasone, *Acta Neuropathol.*, 77, 576, 1989.
92. **Ellis, E. F., Holt, S. A., Wei, E. P., and Kontos, H. A.,** Kinins induce abnormal vascular reactivity, *Am. J. Physiol.*, 255, H397, 1988.
93. **Unterberg, A., Wahl, M., and Baethmann, A.,** Effects of free radicals on permeability and vasomotor response of cerebral vessels, *Acta Neuropathol.*, 76, 238, 1988.
94. **Marshall, J. and Kontos, H. A.,** Endothelium-derived relaxing factors. A perspective from in vivo data, *Hypertension*, 16, 371, 1990.
95. **Rosenblum, W. I.,** Endothelial dependent relaxation demonstrated in vivo in cerebral arterioles, *Stroke*, 17, 494, 1986.
96. **Ignarro, L. J., Buga, G. M., Wood, K. S., Burns, R. E., and Chaudhuri, G.,** Endothelium-derived relaxing factor produced and released from artery and vein is nitric oxide, *Proc. Natl. Acad. Sci. U.S.A.*, 84, 9265, 1987.
97. **Palmer, R. M. J., Ferrige, A. G., and Moncada, S.,** Nitric oxide release accounts for the biological activity of endothelium-derived relaxing factor, *Nature*, 327, 524, 1987.
98. **Moncada, S., Palmer, R. M. J., and Higgs, E. A.,** Biosynthesis of nitric oxide from L-arginine. A pathway for the regulation of cell function and communication, *Biochem. Pharmacol.*, 38, 1709, 1989.
99. **Förstermann, U., Mulsch, A., and Busse, R.,** Stimulation of soluble guanylate cyclase by an acetylcholine-induced endothelium-derived factor from rabbit and canine arteries, *Circ. Res.*, 58, 531, 1986.
100. **Eggermont, J. A., Raeymaekers, L., and Casteels, R.,** Ca^{2+} transport by smooth muscle membrane and its regulation, *Biomed. Biochim. Acta*, 48, S370, 1989.

101. **Yanagisawa, T., Kawada, M., and Taira, N.,** Nitroglycerin relaxes canine coronary arterial smooth muscle without reducing intracellular Ca^{2+} concentrations measured with fura-2, *Br. J. Pharmacol.*, 98, 469, 1989.
102. **Busse, R. and Lamontagne, D.,** Endothelium-derived bradykinin is responsible for the increase in calcium produced by angiotensin-converting enzyme inhibitors in human endothelial cells, *Naunyn-Schmiedebergs Arch. Pharmakol.*, 344, 126, 1991.
103. **Bogle, R. G., Coade, S. B., Moncada, S., Pearson, J. D., and Mann, G. E.,** Bradykinin and ATP stimulate L-arginine uptake and nitric oxide release in vascular endothelial cells, *Biochem. Biophys. Res. Commun.*, 180, 926, 1991.
104. **Rosenblum, W. I.,** Hydoxyl radical mediates the endothelium-dependent relaxation produced by bradykinin in mouse cerebral arterioles, *Circ. Res.*, 61, 601, 1987.
105. **Mullane, K. M. and Moncada, S.,** Prostacyclin mediates the potentiated hypotensive effect of bradykinin following captopril treatment, *Eur. J. Pharmacol.*, 66, 355, 1980.
106. **Nwator, I. A. A., Parsons, A. A., and Whalley, E. T.,** Prostanoid involvement in the relaxation of in vitro mesenteric artery by bradykinin and desArg^9-bradykinin, *Eur. J. Pharmacol.*, 170, 29, 1989.
107. **Regoli, D.,** Neurohumoral regulation of precapillary vessels: the kallikrein-kinin system, *J. Cardiovasc. Pharmacol.*, 6(Suppl. 2), S401, 1984.
108. **Unterberg, A. and Baethmann, A.,** The kallikrein-kinin system as mediator in vasogenic brain edema. I. Cerebral exposure to bradykinin and plasma, *J. Neurosurg.*, 61, 87, 1984.
109. **Xu, J., Hsu, C. Y., Junker, H., Chao, S., Hogan, E. L., and Chao, J.,** Kininogen and kinin in experimental spinal cord injury, *J. Neurochem.*, 57, 975, 1991.
110. **Unterberg, A., Dautermann, C., Baethmann, A., and Müller-Esterl, W.,** The kallikrein-kinin system as mediator in vasogenic brain edema, *J. Neurosurg.*, 64, 269, 1986.

V. Trophic Influences on Cerebral Blood Flow Regulation

Chapter 21

HYPERTENSION AND THE AUTOREGULATION OF CEREBRAL BLOOD FLOW

Seizo Sadoshima and Masatoshi Fujishama

TABLE OF CONTENTS

I. Cerebral Blood Flow Regulation in Hypertension 332

II. Vascular Changes in Hypertension 332

III. Trophic Influences on Vascular Wall 334

IV. Conclusions 337

References 339

0-8493-5096-0/93/$0.00 + $.50

I. CEREBRAL BLOOD FLOW REGULATION IN HYPERTENSION

Cerebral blood flow is regulated by the following four well-known factors: metabolic stimuli, autonomic nerves, chemical stimuli (blood gases and pH), and autoregulation.[1-3] Among them, the autoregulatory mechanism is particularly well developed in small arteries in the brain, although it is a property of many peripheral vascular beds. Autoregulation of blood flow denotes an intrinsic ability of the brain's vascular bed to maintain a constant perfusion over a wide range of blood pressure changes (60 to 150mmHg of mean arterial pressure in the normotensive individual).[4] Alternatively, the autoregulatory mechanism can be defined in terms of vascular changes or simply as arteriolar caliber changes as blood pressure or perfusion pressure varies. It also implies that blood flow remains constant and that vascular resistance changes proportionally to changes in perfusion pressure (which is mean arterial pressure minus intracranial pressure in the brain[5]).

Previous studies in humans[6-9] and also in experimental models[10-12] have revealed that autoregulatory function of cerebral arteries is relatively well maintained in chronic as well as acute hypertension. In essential hypertension, toxemia of pregnancy, glomerulonephritis with hypertension, drug-induced hypertension, and even during psychological excitation, cerebral blood flow is kept constant within the normal range until arterial pressure becomes excessively elevated beyond a certain level, after which cerebral blood flow increases passively with further increases in mean arterial pressure, indicating the upper limit of autoregulation.[13-15]

Encroachment of the vessel wall on the vascular lumen and a reduction of vascular distensibility with inhibited vasodilatation, both of which raise vascular resistance, play important roles in maintaining perfusion pressure within the normal range in downstream vessels, when the autoregulatory plateau is shifted to higher blood pressure levels. Thus, hypertrophy of cerebral vessels is a structural, as well as functional, adaptation, which attenuates cerebral microvascular perfusion pressure and regulates blood flow in hypertension.

II. VASCULAR CHANGES IN HYPERTENSION

Both morphometric and hemodynamic studies have reported that cerebral, as well as other peripheral, arteries undergo structural changes during prolonged hypertension.[5,12,16-21] A sequence of changes involving damage to endothelial cells, increases in endothelial permeability, activation and proliferation of smooth muscle cells in the media (the tunica media, an intermedial coat of arteries), and increases in the extracellular matrix are characteristic findings induced by increases in intraluminal pressure, accompanied by enhanced wall stress.[16,20] These changes lead to abnormally high peripheral artery resistance, even if the vessels are maximally relaxed. Distensibility of the arterial wall is also reduced.

In an experimental setting, these hypertensive structural changes can develop over a few weeks to a few months and may revert to close to normal in a similar relatively short period following effective antihypertensive treatment.[12,19] Folkow et al.[21] have described a rapid and considerable regression of the vascular hypertrophy that takes place when the pressure load is reduced to a normal level for 8 weeks or less. Easily reversible components would be expected to include muscular hypertrophy and the accumulation of salt and water in the vessel wall.[5,20] With longstanding hypertension, irreversible factors may contribute to vascular adaptation in the form of vessel wall connective tissue proliferation, muscular hyperplasia, and degenerative changes, such as calcium deposition and lipohyalinosis.[5,20]

Recently, several morphometric studies on cerebral arteries have been performed in hypertensive animals with or without antihypertensive treatment.[15-19] Warshaw et al.,[16] Hart et al.,[17] and Ibayashi et al.[19] have shown that medial smooth muscle cell hypertrophy of small mesenteric[16] and cerebral[17-19] arteries is greater in spontaneously hypertensive rats than age-matched normotensive Wistar-Kyoto rats. The response to hypertension within the cardiovascular system reaches its plateau by 5 months, and thus, antihypertensive treatment by Ibayashi et al.[19] was started in SHR at 10 weeks of age and continued for the following 10 weeks. At the age of 20 weeks, mean arterial pressure of experimental treated SHR was 177 $\pm$ 9 mmHg (mean $\pm$ SD), being significantly lower than 195 $\pm$ 12 ($p < 0.05$) in the controls, and medial thickness, cross-sectional area, and the ratio of medial thickness per external diameter were also significantly smaller in rats receiving antihypertensive treatment (Figure 1).[19]

An impressive recent finding by Baumbach et al.[15,22] is the "remodeling" of resistance vessels during chronic hypertension. They have demonstrated a reduction of both external and internal diameters, without any increase in medial size, in cerebral arterioles. Remodeling causes encroachment on the vessel wall, increasing the wall/lumen ratio and thus the vascular resistance, which may play an important role in the elevation of vascular resistance in hypertension and also in aging.

Many factors for the development of systemic and chronic hypertension have been suggested and disputed. Abnormalities in the central nervous system, hormonal or hemodynamic disturbances, alterations in renal function, etc. are proposed to be involved.[23] Although the mechanisms sustaining high blood pressure are indigenous to each patient and animal model, the structural as well as functional changes in the vessels in response to increased intraluminal pressure or wall stress are similar.[5,20,24] Thus it is speculated that some nonspecific factors, other than increases in intraluminal pressure, could contribute to the development of morphometric and functional changes in the vessels. Trophic effects of innervation by sympathetic nerves have been

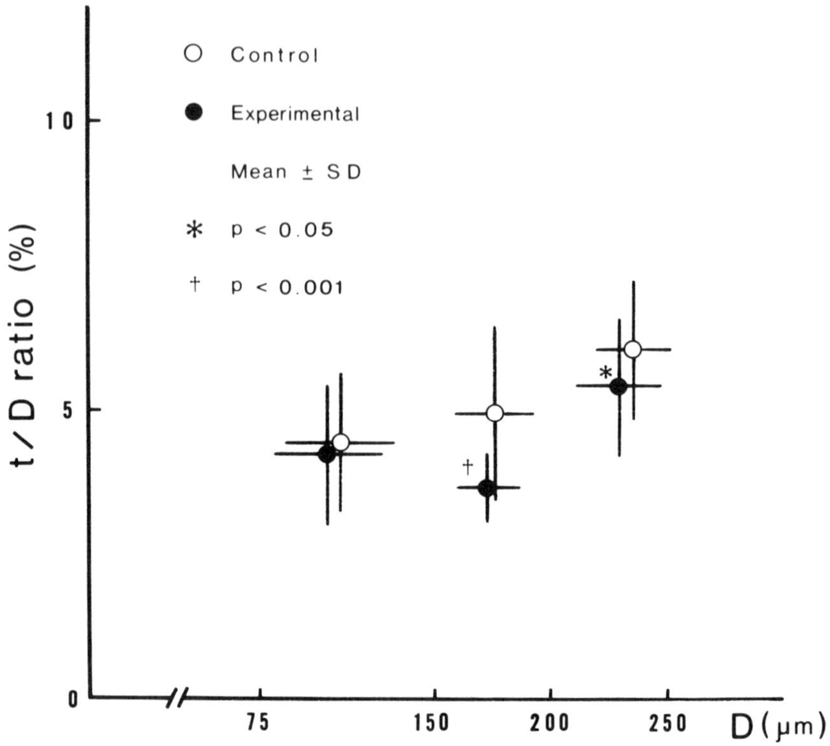

FIGURE 1. Relationship between average of medial thickness to external diameter ratio (t/D ratio) and external diameter. In the experimental group, t/D ratios of the medium and large middle cerebral arteries were significantly smaller than those of the corresponding vessels in the control group. Each circle with bars indicates mean ± SD; t, thickness of the media and D, external diameter. (From Ibayashi, S., et al., *Stroke,* 17, 515, 1986. With permission.)

considered to be one of these.[3] Remodeling is also suggested to be, in part, due to trophic effects of sympathetic nerves on the cerebral vessels.[15,22,25]

III. TROPHIC INFLUENCES ON VASCULAR WALL

The cerebral circulation has been proposed to be regulated, in part, by neurogenic and peptidergic factors. Several vasoactive substances, such as vasoactive intestinal peptide, substance P, neuropeptide Y, and even acetylcholine, have been demonstrated in the cerebral arterial wall by histological and histochemical methods.[3,5,26] In spite of intensive studies in this area, the physiological importance of these peptides on the cerebral arteries has long been debated.

The cerebral arteries are innervated by a rather dense plexus of sympathetic nerve fibers, originating from the ipsilateral superior cervical ganglion.

A number of investigations have been performed to evaluate the possible significance of this sympathetic innervation, by examining the responses of cerebral blood flow to the stimulation of sympathetic nerves. Acute or chronic sympathetic denervation has minimal effect on cerebral blood flow under normal conditions.[2,27] Also, acute denervation,[27-29] or denervation for 1 to 3 weeks,[27,30] has been observed to exert little effect on cerebral blood flow during hypotension. Thus, the role of sympathetic tone in cerebral vascular responses to an acute reduction of blood pressure appears to be small. In contrast, in recent years, several observations have suggested the importance of sympathetic vasoconstriction in regulating cerebral blood flow during acute increases in systemic arterial pressure. Bill and Linder[31] and Heistad et al.[32] found that electric stimulation of sympathetic nerves (5 to 10 V and 10 to 20 Hz) attenuates increases in cerebral blood flow during acute elevations of systemic arterial pressure in experimental animals such as cat,[31,32] dog,[28,32] and monkey.[32] Also, sympathetic stimulation decreases resting cerebral blood flow transiently (i.e., escape phenomenon) but profoundly by 15 to 20% in the baboon, goat, and dog.[3,32] Sadoshima et al.[33] examined the changes in the upper limits of cerebral blood flow autoregulation after acute denervation of sympathetic nerves in spontaneously hypertensive rats. They found that blood pressure levels of the upper limits of autoregulation shifted to the left and were 18 to 23 mmHg lower in denervated than innervated hemispheres.[35] Acute sympathetic denervation leads to a larger increase in cerebral blood flow beyond the upper limits of autoregulation, and, moreover, causes enhanced blood-brain barrier permeability during abrupt elevations of arterial pressure. Although some investigations have failed to show any effect on the cerebral blood flow of electrical sympathetic stimulation, these discrepancies in the results may be attributed in part to the different methods that have been used to measure cerebral blood flow.[3,27-29] It would be reasonable to assume that sympathetic nerves can affect the responsiveness of cerebral vessels to an extreme stress.

Apart from such a vasotonic effect, the trophic influence of sympathetic nerves over vascular smooth muscle has attracted attention very recently. The trophic influence has been examined in situations of denervation and innervation and where the smooth muscle component of the vascular wall has been reported to increase or decrease.[34] Mendez et al.[35] and Luco and Luco[36] examined the action of a normal sympathetic innervation on the fibrillary activity of skeletal muscles in cats and proposed the existence of a hypothetical trophic factor, or mediator, released by sympathetic nerves. Bevan and Tsuru[34] have shown that chronic sympathetic denervation of the arterial wall results in inhibition of smooth muscle cell proliferation and thus a reduction in smooth muscle cells with increases in interstitial fibrous connective tissue (Figure 2). Bevan and Bevan[37] observed that innervation by sympathetic nerves promotes the normal development of ear arteries in normotensive rabbits. The trophic influences also contribute significantly to altered membrane properties in hypertension.[38] Scott and Pang[39] reported that hyperinnervation of small

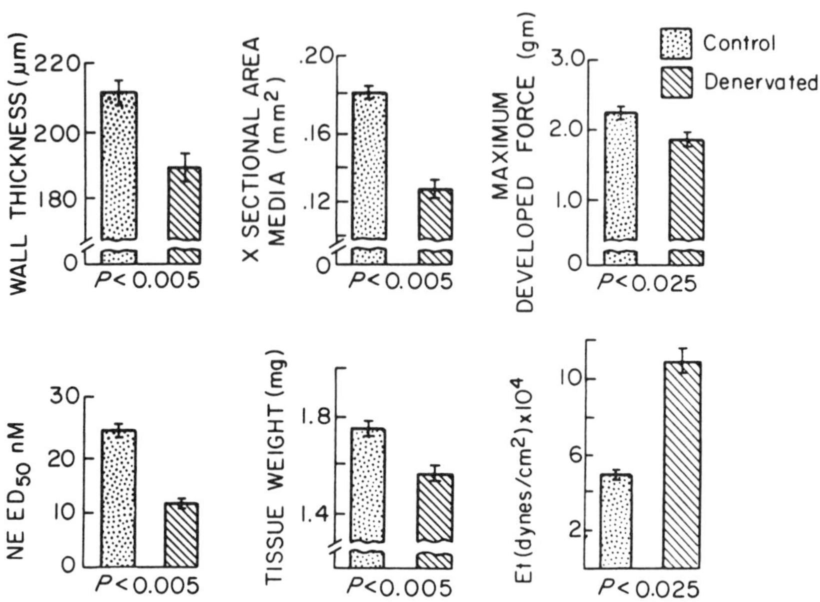

FIGURE 2. Comparison of measurement of paired innervated and denervated ear arteries of growing rabbits, denervated at 3 to 4 weeks of age, 8 weeks after unilateral cervical ganglionectomy. The denervated arteries showed mean decreases in tissue weight (11%), total wall thickness (12%), cross-sectional area of media (27%), contractility (16%), and increases in the tangential modulus of elasticity (Et) and sensitivity to norepinephrine (2.3-fold). All values are mean ± SEM. (From Bevan, D. and Tsuru, H., *Circ. Res.*, 49, 478, 1981. With permission.)

arteries, before significant elevation of blood pressure, may be causally related to the hypertrophy of the media in arteries in hypertensive animals. It might be anticipated, therefore, that sympathetic nerves contribute significantly to the development of cerebral hypertrophy in chronic hypertension.

Hart et al.[17] removed the superior cervical ganglion on one side in stroke-prone, spontaneously hypertensive rats at 8 weeks and morphometric studies on cerebral small arteries were undertaken at 13 weeks of age (systolic blood pressure 253 ± 10 mmHg, mean ± SEM). Wall/lumen ratio was 0.14 in the innervated parenchymal, but not pial vessels, and 0.10 in denervated vessels (Figure 3). Wall/lumen ratio in Wistar-Kyoto rats at the same age was 0.08 (systolic blood pressure; 142 ± 4 mmHg). They concluded that cerebral vessels undergo hypertrophy during hypertension and that sympathetic nerves appear to exert a trophic effect on cerebral vascular muscle in response to hypertension. Sadoshima et al.[33] also demonstrated an increase in the wall per lumen ratio of cerebral arteries during the development of hypertension

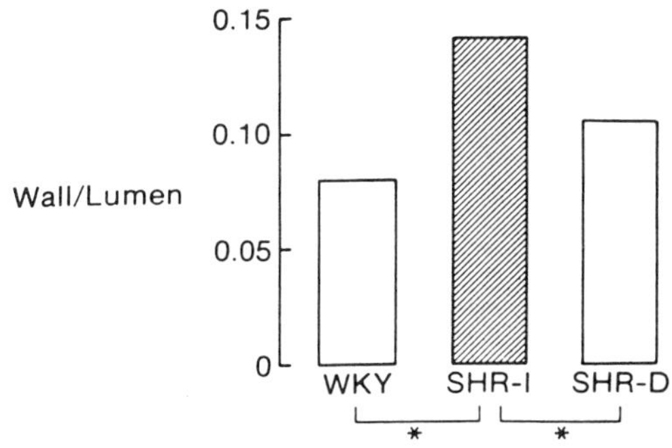

FIGURE 3. Wall/lumen ratio in intraparenchymal arteries of the cerebrum. Asterisk (*) = $p < 0.05$. Wall/lumen ratio was 0.060 ± 025 (mean ± SEM), larger in SHR-I than in WKY. Wall/lumen ratio was 0.037 ± 0.012 larger in SHR-I than SHR-D. SHR, spontaneously hypertensive rat; WKY, Wistar-Kyoto rat; I, innervated; and D, denervated hemisphere. (From Hart, M. N., et al., *Hypertension,* 2, 419, 1980. With permission.)

in spontaneously hypertensive rats: 0.139 ± 0.007(mean ± SEM) and mean arterial pressure 89 ± 3 mmHg(mean ± SEM); 0.170 ± 0.005 and 140 ± 6; and 0.223 ± 0.007 and 165 ± 5 at 4 weeks, 3, and 6 months old, respectively. Chronic cervical ganglionectomy at 4 weeks of age attenuated the development of vascular hypertrophy: 0.128 ± 0.004 at 3 months of age and 0.196 ± 0.007 at 6 months ($p < 0.05$ vs. innervated, respectively). Moreover, the upper limit of cerebral blood flow autoregulation was 13 mmHg lower in denervated than innervated hemispheres: 165 ± 5 and 178 ± 6 mmHg, respectively, at 3 months and 208 ± 8 and 215 ± 8, respectively, at 6 months (Figure 4 and 5). All these results suggest that cerebral vascular hypertrophy may be protective against a breakthrough of blood flow and disruption of the blood brain barrier in acute and chronic hypertension. Trophic, as well as tonic, effects of sympathetic innervation appear to play an important role in the regulation of cerebral blood flow in response to elevation of systemic arterial pressure.

IV. CONCLUSION

This chapter focuses on the trophic effects of sympathetic nerves on cerebral blood vessels. These trophic actions appear to have an important role in the regulation of cerebral blood flow and in the protection of cerebral vessels from damage during hypertension. Further studies are desired to clarify the mechanism of action of trophic effects on the development of vascular hypertrophy.

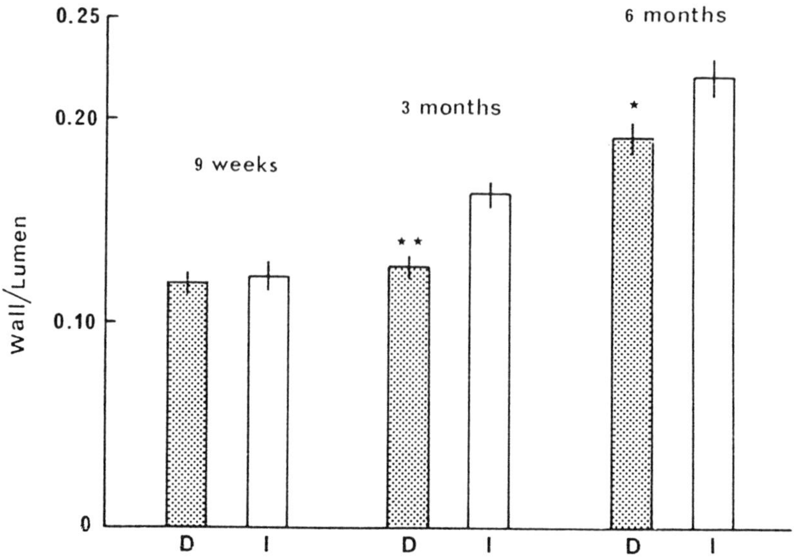

FIGURE 4. Effect of denervation on wall to lumen ratio at 4 weeks, 3 months, and 6 months of age in SHR, in which unilateral cervical ganglionectomy was performed at 4 weeks of age. The ratio is significantly attenuated by chronic denervation. See text for details. SHR, spontaneously hypertensive rat; D, denervated; and I, innervated vessels. $*p < 0.05$, $**p < 0.02$ vs. innervated vessels. (From Sadoshima, S., et al., *Stroke,* 16, 477, 1985. With permission.)

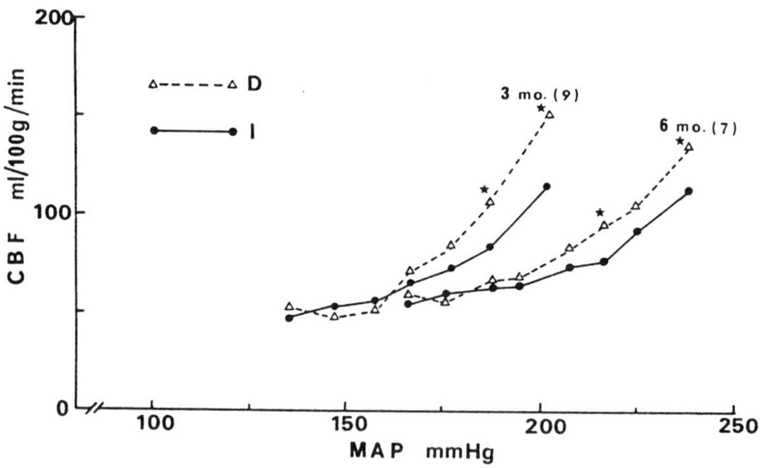

FIGURE 5. Effect of chronic sympathectomy on CBF autoregulation in 3 and 6 months old SHR, in which unilateral cervical ganglionectomy was made at 4 weeks of age. A greater increase in CBF is observed in denervated hemispheres during an acute rise in arterial pressure. See text for details. SHR, spontaneously hypertensive rat; CBF, cerebral blood flow; MAP, mean arterial pressure; D, denervated; and I, innervated hemisphere. $*p < 0.05$ vs. innervated hemisphere. (From Sadoshima, S., et al., *Stroke,* 16, 477, 1985. With permission.)

REFERENCES

1. **Lassen, N. A.,** Control of cerebral circulation in health and disease, *Circ. Res.*, 34, 749, 1974.
2. **Heistad, D. D. and Marcus, M. L.,** Evidence that neuronal mechanisms do not have important effects on cerebral blood flow, *Circ. Res.*, 42, 295, 1978.
3. **Busija, D. W., Sadoshima, S., Marcus, M. L., and Heistad, D. D.,** Functional significance of sympathetic innervation of cerebral vessels: can the issue now be resolved?, in *Trends in Autonomic Pharmacology,* Vol. 2, Kalsner, S., Ed., Urban & Schwarzenberg, Baltimore, 1982, 187.
4. **Lassen, N. A.,** Cerebral blood flow and oxygen consumption in man, *Physiol. Rev.*, 39, 183, 1959.
5. **Paulson, O. B., Strandgaard, S., and Edvinsson, L.,** Cerebral autoregulation, *Cerebrovasc. Metab. Rev.*, 2, 161, 1990.
6. **Strandgaard, S., Olesen, J., Skinhof, E., and Lassen, N. A.,** Autoregulation of brain circulation in severe arterial hypertension, *Br. Med. J.*, 1, 507, 1973.
7. **McHenry, L. C., Jr., West, J. W., Cooper, E. S., Goldberg, H. I., and Jaffe, M. E.,** Cerebral autoregulation in man, *Stroke,* 5, 695, 1974.
8. **Strandgaard, S.,** Autoregulation of cerebral circulation in hypertension, *Acta Neurol. Scand.*, 57(Suppl.), 1, 1978.
9. **Hoffman, W. E., Albrecht, R. F., and Miletich, D. J.,** The influence of aging and hypertension in cerebral autoregulation, *Brain Res.*, 214, 196, 1981.
10. **Sadoshima, S., Fujishima, M., Yoshida, F., Ibayashi, S., Shiokawa, O., and Omae, T.,** Cerebral autoregulation in young spontaneously hypertensive rats. Effect of sympathetic denervation, *Hypertension,* 7, 392, 1985.
11. **Sadoshima, S., Fujii, K., Kusuda, K., Shiokawa, O., Yao, H., Ibayashi, S., and Fujishima, M.,** Importance of bilateral sympathetic innervation on cerebral blood flow autoregulation in the thalamus, *Brain Res.*, 413, 297, 1987.
12. **Tanaka, S., Tanaka, M., and Akashi, A.,** Influence of antihypertensive treatment with budralazine on autoregulation of cerebral blood flow in spontaneously hypertensive rats, *Stroke,* 20, 1724, 1989.
13. **Barry, D. I.,** Cerebral blood flow in hypertension, *J. Cardiovasc. Pharmacol.*, 7, S94, 1985.
14. **Reed, G. and Devous, M.,** Southwestern internal medicine conference: Cerebral blood flow autoregulation and hypertension, *Am. J. Med. Sci.*, 289, 37, 1985.
15. **Baumbach, G. L. and Heistad, D. D.,** Cerebral circulation in chronic arterial hypertension, *Hypertension,* 12, 89, 1988.
16. **Warshaw, D. M., Root, D. T., and Halpern, W.,** Effects of antihypertensive drug therapy on the morphology and mechanics of resistance arteries from spontaneously hypertensive rats, *Blood Vessels,* 17, 257, 1980.
17. **Hart, M. N., Heistad, D. D., and Brody, M. J.,** Effect of chronic hypertension and sympathetic denervation on wall/lumen ratio of cerebral vessels, *Hypertension,* 2, 419, 1980.
18. **Harper, S. L. and Bohlen, H. G.,** Microvascular adaptation in the cerebral cortex of adult spontaneously hypertensive rats, *Hypertension,* 6, 408, 1984.
19. **Ibayashi, S., Ogata, J., Sadoshima, S., Fujii, K., Yao, H., and Fujishima, M.,** The effect of long-term antihypertensive treatment on medial hypertrophy of cerebral arteries in spontaneously hypertensive rats, *Stroke,* 17, 515, 1986.
20. **Chobanian, A. V.,** 1989 Corcoran lecture: adaptive and maladaptive responses of the arterial wall to hypertension, *Hypertension,* 15, 666, 1990.
21. **Folkow, B., Hallbäck, M., Lungren, Y., and Weiss, L.,** The effect of intense treatment with hypertensive drugs on structural design of the resistance vessels in spontaneously hypertensive rats, *Acta Physiol. Scand.*, 83, 280, 1971.

22. **Baumbach, G. L. and Heistad, D. D.,** Adaptive changes in cerebral blood vessels during chronic hypertension, *J. Hyperten.*, 9, 987, 1991.
23. **Warshaw, D. M., Mulvany, M. J., and Halpern, W.,** Mechanical and morphological properties of arterial resistance vessels in young and old spontaneously hypertensive rats, *Circ. Res.*, 45, 250, 1979.
24. **Chobanian, A.,** Overview: hypertension and atherosclerosis, *Am. Heart J.*, 116, 319, 1988.
25. **Faraci, F. M. and Heistad, D. D.,** Regulation of large cerebral arteries and cerebral microvascular pressure, *Circ. Res.*, 66, 8, 1990.
26. **Edvinsson, L. and McCulloch, J.,** Peptidergic mechanisms in the cerebral circulation, Ellis Horwood, Chichester, 1987.
27. **Mueller, S. M., Heistad, D. D., and Marcus, M. L.,** Total and regional cerebral blood flow during hypotension, hypertension and hypocapnia: effect of sympathetic denervation in dogs, *Circ. Res.*, 41, 350, 1977.
28. **Marcus, M. L. and Heistad, D. D.,** Effect of sympathetic nerves on cerebral blood flow in awake dogs, *Am. J. Physiol.*, 238, H549, 1979.
29. **Sadoshima, S. and Heistad, D. D.,** Regional cerebral blood flow during hypotension in normotensive and stroke-prone spontaneously hypertensive rats: effect of sympathetic denervation, *Stroke,* 14, 575, 1983.
30. **Fitch, W., MacKenzie, E. T., and Harper, A. M.,** Effects of decreasing arterial blood pressure on cerebral blood flow in the baboon, *Circ. Res.*, 37, 550, 1975.
31. **Bill, A. and Linder, J.,** Sympathetic control of cerebral blood flow in acute arterial hypertension, *Acta Physiol. Scand.*, 96, 114, 1976.
32. **Heistad, D. D., Marcus, M. L., and Gross, P. M.,** Effect of sympathetic nerves on cerebral vessels in dog, cat and monkey, *Am. J. Physiol.*, 235, H544, 1978.
33. **Sadoshima, S., Yoshida, F., Ibayashi, S., Shiokawa, O., and Fujishima, M.,** Upper limit of cerebral autoregulation during development of hypertension in spontaneously hypertensive rats — effect of sympathetic denervation, *Stroke,* 16, 477, 1985.
34. **Bevan, R. D. and Tsuru, H.,** Functional and structural changes in the rabbit ear artery after sympathetic denervation, *Circ. Res.*, 49, 478, 1981.
35. **Mendez, J., Arenda, L. C., and Luco, J. V.,** Antifibrillary effect of adrenergic fibers on denervated striated muscles, *J. Neurophysiol.*, 33, 882, 1970.
36. **Luco, C. F. and Luco, J. V.,** Sympathetic effects on fibrillary activity of denervated striated muscles, *J. Neurophysiol.*, 34, 1066, 1971.
37. **Bevan, J. A. and Bevan, R. D.,** Sympathetic control of the rabbit basilar artery, in *Neurogenic Control of the Brain Circulation,* Owman, C. and Edvinsson, L., Eds., Pergamon Press, New York, 1977, 285.
38. **Abel, P. W. and Hermsmyer, K.,** Sympathetic cross innervation of SHR and genetic controls suggest a trophic influence on vascular muscle membranes, *Circ. Res.*, 49, 1311, 1981.
39. **Scott, T. M. and Pang, S. C.,** The correlation between the development of sympathetic innervation and the development of medial hypertrophy in jejunal arteries in normotensive and spontaneously hypertensive rats, *J. Autonomic Nerv. Syst.*, 8, 25, 1983.

Chapter 22

CEREBRAL CIRCULATION DURING AGING

Frank M. Faraci

TABLE OF CONTENTS

I. Introduction 342

II. Vascular Morphology and Mechanics 342

III. Cerebral Blood Flow and Metabolism 342

IV. Neural Influence on Cerebral Circulation 343

V. Vascular Responses 344

VI. Endothelium-Dependent Responses 345
- A. Prostacyclin 345
- B. Endothelium-Derived Relaxing Factor 346
- C. Aging and EDRF 346

VII. Summary and Implications 347

Acknowledgments 348

References 349

0-8493-5096-0/93/$0.00 + $.50

I. INTRODUCTION

Aging is associated with a variety of alterations in the cardiovascular system.[1] These alterations include morphological and functional changes in cerebral blood vessels. Abnormalities in regulation of the cerebral circulation are associated with, and may contribute to, an increased incidence of stroke during aging.

This chapter will summarize some of the structural and functional changes that occur in blood vessels of the brain during aging. The review will focus on the following alterations in cerebral blood vessels that occur with aging: (1) vascular morphology and mechanics, (2) resting levels of cerebral blood flow, (3) innervation of cerebral blood vessels, (4) vascular responses, and (5) endothelium-dependent mechanisms (Figure 1). When possible, data obtained in human cerebral blood vessels will be presented. The discussion will deal with changes in the cerebral circulation during aging and will not address changes that occur during normal development (fetal vs. newborn vs. adult).

II. VASCULAR MORPHOLOGY AND MECHANICS

Vascular structure and mechanics appear to change during aging in the cerebral circulation. Studies of both the basilar artery in humans and pial arterioles in Fischer rats indicate that cerebral blood vessels become less distensible with age.[2,3] Increased stiffness of cerebral arterioles appears to be due to a decrease in the relative amount of distensible elements of the vessel wall, smooth muscle, and elastin.[3] Measurements of the cross-sectional area of the vessel wall indicate that cerebral arterioles atrophy with aging.[3] The amount of collagen, a nondistensible component of the vessel wall, increases with age in the basilar artery in humans.[2] Such changes in the composition and mechanical properties of the vessel wall may influence vascular responses. Decreased distensibility of cerebral blood vessels may contribute to impaired vascular responses that have been described with aging.

III. CEREBRAL BLOOD FLOW AND METABOLISM

Do resting levels of cerebral blood flow change during normal aging? Results from most studies in the rat suggest that cerebral blood flow is stable during aging.[4-8] In contrast, in many studies in humans, a reduction in cerebral blood flow with aging has been observed. For example, a negative correlation of local blood flow with age has been described in regions associated with memory and behavior such as the cingulate gyrus[9] and in gray matter of the cerebrum.[10-12] Blood flow to gray matter has been estimated to decrease at a rate of 0.5%/year in humans.[10] This gradual decline in cerebral blood flow is associated with a similar decrease in cerebral oxygen metabolism and an increase in oxygen extraction.[10] In contrast to gray matter, blood flow to subcortical white matter may not decrease with age in humans.[12] Although

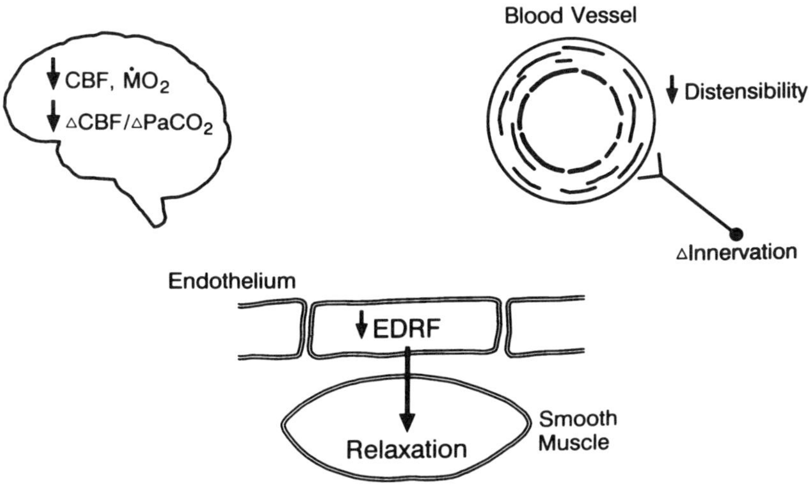

FIGURE 1. Schematic diagram of changes that occur in the cerebral circulation with aging. Compared to the adult, there is a decrease in cerebral blood flow (CBF), a decrease in cerebral metabolic rate for oxygen ($\dot{M}O_2$), a reduction in the sensitivity of cerebral blood vessels to changes in arterial PCO_2 ($PaCO_2$) ($\Delta CBF/\Delta PaCO_2$), a decrease in vascular distensibility, changes in perivascular innervation, and impairment in endothelium-dependent responses. EDRF = endothelium-derived relaxing factor.

some studies describe no decrease in cerebral blood flow with aging,[13] a majority of studies do suggest that cerebral blood flow tends to decrease with age in humans.[12,14,15] The decrease in cerebral blood flow with age in humans, but not rats, may be related to neuronal loss and development of dementia in humans.[15]

IV. NEURAL INFLUENCE ON CEREBRAL CIRCULATION

Large cerebral arteries and pial arterioles are richly innervated by autonomic nerve fibers containing vasodilator and vasoconstrictor neurotransmitters.[16,17] In general, sympathetic nerve fibers arise from the superior cervical ganglion and contain norepinephrine and neuropeptide Y. Although the source of the amine remains a point of controversy, sympathetic fibers innervating cerebral arteries may also contain serotonin.[18] Parasympathetic fibers (from several possible sources) contain acetylcholine and vasoactive intestinal peptide (VIP). Sensory fibers that innervate cerebral blood vessels arise primarily from the trigeminal ganglion and contain substance P, neurokinin A, and calcitonin gene-related peptide (CGRP).

The pattern of innervation by perivascular fibers changes with aging. In the aged rat, there is a decreased expression of vasoconstrictor (norepinephrine and serotonin) fibers and increased expression of vasodilator fibers (VIP and

CGRP) compared to the adult animal.[19] There is also evidence for reduced accumulation of serotonin and decreased density of cerebrovascular nerves in aged rats.[20] A somewhat different pattern of change in perivascular nerve fibers has been observed in human pial arteries.[21] The relative density of neuropeptide Y, VIP, and substance P containing fibers in these blood vessels all decrease with age.

The functional significance of changes in vascular innervation with age is not clear. Alterations in innervation of cerebral blood vessels and subsequent changes in trophic influences by nerves might contribute to structural changes that occur with aging.[3] One functional response, the change in cerebral blood flow that occurs during stimulation of sympathetic nerves, is similar in adult and aged rats.[4]

In addition to peripheral neural influences, central neural mechanisms may also participate in regulation of the cerebral circulation. Activation of cholinergic neurons of the basal forebrain produces vasodilation in the frontal and parietal cortex under normal conditions.[5] Marked impairment of the increase in local cerebral blood flow in the parietal cortex during stimulation of the basal forebrain has been observed in aged rats.[5] Thus, central neural influences on the cerebral circulation may be altered with aging.

V. VASCULAR RESPONSES

Impairment of some vasodilator responses occur in the cerebral circulation with aging. Hypercapnia is a potent dilator of cerebral blood vessels.[22] In both aged rats and humans, compared to adult controls, the normal increase in cerebral blood flow that occurs during increases in arterial PCO_2 is impaired.[8,11,12] Cerebral vasodilatation during hypoxia also appears to be impaired with aging.[6] It has been suggested that decreases in cerebral vascular resistance during reductions in systemic blood pressure (autoregulation) are also impaired in aged humans.[23]

In the basilar artery of 5- to 30-month old rats, impairment of contractile responses to serotonin and prostaglandin $F_{2\alpha}$, but not KCl, has been observed, suggesting that impairment of vascular responses is specific for certain agonists.[24] Submaximal concentrations of the thromboxane analogue U46619 produce similar constrictions of pial arterioles in adult and aged rats.[25]

In contrast, some studies suggest a generalized impairment of cerebral vasoconstrictor responses occur with aging. Aging is associated with no change in sensitivity, but a decrease in maximum contractile responses of the human basilar artery to several vasoconstrictors.[26] Because contraction of the basilar artery to both receptor-mediated and nonreceptor-mediated agonists were reduced to a similar extent, reductions in vascular contraction appear to be nonspecific. Decreases in vascular distensibility that occur with aging[2,3] may contribute to nonspecific impairment of maximum contractile responses in cerebral blood vessels. The normal decrease in cerebral blood flow that occurs during hypocapnia also appears to be impaired in aged humans.[27]

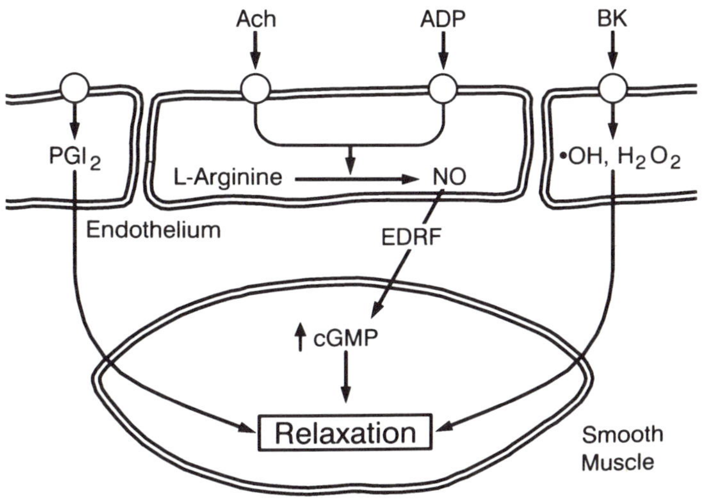

FIGURE 2. Schematic diagram of synthesis of vasoactive factors from endothelium of cerebral arterioles. Endothelium produces prostacyclin (PGI_2) and nitric oxide (NO) in response to receptor mediated agonists. Both hydroxyl radical (· OH) and hydrogen peroxide (H_2O_2) may mediate relaxation in response to bradykinin (BK). cGMP = cyclic GMP; Ach = acetylcholine; ADP = adenosine diphosphate; EDRF = endothelium-derived relaxing factor.

VI. ENDOTHELIUM-DEPENDENT RESPONSES

A. PROSTACYCLIN

Endothelium produces several potent vasoactive factors including prostacyclin and endothelium-derived relaxing factor (EDRF) (Figure 2).[28-30] Prostacyclin, a metabolite of arachidonic acid, produces relaxation of blood vessels including cerebral arteries[31,32] and is a powerful inhibitor of platelet aggregation.[28,33] Relaxation of vascular muscle in response to prostacyclin appears to be due to activation of adenylate cyclase and accumulation of cyclic AMP.[28]

Factors that regulate prostacyclin production in cerebral vessels under normal conditions are not well defined. Although vascular muscle may synthesize prostacyclin, endothelium is presumably the major source of prostacyclin produced by cerebral arteries *in vitro*.[34-36] Both bradykinin and thrombin increase prostacyclin production in human basilar arteries *in vitro*.[34] Using cultured cells, bradykinin, thrombin, and A23187 have been shown to be potent stimuli for production of prostacyclin in cerebral endothelium.[37,38]

Reduction in synthesis of prostacyclin appears to occur during aging. An age-related decrease in prostacyclin formation has been observed in human aortic endothelium in culture.[39] In studies of platelet-endothelial interaction in the aorta, the inhibitory effect of the vessel wall on platelet aggregation is reduced in vessels from aged animals suggesting that prostacyclin (or EDRF) formation is decreased.[40] Similar decreases in formation of prostacyclin may also occur with aging in cerebral endothelium.

B. ENDOTHELIUM-DERIVED RELAXING FACTOR

Endothelium-derived relaxing factor has been identified as nitric oxide (NO) or a related NO-containing compound.[41,42] Nitric oxide is produced from the amino acid L-arginine by NO synthase. After release by endothelium, nitric oxide stimulates soluble guanylate cyclase in vascular muscle which results in a rise in cyclic cGMP and relaxation.[41,43]

In vitro and *in vivo* studies of blood vessels from both animals and humans have demonstrated that relaxation of large cerebral arteries in response to acetylcholine and a number of other agonists is endothelium-dependent and mediated by EDRF.[44-51] Dilatation of cerebral arterioles in response to acetylcholine and ADP *in vivo* is also dependent on formation of nitric oxide (Figure 2).[52-56]

L-arginine, the substrate for NO synthase, has no significant effect on tone of large cerebral arteries *in vitro* or *in vivo*[44,51,52] suggesting that availability of L-arginine for NO synthase is not limiting under normal conditions. In pial arterioles, L-arginine has been observed to have no effect[54,56] or to produce small dilator responses *in vivo.*[55]

Several lines of evidence including measurements of cyclic GMP levels in vascular muscle, changes in vessel diameter or tension, and decreases in cerebral blood flow in response to administration of inhibitors of NO synthase suggest that EDRF influences resting tone of cerebral blood vessels.[57-63] In addition to an influence on vascular tone, EDRF may also be important as an inhibitor of platelet and leukocyte adherence to cerebral endothelium.[64,65]

There appears to be more than one EDRF in the cerebral microcirculation. For example, although responses of cerebral arterioles to bradykinin and acetylcholine are both endothelium-dependent, the mechanisms that mediate dilatation in response to these agonists are different (Figure 2).[66-69] Dilatation of cerebral arterioles in response to acetylcholine is mediated by nitric oxide (EDRF) and not inhibited by indomethacin or scavengers of oxygen radicals.[54,68] In contrast, responses of pial arterioles to bradykinin are inhibited by indomethacin, superoxide dismutase (SOD) and catalase, and by deferoxamine.[66,68,69] These findings suggest that the relaxing factor produced by endothelium in cerebral arterioles in response to bradykinin is hydroxyl radical or possibly hydrogen peroxide in some species (Figure 2).[66-69]

C. AGING AND EDRF

Aging is associated with impairment of endothelium-dependent responses in cerebral blood vessels. Dilatation of cerebral arterioles in response to acetylcholine and bradykinin is less in aged than in adult rats.[25] Because bradykinin and acetylcholine produce dilatation of pial arterioles through different mechanisms (Figure 2), these findings suggest that more than one endothelium-dependent mechanism is impaired in cerebral arterioles with aging. Responses to products released by platelets are also impaired in aged rats. Dilatation of pial arterioles in response to ADP and serotonin is reduced in aged rats.[25] In contrast, vasodilatation in response to nitroglycerin is similar in adult and aged rats suggesting that impaired responses were specific for endothelium-dependent mechanisms and did not involve reduced activity of guanylate cyclase or other impairment of vascular muscle.[25]

Similar to findings in the cerebral microcirculation of rats, aging is associated with impaired endothelium-dependent relaxation of the human basilar artery to thrombin.[49] Relaxation of the basilar artery in response to the endothelium-independent agonist, sodium nitroprusside, is not altered by age, suggesting that activity of guanylate cyclase and accumulation of cGMP are not impaired with aging in human cerebral arteries.[49]

Mechanisms which account for impaired endothelium-dependent responses in cerebral blood vessels during aging are not clear. Impaired responses may be due to the simultaneous production of a contracting factor produced by endothelium as has been described in the aorta of aged rats.[70] However, indomethacin does not restore impaired responses of cerebral arterioles to ADP, serotonin, and acetylcholine toward normal in aged rats.[25] Thus, impaired endothelium-dependent dilatation in the cerebral microcirculation does not appear to be related to production of an endothelium-derived contracting factor that is cyclooxygenase-dependent.[25]

Impaired endothelium-dependent responses in cerebral blood vessels with aging may be due to decreased availability of L-arginine or reduced activity of NO synthase. Such a mechanism appears to be present in atherosclerotic blood vessels because treatment with L-arginine restores impaired endothelium-dependent relaxation toward normal.[71]

In addition to endothelium, both neurons and astrocytes can produce nitric oxide.[72-74] Excitatory amino acids such as the glutamate analogue *N*-methyl-D-aspartate (NMDA) result in increased neuronal synthesis of nitric oxide and marked increases in cyclic GMP in brain tissue.[73] Recent studies suggest that nitric oxide produced by neurons in response to activation of glutamate receptors produces local vasodilation in brain.[75] Because increases in cGMP in brain tissue in response to NMDA are impaired in aged rats,[76] it seems likely that the influence of neuronally derived nitric oxide on the microcirculation may also diminish with age.

VII. SUMMARY AND IMPLICATIONS

Aging is associated with several alterations in blood vessels of the cerebral circulation. Included in these alterations are decreased vascular distensibility, changes in innervation by perivascular nerve fibers, decreases in resting levels of blood flow, changes in vascular responses, and impairment of endothelium-dependent mechanisms (Figure 1).

In the presence of endothelial dysfunction, platelet-endothelial interactions may be altered during aging in cerebral blood vessels (Figure 3). Platelets from aged humans exhibit increased aggregability and produce increased

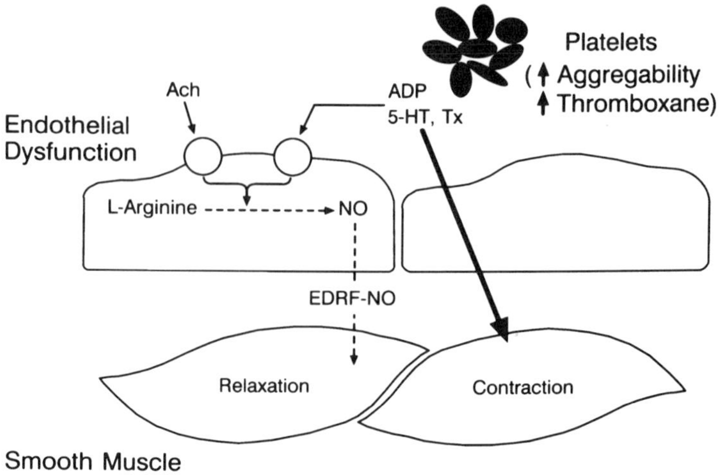

FIGURE 3. Schematic diagram of possible interaction of platelets and endothelium in aged blood vessels. Production of nitric oxide (NO) or endothelium-derived relaxing factor (EDRF) is impaired with aging (indicated by broken line). Aggregability and thromboxane (Tx) formation is increased in aged platelets. In the presence of impaired production of NO, the direct constrictor effects of serotonin (5-HT) and thromboxane predominate (indicated by heavy line).

amounts of thromboxane, a potent vasoconstrictor.[77,78] Impaired formation of inhibitors of platelet aggregation (prostacyclin and nitric oxide) and increased platelet aggregability may increase the incidence of platelet activation and adherence and thus thrombotic events with age. In the presence of impaired formation of nitric oxide, direct constrictor effects of serotonin and thromboxane on cerebral blood vessels predominate (Figure 3), and the balance of vascular tone is shifted toward vasoconstriction with aging.

ACKNOWLEDGMENTS

The author thanks Dr. Donald Heistad for critical review of the manuscript. Original studies summarized in this review from the author's laboratory were supported by National Institutes of Health grants HL-38901 and NS-24621. F. M. Faraci is an Established Investigator of the American Heart Association.

REFERENCES

1. **Docherty, J. R.,** Cardiovascular responses in ageing: a review, *Pharmacol. Rev.,* 42, 103, 1990.
2. **Nagasawa, S., Handa, H., Okumura, A., Naruo, Y., Moritake, K., and Hayashi, K.,** Mechanical properties of human cerebral arteries. I. Effects of age and vascular smooth muscle activation, *Surg. Neurol.,* 12, 297, 1979.
3. **Hajdu, M. A., Heistad, D. D., Siems, J. E., and Baumbach, G. L.,** Effects of aging on mechanics and composition of cerebral arterioles in rats, *Circ. Res.,* 66, 1747, 1990.
4. **Hervonen, A., Kimura, A., Sato, A., and Sato, Y.,** Responses of cortical cerebral blood flow produced by stimulation of cervical sympathetic trunks are well maintained in aged rats, *Neurosci. Lett.,* 120, 55, 1990.
5. **Linville, D. G. and Arneric, S. P.,** Cortical cerebral blood flow governed by the basal forebrain: age-related impairments, *Neurobiol. Aging,* 12, 503, 1991.
6. **Hoffman, W. E., Albrecht, R. F., and Miletich, D. J.,** The role of adenosine in CBF increases during hypoxia in young vs aged rats, *Stroke,* 15, 124, 1984.
7. **Buchweitz-Milton, E. and Weiss, H. R.,** Cerebral oxygen consumption and blood flow in Fischer-344 rats of different ages, *Neurobiol. Aging,* 8, 55, 1987.
8. **Hoffman, W. E., Miletich, D. J., and Albrecht, R. F.,** Cerebrovascular and cerebral metabolic responses of aged rats to changes in arterial PCO_2, *Neurobiol. Aging,* 3, 141, 1982.
9. **Martin, A. J., Friston, K. J., Colebatch, J. G., and Frackowiak, R. S. J.,** Decreases in regional cerebral blood flow with normal aging, *J. Cereb. Blood Flow Metab.,* 11, 684, 1991.
10. **Leenders, K. L., Perani, D., Lammertsma, A. A., Heather, J. D., Buckingham, P., Healy, M. J. R., Gibbs, J. M., Wise, R. J. S., Hatazawa, J., Herold, S., Beaney, R. P., Brooks, D. J., Spinks, T., Rhodes, C., Frackowiak, R. S. J., and Jones, T.,** Cerebral blood flow, blood volume and oxygen utilization. Normal values and effect of age, *Brain,* 113, 27, 1990.
11. **Yamamoto, M., Meyer, J. S., Sakai, F., and Yamaguchi, F.,** Aging and cerebral vasodilator responses to hypercapnia, *Arch. Neurol.,* 37, 489, 1980.
12. **Reich, T. and Rusinek, H.,** Cerebral cortical and white matter reactivity to carbon dioxide, *Stroke,* 20, 453, 1989.
13. **Itoh, M., Hatazawa, J., Miyazawa, H., Matsui, H., Meguro, K., Yanai, K., Watanuki, S., Ido, T., and Matsuzawa, T.,** Stability of cerebral blood flow and oxygen metabolism during normal aging, *Gerontology,* 36, 43, 1990.
14. **Lacombe, P. and Sercombe, R.,** Cerebral circulation and intracerebral systems in the aging brain, in *Neurotransmission and Cerebrovascular Function,* Vol. 1, Excerpta Medica, Amsterdam, 1989, 29.
15. **Lassen, N. A.,** Control of cerebral circulation in health and disease, *Circ. Res.,* 34, 749, 1974.
16. **Edvinsson, L. and McCulloch, J.,** *Peptidergic Mechanisms in the Cerebral Circulation,* Ellis Horwood, Chichester, 1987, 1.
17. **MacKenzie, E. T. and Scatton, B.,** Cerebral circulatory and metabolic effects of perivascular neurotransmitters, *Crit. Rev. Clin. Neurol.,* 2, 357, 1987.
18. **Bonvento, G., MacKenzie, E. T., and Edvinsson, L.,** Serotonergic innervation of the cerebral vasculature: relevance to migraine and ischaemia, *Brain Res. Rev.,* 16, 257, 1991.
19. **Mione, M. C., Dhital, K. K., Amenta, F., and Burnstock, G.,** An increase in the expression of neuropeptide vasodilator, but not vasoconstrictor, cerebrovascular nerves in aging rats, *Brain Res.,* 460, 103, 1988.
20. **Cowen, T. and Thrasivoulou, C.,** Cerebrovascular nerves in old rats show reduced accumulation of 5-hydroxytryptamine and loss of nerve fibers, *Brain Res.,* 513, 237, 1990.

21. **Edvinsson, L., Ekman, R., and Ottosson, A.,** Demonstration of perivascular peptides and changes in concentration with age in man, *Gerontology,* 32(Suppl. 1), 50, 1986.
22. **Busija, D. W. and Heistad, D. D.,** Factors involved in the physiological regulation of the cerebral circulation, *Rev. Physiol. Biochem. Pharmacol.,* 101, 161, 1984.
23. **Jones, J. V. and Graham, D. I.,** Hypertension and the cerebral circulation — its relevance to the elderly, *Am. Heart J.,* 96, 270, 1978.
24. **Hamel, E., Assumel-Lurdin, C., Bouloy, M., and Mackenzie, E. T.,** Selective age-related changes in neuronal markers and smooth muscle reactivity in cerebrovascular beds of Fischer 344 rats, *Neurobiol. Aging,* 11, 631, 1990.
25. **Mayhan, W. G., Faraci, F. M., Baumbach, G. L., and Heistad, D. D.,** Effects of aging on responses of cerebral arterioles, *Am. J. Physiol.,* 258, H1138, 1990.
26. **Hatake, K., Wakabayashi, I., Kakishita, E., and Hishida, S.,** Effect of aging on contractile response to KCl, norepinephrine and 5-hydroxytryptamine in isolated human basilar artery, *Gen. Pharmacol.,* 23, 417, 1992.
27. **Yamaguchi, F., Meyer, J. S., Sakai, F., and Yamamoto, M.,** Normal human aging and cerebral vasoconstrictive responses to hypocapnia, *J. Neurol. Sci.,* 44, 87, 1979.
28. **Gryglewski, R. J., Botting, R. M., and Vane, J. R.,** Prostacyclin: from discovery to clinical application, in *Cardiovascular Significance of Endothelium-Derived Vasoactive Factors,* Rubanyi, G. M., Ed., Futura, Mt. Kisco, NY, 1991, 3.
29. **Vane, J. R., Anggard, E. E., and Botting, R. M.,** Regulatory functions of the vascular endothelium, *New Engl. J. Med.,* 323, 27, 1990.
30. **Luscher, T. F. and Vanhoutte, P. M.,** *The Endothelium: Modulator of Cardiovascular Function,* CRC Press, Boca Raton, FL, 1990.
31. **Parsons, A. A. and Whalley, E. T.,** Effects of prostanoids on human and rabbit basilar arteries precontracted in vitro, *Cephalalgia,* 9, 165, 1989.
32. **Ellis, E. F., Wei, E. P., and Kontos, H. A.,** Vasodilation of cat cerebral arterioles by prostaglandins D_2, E_2, G_2, and I_2, *Am. J. Physiol.,* 237, H381, 1979.
33. **Moncada, S., Gryglewski, R., Bunting, S., and Vane, J. R.,** An enzyme isolated from arteries transforms prostaglandin endoperoxidase to an unstable substance that inhibits platelet aggregation, *Nature,* 263, 663, 1976.
34. **Okumura, R., Hatake, K., Wakabayashi, I., Suehiro, A., Hishida, S., and Kakishita, E.,** Vasorelaxant effect of trapidil on human basilar artery, *J. Pharm. Pharmacol.,* 44, 425, 1992.
35. **Goehlert, U. G., Ng Ying Kin, N. M. K., and Wolfe, L. S.,** Biosynthesis of prostacyclin in rat cerebral microvessels and the choroid plexus, *J. Neurochem.,* 36, 1192, 1981.
36. **Nosko, M., Schulz, R., Weir, B., Cook, D. A., and Grace, M.,** Effects of vasospasm on levels of prostacyclin and thromboxane A_2 in cerebral arteries of the monkey, *Neurosurgery,* 22, 45, 1988.
37. **Moore, S. A., Spector, A. A., and Hart, M. N.,** Eicosanoid metabolism in cerebromicrovascular endothelium, *Am. J. Physiol.,* 254, C37, 1988.
38. **Xu, J., Qu, Z.-X., Moore, S. A., Hsu, C. Y., and Hogan, E. L.,** Receptor-linked hydrolysis of phosphoinositides and production of prostacyclin in cerebral endothelial cells, *J. Neurochem.,* 58, 1930, 1992.
39. **Tokunaga, O., Yamada, T., Fan, J., and Watanabe, T.,** Age-related decline in prostacyclin synthesis by human aortic endothelial cells, *Am. J. Pathol.,* 138, 941, 1991.
40. **Vericel, E., Sedivy, P., and Lagarde, M.,** Decrease of the vessel wall antiaggregating activity in aged rabbits, *Age,* 14, 1, 1991.
41. **Moncada, S., Palmer, R. M. J., and Higgs, E. A.,** Nitric oxide: physiology, pathophysiology, and pharmacology, *Pharmacol. Rev.,* 43, 109, 1991.
42. **Myers, P. R., Minor, R. L., Guerra, R., Bates, J. N., and Harrison, D. G.,** Vasorelaxant properties of the endothelium-derived relaxing factor more closely resemble S-nitrosocysteine than nitric oxide, *Nature,* 345, 161, 1990.
43. **Waldman, S. A. and Murad, F.,** Cyclic GMP synthesis and function, *Pharmacol. Rev.,* 39, 163, 1987.

44. **Faraci, F. M.,** Role of nitric oxide in regulation of basilar artery tone in vivo, *Am. J. Physiol.,* 259, H1216, 1990.
45. **Katusic, Z. S.,** Endothelial L-arginine pathway and regional cerebral arterial reactivity to vasopressin, *Am. J. Physiol.,* 262, H1557, 1992.
46. **Katusic, Z. S., Shepherd, J. T., and Vanhoutte, P. M.,** Vasopressin causes endothelium-dependent relaxations of the canine basilar artery, *Circ. Res.,* 55, 575, 1984.
47. **Katusic, Z. S., Marshall, J. J., Kontos, H. A., and Vanhoutte, P. M.,** Similar responsiveness of smooth muscle of the canine basilar artery to EDRF and nitric oxide, *Am. J. Physiol.,* 257, H1235, 1989.
48. **Whalley, E. T., Amure, Y. O., and Lye, R. H.,** Analysis of the mechanism of action of bradykinin on human basilar artery in vitro, *Naunyn-Schmiedebergs Arch. Pharmakol.,* 335, 433, 1987.
49. **Hatake, K., Kakishita, E., Wakabayashi, I., Sakiyama, N., and Hishida, S.,** Effect of aging on endothelium-dependent vascular relaxation of isolated human basilar artery to thrombin and bradykinin, *Stroke,* 21, 1039, 1990.
50. **Kanamura, K., Waga, S., Fujimoto, K., Itoh, H., and Kubo, Y.,** Endothelium-dependent relaxation of human basilar arteries, *Stroke,* 20, 1208, 1989.
51. **Alonso, M. J., Salaices, M., Sanchez-Ferrer, C. F., and Marin, J.,** Predominant role of nitric oxide in the relaxation induced by acetylcholine in cat cerebral arteries, *J. Pharmacol. Exp. Ther.,* 261, 12, 1992.
52. **Faraci, F. M.,** Role of endothelium-derived relaxing factor in cerebral circulation: large arteries vs. microcirculation, *Am. J. Physiol.,* 261, H1038, 1991.
53. **Mayhan, W. G.,** Endothelium-dependent responses of cerebral arterioles to adenosine 5′diphosphate, *J. Vasc. Res.,* 29, 353, 1992.
54. **Mayhan, W. G., Simmons, L. K., and Sharpe, G. M.,** Mechanism of impaired responses of cerebral arterioles during diabetes mellitus, *Am. J. Physiol.,* 260, H319, 1991.
55. **Rosenblum, W. I., Nishimura, H., and Nelson, G. H.,** Endothelium dependent L-arg- and L-NMMA-sensitive mechanisms regulate tone of brain microvessels, *Am. J. Physiol.,* 259, H1396, 1990.
56. **Bauknight, C., Faraci, F. M., and Heistad, D. D.,** Endothelium-derived relaxing factor modulates noradrenergic constriction of cerebral arterioles in rabbits, *Stroke,* 23, 1522, 1992.
57. **Kovach, A. G. B., Szabo, C., Benyo, Z., Csaki, C., Greenberg, J. H., and Reivich, M.,** Effects of N^G-nitro-L-arginine and L-arginine on regional cerebral blood flow in the cat, *J. Physiol. (London),* 449, 183, 1992.
58. **Kim, P., Schini, V. B., Sundt, T. M., and Vanhoutte, P. M.,** Reduced production of cGMP underlies the loss of endothelium-dependent relaxations in the canine basilar artery after subarachnoid hemorrhage, *Circ. Res.,* 70, 248, 1992.
59. **Lee, T. J. F. and Sarwinski, S. J.,** Nitric oxidergic neurogenic vasodilation in the porcine basilar artery, *Blood Vessels,* 28, 407, 1991.
60. **Edwards, D. H., Byrne, J. V., and Griffith, T. M.,** The effect of chronic subarachnoid hemorrhage on basal endothelium-derived relaxing factor activity in intrathecal cerebral arteries, *J. Neurosurg.,* 76, 830, 1992.
61. **Faraci, F. M. and Heistad, D. D.,** Endothelium-derived relaxing factor inhibits constrictor responses of large cerebral arteries to serotonin, *J. Cereb. Blood Flow Metab.,* 12, 500, 1992.
62. **Tanaka, K., Gotoh, F., Gomi, S., Takashima, S., Mihara, B., Shirai, T., Nogawa, S., and Nagata, E.,** Inhibition of nitric oxide synthesis induces a significant reduction in local cerebral blood flow in the rat, *Neurosci. Lett.,* 127, 129, 1992.
63. **Kozniewska, E., Oseka, M., and Stys, T.,** Effects of endothelium-derived nitric oxide on cerebral circulation during normoxia and hypoxia in the rat, *J. Cereb. Blood Flow Metab.,* 12, 311, 1992.

64. **Bath, P. M. W., Hassall, D. G., Gladwin, A. M., Palmer, R. M. J., and Martin, J. F.,** Nitric oxide and prostacyclin. Divergence of inhibitory effects on monocyte chemotaxis and adhesion to endothelium in vitro, *Arteriosclerosis Thromb.*, 11, 254, 1991.
65. **Nishimura, H., Rosenblum, W. I., Nelson, G. H., and Boynton, S.,** Agents that modify EDRF formation alter antiplatelet properties of brain arteriolar endothelium in vivo, *Am. J. Physiol.*, 261, H15, 1991.
66. **Rosenblum, W. I.,** Hydroxyl radical mediates the endothelium-dependent relaxation produced by bradykinin in mouse cerebral arterioles, *Circ. Res.*, 61, 601, 1987.
67. **Yang, S. T., Mayhan, W. G., Faraci, F. M., and Heistad, D. D.,** Mechanisms of impaired endothelium-dependent cerebral vasodilatation in response to bradykinin during chronic hypertension, *Stroke*, 22, 1177, 1991.
68. **Kontos, H. A., Wei, E. P., Kukreja, R. C., Ellis, E. F., and Hess, M. L.,** Differences in endothelium-dependent cerebral dilation by bradykinin and acetylcholine, *Am. J. Physiol.*, 258, H1261, 1990.
69. **Kontos, H. A., Wei, E. P., Povlishock, J. T., and Christman, C. W.,** Oxygen radicals mediate the cerebral arteriolar dilation from arachidonate and bradykinin in cats, *Circ. Res.*, 55, 295, 1984.
70. **Koga, T., Takata, Y., Kobayashi, K., Takishita, S., Yamashita, Y., and Fujishima, M.,** Age and hypertension promote endothelium-dependent contractions to acetylcholine in the aorta of the rat, *Hypertension*, 14, 542, 1989.
71. **Drexler, H., Zeiher, A. M., Meinzer, K., and Just, H.,** Correction of endothelial dysfunction in coronary microcirculation of hypercholesterolaemic patients by L-arginine, *Lancet*, 338, 1546, 1991.
72. **Bredt, D. S. and Snyder, S. H.,** Nitric oxide, a novel neuronal messenger, *Neuron*, 8, 3, 1992.
73. **Garthwaite, J.,** Glutamate, nitric oxide and cell-cell signaling in the nervous system, *Trends Neurosci.*, 14, 60, 1991.
74. **Murphy, S., Minor, R. L., Welk, G., and Harrison, D. G.,** Evidence for an astrocyte-derived vasorelaxing factor with properties similar to nitric oxide, *J. Neurochem.*, 55, 349, 1990.
75. **Faraci, F. M. and Breese, K. R.,** Nitric oxide mediates vasodilatation in response to activation of *N*-methyl-D-aspartate receptors in brain, *Circ. Res.*, 72, 426, 1993.
76. **de Vente, J., Bol, J. G. J. M., Berkelmans, H. S., Schipper, J., and Steinbusch, H. M. W.,** Immunocytochemistry of cGMP in the cerebellum of the immature, adult, and aged rat: the involvement of nitric oxide. A micropharmacological study, *Eur. J. Neurosci.*, 2, 845, 1990.
77. **Vericel, E., Croset, M., Sedivy, P., Courpron, Ph., Dechavanne, M., and Lagarde, M.,** Platelets and aging. I. Aggregation, arachidonate metabolism and antioxidant status, *Thromb. Res.*, 49, 331, 1988.
78. **Notarbartolo, A., Catalano, I., and Davi, G.,** Platelets, eicosanoids and aging, *Aging Clin. Exp. Res.*, 4, 13, 1992.

Chapter 23

RESPONSES OF CEREBRAL BLOOD VESSELS DURING DIABETES MELLITUS

William G. Mayhan

TABLE OF CONTENTS

I. Introduction 354

II. Morphology of the Endothelium during Diabetes Mellitus 354

III. Endothelium-Dependent Responses of Cerebral Blood Vessels during Diabetes Mellitus 355
- A. Responses of Pial Arterioles 355
- B. Responses of the Basilar Artery 357

IV. Mechanisms of Impaired Endothelium-Dependent Responses of Cerebral Blood Vessels during Diabetes Mellitus 358
- A. Mechanism of Impaired Responses in Pial Arterioles 360
- B. Mechanism of Impaired Responses of the Basilar Artery 360

V. Summary and Implications 362

Acknowledgments 363

References 363

0-8493-5096-0/93/$0.00 + $.50

I. INTRODUCTION

Diabetes mellitus produces abnormalities of the microcirculation in many vascular beds, including the cerebral circulation. Diabetes mellitus appears to be a contributing factor in the pathogenesis of many cerebrovascular events, including stroke.[1-4] The mechanisms by which diabetes mellitus contributes to the pathogenesis of stroke, however, are not clear.

Since the studies of Furchgott and Zawadski[5] it has become apparent that endothelial cells participate actively in the dilatation of large and small blood vessels by releasing an endothelium-derived relaxing factor (EDRF). Recent studies have identified EDRF as nitric oxide or a compound with the pharmacological properties of nitric oxide.[6-8] In addition, we and others have found that cerebral arteries and arterioles dilate in response to agonists which are known to release EDRF, and these responses can be modulated by inhibitors of nitric oxide formation.[9-18] Thus, endothelium of cerebral arteries and arterioles contributes to cerebral vascular responses to many important agonists.

We have suggested that the pathogenesis of cerebrovascular abnormalities during diabetes mellitus may be related to altered endothelium-dependent responses of cerebral blood vessels.[12,19] This may be particularly critical for responses of cerebral blood vessels to products released by platelets. Platelets contain large amounts of serotonin, adenosine 5′-diphosphate (ADP), and thromboxane which are released during platelet aggregation. Aggregation and adherence of platelets to endothelium is increased during diabetes mellitus.[20-24] Responses of blood vessels to products released by platelets may be modulated by the endothelium, and thus if the endothelium is altered during diabetes mellitus, impaired responses of cerebral blood vessels to endothelium-dependent products released by platelets may have important implications for the pathogenesis of stroke during diabetes mellitus.

This chapter reviews the current understanding of the effects of diabetes mellitus on endothelium-dependent responses of cerebral blood vessels and possible mechanisms by which diabetes mellitus impairs endothelium-dependent responses of cerebral blood vessels.

II. MORPHOLOGY OF THE ENDOTHELIUM DURING DIABETES MELLITUS

Diabetes mellitus produces morphological alterations in the vascular wall, i.e., smooth muscle and endothelium, of cerebral blood vessels.[25-28] During diabetes mellitus, smooth muscle cells of cerebral arterioles undergo changes in shape and in internal cellular elements, demonstrated by swelling of mitochondria and cisternae of the endoplasmic reticulum.[25,26] Similar to that observed for vascular smooth muscle, the endothelium of cerebral arterioles also exhibits changes in appearance during diabetes mellitus. In addition, there is a loss and/or degeneration of endothelium from cerebral arterioles during diabetes mellitus.[25,26]

The relationship between morphological changes in vascular smooth muscle and endothelium to functional changes in reactivity of the cerebral circulation during diabetes mellitus is not known. It is possible that morphological changes and/or loss of endothelium may contribute to impaired endothelium-dependent responses of cerebral blood vessels during diabetes mellitus.

III. ENDOTHELIUM-DEPENDENT RESPONSES OF CEREBRAL BLOOD VESSELS DURING DIABETES MELLITUS

Endothelium-dependent relaxation of peripheral arteries to acetylcholine, histamine, the calcium ionophore (A23187), and ADP *in vitro* is impaired in animal models of diabetes mellitus[29-34] and in humans with diabetes mellitus.[35] In addition, dilatation of peripheral arterioles *in vivo* in response to acetylcholine is altered during diabetes mellitus.[36] Thus, it appears that diabetes mellitus alters endothelium-dependent responses of large and small peripheral blood vessels. Our discussion will focus on studies which have examined responses of cerebral blood vessels during diabetes mellitus.

A. RESPONSES OF PIAL ARTERIOLES

We and others have examined responses of pial arterioles *in vivo* during diabetes mellitus. Studies of Rosenblum and Levasseur,[37] although not specifically designed to examine the role of the endothelium in responses of cerebral blood vessels during diabetes mellitus, found similar vasodilatation to papaverine and similar vasoconstriction to norepinephrine, serotonin, and prostaglandin $F_{2\alpha}$ in nondiabetic and diabetic mice.[37] Thus, these studies suggest that diabetes mellitus does not alter responses of pial arterioles in mice.

Recently, we examined the role of the endothelium in responses of pial arterioles in rats during diabetes mellitus. Dilatation of pial arterioles in response to acetylcholine was significantly impaired in diabetic compared to nondiabetic rats[12] (Figure 1). Impaired dilatation of pial arterioles in diabetic rats in response to acetylcholine was not related to a nonspecific effect of diabetes mellitus on vasodilatation since nitroglycerin produced similar dose-related dilatation of pial arterioles in diabetic and nondiabetic rats.[12] Thus, it appears that diabetes mellitus impairs endothelium-dependent dilatation of pial arterioles in response to acetylcholine by altering endothelial cell function.

In addition to examining responses of pial arterioles to acetylcholine during diabetes mellitus, we examined responses of pial arterioles to products released by platelets.[12,19] ADP produced marked dilatation of pial arterioles in nondiabetic rats, but only minimal dilatation in diabetic rats (Figure 2).[12,19]

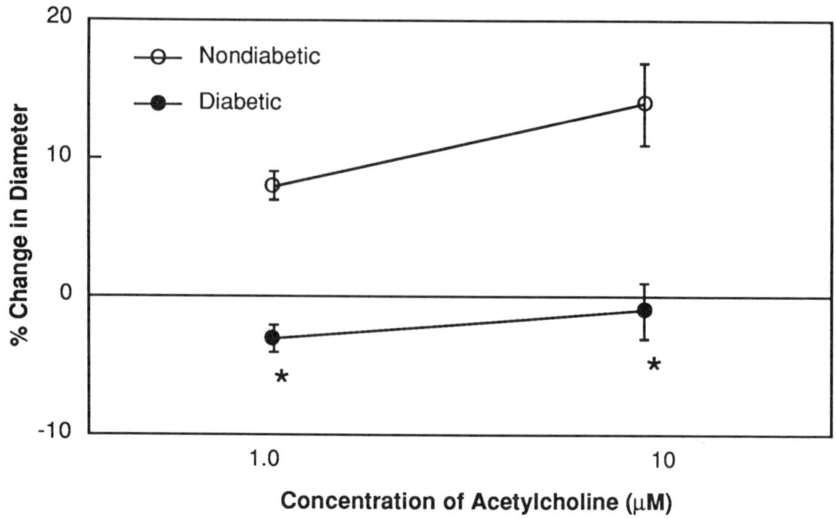

FIGURE 1. Responses of pial arterioles to acetylcholine in nondiabetic (open circle) and diabetic (closed circle) rats. Values are mean ± SE. $*p < 0.05$ vs. response in nondiabetic rats. (From Mayhan, W. G., et al., *Am. J. Physiol.*, 260, H319, 1991. With permission.)

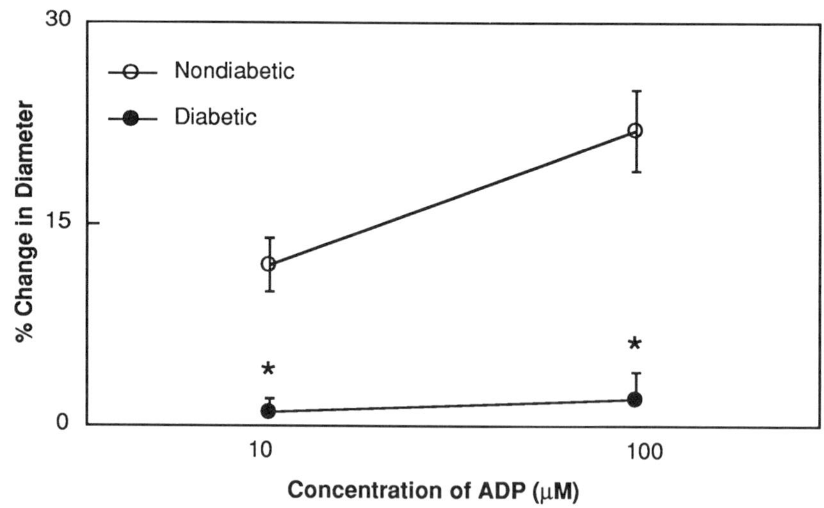

FIGURE 2. Responses of pial arterioles to ADP in nondiabetic (open circles) and diabetic (closed circles) rats. Values are mean ± SE. $*p < 0.05$ vs. response in nondiabetic rats. (Data from Mayhan, W. G., et al., and Mayhan, W. G., *Am. J. Physiol.*, 260, H319, 1991 and 256, H621, 1989. With permission.)

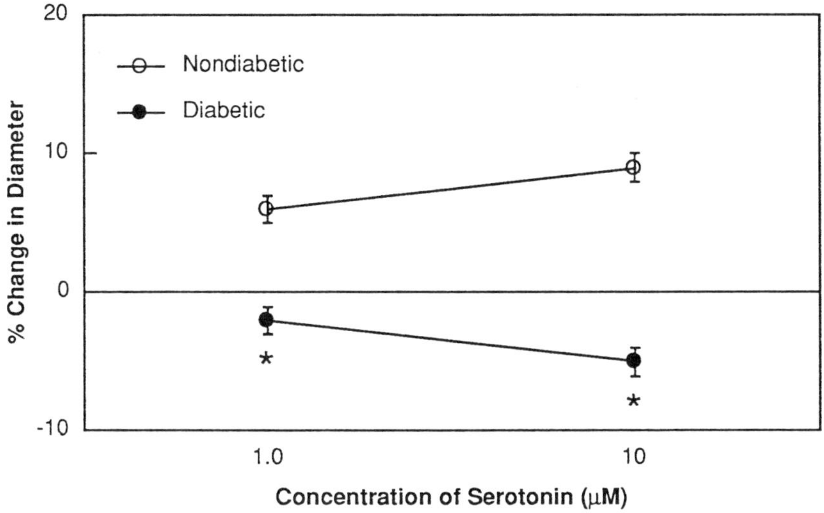

FIGURE 3. Responses of pial arterioles to serotonin in nondiabetic (open circles) and diabetic (closed circles) rats. Values are mean ± SE. $^{*}p < 0.05$ vs. response in nondiabetic rats. (Data from Mayhan, W. G., *Am. J. Physiol.*, 256, H621, 1989. With permission.)

Serotonin dilated pial arterioles in nondiabetic rats, but constricted pial arterioles in diabetic rats[19] (Figure 3). The thromboxane analogue (U46619) produced similar constriction of pial arterioles in nondiabetic and diabetic rats.[12,19] Thus, endothelium-dependent dilatation of pial arterioles in response to products released by platelets (ADP and serotonin) is impaired in diabetic rats.

We suggest that when platelets aggregate and release ADP, serotonin, and thromboxane, impairment of dilator responses to ADP and serotonin coupled with preservation of constrictor responses to thromboxane may contribute to the pathogenesis of cerebral ischemia and perhaps stroke during diabetes mellitus.

B. RESPONSES OF THE BASILAR ARTERY

Evidence suggests that there are important regional differences in responses of cerebral blood vessels to endothelium-dependent agonists. In contrast to studies of pial arterioles, in which acetylcholine produces dilatation by releasing an EDRF, studies *in vitro* suggest that acetylcholine has either no effect, constricts, or relaxes the basilar artery.[38-42] We[43] and others[10,11] have shown that acetylcholine dilates the basilar artery in rats by releasing nitric oxide or a compound with the pharmacological properties of nitric oxide. Furthermore, in contrast to pial arterioles in which bradykinin produces dilation by the production of oxygen radicals generated via the cyclooxygenase pathway,[44-46] studies suggest that bradykinin relaxes the basilar artery independent of the release of oxygen radicals and the cyclooxygenase pathway.[43,47,48]

There also appear to be important regional differences in responses of cerebral blood vessels to products released by platelets. ADP produces relaxation of large cerebral arteries *in vitro*[49] and we have shown that ADP produces endothelium-dependent dilatation of pial arterioles in rats *in vivo*.[12,13,19,50,51] In contrast, ADP produces only minimal dilation of the rat basilar artery *in vivo*,[52-54] and ADP has been reported to produce both relaxation and contraction of the canine basilar artery *in vitro*.[55,56] Serotonin produces constriction of large pial arteries and dilatation of small pial arterioles[57-59] *in vivo* and endothelium-dependent constriction of pial arterioles in mice *in vivo*.[60] We have reported that serotonin produces modest dilatation of pial arterioles in rats *in vivo*,[50,51] but constriction of the basilar artery in rats *in vivo*.[52-54]

Since there appear to be important regional differences in responses of cerebral vessels to many vasoactive agonists, we examined the effects of diabetes mellitus on endothelium-dependent responses of the basilar artery.

Acetylcholine and bradykinin produced marked dilatation of the basilar artery in nondiabetic rats, but only minimal dilatation of the basilar artery in diabetic rats (Figure 4).[61] Dilatation of the basilar artery in response to nitroglycerin, however, was similar in nondiabetic and diabetic rats suggesting that impaired dilatation of the basilar artery in response to acetylcholine and bradykinin was specific for endothelium-dependent agonists.[61] Thus, similar to that reported for pial arterioles, diabetes mellitus impairs endothelium-dependent responses of the basilar artery.

Next, we examined the effects of diabetes mellitus on responses of the basilar artery to products released by platelets.[53] Adenosine 5′-diphosphate produced only minimal changes in diameter of the basilar artery which was similar in nondiabetic and diabetic rats.[53] In addition, constriction of the basilar artery in response to serotonin and the thromboxane analogue (U46619) was similar in nondiabetic and diabetic rats.[53] Thus, in contrast to that observed for pial arterioles, responses of the basilar artery to products released by platelets (ADP and serotonin) do not appear to be altered during diabetes mellitus.

IV. MECHANISMS OF IMPAIRED ENDOTHELIUM-DEPENDENT RESPONSES OF CEREBRAL BLOOD VESSELS DURING DIABETES MELLITUS

Previous studies using *in vitro* methodology have examined mechanisms of impaired endothelium-dependent responses of the thoracic aorta in diabetic rabbits[30,62] and rats.[63] Tesfamariam et al.[30] suggest that impaired endothelium-

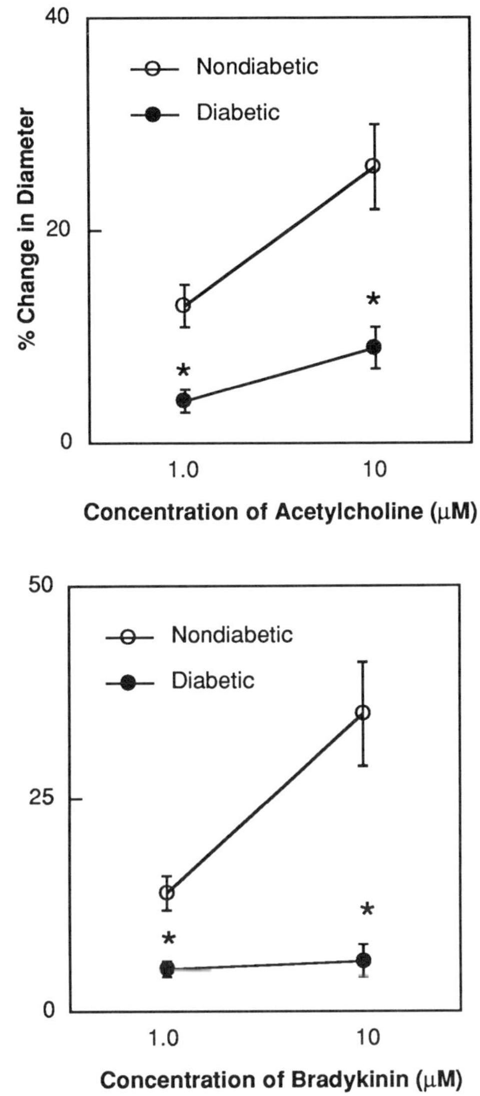

FIGURE 4. Responses of the basilar artery to acetylcholine and bradykinin in nondiabetic (open circles) and diabetic (closed circles) rats. Values are mean ± SE. $^*p < 0.05$ vs. response in nondiabetic rats. (Data from Mayhan, W. G., *Brain Res.*, 580, 297, 1992. With permission.)

dependent relaxation of the aorta during diabetes mellitus may be related to the production of a cyclooxygenase constrictor substance and presumably related to activation of the thromboxane A_2/prostaglandin H_2 receptor.[30] These investigators found that indomethacin and/or SQ 29548 (a specific thromboxane A_2/prostaglandin H_2 receptor antagonist) restored relaxation of the thoracic aorta to acetylcholine in diabetic rabbits to that observed in nondiabetic rabbits.[30] Additional studies by Tesfamariam et al.[62] suggest that acute exposure of the thoracic aorta to elevated levels of glucose impairs acetylcholine-induced endothelium-dependent relaxation, which can be restored towards that observed in nondiabetic rabbits by treatment with protein kinase C inhibitors (H-7 and sphingosine). These investigators concluded that impaired endothelium-dependent relaxation of the aorta during acute elevations in glucose was related to a increased production of a prostanoid constrictor substance, due to the activation of protein kinase C.[62] Finally, studies by Hattori et al.[63] have suggested that impaired endothelium-dependent relaxation of the thoracic aorta in rats during diabetes mellitus may be related to an increased production of superoxide anion. Treatment of the thoracic aorta with superoxide dismutase restored the profile for relaxation of the aorta in response to acetylcholine, histamine, and ADP towards that observed in nondiabetic rats.[63] Thus, previous studies have examined mechanisms of impaired endothelium-dependent responses of large peripheral blood vessels during diabetes mellitus. We have recently extended studies of peripheral blood vessels to studies which have examined the mechanism of impaired responses of cerebral blood vessels during diabetes mellitus.

A. MECHANISM OF IMPAIRED RESPONSES IN PIAL ARTERIOLES

To determine whether impaired responses of pial arterioles in diabetic rats may be related to the production of a cyclooxygenase constrictor substance, we examined responses of pial arterioles to agonists before and after treatment with indomethacin.[12] Indomethacin restored dilator responses of pial arterioles to acetylcholine and ADP in diabetic rats towards that observed in nondiabetic rats.[12]

We also have investigated the precise nature of the constrictor substance responsible for impaired responses of pial arterioles in diabetic rats.[12] The thromboxane A_2/prostaglandin H_2 receptor antagonist, SQ 29548, restored dilatation of pial arterioles in response to acetylcholine and ADP in diabetic rats towards that observed in nondiabetic rats (Figure 5).[12]

These findings suggest that synthesis and release of a cyclooxygenase constrictor substance, presumably a substance which activates the thromboxane A_2/prostaglandin H_2 receptor, are responsible for impaired endothelium-dependent dilatation of pial arterioles during diabetes mellitus.

B. MECHANISM OF IMPAIRED RESPONSES OF THE BASILAR ARTERY

We examined the possibility that impaired responses of the basilar artery in diabetic rats may be related to the activation of the thromboxane A_2/prostaglandin H_2 receptor.[61] We found that treatment with SQ 29548 did not alter responses of the basilar artery to acetylcholine and bradykinin in diabetic

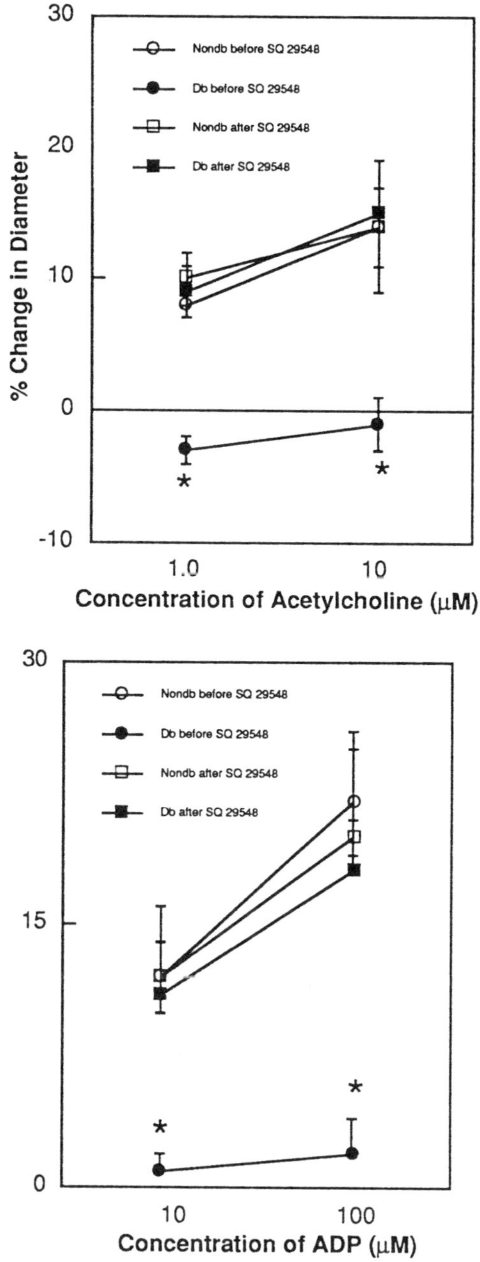

FIGURE 5. Responses of pial arterioles to acetylcholine and ADP in nondiabetic (open circles) and diabetic (closed circles) rats before SQ 29548 and to acetylcholine and ADP in nondiabetic (open squares) and diabetic (closed squares) after SQ 29548. Values are mean ± SE. $*p < 0.05$ vs. response in nondiabetic rats. (Data from Mayhan, W. G., et al., *Am. J. Physiol.*, 260, H319, 1991. With permission.)

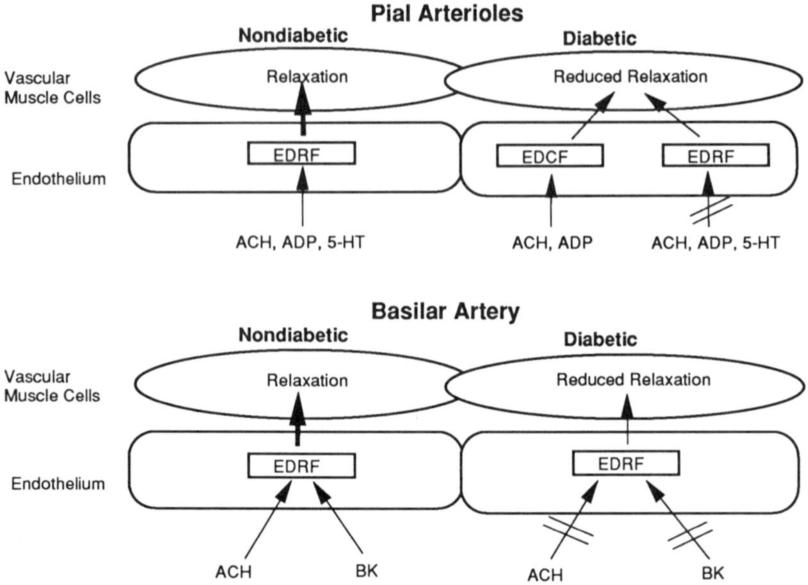

FIGURE 6. Schematic illustration of the proposed effects of diabetes mellitus on endothelium-dependent responses of cerebral blood vessels, and possible mechanisms by which diabetes mellitus impairs endothelium-dependent responses of cerebral blood vessels.

rats.[61] Thus, it appears that the mechanism of impaired dilatation of the basilar artery in diabetic rats in response to endothelium-dependent agonists, unlike that found for pial arterioles,[12] is not related to the activation of the thromboxane A_2/prostaglandin H_2 receptor.

V. SUMMARY AND IMPLICATIONS

Diabetes mellitus produces morphological and functional alterations of the endothelium in many vascular beds, including the cerebral circulation. Diabetes mellitus also appears to be an important contributing factor to the pathogenesis of stroke. We have investigated the role of the endothelium in modulating reactivity of cerebral blood vessels during diabetes mellitus and possible mechanisms for impaired responses of cerebral blood vessels during diabetes mellitus. We found that diabetes mellitus impairs endothelium-dependent responses of cerebral blood vessels. The mechanism of impaired responses of cerebral blood vessels during diabetes mellitus, however, appears to be different for large and small cerebral blood vessels (Figure 6). In nondiabetic animals, acetylcholine and endothelium-dependent products released by platelets produce relaxation of vascular muscle by releasing EDRF. Impaired responses of pial arterioles during diabetes mellitus appear to be related to the production of a cyclooxygenase constrictor substance (EDCF) and are presumably related to activation of the thromboxane A_2/prostaglandin

H_2 receptor (Figure 6). The mechanism of impaired responses of the basilar artery to endothelium-dependent agonists appears to be different than for pial arterioles (Figure 6). In nondiabetic animals, acetylcholine and bradykinin produce relaxation of vascular muscle by releasing EDRF. In contrast to pial arterioles, impaired responses of the basilar artery during diabetes mellitus do not appear to be related to the release of an EDCF, but may involve impaired synthesis and/or release of EDRF (Figure 6). We suggest that altered endothelial cell function may have important implications for the pathogenesis of stroke during diabetes mellitus.

ACKNOWLEDGMENTS

Original studies were supported by funds from the National Heart, Lung, and Blood Institute Grant HL-40781, Research Career Development Award HL02124, Grant-in-Aid from the American Heart Association (National Affiliate; 91006230), Grant-in-Aid from the American Heart Association (Nebraska Affiliate; NE-89-G-21), Grant-in-Aid from the American Heart Association (Iowa Affiliate; IA-87-G-22), and from the Nebraska Cancer and Smoking Disease Research Program (92-32).

REFERENCES

1. **Abbott, R. D., Donahue, R. P., MacMahon, S. W., Reed, D. M., and Yano, K.,** Diabetes and the risk of stroke, *JAMA,* 257, 949, 1987.
2. **Kannel, W. B. and McGee, D. L.,** Diabetes and cardiovascular disease, *JAMA,* 241, 2035, 1979.
3. **Hingorani, V. and Brecher, P.,** Glucose and fatty acid metabolism in normal and diabetic rabbit cerebral microvessels, *Am. J. Physiol.,* 252, E648, 1987.
4. **Wolf, P. A., Kannel, W. B., and Verter, J.,** Current status of risk factors for stroke, *Neurol. Clin.,* 1, 317, 1983.
5. **Furchgott, R. F. and Zawadski, J. V.,** The obligatory role of endothelial cells in the relaxation of arterial smooth muscle by acetylcholine, *Nature,* 288, 373, 1980.
6. **Rees, D. D., Palmer, R. M. J., Hodson, H. F., and Moncada, S.,** A specific inhibitor of nitric oxide formation from L-arginine attenuates endothelium-dependent relaxation, *Br. J. Pharm.,* 96, 418, 1989.
7. **Palmer, R. M. J., Ferrige, A. G., and Moncada, S.,** Nitric oxide release accounts for the biological activity of endothelium derived relaxing factor, *Nature,* 327, 524, 1987.
8. **Ignarro, L. J.,** Biosynthesis and metabolism of endothelium-derived nitric oxide, *Annu. Rev. Pharmacol. Toxicol.,* 30, 535, 1990.
9. **Faraci, F. M., Mayhan, W. G., and Heistad, D. D.** Endothelium-dependent responses of cerebral blood vessels in vivo, in *Endothelium-Derived Relaxing Factors,* Rubanyi, G. M. and Vanhoutte, P. M., Eds., S. Karger, Basel, 1990, 185.
10. **Faraci, F. M.,** Role of nitric oxide in regulation of basilar artery tone in vivo, *Am. J. Physiol.,* 259, H1216, 1990.
11. **Faraci, F. M.,** Role of endothelium-derived relaxing factor in cerebral circulation: large arteries vs. microcirculation, *Am. J. Physiol. Heart Circ. Physiol.,* 261, H1038, 1991.

12. **Mayhan, W. G., Simmons, L. K., and Sharpe, G. M.,** Mechanism of impaired responses of cerebral arterioles during diabetes mellitus, *Am. J. Physiol.,* 260, H319, 1991.
13. **Mayhan, W. G.,** Endothelium-dependent responses of cerebral arterioles to adenosine 5′-diphosphate, *J. Vasc. Res.,* 29, 353, 1992.
14. **Rosenblum, W. I. and Nelson, G. H.,** Endothelium dependence of dilation of pial arterioles in mouse brain by calcium ionophore, *Stroke,* 19, 1379, 1988.
15. **Rosenblum, W. I.,** Endothelial dependent relaxation demonstrated in vivo in cerebral arterioles, *Stroke,* 17, 494, 1986.
16. **Rosenblum, W. I., Nishimura, H., and Nelson, G. H.,** Endothelium-dependent L-arg- and L-NMMA-sensitive mechanisms regulate tone of brain microvessels, *Am. J. Physiol.,* 259, H1396, 1990.
17. **Marshall, J. J. and Kontos, H. A.,** Endothelium-derived relaxing factors. A perspective from in vivo data, *Hypertension,* 16, 371, 1990.
18. **Kontos, H. A., Wei, E. P., Kukreja, R. C., Ellis, E. F., and Hess, M. L.,** Differences in endothelium-dependent cerebral dilation by bradykinin and acetylcholine, *Am. J. Physiol.,* 258, H1261, 1990.
19. **Mayhan, W. G.,** Impairment of endothelium-dependent dilatation of cerebral arterioles during diabetes mellitus, *Am. J. Physiol.,* 256, H621, 1989.
20. **Alessandrini, P., McRae, J., Feman, S., and FitzGerald, G. A.,** Thromboxane biosynthesis and platelet function in type I diabetes mellitus, *New Engl. J. Med.,* 319, 208, 1988.
21. **Heath, H., Brigden, W. D., and Canever, J. V.,** Platelet adhesiveness and aggregation in relation to diabetic retinopathy, *Diabetologia,* 7, 308, 1971.
22. **Dunbar, J. C., Reinholt, L., Henry, R. L., and Mammen, E.,** Platelet aggregation and disaggregation in the streptozotocin induced diabetic rat: the effect of sympathetic inhibition, *Diab. Res. Clin. Prac.,* 9, 265, 1990.
23. **Mayne, E. C., Bridges, J. M., and Weaver, J. A.,** Platelet adhesiveness, platelet fibrinogen, and factor VIII levels in diabetes mellitus, *Diabetologia,* 36, 978, 1970.
24. **Sagel, J., Colwell, J. A., and Crook, L.,** Increased platelet aggregation in early diabetes mellitus, *Ann. Int. Med.,* 82, 733, 1975.
25. **Moore, S. A., Bohlen, H. G., Miller, B. G., and Evan, A. P.,** Cellular and vessel wall morphology of cerebral cortical arterioles after shortterm diabetes in adult rats, *Blood Vessels,* 22, 265, 1985.
26. **Bohlen, H. G.,** Cerebral microvascular control in normal, hypertensive and diabetic conditions, in *Microvascular Perfusion and Transport in Health and Disease,* McDonagh, P. F., Ed., S. Karger, Basel, 1987, 80.
27. **Johnson, P. C., Brendel, K., and Meezan, E.,** Thickened cerebral cortical capillary basement membranes in diabetes, *Arch. Pathol. Lab. Med.,* 106, 214, 1982.
28. **Lorenzi, M.,** The blood-brain barrier in diabetes mellitus, *Adv. Exp. Biol. Med.,* 274, 381, 1990.
29. **Oyama, Y., Kawasaki, H., Hattori, Y., and Kanno, M.,** Attenuation of endothelium dependent relaxation in aorta from diabetic rats, *Eur. J. Pharmacol.,* 131, 75, 1986.
30. **Tesfamariam, B., Jakubowski, J. A., and Cohen, R. A.,** Contraction of diabetic rabbit aorta caused by endothelium-derived PGH2-TxA2, *Am. J. Physiol.,* 257, H1327, 1989.
31. **Wakabayashi, I., Hatake, K., Kimura, N., Kakishita, E., and Nagai, K.,** Modulation of vascular tonus by the endothelium in experimental diabetes, *Life Sci.,* 40, 643, 1987.
32. **Durante, W., Sen, A. K., and Sunahara, F. A.,** Impairment of endothelium dependent relaxation in aortae from spontaneously diabetic rats, *Br. J. Pharmacol.,* 94, 463, 1988.
33. **Meraji, S., Jayakody, L., Senartine, M. P. J., Thomson, A. B. R., and Kappagada, T.,** Endothelium dependent relaxation in aorta of BB rat, *Diabetes,* 36, 978, 1987.
34. **Pieper, G. M. and Gross, G. J.,** Oxygen free radicals abolish endothelium dependent relaxation in diabetic rat aorta, *Am. J. Physiol.,* 255, H825, 1988.

35. **Saenz De Tejada, I., Goldstein, I., Azadzoi, K., Krane, R. J., and Cohen, R. A.,** Impaired neurogenic and endothelium-mediated relaxation of penile smooth muscle from diabetic men with impotence, *New Engl. J. Med.,* 320, 1025, 1989.
36. **Lash, J. M. and Bohlen, H. G.,** Structural and functional origins of suppressed acetylcholine vasodilation in diabetic rat intestinal arterioles, *Circ. Res.,* 69, 1259, 1991.
37. **Rosenblum, W. I. and Levasseur, J. E.,** Microvascular responses of intermediate size arterioles on the cerebral surface of diabetic mice, *Microvasc. Res.,* 28, 368, 1984.
38. **Kanamura, K., Waga, S., Kojima, T., Fujimoto, K., and Itoh, H.,** Endothelium dependent relaxation of canine basilar arteries, *Stroke,* 18, 932, 1987.
39. **Katusic, Z. S., Shepherd, J. T., and Vanhoutte, P. M.,** Endothelium dependent contractions to calcium ionophore A23187, arachidonic acid, and acetylcholine in canine basilar arteries, *Stroke,* 19, 476, 1988.
40. **Kanamaru, K., Waga, S., Fujimoto, K., Itoh, H., and Kubo, Y.,** Endothelium-dependent relaxation of human basilar arteries, *Stroke,* 20, 1208, 1989.
41. **Nakagomi, T., Kassell, N. F., Sasaki, T., Fujiwara, S., Lehman, R. M., and Torner, J. C.,** Impairment of endothelium dependent vasodilation induced by acetylcholine and adenosine triphosphate following experimental subarachnoid hemorrhage, *Stroke,* 18, 482, 1987.
42. **Chiba, S., Itoh, N., and Tsuji, T.,** Vascular responses to intraluminal acetylcholine in isolated, perfused canine and simian basilar arteries, *J. Auton. Pharmacol.,* 6, 101, 1986.
43. **Mayhan, W. G.,** Impairment of endothelium-dependent dilatation of basilar artery during chronic hypertension, *Am. J. Physiol.,* 259, H1455, 1990.
44. **Kontos, H. A., Wei, E. P., Povlishock, J. T., and Christman, C. W.,** Oxygen radicals mediate the cerebral arteriolar dilation from arachidonate and bradykinin in cats, *Circ. Res.,* 55, 295, 1984.
45. **Rosenblum, W. I.,** Hydroxyl radical mediates the endothelium dependent relaxation produced by bradykinin in mouse cerebral arterioles, *Circ. Res.,* 61, 601, 1987.
46. **Yang, S. T., Mayhan, W. G., Faraci, F. M., and Heistad, D. D.,** Mechanisms of impaired endothelium-dependent cerebral vasodilatation in response to bradykinin in hypertensive rats, *Stroke,* 22, 1177, 1991.
47. **Katusic, Z. S., Marshall, J. J., Kontos, H. A., and Vanhoutte, P. M.,** Similar responsiveness of smooth muscle of the canine basilar artery to EDRF and nitric oxide, *Am. J. Physiol.,* 257, H1235, 1989.
48. **Whalley, E. T., Amure, Y. O., and Lye, R. H.,** Analysis of the mechanism of action of bradykinin on human basilar artery in vitro, *Arch. Pharmacol.,* 335, 433, 1987.
49. **Hardebo, J. E., Kahrstrom, J., and Owman, Ch.,** P1 and P2 purine receptors in brain circulation, *Eur. J. Pharmacol.,* 144, 343, 1987.
50. **Mayhan, W. G., Faraci, F. M., and Heistad, D. D.,** Impairment of endothelium dependent responses of cerebral arterioles in chronic hypertension, *Am. J. Physiol.,* 253, H1435, 1987.
51. **Mayhan, W. G., Faraci, F. M., and Heistad, D. D.,** Responses of cerebral arterioles to adenosine 5′-diphosphate, serotonin, and the thromboxane analogue U-46619 during chronic hypertension, *Hypertension,* 12, 556, 1988.
52. **Mayhan, W. G.,** Responses of the basilar artery to products released by platelets during chronic hypertension, *Brain Res.,* 545, 97, 1991.
53. **Mayhan, W. G.,** Effect of diabetes mellitus on responses of the basilar artery in rats to products released by platelets, *Stroke,* 23, 1499, 1992.
54. **Faraci, F. M., Mayhan, W. G., and Heistad, D. D.,** Responses of rat basilar artery to acetylcholine and platelet products in vivo, *Stroke,* 22, 56, 1991.
55. **Shirahase, H., Usui, H., Manabe, K., Kurahashi, K., and Fujiwara, M.,** Endothelium-dependent contraction and -independent relaxation induced by adenine nucleotides and nucleoside in the canine basilar artery, *J. Pharmacol. Exp. Ther.,* 247, 1152, 1988.
56. **Katusic, Z. S., Shepherd, J. T., and Vanhoutte, P. M.,** Vasopressin causes endothelium dependent relaxations of the canine basilar artery, *Circ. Res.,* 55, 575, 1984.

57. **Thompson, L. P. and Webb, R. C.,** Vascular responsiveness to serotonin metabolites in mineralocorticoid hypertension, *Hypertension,* 9, 277, 1987.
58. **Auer, L. M., Leber, K., and Sayama, I.,** Effect of serotonin and its antagonist ketanserin on pial vessels, *J. Cereb. Blood Flow Metab.,* 5, 517, 1985.
59. **Harper, A. M. and MacKenzie, E. T.,** Effects of 5-hydroxytryptamine on pial arteriolar calibre in anaesthetized cats, *J. Physiol.,* 735, 746, 271.
60. **Rosenblum, W. I. and Nelson, G. H.,** Endothelium dependent constriction demonstrated in vivo in mouse cerebral arterioles, *Circ. Res.,* 63, 837, 1988.
61. **Mayhan, W. G.,** Impairment of endothelium-dependent dilatation of the basilar artery during diabetes mellitus, *Brain Res.,* 580, 297, 1992.
62. **Tesfamariam, B., Brown, M. L., and Cohen, R. A.,** Elevated glucose impairs endothelium-dependent relaxation by activating protein kinase C, *J. Clin. Invest.,* 87, 1643, 1991.
63. **Hattori, Y., Kawasaki, H., Abe, K., and Kanno, M.,** Superoxide dismutase recovers altered endothelium-dependent relaxation in diabetic rat aorta, *Am. J. Physiol.,* 261, H1086, 1991.

Chapter 24

EFFECTS OF TRAUMATIC BRAIN INJURY ON CEREBRAL BLOOD FLOW

Koichi Okiyama and Tracy K. McIntosh

TABLE OF CONTENTS

I. Ischemia 368

II. Hyperemia 371

III. Disturbances of Cerebrovascular Reactivity 372
- A. Autoregulation 372
- B. CO_2 Reactivity 372
- C. Metabolic Regulation 374

IV. Conclusion 375

Acknowledgment 375

References 375

0-8493-5096-0/93/$0.00 + $.50

It is generally believed that abnormalities in the cerebral circulation exist following traumatic brain injury.[1] These changes in the cerebral circulation may play an important role in the pathophysiology of traumatic brain injury and may contribute to the development of secondary or delayed brain damage. Recent studies on acute head injury have revealed wide variations of derangements in the cerebral circulation, including ischemia, hyperemia, and impaired cerebrovascular reactivity. Since these studies have utilized various methods and protocols to evaluate cerebral blood flow (CBF), one must consider several factors which might influence the CBF data, including: (1) the timing of CBF measurements, (2) type of lesions (focal or diffuse brain injury), (3) the method of measurement (global and regional CBF measurements), (4) treatment and management of the patient (e.g., hyperventilation, treatment with mannitol and/or barbiturates, surgery), and (5) the patient population with regard to age, injury severity, and general systemic factors. Alterations in CBF following traumatic brain injury observed in recent clinical and experimental studies are summarized in Table 1 and 2.

I. ISCHEMIA

It has been suggested that cerebral ischemia may be one of the most important mechanisms in the production of secondary brain damage after severe brain trauma.[2] Post-mortem studies have indicated that there is a high incidence of histopathologic ischemic brain damage after severe head injury.[3,4] In addition, experimental studies have demonstrated that an acute but global decrease in CBF occurs after traumatic brain injury, which might lead to secondary brain damage, although the fall in CBF does not approach the ischemic flow threshold of infarction.[5-7] Nevertheless, most of earlier clinical studies on acute head injury failed to demonstrate the evidence for cerebral ischemia.[8-10]

Similar to studies of acute spinal cord trauma, which have shown a linear dose-dependent relationship between the reduction in spinal cord blood flow and the severity of injury during the first few hours after trauma,[11,12] it can be speculated that ischemia, if present, may occur in the first few hours after clinical brain injury and may not have been detected at the time the first CBF study was performed.[10,13] This possibility is supported by experimental studies, generally showing that the most profound decrease in regional CBF occurs in the first few hours after brain injury.[5-7,14] In studies of clinical head injury, a depression of CBF is often seen in the early hours after injury.[13,15] Bouma et al.[16] reported that CBF was low during the first 6 h after injury and found CBF below the threshold for infarction (CBF $\leq$ 18 ml/100 g/min) in one third of the CBF values obtained within 6 h, suggesting that an acute period of ischemia does occur in a subset of severely head-injured patients. These investigators also demonstrated that a significant correlation exists between motor score and CBF in the first 8 h after injury. Using stable xenon-133

TABLE 1
Alterations in CBF Following Traumatic Brain Injury: Recent Clinical Studies

Author	Number of Patients	Technique	Observation
Bouma and Muizelaar, 1992[37]	161	^{133}Xe (Inhalation/ intravenous)	Early ischemia (0–12 h postinjury)
Marion et al., 1991[17]	61	^{133}Xe/CT CBF	Early reduced flow (0–24 h postinjury)
Muizelaar et al., 1989[9]	32	^{133}Xe (Inhalation/ intravenous)	Reduced flow/relative & absolute hyperemia
Obrist et al., 1984[10]	186	^{133}Xe (Intravenous)	Reduced flow/relative & absolute hyperemia
Robertson et al., 1992[68]	102	N_2O Saturation method	Reduced flow/normal/ hyperemia

TABLE 2
Alterations in CBF Following Traumatic Brain Injury: Experimental Studies

Author	Species	Technique	Observation
DeWitt et al., 1986[57]	Cat	Microspheres	Transient increase (1 min)
Lewelt et al., 1980[40]	Cat	Hydrogen clearance	Disturbed autoregulation (1–6 h)
Lewelt et al., 1982[42]	Cat	Hydrogen clearance	Impaired CO_2 reactivity (1–3 h)
Nilsson and Nordstrom, 1977[60]	Rat	^{14}Cethanol ^{133}Xe inhalation	Reduced flow (2–4, 10–20, 40 min)
Pfenninger et al., 1989[14]	Piglet	Microspheres	Reduced flow/ischemia (5, 30, 90 min)
Yamakami and McIntosh, 1989[5]	Rat	Microspheres	Reduced flow (15, 30 min; 1, 2 h)
Yamakami and McIntosh, 1990[6]	Rat	Microspheres	Reduced flow (15, 30 min; 1, 2 h)
Yuan et al., 1988[7]	Rat	Microspheres	Reduced flow (5, 15, 30, 60 min)

Note: Numbers in parentheses represent time postinjury.

computerized tomography CBF measurements (xenon-CT CBF), Marion et al.[17] recently found that during the first 4 h posttrauma, patients without surgical mass lesions showed a trend toward low initial flows with subsequent increase in CBF at 24 h, and that low CBF in the first 24 h postinjury was significantly correlated with a low initial Glasgow coma scale (GCS) score in patients without mass lesions. On the other hand, using Technetium-99m-hexamethylpropyleneamine (HMPAO) single photon emission computed tomography (SPECT), focal decreased perfusion (which may not be detected by global CBF measurement such as the ^{133}Xe technique) has been reported in the acute stage of head injury.[18,19] Taken together, these recent data indicate that either regional or global CBF reduction with subsequent ischemia might occur within the first few hours after severe brain injury, and the decreased perfusion might have important effects on neurologic status and outcome.

Global cerebral metabolic rate of oxygen ($CMRO_2$) is often decreased after brain trauma and has shown to be inversely related to the severity of coma as defined by the GCS.[10] Therefore, posttraumatic oligemia might be a secondary result of impaired metabolism via normal flow-metabolism coupling, and reduced blood flow may not necessarily indicate ischemia. It has also been reported that depressed CBF later in the posttraumatic course usually reflects either low metabolic demands or brain energy failure.[16] It should be noted, however, that determination of $CMRO_2$ involves the measurement of global CBF and arterio-jugular venous difference in oxygen content ($AVDO_2$) in most studies of acute head injury.[10,16] In addition to the argument that jugular venous blood may not accurately represent oxygen content throughout the brain,[20] these global measurements may not detect regional heterogenous blood flow and metabolic alterations, which might occur in pathological states such as traumatic brain injury.

Although the suggested presence of true ischemia in the acute posttraumatic period remains controversial, it is conceivable that the early postinjury period is associated with concomitant metabolic alterations which may create a "relative" ischemia in vulnerable brain regions. Using [^{14}C]2-deoxyglucose autoradiography, Yoshino et al.[21] have reported that following experimental fluid percussion brain injury in the rat, a hypermetabolic response occurs as early as 30 min postinjury which is resolved by 6 h. This acute increase in glucose utilization and energy demand, coupled with a global hypoperfusion or oligemia, may therefore reflect a state of "relative" ischemia which may adversely affect ion homeostasis, membrane function and neuronal survival.

A number of studies suggest that traumatic and ischemic brain injury share common pathological sequelae that contribute to delayed neuronal damage, including an activation of excitatory amino acid neurotransmitters.[22-24] It has also been shown that experimental brain injury increases the vulnerability of traumatized brain to secondary ischemia, which may be mediated through synaptic modifications induced by excitatory neurotransmitters.[23] Consequently, alterations in CBF, even those above the ischemic flow threshold, could provoke infarction if the insult is associated with brain trauma.

Several factors have been postulated to contribute to the posttraumatic reduction in CBF which may lead to cerebral ischemia and infarction. These include stretching and distortion of the brain vessels resulting from mechanical displacement of brain structures (e.g., brain shift or herniation caused by intracranial hypertension), arterial hypotension following multiple injuries, vasospasm, and posttraumatic changes in cerebral microvasculature.[2,25,26]

Cerebral vasospasm has been angiographically observed after severe head injury and is implicated in the etiology of posttraumatic ischemia.[27,28] Recently, using transcranial Doppler ultrasonography, several authors have demonstrated that a significant percentage of patients with severe head injury develop cerebral vasospasm.[29,30] Consequently, cerebrovascular spasm is probably one of the potential mechanisms underlying the development of posttraumatic hypoperfusion states. Recently, McIntosh and Ferriero have reported that a regional increase in the vasoconstrictor neuropeptide Y occurs following experimental fluid percussion brain injury in the rat, specifically in those brain regions showing the greatest decline in CBF following injury.[31] These authors suggest that a posttraumatic increase in neuropeptide Y may be associated with the development of regional posttraumatic vasospasm.

Pathological changes in the microvasculature may also be associated with posttraumatic hypoperfusion. It has been shown that, following acute head trauma in the nonhuman primate[26] and in humans,[32] microvascular collapse occurs due to astrocytic perivascular podocytic process swelling, suggesting that the compression of the microcirculation may cause a reduction in local tissue perfusion. With cerebral angiography, a "non-filling" phenomenon has been observed in severely head-injured patients, and a diffuse vascular collapse produced by high intracranial pressure (ICP) has been implicated in the development of such phenomena.[20]

II. HYPEREMIA

A number of clinical studies of severe head injury have demonstrated the existence of posttraumatic hyperemia.[10,33,34] However, the role of brain hyperemia in the pathophysiological cascade following head injury has not been clarified. Although cerebral hyperemia has been implicated in the development of intracranial hypertension following brain injury,[10] no strong evidence for the relationship between CBF and ICP has been found. Muizelaar et al.[9] failed to demonstrate the correlation between hyperemia and ICP and suggested that increased cerebral blood volume (CBV) may play an important role in intracranial hypertension, even though this is not always reflected in a high CBF. It has also been shown that CBV may increase while CBF may remain unchanged or even decrease.[35] These results indicate that a state of cerebrovascular congestion without a fast flow exists following brain injury, suggesting that high CBF may not necessarily indicate high ICP, and that increased CBV might contribute to the development of posttraumatic elevated ICP. The existence of this hemodynamic state of cerebral congestion is supported by positron emission tomography (PET) study, indicating that a low perfusion hyperemia (in which regional CBF [rCBF] is decreased while regional CBV [rCBV] is increased) exists in the subacute stage of cerebral contusion.[36] It has also been reported that no correlation exists between CBF and CBV, and that CBV correlated well with the pressure-volume index, which represents brain stiffness.[37] Taken in concert, increased CBV may primarily contribute to hyperemia, high ICP, as well as diffuse brain swelling following head injury.[37,38]

Since an increase in rCBV suggests an increase in the vascular beds, hyperemia has been explained as a consequence of vasomotor paralysis, i.e., acute reduction in vasomotor tone resulting in cerebral vasodilatation.[48] In addition to the impaired autoregulation, flow resistance in this instance would remain shifted to the venous side, associated with compressed venous drainage due to increased ICP. Accordingly, these factors may lead to increased vascular beds, and intracerebral congestion of the blood.

III. DISTURBANCES OF CEREBROVASCULAR REACTIVITY

A. AUTOREGULATION

Autoregulation of CBF can be defined as the physiological regulatory mechanism that maintains a constant flow over wide ranges of arterial blood pressure or cerebral perfusion pressure.[39] Despite the experimental studies suggesting that traumatic brain injury causes an impairment of cerebral autoregulation,[40] pressure autoregulation after brain trauma has been reported to be either defective or intact following clinical brain trauma.[34,41] It has also been shown that pressure autoregulation is still intact in a significant number of patients with severe head injury and that no significant relationship exists between autoregulation and posttraumatic CBF, time after injury, clinical severity, and outcome.[37]

B. CO_2 REACTIVITY

Although reduced or abolished CO_2 reactivity has been reported in the acute period following experimental brain injury,[42] reactivity of cerebrovasculature to changes in CO_2 is preserved in most head-injured patients, and, when found to be abolished (mostly in comatose patients), is associated with poor clinical prognosis.[34,41] The rationale of hyperventilation therapy, accordingly, is that elevated ICP can be improved by hyperventilation, through cerebrovascular vasoconstriction (if CO_2 reactivity is not defective), with subsequent reduction in blood volume.[10] Sustained hyperventilation, however, has been reported to be ineffective after 24 h, since cerebral arteriolar diameter, which decreases shortly after commencement of hyperventilation, returns to the baseline within 24 h.[43]

Several possible explanations for the impairment of autoregulation have been postulated. First, an accumulation of acid metabolites (e.g., lactic acid, arachidonic acid metabolites) in the brain under the conditions of either ischemia, suppressed oxidative metabolism, or increased glycolysis has been reported, resulting in the flaccidity of the vessel walls and vasoparalysis.[44] Lactic acid accumulation within the brain tissues following experimental brain trauma has been reported and implicated in brain acidosis.[45] In addition, cerebrospinal fluid lactic acidosis has been shown to correlate with cerebral hyperemia in severely head-injured patients.[33] However, a significant degree of generalized cerebral acidosis is still controversial in cerebral ischemia[46] and in brain trauma,[47,48] and diffuse loss of autoregulation cannot be explained only by tissue acidosis. Second, an increase in extracellular potassium, which has also been reported after experimental brain injury,[49] has been shown to contribute to postischemic loss of autoregulation.[50] Third, brainstem lesions have been implicated in impaired autoregulation after head injury,[41] although the role of the brainstem in the regulation of cerebrovascular reactivity is not fully understood. Finally, endothelial dysfunction may also be of major significance for defective autoregulation.[46] Recent attention has been focused on the possible involvement of endothelial cells in cerebrovascular regulation.[51] Endothelial cells may play a major role in coordinating integral responses within the vasculature.[52] The endothelium can serve as a mechanoreceptor, sensing and transducing physical stimuli into changes in vascular tone by the release of endothelium-derived contracting or relaxing factors, and may contribute to the myogenic mechanism of autoregulation of blood flow.[46,51] Accordingly, disturbances in cerebrovascular autoregulation and reactivity following trauma may be, in part, mediated by endothelial abnormalities, which have been reported after head injury.[26,32,53]

In clinical studies, several authors have found a dissociation between pressure autoregulation and CO_2 responsiveness (i.e., impaired autoregulation and preserved CO_2 reactivity, and vice versa).[41,54] This dissociative impairment may indicate that differential regulatory mechanisms of the cerebral vasculature are activated following trauma. It has been shown that autoregulatory adjustments to changes in arterial pressures occur in pial arteries between 200 and 400 μm in diameter.[55] On the other hand, while responses of pial vessels to hypocapnia are size independent, the responsiveness to hypercapnia is size dependent, with the smaller vessels (<100 μm) responding more markedly than the larger ones (>100 μm), presumably due to neurologically induced vasoconstriction of the larger vessels, which partially offsets the vasodilator effect of CO_2.[56] Differences in pial arteriolar diameter have also been demonstrated to influence the reactivity to experimental brain injury; smaller arterioles (<100 μm) exhibit a greater degree of vasodilation.[57] Abnormalities in the pial vessels, including endothelial damage, have been observed after experimental brain injury, suggesting that the sudden dilatation of the cerebral arteries and arterioles, produced by a transient rise in arterial blood pressure due to increased sympathetic activity, causes multiple endothelial lesions.[53] These authors have also shown that endothelial lesions are responsible for absent or reduced responses to hypocapnia following brain injury. In addition, the endothelial injury and dysfunction may also lead to impaired endothelium-dependent vasodilatation, resulting in hyperreactivity of underlying vascular smooth muscle and pathophysiologically elevated vascular tone (i.e., vasospasm).[68] Taken together, traumatic brain injury could cause disturbances in cerebrovascular reactivity to changes in perfusion pressure or CO_2 content through effects on the cerebral microvasculature, especially endothelial cells.

C. METABOLIC REGULATION

Although $CMRO_2$ is decreased in proportion to the level of coma after severe head injury, CBF does not necessarily decrease postinjury, indicating that an uncoupling between CBF and $CMRO_2$ occurs following severe head injury.[10] Such a loss of metabolic autoregulation, often associated with hyperemia, has been attributed, in part, to disturbances of oxidative metabolism.[37]

Experimental studies have demonstrated that traumatic brain injury produces a variety of changes in local cerebral glucose utilization (CMR_{glu}) and have suggested that the comatose state produced by experimental brain injury is not necessarily associated with a marked decrease in overall cerebral metabolism.[58-60] In addition, although it has been suggested that brain trauma may produce disturbances of oxidative metabolism,[61,62] no compelling evidence for mitochondrial dysfunction has been found.[63] Recent studies have indicated that a transient hypermetabolic response occurs following fluid percussion brain injury[21] and experimental subdural hematoma,[64] and that excitatory neurotransmission may play a major role in the development of posttraumatic hypermetabolism.[21,64] Taken together with the observation of $CMRO_2$ described above, $CMRO_2$ and CMR_{glu} do not appear to change in parallel following brain injury.

Recent studies have shown that a transient increase in physiological neuronal activity dramatically increases both glucose uptake and brain blood flow while causing minimal changes in oxygen consumption and reducing regional oxygen extraction, suggesting that neural activity regulates local blood flow for purposes other than oxidative metabolism.[65,66] The disproportionate changes in CBF and CMR_{glu} compared to $CMRO_2$ might also take place in pathological situations such as traumatic brain injury. In this case, classical tight coupling between CBF and $CMRO_2$ might be reset, and adequate CBF to support brain metabolism may not be predicted by $CMRO_2$ measurements alone.

CBF and metabolism are normally coupled statically or dynamically. Statically, rCBF is thought to be set in relation to a heterogenous distribution of regional metabolic rates.[67] In contrast to the static coupling, however, dynamic coupling is mediated through the normal coupling sequence (i.e., neuronal activity-metabolism-blood flow) as well as via direct neuronal activity.[67] Neuronal-glial activity may directly influence CBF through putative intercellular messengers. In the case of excessive activation of the neuron, a greater increase in neuronal activity than in metabolism would result in greater increase in blood flow than in metabolism, namely regional hyperperfusion.

IV. CONCLUSION

From both experimental and clinical studies, it can be concluded that either a regional or global reduction in CBF might occur within the first few hours after injury, and this decreased perfusion, including a ''relative'' ischemia, might have important effects on posttraumatic outcome. Hyperemia after brain injury may be secondary to the increased CBV, which may be primarily responsible for the development of intracranial hypertension. Functional impairment of cerebrovascular reactivity, namely cerebral vasoparalysis, may also contribute to the increased CBV.

Serial measurements of CBF beginning in the acute period following injury allow for more accurate detection of changes in CBF or abnormal cerebrovascular reactivity and should contribute to the elucidation of the pathophysiological mechanisms that occur early after traumatic brain injury. This intensive clinical intervention may assist in the development of novel and effective therapeutic strategies to prevent secondary irreversible neuronal damage and may lead to improved outcome following severe head injury. It is important to recognize the necessity of developing new pharmacologic agents which will normalize posttraumatic CBF changes and reduce the apparent pathologic hypoperfusion which may contribute to posttraumatic neuronal damage and death.

ACKNOWLEDGMENT

A portion of this work was supported, in part, by Public Health Service Grant from the National Institutes of Health (RO1-NS26818), Veterans Administration Merit Review Grant (74R), and the Brain Trauma Research Foundation.

REFERENCES

1. **Langfitt, T. W., Weinstein, J. D., and Kassell, N. F.,** Vascular factors in head injury, in *Head Injury,* Caveness, W. F. and Walker, A. E., Eds., Lippincott, Philadelphia, 1966, 172.
2. **Miller, J. D.,** Head injury and brain ischemia — Implications for therapy, *Br. J. Anaesth,* 57, 120, 1985.
3. **Graham, D. I., Adams, J. H., and Doyle, D.,** Ischaemic brain damage in fatal nonmissile head injuries, *J. Neurol. Sci.,* 39, 213, 1978.
4. **Graham, D. I., Ford, I., Adams, J. H., Doyle, D., Teasdale, G. M., Lawrence, A., and McLellan, D. R.,** Ischemic brain damage is still common in fatal nonmissile head injury, *J. Neurol. Neurosurg. Psychiatry,* 52, 346, 1989.
5. **Yamakami, I. and McIntosh, T. K.,** Effects of traumatic brain injury on regional cerebral blood flow in rats as measured with radiolabeled microspheres, *J. Cereb. Blood Flow Metab.,* 9, 117, 1989.

6. **Yamakami, I. and McIntosh, T. K.,** Alterations in regional cerebral blood flow following brain injury in the rat, *J. Cereb. Blood Flow Metab.*, 11, 655, 1991.
7. **Yuan, X.-Q., Prough, D. S., Smith, T. L., and Dewitt, D. S.,** The effects of traumatic brain injury on regional cerebral blood flow in rats, *J. Neurotrauma,* 5, 289, 1988.
8. **Enevoldsen, E. M., and Jensen, F. T.,** Compartmental analysis of regional cerebral blood flow in patients with severe head injuries, *J. Neurosurg.*, 47, 699, 1977.
9. **Mulizelaar, J. P., Marmarou, A., DeSalles, A. A. F., Ward, J. D., Zimmerman, R. S., Li, Z., Choi, S. C., and Young, H. F.,** Cerebral blood flow and metabolism in severely head-injured children. I. Relationship with GCS score, outcome, ICP, and PVI, *J. Neurosurg.*, 71, 63, 1989.
10. **Obrist, W. D., Langfitt T. W., Jaggi, J. L., Cruz, J., and Gennarelli, T. A.,** Cerebral blood flow and metabolism in comatose patients with acute head injury: Relationship to intracranial hypertension, *J. Neurosurg.*, 61, 241, 1984.
11. **Fehlings, M. G., Tator, C. H., and Linden, R. D.,** The relationships among the severity of spinal cord injury, motor and somatosensory evoked potentials and spinal cord blood flow, *Electroencephalogr. Clin. Neurophysiol.*, 74, 241, 1989.
12. **Tator, C. H. and Fehlings, M. G.,** Review of the secondary injury theory of acute spinal cord trauma with emphasis on vascular mechanisms, *J. Neurosurg,* 75, 15, 1991.
13. **Mendelow, A. D., Teasdale, G. M., Russel, T., Flood, J., Patterson, J., and Murray, G. D.,** Effect of mannitol on cerebral blood flow and cerebral perfusion pressure in human head injury, *J. Neurosurg.*, 63, 43, 1985.
14. **Pfenninger, E. G., Reith, A., Breitig, D., Grunert, A., and Ahnefeld, F. W.,** Early changes of intracranial pressure, perfusion pressure, and blood flow after acute head injury. I. An experimental study of the underlying pathophysiology, *J. Neurosurg.*, 70, 774, 1989.
15. **Overgaad, J., Mosdal, C., and Tweed, W. A.,** Cerebral circulation after head injury. III. Does reduced regional cerebral blood flow determine recovery of brain function after blunt head injury?, *J. Neurosurg.*, 55, 63, 1981.
16. **Bouma, G. J., Muizelaar, J. P., Choi, S. C., Newlon, P. G., and Young, H. F.,** Cerebral circulation and metabolism after severe traumatic brain injury: the elusive role of ischemia, *J. Neurosurg.*, 75, 685, 1991.
17. **Marion, D. W., Darby, J., and Yonas, H.,** Acute regional cerebral blood flow changes caused by severe head injuries, *J. Neurosurg.*, 74, 407, 1991.
18. **Abdel-Dayem, H. M., Sadek, S. A., Kouris, K., Bahar, R. H., Higazi, I., Eriksson, S., Englesson, S. H., Berntman, L., Sigurdsson, G. H., Foad, M., and Olivecrona, H.,** Changes in cerebral perfusion after acute head injury: comparison of CT with Tc-99m HM-PAO SPECT, *Radiology,* 165, 221, 1987.
19. **Newton, M. R., Greenwood, R. J., Britton, K. E., Charlesworth, M., Nimmon, C. C., Carroll, M. J., and Dolke, G.,** A study comparing SPECT with CT and MRI after closed head injury, *J. Neurol. Neurosurg. Psychiatry,* 55, 92, 1992.
20. **Bruce, D. A., Langfitt, T. W., Miller, J. D., Schutz, H., Vapalahti, M. P., Stanek, A., and Goldberg, H. I.,** Regional cerebral blood flow, intracranial pressure, and brain metabolism in comatose patients, *J. Neurosurg.*, 38, 131, 1973.
21. **Yoshino, A., Hovda, D. A., Kawamata, T., Katayama, Y., and Becker, D. P.,** Dynamic changes in local cerebral glucose utilization following cerebral concussion in rats: evidence of a hyperand subsequent hypometabolic state, *Brain Res.*, 561, 106, 1991.
22. **Faden, A. I., Demediuk, P., Painter, S. S., and Vink, R.,** The role of excitatory amino acids and NMDA receptors in traumatic brain injury, *Science,* 244, 798, 1989.
23. **Jenkins, L. W., Moszynski, K., Lyeth, B. G., Lewelt, W., DeWitt, D. S., Allen, A., Dixon, C. E., Povlishock, J. T., Majewski, T. J., Clifton, G. L., Young, H. F., Becker, D. P., and Hayes, R. L.,** Increased vulnerability of the mildly traumatized rat brain to cerebral ischemia: the use of controlled secondary ischemia as a research tool to identify common or different mechanisms contributing to mechanical and ischemic brain injury, *Brain Res.*, 477, 211, 1989.

24. **McIntosh, T. K., Smith, D. H., Hayes, R. L., Vink, R., and Simon, R. P.,** Role of excitatory amino acid neurotransmitters in the pathogenesis of traumatic brain injury, in *Excitatory Amino Acids,* Simon, R. P., Ed., Georg Thiem Verlag, Stuttgart, 1992, 247.
25. **Bruce, D. A. and Langfitt, T. W.,** The prognostic value of ICP, CCP, CBF, and $CMRO_2$ in head injury, in *Head Injuries. Second Chicago Symposium on Neural Trauma,* McLaurin, R. L., Ed., Grune & Stratton, New York, 1976, 23.
26. **Maxwell, W. L., Irvine, A., Adams, J. H., Graham, D. I., and Gennarelli, T. A.,** Response of cerebral microvasculature to brain injury, *J. Pathol.,* 155, 327, 1988.
27. **MacPheson, P. and Graham, D. I.,** Correlation between angiographic findings and the ischaemia of head injury, *J. Neurol. Neurosurg. Psychiatry,* 41, 122, 1978.
28. **Suwanwela, C. and Suwanwela, N.,** Intracranial arterial narrowing and spasm in acute head injury, *J. Neurosurg.,* 36, 314, 1972.
29. **Compton, J. S. and Teddy, P. J.,** Cerebral arterial vasospasm following severe head injury: a transcranial Doppler study, *Br. J. Neurosurg.,* 1, 435, 1987.
30. **Weber, M., Grolimund, P., and Seller, R. W.,** Evaluation of posttraumatic cerebral blood flow velocities by transcranial Doppler ultrasonography, *Neurosurgery,* 27, 106, 1990.
31. **McIntosh, T. K. and Ferriero, D.,** Changes in neuropeptide Y after experimental traumatic brain injury in the rat, short communication, *J. Cereb. Blood Flow Metab.,* 12, 697, 1992.
32. **Bullock, R., Maxwell, W. L., Graham, D. I., Teasdale, G. M., and Adams, J. H.,** Glial swelling following human cerebral contusion: an ultrastructural study, *J. Neurol. Neurosurg. Psychiatry,* 54, 427, 1991.
33. **Enevoldsen, E. M., Cold, G. E., Jensen, F. T., and Malmros, R.,** Dynamic changes in regional CBF, intraventricular pressure, CSF pH and lactate levels during the acute phase of head injury, *J. Neurosurg.,* 44, 191, 1976.
34. **Overgaad, J. and Tweed, W. A.,** Cerebral circulation after head injury. I. Cerebral blood flow and its regulation after closed head injury with emphasis on clinical correlations, *J. Neurosurg.,* 41, 531, 1974.
35. **Grubb, R. L., Raichle, M. E., Higgins, C. S., and Eichling, J. O.,** Measurement of regional cerebral blood volume by emission tomography, *Ann. Neurol.,* 4, 322, 1978.
36. **Tenjin, H., Ueda, S., Mizukawa, N., Imahori, Y., Hino, A., Yamaki, T., Kuboyama, T., Ebisu, T., Hirakawa, K., Yamashita, M., and Nakahashi, H.,** Positron emission tomographic studies on cerebral hemodynamics in patients with cerebral contusion, *Neurosurgery,* 26, 971, 1990.
37. **Bouma, G. J. and Muizelaar, J. P.,** Cerebral blood flow, cerebral blood volume, and cerebrovascular reactivity after severe head injury, *J. Neurotrauma,* 9, S333, 1992.
38. **Langfitt, T. W., Tannanbaum, H. K., and Kassell, N. F.,** The etiology of acute brain swelling following experimental head injury, *J. Neurosurg.,* 24, 172, 1966.
39. **Lassen, N. A.,** Cerebral blood flow and oxygen consumption in man, *Physiol. Rev.,* 39, 183, 1959.
40. **Lewelt, W., Jenkins, L. W., and Miller, J. D.,** Autoregulation of cerebral blood flow after experimental fluid percussion injury of the brain, *J. Neurosurg.,* 53, 500, 1980.
41. **Enevoldsen, E. M., and Jensen, F. T.,** Autoregulation and CO_2 responses of cerebral blood flow in patients with acute severe head injury, *J. Neurosurg.,* 48, 689, 1978.
42. **Lewelt, W., Jenkins, L. W., and Miller, J. D.,** Effects of experimental fluid-percussion injury of the brain on cerebrovascular reactivity to hypoxia and hypercapnia, *J. Neurosurg.,* 56, 332, 1982.
43. **Muizelaar, J. P., van der Poel, H. G., Li, Z. C., Kontos, H. A., and Levasseur, J. E.,** Pial arteriolar vessel diameter and CO_2 reactivity during prolonged hyperventilation in the rabbit, *J. Neurosurg.,* 69, 923, 1988.
44. **Lassen, N. A.,** The luxury-perfusion syndrome and possible relation to acute metabolic acidosis localized within the brain, *Lancet,* 2, 1113, 1966.

45. **Yang, M. S., DeWitt, D. S., Becker, D. P., and Hayes, R. L.,** Regional brain metabolite levels following mild experimental head injury in the cat, *J. Neurosurg.*, 63, 617, 1985.
46. **Paulson, O. B., Strandgaard, S., and Edvinsson, L.,** Cerebral autoregulation, *Cerebrovasc. Brain Metab. Rev.*, 2, 161, 1990.
47. **Rango, M. R., Lenkinski, R. E., Alves, W. M., and Gennarelli, T. A.,** Brain pH in head injury: an image-guided ^{31}P magnetic resonance spectroscopy study, *Ann. Neurol.*, 28, 661, 1990.
48. **Marmarou, A.,** Intracellular acidosis in human and experimental brain injury, *J. Neurotrauma*, 9, S551–S562, 1992.
49. **Katayama, Y., Becker, D. P., Tamura, T., and Hovda, D. A.,** Massive increase in extracellular potassium and the indiscriminate release of glutamate following concussive brain injury, *J. Neurosurg.*, 73, 889, 1990.
50. **Harris, R. J. and Symon, L.,** Extracellular pH, potassium, and calcium activities in progressive ischaemia of rat cortex, *J. Cereb. Blood Flow Metab.*, 4, 178, 1984.
51. **Rubanyi, G. M.,** Endothelium-derived relaxing and contracting factors, *J. Cell. Biochem.*, 46, 27, 1991.
52. **Davies, P. F., Olesen, S. P., Clapham, D. E., Morrel, E. M., and Schoen, F. J.,** Endothelial communication, *Hypertension*, 11, 563, 1988.
53. **Wei, E. P., Dietrich, W. D., Povlishock, J. T., Navari, R. M., and Kontos, H. A.,** Functional, morphological, and metabolic abnormalities of the cerebral microcirculation after concussive brain injury in cats, *Circ. Res.*, 46, 37, 1980.
54. **Harper, A. M.,** Autoregulation of cerebral blood flow: influence of the arterial blood pressure on the flow through the cerebral cortex, *J. Neurol. Neurosurg. Psychiatry*, 29, 398, 1966.
55. **Kontos, H. A., Wei, E. P., Navari, R. M., Levasseur, J. E., Rosenblum, W. I., and Patterson, J. L., Jr.,** Responses of cerebral arteries to acute hypotension and hypertension, *Am. J. Physiol.*, 234, H371, 1978.
56. **Wei, E. P., Kontos, H. A., and Patterson, J. L., Jr.,** Dependence of pial response to hypercapnia on vessel size, *Am. J. Physiol.*, 238, H697, 1980.
57. **DeWitt, D. S., Jenkins, L. W., Wei, E. P., Lutz, H., Becker, D. P., and Kontos, H. A.,** Effects of fluid-percussion brain injury on regional cerebral blood flow and pial arteriolar diameter, *J. Neurosurg.*, 64, 787, 1986.
58. **Andersen, B. J. and Marmarou, A.,** Isolated stimulation of glycolysis following traumatic brain injury, in *Intracranial Pressure VII*, Hoff, J. T. and Betz, A. L., Eds., Springer, Berlin, 1989, 575.
59. **Hayes, R. L., Katayama, Y., Jenkins, L. W., Lyeth, B. G., Clifton, G. L., Gunter, J., Povlishock, J. T., and Young, H. F.,** Regional rates of glucose utilization in the cat following concussive head injury, *J. Neurotrauma*, 5, 121, 1988.
60. **Nilsson, B. and Nordstrom, C.H.,** Rate of cerebral energy consumption in concussive head injury in the rat, *J. Neurosurg.*, 47, 274, 1977.
61. **Hovda, D. A., Yoshino, A., Kawamata, T., Katayama, Y., and Becker, D. P.,** Diffuse prolonged depression of cerebral oxidative metabolism following concussive brain injury in the rat: a cytochrome oxidase histochemistry study, *Brain Res.*, 567, 1, 1991.
62. **Unterberg, A. W., Andersen, B. J., Clarke, G. D., and Marmarou, A.,** Cerebral energy metabolism following fluid-percussion brain injury in cats, *J. Neurosurg.*, 68, 594, 1988.
63. **Vink, R., Head, V. A., Rogers, P. J., McIntosh, T. K., and Faden, A. I.,** Mitochondrial metabolism following traumatic brain injury in rats, *J. Neurotrauma*, 7, 21, 1990.
64. **Kuroda, Y., Ingris, F. M., Miller, J. D., McCulloch, J., Graham, D. I., and Bullock, R.,** Transient glucose hypermetabolism after acute subdural hematoma in the rat, *J. Neurosurg.*, 76, 471, 1992.

65. **Fox, P. T. and Raichle, M. E.,** Focal physiological uncoupling of cerebral blood flow and oxidative metabolism during somatosensory stimulation in human subjects, *Proc. Natl. Acad. Sci. U.S.A.,* 83, 1140, 1986.
66. **Fox, P. T., Raichle, M. E., Mintun, M. A., and Dence, C.,** Nonoxidative glucose consumption during focal physiologic neural activity, *Science,* 241, 462, 1988.
67. **Kuschinsky, W.,** Physiology of cerebral blood flow and metabolism, *Arzneim. Forsch./ Drug Res.,* 41, 284, 1991.
68. **Robertson, C. S., Contant, C. F., Narayan, R. K., and Grossman, R. G.,** Cerebral blood flow, $AVDO_2$, and neurologic outcome in head-injured patients, *J. Neurotrauma,* 9, S349, 1992.

Chapter 25

CEREBROVASCULAR REGULATION IN THE FETUS AND NEONATE

William J. Pearce

TABLE OF CONTENTS

I. Introduction 382

II. Cerebrovascular Reactivity During the Perinatal Period 382

III. Prostaglandins and the Neonatal Cerebral Circulation 383

IV. Neonatal Cerebral Endothelium 384

V. Cerebrovascular Innervation 385

VI. Age-Related Changes in Cerebral Perfusion and Metabolism 386

VII. Cerebral Autoregulation in the Neonate 387

VIII. Hypercapnic and Hypoxic Cerebral Vasodilatation 389

IX. Cerebral Pathophysiology During the Perinatal Period 390

X. Summary 391

References 392

0-8493-5096-0/93/$0.00 + $.50

I. INTRODUCTION

In the brain of a newborn infant, myelination is incomplete, synapses are still forming, and motor coordination is rudimentary at best. Correspondingly, the blood vessels of the brain are also immature at birth, particularly in preterm infants. At about 26 weeks of gestational age, human cerebral blood vessels begin to grow rapidly, increasing in both density and diameter, and reach peak numbers and sizes by 35 weeks.[1] Thereafter, it is the composition and function of the arteries that begins to change most dramatically; their numbers and sizes change relatively little.

One of the key compositional changes in cerebral arteries characteristic of postnatal maturation is a progressively increasing mechanical stiffness.[2,3] This increasing stiffness is due, in part, to decreases in extracellular water which are rapid during the first few days of extrauterine life and then proceed more slowly during the remainder of maturation. Simultaneously, the artery walls quickly thicken, due largely to the synthesis and extracellular deposition of collagen and elastin. As maturation proceeds, connective tissue turnover continues with the production of relatively more Type III and less Type I collagen, and increases in the collagen to elastin ratio which are greatest in the largest arteries.[4] It is these changes in connective tissue makeup that dominate increases in cerebral artery stiffness during the perinatal period.

Accompanying these changes in stiffness and composition are important changes in cerebrovascular reactivity, many of which are coincidental with changes in the circulating hormone levels that occur during the perinatal period. For example, plasma renin activity and concentrations of angiotensin II, arginine vasopressin, T3, and T4 are all higher in newborns than adults.[5] Although a causal link between changes in circulating hormone levels and changes in cerebrovascular reactivity has yet to be demonstrated, the connection seems probable in light of the well-documented ability of steroid hormones to change tissue levels of key enzymes such as sodium-potassium ATPase and guanylate cyclase.[6]

II. CEREBROVASCULAR REACTIVITY DURING THE PERINATAL PERIOD

At all ages, the contractile characteristics of cerebral arteries are heterogeneously distributed throughout the cerebrovascular tree. Such differences exist not only between arteries and veins, but also between large and small arteries, between arteries of the brainstem and those of the cortex, and between pial and parenchymal arterioles. Species differences further contribute to this heterogeneity. Thus, it is important to bear in mind both the species and the artery under study when considering cerebrovascular reactivity.[2]

Perinatal studies of the cerebral circulation have employed three main species in the majority of work published to date: the puppy, the piglet, and the lamb. Of these, cerebral development at birth is least mature in the puppy and most mature in the term lamb. Nonetheless, certain characteristics are common to the cerebral arteries of all three species. First, maximum contractile force increases with advancing age. Second, sensitivity to the nitrogenous vasodilators, such as nitroglycerine and nitroprusside, is present at birth. Third, sensitivity to the vasodilating effects of adenosine is also present at birth. In general, each of these characteristics is also present in cerebral arteries of all sizes from term human infants.[7,8]

Another characteristic common to most species is that the reactivity of the cerebral arteries to receptor-dependent agonists changes dramatically between fetal and newborn life.[3,9,10] For example, cerebral artery contractile responses to serotonin are larger in the term fetus than in the newborn lamb, and both are greater than in adult sheep. Similar changes have been reported in a wide variety of species for many different agents including norepinephrine, acetylcholine, vasoactive peptides, and others. Such changes suggest that the type and number of receptors populating the cerebral arteries are dynamic and under developmental, and, probably, hormonal control. Equally important, these populations appear subject to environmental modulation, as suggested by the finding of different patterns of receptor dependent cerebrovascular reactivity in lambs carried *in utero* at sea level and those carried at high altitude.[11]

III. PROSTAGLANDINS AND THE NEONATAL CEREBRAL CIRCULATION

One group of receptor-dependent vasoactive compounds which has been well characterized during the perinatal period is the prostaglandin family. These compounds are of major perinatal importance not only because they maintain patency of the ductus arteriosus, but also because they influence hemodynamic resistance in many vascular beds.[5,12] In addition, total prostaglandin concentrations are higher in cortical subarachnoid cerebrospinal fluid than in either the cisterna magna or arterial blood, suggesting a cortical site of synthesis.[12] Because perinatal administration of inhibitors of cyclooxygenase, a key enzyme in the synthesis of prostaglandins, can reduce cerebral perfusion in multiple species including puppies, piglets, lambs, and human infants, it appears that prostaglandins have a net vasodilating effect in the cerebral circulation during the perinatal period.[12,13]

One of the most important vasodilating prostaglandins during the perinatal period is PGE_2, a compound with potent vasodilating effects in both the piglet and the fetal baboon.[10,12] Because plasma PGE_2 is higher in the baboon fetus than in the mother, and its vasodilator potency is greater in newborns than adults, PGE_2 has been proposed to contribute to the lower cerebrovascular resistance characteristic of fetal life.[10] PGE_1 is also a potent vasodilator of cerebral, but not mesenteric, arteries of the fetal baboon. And as for PGE_2, sensitivity to PGE_1 appears to diminish with maturity.[14]

Another important vasodilating prostaglandin is prostacyclin (PGI_2). During the perinatal period, PGI_2 can reduce tone in cerebral, mesenteric, and pulmonary arteries of both piglets and baboons.[10,12,14] Prostaglandin $F_{2\alpha}$ has also been reported to promote vasodilation, but only at very low concentrations in the fetal baboon middle cerebral artery.[10] Contractile responses to $PGF_{2\alpha}$ predominate in adult baboons and in pigs of all ages.[14,15] At least in newborn piglets, the leukotrienes C_4, D_4, and E_4 all promote cerebral vasoconstriction.[16] Similarly, thromboxane analogues also promote vasoconstriction in the cerebral arteries of newborn piglets.[15]

An important feature of prostanoid metabolism, at least in the newborn piglet, is that it mediates and/or modulates the cerebrovascular responses to a wide variety of both physiological and pharmacological stimuli. For example, opioids such as enkephalins and dynorphins elicit the synthesis and release of vasodilator prostaglandins which mediate the vasodilator components of response to these opioids.[17] Lysine vasopressin is another agent that appears to promote the release of vasodilator prostanoids.[18] Conversely, the contractile responses of piglet cerebral arteries to the free radicals released by hydrogen peroxide appear to involve the synthesis and release of vasoconstrictor prostanoids.[19] However, not all cerebrovascular responses in newborn piglets involve prostanoid release; cerebral vasodilator responses to the amino acids NMDA, glutamate, aspartate, and taurine, for example, all appear independent of prostanoid release.[20]

IV. NEONATAL CEREBRAL ENDOTHELIUM

The vascular endothelium is another source of vasodilator prostanoids, particularly PGI_2, in the neonatal cerebral circulation. The cerebral endothelium of most species, including humans, is also capable at birth of synthesizing and releasing endothelium-derived relaxing factor.[8] This factor, known as EDRF, is widely held to be nitric oxide synthesized from L-arginine by the enzyme nitric oxide synthetase.[21] Nitric oxide released by the cerebral endothelium readily diffuses into the adjacent vascular smooth muscle where it activates guanylate cyclase, elevates vascular levels of cyclic GMP, and precipitates vasodilatation through the actions of cGMP-dependent protein kinase. This pathway appears fully intact at birth in multiple species, including humans, although the magnitude of endothelium-dependent relaxation may be less in neonates than in the adults of some species.[8] Cerebral endothelium can also release the peptide endothelin, which in the newborn piglet causes vasoconstriction at maximum physiological concentrations.[22] At present, however, the physiological stimuli which promote the release and action of vasoactive endothelial factors from cerebral arteries during the perinatal period remain uncertain. Current candidates include hypoxia, flow-induced shear stress, and stretch of the cerebral arterial wall.[23-25]

Aside from its potential influence on cerebrovascular tone, the cerebral endothelium also serves another important function, that of the blood brain barrier. The tight junctions typical of cerebral endothelium develop early in fetal life and then undergo active modifications during the late prenatal period in both the puppy and the lamb.[26,27] At birth, the cerebral endothelium is slightly more permeable than at maturity, and this "leaky" endothelium allows a higher serum protein concentration in the cerebrospinal fluid of neonates than in adults, and certain dyes penetrate the brain more easily in fetuses and newborns than in adults.[28] Nonetheless, the blood-brain barrier of newborns is largely impermeable to norepinephrine, angiotensin II, and hydrogen ion, suggesting that the most important aspects of blood brain barrier function are intact at birth.[26,29]

V. CEREBROVASCULAR INNERVATION

In adults, the cerebral arteries are innervated by fibers containing adrenergic, cholinergic, and peptidergic neurotransmitters. For all of these nerve types, there are three general phases of nerve development: (1) the outgrowth of new axons; (2) the development of transmitter synthesis and storage capacity; and (3) the growth and differentiation of nerve varicosities.[2] In general, postsynaptic function, reflecting the presence of appropriately coupled receptors, can usually be demonstrated before presynaptic elements are fully functional. As for contractility in general, the rate and timing of the development of the cerebrovascular innervation vary considerably among species and among different neurotransmitter systems.

The neurovascular system best characterized in cerebral arteries during the perinatal period is the adrenergic sympathetic innervation. In human fetuses, immature adrenergic nerves with few varicosities can be demonstrated at 19 to 23 weeks of gestational age and their density is greatest in the more rostral vessels.[30] In the baboon, cerebral arteries contract in response to norepinephrine and the strength of these contractions is greatest in the fetus and diminishes with age.[31] Similarly, the cerebral arteries of the newborn puppy, piglet, and lamb have all been shown to contract in response to norepinephrine.[16,32,33] In the newborn piglet, norepinephrine appears to act predominantly on alpha-1 adrenergic receptors in cerebral resistance vessels[34] and on alpha-2 adrenergic receptors in pial arterioles.[16] In the newborn piglet, norepinephrine also stimulates the release of PGE_2, which apparently limits the magnitude of the vasoconstrictor response to norepinephrine.[35] In addition, electrical stimulation of the cerebrovascular sympathetic innervation can decrease cerebral blood flow by up to 25% in the newborn lamb[36] and 15% in the newborn piglet.[37] In the lamb, as in the baboon, the responsiveness to norepinephrine is greatest in the fetus and diminishes with age, suggesting that the functional importance of the adrenergic cerebrovascular innervation is probably greater during fetal, than during adult, life.[33]

Nerves containing acetylcholine can also be demonstrated in fetal human cerebral arteries between 19 and 23 weeks of gestational age, and as for the adrenergic fibers, the fibers generally lack varicosities and are probably functionally immature.[30] In fetal and newborn baboon cerebral arteries, acetylcholine elicits a contractile response which is absent in corresponding arteries from adults.[31] In newborn piglet pial arteries, low concentrations of acetylcholine produce dilation whereas higher concentrations (100 μM) produce vasoconstriction.[29] Interestingly, indomethacin at 5 mg/kg can block pial artery contractile responses to 100 μM acetylcholine, suggesting that vasoconstrictor prostanoids, such as $PGF_{2\alpha}$ and thromboxane A_2, somehow mediate the response.[15]

Although there is some evidence of a serotonergic innervation supplying arteries of the circle of Willis in term human infants,[38] these findings remain controversial and difficult to corroborate. Certainly, receptors for serotonin are present in the cerebral arteries of most species at birth, but the pharmacological identity and cross reactivity of serotonin with these receptors and alpha adrenergic receptors in the neonatal cerebral circulation remains uncertain. On the other hand, the presence of a peptidergic innervation supplying human fetal cerebral arteries is more widely accepted.[39] These peptidergic systems supply separate nerves containing neuropeptide Y and vasoactive intestinal polypeptide to the major arteries of the circle of Willis and the large pial arteries. In fetal rats, the cerebral arteries are innervated by sensory fibers from the trigeminal ganglion which contain substance P, vasoactive intestinal polypeptide, cholecystokinin, somatostatin, and calcitonin gene-related peptide.[40] In adults, these peptides are all vasodilators. Their effects on cerebral arteries during the perinatal period, however, remain largely undocumented, as do the physiological stimuli which elicit their release.

VI. AGE-RELATED CHANGES IN CEREBRAL PERFUSION AND METABOLISM

In all mammalian species, cerebral perfusion and cerebral metabolic rate are closely coupled. Although the exact mechanisms responsible for this coupling remain elusive, the fact remains that this matching between flow and metabolism is a characteristic feature of cerebrovascular regulation, even during the perinatal period. Thus, the key to understanding age-related changes in cerebral blood flow is to focus first on the developmental changes which occur in the cerebral metabolic rate. In the newborn puppy, the brain is relatively immature at birth, cerebral metabolic rate is low, and so is cerebral perfusion. With postnatal maturation in the puppy, both cerebral metabolic rate and cerebral blood flow rise to reach adult levels.[26,41] In contrast, the lamb cerebrum is largely mature at birth, the reticular activating system is fully functional, and cerebral blood flow is higher than in adults.[42,43] For term human infants, the pattern is somewhere between these two animal models. At birth, human cerebral blood flow and cerebral metabolic rate are low, and both variables increase steadily through the first 6 years of life, after which cerebral flow and metabolism gradually decline throughout the remainder of life.[41]

Without doubt, cerebral metabolic rate is not the only factor influencing cerebral perfusion in the neonate. As shown in an extensive series of studies carried out in fetal and newborn lambs, it appears that cerebral oxygen delivery (the product of cerebral blood flow and arterial oxygen content) is an actively regulated variable.[44-47] Because the position of the oxyhemoglobin dissociation curve directly determines the amount of oxygen which can be extracted from blood by the tissue, shifts in the hemoglobin P_{50} produce corresponding shifts in the rate of cerebral perfusion; leftward shifts in the curve decrease the amount of tissue extractable oxygen and produce an increase in flow.[46,47] Correspondingly, other maneuvers that alter oxygen carrying capacity, such as hemodilution or carbon monoxide poisoning, will also alter the ratio of cerebral perfusion to metabolism.[48] Central to the concept of the regulation of oxygen delivery is the assumption of a feedback mechanism matching tissue oxygen supply and demand.[44,45,49] Although the mechanisms mediating this matching remain elusive, the ''oxygen coupling hypothesis'' remains of great value in predicting the behavior of cerebral perfusion in response to a wide variety of physiological stimuli.

Other stimuli which can influence cerebral perfusion include direct vascular stimuli, such as neurotransmitters or prostaglandins which act primarily on vascular smooth muscle, and metabolic stimuli, such as catabolic hormones or anesthetics, which act primarily to alter cerebral metabolic rate. For both classes of stimuli, their net effect is determined by how they affect the cerebral oxygen supply/demand ratio and how the mechanisms maintaining this coupling compensate. As with most biological control systems, compensation is often not complete and some ''steady state error'' will remain at equilibrium. Thus, the high carbon dioxide and PGE_2 levels typical of fetal life may contribute to a relative overperfusion of the fetal brain, at least in the ovine species.[43,47,50] In human infants, the mechanisms matching tissue oxygen supply and demand appear fully intact at birth.[48,51]

VII. CEREBRAL AUTOREGULATION IN THE NEONATE

Another feature of cerebrovascular regulation in both neonates and adults is autoregulation, defined as the ability to maintain a constant rate of cerebral perfusion despite changes in cerebral perfusion pressure (arterial pressure minus cerebrospinal fluid pressure). A key characteristic of autoregulation is the range of perfusion pressures over which it is effective. In adults, this range extends from a lower limit of approximately 50 or 60 mmHg to an upper limit of approximately 140 to 150 mmHg of cerebral perfusion pressure (Figure 1). In fetuses and neonates, cerebral perfusion pressure is considerably lower than in adults (due largely to a lower mean arterial pressure), and, correspondingly, the lower limit of autoregulation extends to lower perfusion pressures of 30 to 40 mmHg in most species, including human infants.[26,42,52,53] Similarly, the upper limit of autoregulation is also often lower in neonates

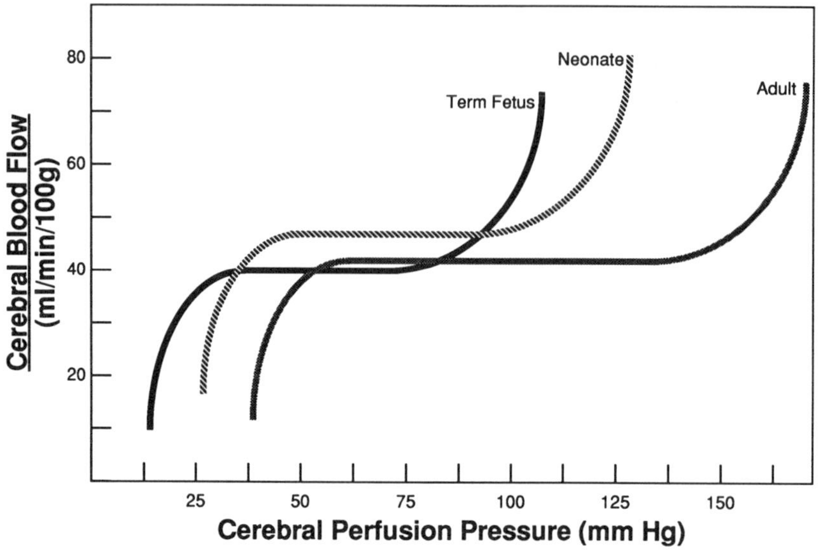

FIGURE 1. Cerebral autoregulation, depicted in an idealized form in this figure, is the integrated ability of cerebrovascular regulatory mechanisms to maintain a relatively constant level of cerebral perfusion at varying perfusion pressures. In adults, cerebral autoregulation occurs over a range of cerebral perfusion pressures between approximately 50 and 150 mmHg. Corresponding to the reduced magnitude of perfusion pressures in fetuses and neonates, the upper and lower limits of autoregulation are greater in adults than in the fetuses and newborns of most species, including humans. At birth, the level of cerebral perfusion often transiently increases, and then returns to adult levels during the first few months of extrauterine life. For additional details, see the text.

(70 to 100 mmHg), rendering the neonates of most species including human infants more vulnerable than adults to hypertensive transients.[53-55] In most species, including humans, cerebral autoregulation is fully functional at birth.[51]

One possible mediator of the autoregulatory cerebral vasodilatation induced by hypotension is tissue adenosine. Cerebral adenosine, an excellent vasodilator, has been shown to increase as cerebral perfusion pressure is lowered.[56] In addition, cerebral adenosine has also been shown to increase as cerebral oxygen supply is decreased, suggesting a possible common mechanism for the coupling of cerebral flow and metabolism, and cerebral autoregulation.[57] However, hypotension also increases the cerebrospinal fluid concentrations of a variety of other compounds including both vasodilator and vasoconstrictor prostaglandins[58-60] and opioids.[61] At the other end of the autoregulatory range, sympathetic vasoconstriction limits the increases in cerebral perfusion caused by elevated perfusion pressure in newborn piglets and thus extends the upper limit of cerebral autoregulation.[62,63] Clearly, cerebral autoregulation is a complex response involving multiple mechanisms, which may explain why it is vulnerable to a wide variety of insults including metabolic acidosis,[64] severe hypoxia or asphyxia,[65,66] cerebral ischemia,[58] and intracranial hemorrhage.[67]

VIII. HYPERCAPNIC AND HYPOXIC CEREBRAL VASODILATATION

One of the oldest known cerebral vasodilators in adults is carbon dioxide. Hypercapnia can also increase cerebral perfusion in both newborn[65] and preterm fetal lambs,[42] as well as in newborn[51] and preterm[68] human infants. In general, hypercapnia is a less potent vasodilator in newborns and infants than in adults,[69-71] although the reasons for this difference are unclear. Some of this difference may arise from the possibility that acidosis, in the range which typically accompanies hypercapnia, may be a better vasodilator in adult than in newborn cerebral arteries.[42] Alternatively, age-related changes in hematocrit may be involved, given that hematocrit has been reported to be inversely proportional to cerebral CO_2 reactivity in the newborn baboon.[72] In newborn piglets, vasodilator prostanoids mediate up to 50% of the cerebral response to hypercapnia,[12,73-75] suggesting that, at least in this species, age-related differences in prostanoid metabolism may contribute to age-related differences in hypercapnic sensitivity. In any case, hypercapnic vasodilatation in newborns apparently does not involve reflex changes in sympathetic discharge[76] or changes in cerebral metabolic rate.[70,77,78]

Acute hypoxia also elicits cerebral vasodilatation in neonates of most mammalian species, including newborn rats,[79] fetal and newborn lambs,[36,42,80] piglets,[81,82] and newborn puppies.[83-85] In newborn lambs, the response is greater than in adults, but in newborn puppies it is less, suggesting that the magnitude of the response may be related to the extent of cerebral maturation and/or cerebral metabolic rate.[43,86] Consistent with this view, the brainstem regions of both lambs and puppies, which are generally the most mature of any brain region at birth and have the highest metabolic rates, also exhibit greater responsiveness to hypoxia than other brain regions.[26,87,88]

With the onset of cerebral hypoxia, the cerebrovascular response first involves a pronounced vasodilatation which serves to increase cerebral perfusion and maintain oxygen delivery with little change in the oxygen extraction fraction (oxygen uptake/oxygen delivery). With an increasing severity of hypoxia, the cerebral oxygen extraction fraction begins to increase until maximum oxygen extraction is attained. If hypoxia becomes even more severe, then the cerebral oxygen consumption may decrease and anaerobic glycolysis may ensue with the attendant lactic acidosis.[89] Thus, hypoxic vasodilatation may be viewed as an extreme response of the mechanisms coupling cerebral oxygen supply and demand.[90] As stated above, adenosine is a possible mediator of hypoxic cerebral vasodilatation because acute hypoxia increases cerebral adenosine in adults and newborns of both rats[79] and pigs.[81,82] In newborn puppies, however, acute hypoxia also increases vasodilator prostaglandins.[91] Furthermore, hypoxia may also involve a direct effect on the vascular smooth muscle and endothelium of cerebral arteries.[23,92,93] Clearly, hypoxia is a complex stimulus which elicits multiple mechanisms of cerebrovascular response in both neonates and adults.

IX. CEREBRAL PATHOPHYSIOLOGY DURING THE PERINATAL PERIOD

One of the most common of insults to occur during the perinatal period is that of asphyxia which, in essence, is a combined stimulus of both hypercapnia and hypoxia. Thus, asphyxia dramatically increases cerebral perfusion and, at least in piglets, simultaneously increases adenosine and vasodilator prostaglandins.[12] During asphyxia in piglets, blood flow to the brainstem appears to be preferentially maintained, a pattern which may involve reflex sympathetic cerebral vasoconstriction in nonbrainstem areas.[94-96] In newborn lambs and human infants which recover from asphyxia, there is often long-term but reversible interference with both the mechanisms, which match cerebral oxygen supply and demand, and the mechanisms responsible for cerebral autoregulation.[97-100]

Cerebral ischemia is another insult common to the perinatal period which combines the effects of hypercapnia and hypoxia. Ischemia is more severe however, in that it precludes any vascular exchanges of gases, substrates, or wastes. Thus, even short-term cerebral ischemia is often associated with prolonged postrecovery increases in brain water content, inhibition of protein synthesis, disruption of cellular calcium homeostasis, and depressed prostanoid synthetic capacity, in addition to the morbidities associated with asphyxia.[101-104] Fortunately, the tolerance to cerebral ischemia appears to be greater in newborns than adults, as suggested by studies in piglets.[105,106] In human newborns, the threshold rate of cerebral blood flow below which irreversible ischemic damage is certain lies between approximately 10 and 15 ml/min/100 g.[107]

If cerebral asphyxia or ischemia are prolonged or severe enough, intraventricular hemorrhage can result, particularly in premature infants. Indeed, intraventricular hemorrhage is the most common neurological disorder in most neonatal intensive care units, with the incidence of periventricular hemorrhage approaching 40 to 45% in infants less than 35 weeks of gestational age.[108] Furthermore, the probability of periventricular hemorrhage appears inversely related to body weight with up to 60% of neonates weighing less than 1250 grams ultimately experiencing intraventricular hemorrhage.[109,110] Of particular interest is the tendency for intraventricular hemorrhage to occur predominantly in the germinal matrix region, a finding attributed to the relative immaturity of blood vessels located there.[27,108,109,111-113] Although multiple factors, including altered coagulation characteristics, acid-base imbalances, and deranged prostanoid metabolism, are probably involved,[110,114,115] it is clear that once periventricular blood appears, most normal cerebrovascular regulatory mechanisms are compromised. Perivascular blood attenuates adrenergic vasoconstriction, endothelium-mediated relaxation, hypercapnic vasodilatation, autoregulation, and a host of other responses. Clearly, the primary goal for management of periventricular hemorrhage is prevention by minimizing the influences which predispose to increased rates of cerebral perfusion.[108,113] To this end, an understanding of the basic mechanisms governing cerebral blood flow is invaluable.

X. SUMMARY

The contractile characteristics of cerebral blood vessels vary considerably between arteries and veins, between vessels of different size and anatomical location, and certainly between species. Thus it should be no surprise that the characteristics of cerebral vessels also change dramatically during development and maturation. These effects of age involve changes in both vessel composition and reactivity, coordinated by an integration of environmental and endocrinological influences. Compositionally, cerebrovascular water content decreases and connective tissue content increases during the postnatal period of most species, contributing to an overall increase in stiffness with age. In addition to a generalized increase in contractile capacity, there are also numerous changes in the profile of receptors that populate the cerebral vessels, and these changes dominate the age-related changes in reactivity observed in most species. In spite of these numerous postnatal changes, however, cerebral arteries are generally fully capable of mediating cerebrovascular homeostasis at birth in most species. Contractile responses are, on the whole, well-developed for both amines and leukotrienes, as are the mechanisms which mediate relaxations to adenosine, prostaglandins, and increased cyclic nucleotide synthesis. Endothelial function is also present at birth, although barrier function may be a little less restrictive, and the capacity for release of vasoactive factors may be slightly attenuated, relative to the adult. A cerebrovascular innervation also appears present at birth and includes nerves containing norepinephrine, acetylcholine, and various vasoactive peptides. Although the distribution and efficacy of this innervation is generally different than that found in the adult, it is nonetheless functional and may participate in cerebral vasoregulation.

At the organ level, cerebral metabolic rate and cerebral perfusion are closely coupled in the fetus and neonate, as they are in the adult. This coupling persists, even though cerebral metabolic rate usually changes significantly during the immediate postnatal period. Perhaps more importantly, cerebral autoregulation is also intact in the fetus and newborn, although the autoregulatory range is generally shifted toward lower perfusion pressures in correspondence with the lower arterial pressures which obtain in the fetus and neonate. Vasodilatory responses to hypercapnia are also evident in both the fetus and neonate, albeit with a somewhat reduced sensitivity compared to adults in some species. On the other hand, hypoxic increases in cerebral blood flow are generally equal to or greater than those of adults, depending on species. But in all species, the fetal and newborn brain is generally more fragile and less capable of adaptive compensation than the brains of adults, and, for this reason, neonates are particularly vulnerable to cerebrovascular insults such as asphyxia and ischemia, which often result short-term in periventricular hemorrhage and long-term in permanent neurological deficits.

REFERENCES

1. **Mito, T., Konomi, H., Houdou, S., and Takashima, S.,** Immunohistochemical study of the vasculature in the developing brain, *Pediatric Neurol.*, 7, 18, 1991.
2. **Duckles, S. P. and Banner, W. J.,** Changes in vascular smooth muscle reactivity during development, *Annu. Rev. Pharmacol. Toxicol.*, 24, 65, 1984.
3. **Pearce, W. J., Hull, A. D., Long, D. M., and Longo, L. D.,** Developmental changes in ovine cerebral artery composition and reactivity, *Am. J. Physiol.*, 261, R458, 1991a.
4. **Hegedus, K. and Molnar, P.,** Age-related changes in reticulin fibers and other connective tissue elements in the intima of the major intracranial arteries, *Clin. Neuropathol.*, 8, 92, 1989.
5. **Heymann, M. A., Iwamoto, H. S., and Rudolph, A. M.,** Factors affecting changes in the neonatal systemic circulation, *Annu. Rev. Physiol.*, 43, 371, 1981.
6. **Amechi, O. A., Butterworth, P. J., and Thomas, P. J.,** Effects of gonadal steroids on guanylate cyclase activity in the developing and adult brain, *Brain Res.*, 342, 158, 1985.
7. **Laudignon, N., Beharry, K., Rex, J., and Aranda, J. V.,** Effect of adenosine on total and regional cerebral blood flow of the newborn piglet, *J. Cereb. Blood Flow Metab.*, 10, 392, 1990a.
8. **Pearce, W. J. and Longo, L. D.,** Developmental aspects of endothelial function, *Semin. Perinatol.*, 15, 40, 1991b.
9. **Toda, N. and Hayashi, S.,** Age-dependent alteration in the response of isolated rabbit basilar arteries to vasoactive agents, *J. Pharmacol. Exp. Ther.*, 211, 716, 1979.
10. **Hayashi, S., Park, M. K., and Kuehl, T. J.,** Relaxant and contractile responses to prostaglandins in premature, newborn and adult baboon cerebral arteries, *J. Pharmacol. Exp. Ther.*, 233, 628, 1985.
11. **Longo, L. D. and Pearce, W. J.,** Fetal and newborn cerebral vascular responses and adaptations to hypoxia, *Semin. Perinatal Biol.*, 15, 49, 1991.
12. **Leffler, C. W. and Busija, D. W.,** Prostanoids in cortical subarachnoid cerebrospinal fluid and pial arterial diameter in newborn pigs, *Circ. Res.*, 57, 689, 1985.
13. **Saliba, E., Chantepie, A., Autret, E., Gold, F., Pourcelot, L., and Laugier, J.,** Effects of indomethacin on cerebral hemodynamics at rest and during endotracheal suctioning in preterm neonates, *Acta Paediatr. Scand.*, 80, 611, 1991.
14. **Park, M. K., Kuehl, T. J., and Hayashi, S.,** Differential effects of prostaglandins on mesenteric and cerebral arteries isolated from premature newborn baboons, *Eur. J. Pediatr.*, 146, 61, 1987a.
15. **Wagerle, L. C. and Busija, D. W.,** Effect of thromboxane A2/endoperoxide antagonist SQ29548 on the contractile response to acetylcholine in newborn piglet cerebral arteries, *Circ. Res.*, 66, 824, 1990a.
16. **Busija, D. W., Leffler, C. W., and Beasley, D. G.,** Effects of leukotrienes C4, D4, and E4 on cerebral arteries of newborn pigs, *Pediatr. Res.*, 20, 973, 1986.

17. **Armstead, W. M., Mirro, R., Busija, D. W., and Leffler, C. W.,** Prostanoids modulate opioid cerebrovascular responses in newborn pigs, *J. Pharmacol. Exp. Ther.,* 255, 1083, 1990b.
18. **Armstead, W. M., Mirro, R., Busija, D. W., and Leffler, C. W.,** Vascular responses to vasopressin are tone-dependent in the cerebral circulation of the newborn pig, *Circ. Res.,* 64, 136, 1989c.
19. **Leffler, C. W., Busija, D. W., Armstead, W. M., and Mirro, R.,** H_2O_2 effects on cerebral prostanoids and pial arteriolar diameter in piglets, *Am. J. Physiol.,* 258, H1382, 1990a.
20. **Busija, D. W. and Leffler, C. W.,** Dilator effects of amino acid neurotransmitters on piglet pial arterioles, *Am. J. Physiol.,* 257, H1200, 1989.
21. **Moncada, S., Palmer, R. M., and Higgs, E. A.,** Biosynthesis of nitric oxide from L-arginine. A pathway for the regulation of cell function and communication, *Biochem. Pharmacol.,* 38, 1709, 1989.
22. **Armstead, W. M., Mirro, R., Leffler, C. W., and Busija, D. W.,** Influence of endothelin on piglet cerebral microcirculation, *Am. J. Physiol.,* 257, H707, 1989b.
23. **Pearce, W. J., Ashwal, S., and Cuevas, J.,** Direct effects of graded hypoxia on intact and denuded rabbit cranial arteries, *Am. J. Physiol.,* 257, H824, 1989.
24. **Bevan, J. A. and Joyce, E. H.,** Saline infusion into lumen of resistance artery and small vein causes contraction, *Am. J. Physiol.,* 259, H23, 1990.
25. **Ohno, M., Ochiai, M., Taguchi, J., Hara, K., Akatsuka, N., and Kurokawa, K.,** Stretch may enhance the release of endothelium-derived relaxing factor in rabbit aorta, *Biochem. Biophys. Res. Commun.,* 173, 1038, 1990.
26. **Buckley, N. M.,** Maturation of circulatory system in three mammalian models of human development, *Comp. Biochem. Physiol.,* 83, 1, 1986.
27. **Leuschen, M. P. and Nelson, R. M. J.,** Telencephalic microvessels of premature beagle pups, *Anat. Rec.,* 215, 59, 1986.
28. **Stewart, P. A. and Hayakawa, E. M.,** Interendothelial junctional changes underlie the developmental 'tightening' of the blood-brain barrier, *Brain Res.,* 429, 271, 1987.
29. **Wagerle, L. C. and Busija, D. W.,** Cholinergic mechanisms in the cerebral circulation of the newborn piglet: effect of inhibitors of arachidonic acid metabolism, *Circ. Res.,* 64, 1030, 1989.
30. **Edvinsson, L., Owman, C., and Sjoberg, N. O.,** Autonomic nerves, mast cells, and amine receptors in human brain vessels. A histochemical and pharmacological study, *Brain Res.,* 115, 377, 1976.
31. **Hayashi, S., Park, M. K., and Kuehl, T. J.,** Higher sensitivity of cerebral arteries isolated from premature and newborn baboons to adrenergic and cholinergic stimulation, *Life Sci.,* 35, 253, 1984.
32. **Busija, D. W., Leffler, C. W., and Wagerle, L. C.,** Responses of newborn pig pial arteries to sympathetic nervous stimulation and exogenous norepinephrine, *Pediatr. Res.,* 19, 1210, 1985.
33. **Wagerle, L. C., Kurth, C. D., and Roth, R. A.,** Sympathetic reactivity of cerebral arteries in developing fetal lamb and adult sheep, *Am. J. Physiol.,* 258, H1432, 1990b.
34. **Wagerle, L. C. and Delivoria-Papadopoulos, M.,** Alpha-adrenergic receptor subtypes in the cerebral circulation of newborn piglets, *Am. J. Physiol.,* 252, R1092, 1987.
35. **Busija, D. W. and Leffler, C. W.,** Eicosanoid synthesis elicited by norepinephrine in piglet parietal cortex, *Brain Res.,* 403, 243, 1987.
36. **Wagerle, L. C., Heffernan, T. M., Sacks, L. M., and Delivoria-Papadopoulos, M.,** Sympathetic effect on cerebral blood flow regulation in hypoxic newborn lambs, *Am. J. Physiol.,* 245, H487, 1983.
37. **Wagerle, L. C., Kumar, S. P., and Delivoria-Papadopoulos, M.,** Effect of sympathetic nerve stimulation on cerebral blood flow in newborn piglets, *Pediatr. Res.,* 20, 131, 1986.

38. **Griffith, S. G. and Burnstock, G.,** Immunohistochemical demonstration of serotonin in nerves supplying human cerebral and mesenteric blood-vessels. Some speculations about their involvement in vascular disorders, *Lancet,* 1, 561, 1983.
39. **Kawamura, K., Sakata, N., and Takebayashi, S.,** Neuropeptide Y- and vasoactive intestinal polypeptide-containing nerve fibers in the human cerebral arteries: characteristics of distribution, *Angiology,* 42, 35, 1991.
40. **Horgan, K., O'Connor, T. P., and van der Kooy, D.,** Prenatal specification and target induction underlie the enrichment of calcitonin gene-related peptide in the trigeminal ganglion neurons projecting to the cerebral vasculature, *J. Neurosci.,* 10, 2485, 1990.
41. **Kennedy, C., Grave, G. D., Jehle, J. W., and Sokoloff, L.,** Blood flow to white matter during maturation of the brain, *Neurology,* 20, 613, 1970.
42. **Mann, L. I.,** Fetal brain metabolism and function, *Clin. Obstet. Gynecol.,* 13, 638, 1970.
43. **Jones, M. D., Jr. and Traystman, R. J.,** Cerebral oxygenation of the fetus, newborn, and adult, *Semin. Perinat.,* 8, 205, 1984.
44. **Jones, M. D., Jr., Traystman, R. J., Simmons, M. A., and Molteni, R. A.,** Effects of changes in arterial O_2 content on cerebral blood flow in the lamb, *Am. J. Physiol.,* 240, H209, 1981.
45. **Jones, M. D., Jr., Rosenberg, A. A., Simmons, M. A., Molteni, R. A., Koehler, R. C., and Traystman, R. J.,** Oxygen delivery to the brain before and after birth, *Science,* 216, 324, 1982.
46. **Koehler, R. C., Jones, M. D. J., and Traystman, R. J.,** Cerebral circulatory response to carbon monoxide and hypoxic hypoxia in the lamb, *Am. J. Physiol.,* 243, H27, 1982.
47. **Rosenberg, A. A., Harris, A. P., Koehler, R. C., Hudak, M. L., Traystman, R. J., and Jones, M. D. J.,** Role of O_2-hemoglobin affinity in the regulation of cerebral blood flow in fetal sheep, *Am. J. Physiol.,* 251, H56, 1986b.
48. **Ramaekers, V. T. and Casaer, P.,** Defective regulation of cerebral oxygen transport after severe birth asphyxia, *Dev. Med. Child Neurol.,* 32, 56, 1990a.
49. **Koehler, R. C., Traystman, R. J., Rosenberg, A. A., Hudak, M. L., and Jones, M. D. J.,** Role of O_2-hemoglobin affinity on cerebrovascular response to carbon monoxide hypoxia, *Am. J. Physiol.,* 245, H1019, 1983.
50. **Gleason, C. A., Jones, M. D. J., Traystman, R. J., and Notter, R. H.,** Fetal cerebral responses to ventilation and oxygenation in utero, *Am. J. Physiol.,* 255, R1049, 1988.
51. **Pryds, O., Andersen, G. E., and Friis-Hansen, B.,** Cerebral blood flow reactivity in spontaneously breathing, preterm infants shortly after birth, *Acta Paediatr. Scand.,* 79(4), 391, 1990.
52. **Hernandez, M. J., Brennan, R. W., and Bowman, G. S.,** Autoregulation of cerebral blood flow in the newborn dog, *Brain Res.,* 184, 199, 1980.
53. **Ramaekers, V. T., Casaer, P., Daniels, H., and Marchal, G.,** Upper limits of brain blood flow autoregulation in stable infants of various conceptional age, *Early Human Dev.,* 24, 249, 1990b.
54. **Pasternak, J. F. and Groothuis, D. R.,** Autoregulation of cerebral blood flow in the newborn beagle puppy, *Biol. Neonate,* 48, 100, 1985.
55. **Arnold, B. W., Martin, C. G., Alexander, B. J., Chen, T., and Fleming, L. R.,** Autoregulation of brain blood flow during hypotension and hypertension in infant lambs, *Pediatr. Res.,* 29, 110, 1991.
56. **Laudignon, N., Beharry, K., Farri, E., and Aranda, J. V.,** The role of adenosine in the vascular adaptation of neonatal cerebral blood flow during hypotension, *J. Cereb. Blood Flow Metab.,* 11, 424, 1991.
57. **Park, T. S., Van Wylen, D. G., Rubio, R., and Berne, R. M.,** Brain interstitial adenosine and sagittal sinus blood flow during systemic hypotension in piglet, *J. Cereb. Blood Flow Metab.,* 8, 822, 1988.

58. **Leffler, C. W., Busija, D. W., Beasley, D. G., Armstead, W. M., and Mirro, R.,** Postischemic cerebral microvascular responses to norepinephrine and hypotension in newborn pigs, *Stroke,* 20, 541, 1989.
59. **Chemtob, S., Beharry, K., Rex, J., Varma, D. R., and Aranda, J. V.,** Changes in cerebrovascular prostaglandins and thromboxane as a function of systemic blood pressure. Cerebral blood flow autoregulation of the newborn, *Circ. Res.,* 67, 674, 1990.
60. **Armstead, W. M., Leffler, C. W., Busija, D. W., and Mirro, R.,** Vasopressin and prostanoid mechanisms in control of cerebral blood flow in hypotensive newborn pigs, *Am. J. Physiol.,* 258, H408, 1990a.
61. **Armstead, W. M., Mirro, R., Busija, D. W., Desiderio, D. M., and Leffler, C. W.,** Opioids in cerebrospinal fluid in hypotensive newborn pigs, *Circ. Res.,* 68, 922, 1991.
62. **Fletcher, A. M., Leffler, C. W., and Busija, D. W.,** Effects of hypertension and sympathetic denervation on cerebral blood flow in newborn pigs, *Am. J. Vet. Res.,* 50, 754, 1989.
63. **Monin, P., Feillet, F., Hascoet, J. M., and Vert, P.,** Effect of sympathetic nervous system on cerebral blood flow in the newborn piglet, *Biol. Neonate,* 58, 192, 1990.
64. **Ong, B. Y., Greengrass, R., Bose, D., Gregory, G., and Palahniuk, R. J.,** Acidemia impairs autoregulation of cerebral blood flow in newborn lambs, *Can. Anaesth. Soc. J.,* 33, 5, 1986.
65. **Gardiner, R. M.,** Cerebral blood flow and oxidative metabolism during hypoxia and asphyxia in the new-born calf and lamb, *J. Physiol. (London),* 305, 357, 1980.
66. **Tweed, A., Cote, J., Lou, H., Gregory, G., and Wade, J.,** Impairment of cerebral blood flow autoregulation in the newborn lamb by hypoxia, *Pediatr. Res.,* 20, 516, 1986.
67. **Busija, D. W. and Leffler, C. W.,** Selective attenuation by perivascular blood of prostanoid-dependent cerebrovascular dilation in piglets, *Stroke,* 22, 484, 1991.
68. **Wyatt, J. S., Edwards, A. D., Cope, M., Delpy, D. T., McCormick, D. C., Potter, A., and Reynolds, E. O.,** Response of cerebral blood volume to changes in arterial carbon dioxide tension in preterm and term infants, *Pediatr. Res.,* 29, 553, 1991.
69. **Hernandez, M. J., Brennan, R. W., Vannucci, R. C., and Bowman, G. S.,** Cerebral blood flow and oxygen consumption in the newborn dog, *Am. J. Physiol.,* 234, R209, 1978.
70. **Gregoire, N. M., Gjedde, A., Plum, F., and Duffy, T. E.,** Cerebral blood flow and cerebral metabolic rates for oxygen, glucose, and ketone bodies in newborn dogs, *J. Neurochem.,* 30, 63, 1978.
71. **Pryds, O., Greisen, G., Lou, H., and Friis-Hansen, B.,** Heterogeneity of cerebral vasoreactivity in preterm infants supported by mechanical ventilation, *J. Pediatr.,* 115, 638, 1989.
72. **Raju, T. N. and Kim, S. Y.,** The effect of hematocrit alterations on cerebral vascular CO_2 reactivity in newborn baboons, *Pediatr. Res.,* 29, 385, 1991.
73. **DeGiulio, P. A., Roth, R. A., Mishra, O. P., DelivoriaPapadopoulos, M., and Wagerle, L. C.,** Effect of indomethacin on the regulation of cerebral blood flow during respiratory alkalosis in newborn piglets, *Pediatr. Res.,* 26, 593, 1989.
74. **Leffler, C. W., Mirro, R., Thompson, C., Shibata, M., Armstead, W. M., Pourcyrous, M., and Thelin, O.,** Activated oxygen species do not mediate hypercapnia-induced cerebral vasodilation in newborn pigs, *Am. J. Physiol.,* 261, H335, 1991.
75. **Wagerle, L. C., DeGiulio, P. A., Mishra, O. P., and Delivoria-Papadopoulos, M.,** Effect of dexamethasone on cerebral prostanoid formation and pial arteriolar reactivity to CO_2 in newborn pigs, *Am. J. Physiol.,* 260, H1313, 1991.
76. **Massik, J., Jones, M. D. J., Miyabe, M., Tang, Y. L., Hudak, M. L., Koehler, R. C., and Traystman, R. J.,** Hypercapnia and response of cerebral blood flow to hypoxia in newborn lambs, *J. Appl. Physiol.,* 66, 1065, 1989.
77. **Rosenberg, A. A., Jones, M. D. J., Traystman, R. J., Simmons, M. A., and Molteni, R. A.,** Response of cerebral blood flow to changes in P_{CO_2} in fetal, newborn, and adult sheep, *Am. J. Physiol.,* 242, H862, 1982.

78. **Rosenberg, A. A.,** Response of the cerebral circulation to profound hypocarbia in neonatal lambs, *Stroke,* 19, 1365, 1988b.
79. **Aranda, J. V., Beharry, K., Laudignon, N., and Sasyniuk, B. I.,** Ontogeny of adenosine production and degradation and its implications in neonatal cerebral blood flow regulation, *Dev. Pharmacol. Ther.,* 13, 96, 1989.
80. **Hohimer, A. R., Chao, C. R., and Bissonnette, J. M.,** The effect of combined hypoxemia and cephalic hypotension on fetal cerebral blood flow and metabolism, *J. Cereb. Blood Flow Metab.,* 11, 99, 1991.
81. **Park, T. S., Van Wylen, D. G., Rubio, R., and Berne, R. M.,** Increased brain interstitial fluid adenosine concentration during hypoxia in newborn piglet, *J. Cereb. Blood Flow Metab.,* 7, 178, 1987b.
82. **Laudignon, N., Farri, E., Beharry, K., Rex, J., and Aranda, J. V.,** Influence of adenosine on cerebral blood flow during hypoxic hypoxia in the newborn piglet, *J. Appl. Physiol.,* 68, 1534, 1990b.
83. **Camp, D., Kotagal, U. R., and Kleinman, L. I.,** Preservation of cerebral autoregulation in the unanesthetized hypoxemic newborn dog, *Brain Res.,* 241, 207, 1982.
84. **Raju, T. N., Bhat, R., and Vidyasagar, D.,** Age-related difference in cerebral perfusion pressure response to acute hypoxia in neonatal puppies, *Biol. Neonate,* 41, 258, 1982.
85. **Ment, L. R., Stewart, W. B., Duncan, C. C., and Pitt, B. R.,** Beagle puppy model of perinatal cerebral insults. Cerebral blood flow changes and intraventricular hemorrhage evoked by hypoxemia, *J. Neurosurg.,* 65, 847, 1986a.
86. **Szymonowicz, W., Walker, A. M., Cussen, L., Cannata, J., and Yu, V. Y.,** Developmental changes in regional cerebral blood flow in fetal and newborn lambs, *Am. J. Physiol.,* 254, H52, 1988.
87. **Lou, H. C., Tweed, W. A., and Davies, J. M.,** Preferential blood flow increase to the brain stem in moderate neonatal hypoxia: reversal by naloxone, *Eur. J. Pediatr.,* 144, 225, 1985.
88. **McPhee, A. J., Kotagal, U. R., and Kleinman, L. I.,** Cerebrovascular hemodynamics during and after recovery from acute asphyxia in the newborn dog, *Pediatr. Res.,* 19, 645, 1985.
89. **Richardson, B. S., Rurak, D., Patrick, J. E., Homan, J., and Carmichael, L.,** Cerebral oxidative metabolism during sustained hypoxaemia in fetal sheep, *J. Dev. Physiol.,* 11, 37, 1989.
90. **Koehler, R. C., Traystman, R. J., and Jones, M. D. J.,** Influence of reduced oxyhemoglobin affinity on cerebrovascular response to hypoxic hypoxia, *Am. J. Physiol.,* 251, 756, 1986.
91. **Ment, L. R., Stewart, W. B., Duncan, C. C., Pitt, B. R., and Cole, J. S.,** Beagle puppy model of perinatal cerebral infarction. Regional cerebral prostaglandin changes during acute hypoxemia, *J. Neurosurg.,* 65, 851, 1986b.
92. **Pearce, W. J. and Ashwal, S.,** Developmental changes in thickness, contractility, and hypoxic sensitivity of newborn lamb cerebral arteries, *Pediatr. Res.,* 22, 192, 1987.
93. **Gilbert, R. D., Pearce, W. J., Ashwal, S., and Longo, L. D.,** Effects of hypoxia on contractility of isolated fetal lamb cerebral arteries, *J. Dev. Physiol.,* 13, 199, 1990.
94. **Goplerud, J. M., Wagerle, L. C., and Delivoria-Papadopoulos, M.,** Regional cerebral blood flow response during and after acute asphyxia in newborn piglets, *J. Appl. Physiol.,* 66, 2827, 1989.
95. **Pourcyrous, M., Leffler, C., and Busija, D.,** Role of prostanoids in cerebrovascular responses to asphyxia and reventilation in newborn pigs, *Am. J. Physiol.,* 259, H662, 1990.
96. **Goplerud, J. M., Wagerle, L. C., and Delivoria-Papadopoulos, M.,** Sympathetic nerve modulation of regional cerebral blood flow during asphyxia in newborn piglets, *Am. J. Physiol.,* 260, H1575, 1991.
97. **Rosenberg, A. A.,** Cerebral blood flow and O_2 metabolism after asphyxia in neonatal lambs, *Pediatr. Res.,* 20, 778, 1986a.

98. **Rosenberg, A. A.,** Regulation of cerebral blood flow after asphyxia in neonatal lambs, *Stroke,* 19, 239, 1988a.
99. **Levene, M. I., Gibson, N. A., Fenton, A. C., Papathoma, E., and Barnett, D.,** The use of a calcium-channel blocker, nicardipine, for severely asphyxiated newborn infants, *Dev. Med. Child Neurol.,* 32, 567, 1990.
100. **Pryds, O., Greisen, G., Lou, H., and Friis-Hansen, B.,** Vasoparalysis associated with brain damage in asphyxiated term infants, *J. Pediatr.,* 117, 119, 1990b.
101. **Dwyer, B. E., Nishimura, R. N., and Fujikawa, D. G.,** Cerebral hypoxia ischemia in immature rats: methodological considerations, *Exp. Neurol.,* 99(3), 772, 1988.
102. **Schaller, R., Bauer, R., Kluge, H., and Zwiener, U.,** Effects of hypoxic hypoxia on the kinetics of synaptosomal Ca^{2+}ATPase activity in newborn piglets and young rabbits, *Biomedica Biochimica Acta,* 48(2–3): S208, 11, 1989.
103. **Leffler, C. W., Mirro, R., Armstead, W. M., Busija, D. W., and Thelin, O.,** Prostanoid synthesis and vascular responses to exogenous arachidonic acid following cerebral ischemia in piglets, *Prostaglandins,* 40(3), 241, 1990b.
104. **Mujsce, D. J., Christensen, M. A., and Vannucci, R. C.,** Cerebral blood flow and edema in perinatal hypoxic-ischemic brain damage, *Pediatr. Res.,* 27(5), 450, 1990.
105. **Harada, J., Takaku, A., Endo, S., Kuwayama, N., and Fukuda, O.,** Differences in critical cerebral blood flow with age in swine, *J. Neurosurg.,* 75, 103, 1991.
106. **Ichord, R. N., Kirsch, J. R., Helfaer, M. A., Haun, S., and Traystman, R. J.,** Age-related differences in recovery of blood flow and metabolism after cerebral ischemia in swine, *Stroke,* 22, 626, 1991.
107. **Ashwal, S., Schneider, S., and Thompson, J.,** Xenon computed tomography measuring cerebral blood flow in the determination of brain death in children, *Ann. Neurol.,* 25, 539, 1989.
108. **Volpe, J. J.,** Neonatal intraventricular hemorrhage, *N. Engl. J. Med.,* 304, 886, 1981.
109. **Ment, L. R., Stewart, W. B., Duncan, C. C., and Lambrecht, R.,** Beagle puppy model of intraventricular hemorrhage, *J. Neurosurg.,* 57, 219, 1982.
110. **Ment, L. R., Stewart, W. B., and Duncan, C. C.,** Beagle puppy model of intraventricular hemorrhage. Effect of superoxide dismutase on cerebral blood flow and prostaglandins, *J. Neurosurg.,* 62, 563, 1985.
111. **Trommer, B. L., Groothuis, D. R., and Pasternak, J. F.,** Quantitative analysis of cerebral vessels in the newborn puppy: the structure of germinal matrix vessels may predispose to hemorrhage, *Pediatr. Res.,* 22, 23, 1987.
112. **Sotrel, A. and Lorenzo, A. V.,** Ultrastructure of blood vessels in the ganglionic eminence of premature rabbits with spontaneous germinal matrix hemorrhages, *J. Neuropathol. Exp. Neurol.,* 48, 462, 1989.
113. **Ment, L. R., Stewart, W. B., Ardito, T. A., and Madri, J. A.,** Beagle pup germinal matrix maturation studies, *Stroke,* 22, 390, 1991.
114. **Karch, D.,** Hypoxia during the perinatal period and the formation of cerebral lesions, *Klin. Wochenschr.,* 60, 1427, 1982.
115. **Sakuraba, M. and Saling, E.,** Umbilical cord blood coagulability, acidosis and intracranial hemorrhage, *J. Perinat. Med.,* 17, 99, 1989.

Chapter 26

CEREBRAL BLOOD FLOW AND MIGRAINE

Mark J. Gorman and K. M. A. Welch

TABLE OF CONTENTS

I. History of CBF in Migraine 400

II. CBF During the Prodrome and During Headache 401

III. CBF Between Attacks 402

IV. Localization of Headache in Relation to CBF Changes 404

V. Physiologic Blood Flow Changes Observed in Migraine 404

VI. Are Classic and Common Migraine Different Entities?: The CBF Data 405

VII. Varying Results Between Labs: Different Techniques and Compton Scatter 406

VIII. The Contribution of CBF Studies to the Pathogenesis of Migraine: Vascular and Neuronal Theories and the Spreading Depression of Leao 407

IX. CBF Implications for the Vascular and Neuronal Theories of Migraine 408

References 409

0-8493-5096-0/93/$0.00 + $.50

The mechanism underlying migraine has been a source of controversy in the neurologic literature. Despite numerous advances in biomedical technology, the complete story of migraine remains elusive, yet our understanding of the pathophysiology has improved considerably. A large share of this can be attributed to the information gained in the study of cerebral blood flow (CBF).

I. HISTORY OF CBF IN MIGRAINE

The mechanism of migraine has been related to blood vessel and CBF alterations for more than 100 years. Early information of blood flow changes in migraine was derived from both direct and indirect observations of blood vessels during the headache. Goltman[1] reported a surgeon's operative findings and his own postsurgical observations of a young woman who underwent craniotomy during her classic* migraine attack. He stated that first vasomotor spasm was inferred by blanching of the face. Following this, vascular dilation of the dural vessels was observed through the hole in the skull and the CSF was found to be under increased pressure. Later the bulging of the skin overlying the skull defect subsided coincident with the relief from the migraine attack. Depression of the skull defect followed by bulging and subsequent return to baseline was viewed repeatedly during migraines in this patient.

In one of what is now regarded as a classic series of experiments by Wolff and colleagues,[3] the effects of histamine and ergotamine tartrate were assessed using various parameters in 32 attacks of migraine in 16 subjects and compared to nonmigrainous controls. They recorded increased temporal artery pulsations unilateral to head pain in both histamine-induced headaches and spontaneous migraine attacks (recorded after the prodrome). Headaches were induced by mechanical distention of the temporal artery with saline. Following ergotamine administration, the headache pain subsided concomitant with and in proportion to reduction in temporal artery pulsations. Similar findings were seen with direct compression of the common carotid artery unilateral to the headache pain. Information obtained indirectly of the internal carotid circulation during the migraine was inconclusive. They postulated that "the head pain of a migraine attack is produced by the distention of cranial arteries and that the termination of the headache by ergotamine tartrate is due to the capacity of this agent to constrict these cranial arteries and thus reduce the amplitude of their pulsations."[3]

Further evidence that the pain of migraine resulted mainly from distention of the extracerebral arteries and the differentiation of the prodrome of migraine from the headache phase experimentally was published in 1941. This included

* Classic and common migraine will be used interchangeably with the newer terms migraine with aura and migraine without aura, as defined in the headache classification of the International Headache Society.[2] The reason being that many of the references cited used older definitions of migraine and few provided adequate clinical data (except to state that the subjects fit the categories) to determine if they all meet the latest criterion.

the study of a physician with scotoma prior to migraine using the vasodilator, amyl nitrate, to alternately worsen the scotoma or abolish it, depending on the dose (a lower dose dilated the arteries and increased blood flow, abolishing the scotoma; a higher dose decreased the blood pressure with a concomitant presumed drop in CBF and worsening of the scotoma).[4] These studies and others in the series dominated the main body of neurological theory concerning migraine headache for most of the next 40 years.

II. CBF DURING THE PRODROME AND DURING HEADACHE

Early studies of CBF in migraine uniformly revealed hypoperfusion during the prodrome and hyperperfusion of the intracerebral as well as extracerebral cranial circulation during the headache phase.[5-8] Elkind et al., using the ^{24}Na tissue clearance method to study frontotemporal skin blood flow, observed significantly increased flows unilateral to head pain in migraineurs.[9] This was later confirmed by Sakai and Meyer.[10] O'Brien, employing the ^{133}Xe inhalation technique with only a single detector over each hemisphere, found hypoperfusion during prodrome and hyperemia during headache without interhemispheric flow variation.[7] Skinhøj and Paulson, using the ^{133}Xe intracarotid technique found pronounced reduction in flows generally, with regional differences correlating to symptoms and a normal angiogram during the prodromal phase. They suggested that the reduced flows occurred at the arteriolar level, rather than in large vessels.[11] Norris et al., using the same technique, did not find regional differences and felt their readings reflected findings of a basilar system migraine as measured in the carotid system.[6] Simard and Paulson also observed markedly reduced CBF without regional differences and, in addition, found diminished CO_2 reactivity during the prodrome phase.[12] Edmeads was among the first to note that CBF reduction extended beyond the aura symptoms.[13]

A major improvement in the technology and coincidental induction of migraine attacks allowed serial study of several migraine attacks beginning almost immediately at the start of a prodrome and then followed through the early stages of a migrainous episode. Olesen et al.[14] used the ^{133}Xe intracarotid injection method with regional cerebral blood flow (rCBF) with unprecedented resolution measured by 254 collimated detectors spread over a single hemisphere. They observed spontaneous, large decreases in rCBF concomitant with neurologic prodrome symptoms and headache in eight patients, seven of whom were felt to have migraine. Initially thought to be spontaneous migraines, these episodes were later felt to be induced by the intracarotid catheter method that was used.[15] What is most interesting is that they were able to discern a shortlived hyperemia (in four of the eight cases) followed by more widespread hypoperfusion in the posterior parts of the hemisphere which appeared to correspond anatomically with the neurological symptoms of the prodrome. They did not find any evidence of hyperemia (although they only observed their subjects for the first 2 hours of an attack) and observed that in every instance the headache commenced while the rCBF was significantly low. Although the rCBF was significantly low in certain areas, it was almost always well above critical values of ischemia.

Although a groundbreaking report, there have been many criticisms of this paper. One of the most important was that none of the patients had typical migraines, having been studied with angiography because they were unusual, and in fact seven of eight were males. The induced attacks usually varied in some way from their typical migrainous symptoms and due to technical reasons they were only able to measure one hemisphere. Also the method of induction itself may have altered blood flow. They were, however, able to make several consecutive measurements in the same patient over a brief timespan during a single episode with a high degree of accuracy which had not hitherto been done. The results have since been confirmed in subjects with more typical migrainous symptoms and using other techniques.[15-17] The only observation which has not been repeated was the initial transient hyperemia seen in four of the cases.

Lauritzen and Olesen,[17] using the ^{133}Xe inhalation method as measured by SPECT, extended these findings out to about 6 hours postsymptom onset and also found some hyperemia of the basal ganglia in the common migraineurs, despite normal cortical flows in these subjects. Andersen et al. brought the measurements out even further in time and found delayed hyperperfusion in classic migraine subjects which persisted even after the headache pain had resolved.[16]

Using the Xe CT-CBF method which provides higher resolution as well as the ability to measure subcortical blood flow, Kobari et al. found higher CBF during migraine headaches not only in the cerebral cortex but also in the subcortical gray structures, most markedly in the thalamus, followed by basal ganglia, cortical gray, and then subcortical white matter.[18,19] They also found only minor asymmetries from one side to the other, despite laterality of headache pain (none were examined during prodrome).

III. CBF BETWEEN ATTACKS

Observations by Elkind et al.[9] revealed no significant difference in frontotemporal scalp blood flow between asymptomatic migraineurs and controls. O'Brien[7] showed normal resting CBF in 18 migraineurs. Mathew et al.[5] using intracarotid injection of ^{133}Xe and a gamma camera found no significant differences in interictal measures of general CBF, gray matter flow, and cerebral blood volume in classic or common migraine subjects, as compared with normal controls.

Sakai and Meyer,[20] using a ^{133}Xe inhalation model with eight paired collimated NaI detectors, showed that the hyperemia found diffusely during migraine headaches slowly resolved, returning to normal levels over an average 2 day period. This slowly resolving hyperemia was not observed in patients with cluster headache, whose flow levels returned to normal generally within 1 h, despite having a more significant hyperemia on average than the migraine patients. Because the hyperemia was limited to the time period of the headache, they attributed this to pain itself, rather than postischemic hyperemia, and concluded that the cause of the cluster headaches was the profound hyperperfusion of the extracerebral vessels.

In that paper and in a later article,[10] Sakai and Meyer found that cerebral dysautoregulation, as measured by altered CBF during a tilt-table test, observed during and shortly after the headache also slowly resolved concomitant with blood flow changes. CO_2 responsiveness of CBF more than 2 days after migraine in 21 patients (7 classic and 14 common) was significantly higher than normal and was also significantly greater on the headache side than the nonheadache side. CBF response to voluntary hyperventilation and to breathing 100% O_2 did not differ significantly from normal controls. They found no significant differences between common and classic migraineurs with respect to interictal blood flow.

Olesen et al. studied eight patients with classic migraine and found baseline CBF to be normal in seven (the eighth, a patient with a history of head trauma and dementia, had a focal hyperemia).[14] Lauritzen and Olesen studied patients at least 1 week after their last attack, and all except one patient (who showed a mild focal degree of hypoperfusion) showed normal, symmetrical blood flow patterns.[17]

Using an eight probe pair external collimetry system with the ^{133}Xe inhalation method, Levine et al.[21] studied 27 classic/complicated migraineurs, 18 common migraineurs, and 18 controls at least 2 weeks after their last attack in the absence of medications. Although they found no significant difference between mean hemispheric CBF, when comparing the number of asymmetric probe pairs (matched to homologous cortical areas), they found two or more asymmetric probe pairs more frequently in migraine subjects (independent of type) than controls. Posterior probe asymmetries were much more evident in migraineurs.

In a similar study, Lagrèze and colleagues[26] studied 8 subjects with classic, 11 with common, and 20 healthy controls, medication free, at least 6 days after their last attack. The ^{133}Xe inhalation method with 16 paired detectors provided slightly higher resolution than earlier studies. When comparing lumped data for the different groups they found no significant differences in the measured and calculated parameters. When they examined the individuals within each group, however, the classic migraine subjects, not the common migraineurs or controls, had significantly altered CBF, but no consistent pattern of abnormality emerged. This study was hampered by a small subject group and sparse clinical data. They concluded that "the salient feature of classic migraine was a disruption of the intrahemispheric rCBF pattern" and felt that this provided further evidence for the dichotomy between common and classic migraine. They did not speculate as to the etiology for these differences, nor did they attempt to explain why the pattern of blood flow abnormalities varied highly between subjects.

Studying the interictal period of 23 subjects with migraine using ^{123}I-IMP (iodoamphetamine) SPECT, Schlake et al.[22] found significant alterations of CBF. Only 1 of 5 subjects with classic (visual scotomas only) migraine showed decreased tracer uptake (implying low blood flow), but all 15 subjects with hemiplegic (any neurologic symptom in addition to scotoma) migraine showed regional tracer uptake reductions. Most of the reductions correlated to headache site and to the expected topography of the neurologic deficits, and although quantitative correlations were not possible, the more severe cases seemed to have more pronounced reduction in tracer uptake. As SPECT scanning with IMP may reflect metabolism as well, they felt that their results indicate that migraines and especially migraine with neurologic findings other than visual aura are characterized by permanent alterations in blood flow, which may reflect similar changes in metabolism. They confirmed most of these findings in a more recent paper examining a similar group of patients with 99m-Tc-HMPAO SPECT.[23] Using acetazolamide injection as a vasodilator, they were able to improve or correct the blood flow asymmetries in 17 out of 20 of their patients. The 3 who did not correct were all in the older age range (47, 51, 58 years) and they postulated that the lack of reactivity in these patients may have been related to cerebrovascular disease or the aging process.

IV. LOCALIZATION OF HEADACHE IN RELATION TO CBF CHANGES

Many of the early studies did not present adequate clinical information to examine this question. One which did found no strong correlations.[7] Later studies utilizing the intracarotid ^{133}Xe method were limited to unilateral measurements, and although they found rCBF changes, it is unknown what occurred contralateral to the measurements.[6,12,15,24] SPECT and inhalation studies found fairly good correlation of unilateral headache to low flows (8 of 10, 80%, when pooled), but bilateral headache was not helpful in predicting low flows.[16,17] Xe CT-CBF studies did not show any correlation of blood flow changes with headache side.[18]

V. PHYSIOLOGIC BLOOD FLOW CHANGES OBSERVED IN MIGRAINE

Cerebral vessel reactivity under varied circumstances is reported to be altered during attacks of migraine. Cerebral autoregulation to tilt-testing was abnormal during or immediately following migraine headache in 4/12 cases (all migraine with aura, measured early in the attack).[20] Autoregulation as measured by CBF changes during angiotension-induced hypertension was, however, normal.[25] None of the expected rise in blood flow during physiologic activation was seen in the oligemic areas during migraine,[14,25] although non-oligemic areas exhibited a normal increase in blood flow.

Cerebrovascular reactivity to changes in CO_2 concentration, either by CO_2 inhalation or by hyperventilation, were found to be impaired by all groups,[10,12,25] but in some was limited to areas of abnormal flow in classic migraineurs only,[25] and the severity of abnormality seemed to parallel migraine severity and resolved slowly with the attack. Others have found hypersensitivity to CO_2 inhalation interictally, as noted above.[10] Wolff (as quoted by Hachinski[24]) and others have aborted prodromal scotoma with CO_2 inhalation, which may indicate preserved reactivity very early in the migraine attack. Similarly, a vasodilator, amyl nitrate, has also been used to abort prodromal scotoma.[4] Later, during the headache phase of a migraine attack, ergotamine, a vaso-constricting agent, was found to diminish headache pain in conjunction with a parallel decrease in the size and pulsatility of extracerebral cranial vessels.[4] Interestingly, no changes in CBF were seen with ergotamine administration, despite resolution of the headache.[13] All of the above alterations in reactivity seem to indicate a general pattern of abnormality of the resistance vessels during migraine which is not found in normals.

VI. ARE CLASSIC AND COMMON MIGRAINE DIFFERENT ENTITIES?: THE CBF DATA

Mathew et al. found no significant differences in rCBF values obtained during headache between common and classic migraine types; however, a wide range of values were reported.[5] Hachinski et al. reported three cases of migraine, two classic with changes in CBF as described above, and one common without CBF changes.[24] There have, however, been reports of some patients with apparently classic migraine without the blood flow changes that have been ascribed to it.[13,16] Sakai and Meyer found no significant difference between groups of classic and common migraineurs, either during headache or when measured afterward, nor were there differences in CO_2 responsiveness during the headache or interictally.[10,20] These findings were echoed in later publications which found no interictal blood flow differences nor any differences in subcortical and cortical blood flow between classic and common migraine.[18,19,21]

Conversely, Lauritzen and Olesen, using both intracarotid ^{133}Xe and SPECT studies in induced and spontaneous migraines, recorded no CBF alterations in the common migraine group, whereas typical findings were observed in classic migraine.[15,17] In a complex study utilizing ^{133}Xe inhalation technique comparing interictal flows in classic vs. common migraine, Lagrèze et al. found no meaningful differences when comparing group means, but found individuals with classic migraine to have abnormal blood flow patterns which were not seen as often in common migraineurs.[26] It is difficult to reconcile the disparity of results presented, but as most of the data is from two major investigational groups, perhaps the methodology and relatively small numbers studied are responsible. Further information is needed to resolve the issue of whether common and classic migraine represent different pathologic entities.

VII. VARYING RESULTS BETWEEN LABS: DIFFERENT TECHNIQUES AND COMPTON SCATTER

The inhalation technique for measuring CBF has been criticized because of its inability to isolate the intracranial from extracranial circulation and also because the long instrumentation time impedes quick and sequential measurements during a migraine attack.[27] Additionally, the readings are felt to be even less accurate than those using the intracarotid technique because of the contribution of hemispheric crosstalk. It does have the advantages of being noninvasive and able to measure blood flow in all areas of the brain simultaneously.

The intracarotid injection technique is invasive, thought to induce migraine itself, and the blood flow measurements are limited to a single large arterial territory at any one time. The technique, however, affords rapid measurements of well-defined portions of the cerebral circulation, which can be performed many times within a single episode of migraine.

CBF measurements employing ^{133}Xe using either method seem to overestimate the true blood flow in low flow areas because of the phenomenon of Compton scatter. This, briefly, is the actual measurement in the low flow area of scattered radiation from surrounding higher flow areas. The count rate obtained in any particular area is a composite reading, with the strongest component coming from the area directly underneath the probe, and some contribution also from the neighboring areas, those closest exerting the greatest influence, diminishing as the distance increases. This artifactually increases the measurement in the lowest flow areas and led to the, probably inaccurate, conclusion that rCBF in involved areas during early migrainous stages was well above ischemic values.[14]

Skyhøj Olsen et al. using the estimates of the actual data based on the contribution of Compton scatter concluded that ischemia could not be ruled out in the low flow areas, and in fact changes of rCBF by as much as 50% in these areas would go unmeasured because of the Compton scatter from surrounding higher flow areas. They go on to suggest that what appeared to be spreading oligemia may have actually been worsening oligemia in a static area.[28,29] These contentions are supported by other data obtained in studies of focal ischemia in infarction.[30] Donley et al. felt that intracarotid ^{133}Xe method could identify regions of focal ischemia, especially if multiple small collimated detectors were used, but estimated that even with these measures that 35 to 55% of the total activity measured may not come from tissue underneath the probe.[27] Bolsmjö has confirmed the inaccuracies of this method of data collection in focal ischemia using an experimental model and computer simulation of the brain.[31]

VIII. THE CONTRIBUTION OF CBF STUDIES TO THE PATHOGENESIS OF MIGRAINE: VASCULAR AND NEURONAL THEORIES AND THE SPREADING DEPRESSION OF LEAO

Wolff hypothesized that the symptoms of the prodrome in classic migraine were due to cerebral ischemia and that the intracerebral blood vessels responded to this insult by dilating in order to adequately restore CBF. The headache was felt to be an epiphenomenon resulting from dilation of the extracerebral vessels which coincidently accompanied the restorative intracerebral dilatation.

Working independently with rabbit cortex in attempts to further elucidate the physiologic underpinnings of epilepsy, Leao observed an electrical wave of depolarization spreading across the cortex like a ripple in a pond following both mechanical and electrical perturbation of a focal cortical area.[32] This he termed "spreading depression" and he also visually observed that there was a marked pial hyperemia which accompanied this phenomenon.[33,34] Just prior to the spreading electrical depolarization, he documented a strong but short-lived electrical excitability.

Most of the early papers of CBF in migraine seemed to confirm the long-held vascular theories most strongly propounded by Wolff, with their observations that migraine headache was accompanied by a significant, although bilateral cerebral hyperemia. Hypoperfusion observed during the prodrome of the few subjects who were studied lent further credence, and it was widely held that the hyperperfusion observed during the headache phase was reactive to a preceding ischemia.

It was not until the observations of Olesen et al.[14] that these concepts were substantially questioned. Many of their findings were felt to be incongruous with the vascular theory. These included:

1. The observed blood flow changes of hypoperfusion preceded and outlasted the symptoms of prodrome, and in fact, the headache was initiated and at its worst during the hypoperfusion stage of a migrainous attack;
2. The headache resolved while delayed hyperemia was still in effect;
3. The spreading oligemia crossed vascular boundaries and was only limited by cytoarchitectonic and physical barriers;
4. Initial hyperemia was seen just before the hypoperfusion began.

Olesen has taken the viewpoint that these observations represent a spontaneous human phenomenon similar to that observed by Leao in rabbits, and, therefore, migraine attacks are primarily a neuronal abnormality of cortical spreading depression with secondary vascular changes. Further evidence for their theory was the estimate that the speed of spreading oligemia (2 mm/min) very nearly matched that estimated for the electrical spreading depression (3 mm/min) observed by Leao (as quoted by Lauritzen[35]).

There have been many detractors of this theory and they have cited evidence that although spreading depression is easily induced in the smooth cortex of the rabbit brain, it is progressively more difficult to elicit in more highly evolved and convoluted brains and has rarely been seen in monkeys. Gloor added his personal experience with over 1000 exposed brains during epilepsy surgery which were either mechanically or electrically stimulated during the course of the procedure. On not one occasion did he observe, presumably electrically, any phenomenon remotely similar to spreading depression.[36] This is consonant with the experience of others.[37]

Leao himself, although noting the similarity of the slow march of scotomata in migraine to that of his spreading depression, remarked that he observed accompanying vasodilation, while in migraine, scotomata were felt to result from vasoconstriction.[32] Others have pointed out that there have not been any physiologic observations of spreading depression in humans. Proponents felt that this was mainly for technical reasons, and in 1990, Barkley et al. described two unique magnetic field changes only during migraine which they felt were physiologic human correlates of spreading depression.[38] The third wave, originally described as part of the migraine syndrome, may be an artifact of measurement (personal communication).

IX. CBF IMPLICATIONS FOR THE VASCULAR AND NEURONAL THEORIES OF MIGRAINE

The controversy through the years has been whether the primary abnormality (intrinsic pathologic alteration) in migraine is to be found in the blood vessels themselves or in the underlying brain. EEGs have almost always been normal in migraineurs during attacks, and interictally they are sometimes characterized by the seemingly innocent, prolonged driving response to photic stimulation. Magneto encephalographic (MEG) studies have revealed what appear to be some characteristic changes of the migraine attack, but the nature and implications of this need to be further elucidated. Transcranial Doppler studies can show accelerated flows in migraineurs.

CBF studies in migraine, especially those which used high resolution intracarotid techniques, provide us with new insights. Complicating inaccuracies in the detection techniques leave considerable doubt as to the actual blood flow during different phases of migraine with aura, but some clear facts have emerged. Oligemia (and probably ischemia) accompanies the prodrome. The headache usually begins when cerebral blood flow is diminished. Oligemia appears to spread out from the areas correlating with prodromal symptoms. Hyperemia appears afterward, well into the headache phase, and may represent luxury perfusion following ischemia during the initial stages. Cortical hyperemia outlasts headache pain. Blood flow changes cross vascular borders. Interictal CBF studies indicate subtle yet long-standing cortical flow asymmetries and reactivities (although whether these are the remains of severe attacks or related to the etiology remains to be shown).

Whether migraine with and without aura are separate clinical entities is still controversial, but many of the differences seen between the clinical types of migraine may be related to the severity of neurologic findings during the attack. The above conclusions do not present a clear-cut resolution to the dichotomy of the vascular and neuronal theories of migraine, but rather seem to indicate that they are both pieces to the puzzle and that migraine is a complicated disorder involving brain, blood vessels, and the nature of their interaction.

REFERENCES

1. **Goltman, A. M.,** The mechanism of migraine, *J. Allergy,* 7, 351, 1936.
2. Headache classification committee of the International Headache Society, Classification and diagnostic criteria for headache disorders, cranial neuralgias and facial pain, *Cephalalgia,* 8, 1, 1988.
3. **Graham, J. R. and Wolff, H. G.,** Mechanism of migraine headache and action of ergotamine tartrate, *Arch. Neurol. Psychiatry,* 39, 737, 1938.
4. **Schumacher, G. A. and Wolff, H. G.,** Experimental studies on headache. A. Contrast of histamine headache with the headache of migraine and that associated with hypertension. B. Contrast of vascular mechanisms in preheadache and in headache phenomena of migraine, *Arch. Neurol. Psychiatry,* 45, 199, 1941.
5. **Mathew, N. T., Hrastnik, F., and Meyer, J. S.,** Regional cerebral blood flow in the diagnosis of vascular headache, *Headache,* 15, 252, 1976.
6. **Norris, J. W., Hachinski, V. C., and Cooper, P. W.,** Changes in cerebral blood flow during a migraine attack, *Br. Med. J.,* 3, 676, 1975.
7. **O'Brien, M. D.,** Cerebral blood changes in migraine, *Headache,* 10, 139, 1971.
8. **Skinhøj, E.,** Hemodynamic studies within the brain during migraine, *Arch. Neurol.,* 29, 95, 1973.
9. **Elkind, A. H., Friedman, A. P., and Grossman, J.,** Cutaneous blood flow in vascular headaches of the migraine type, *Neurology,* 14, 24, 1964.
10. **Sakai, F. and Meyer, J. S.,** Abnormal cerebrovascular reactivity in patients with migraine and cluster headache, *Headache,* 19, 257, 1979.
11. **Skinhøj, E. and Paulson, O. B.,** Regional blood flow in internal carotid distribution during migraine attack, *Br. Med. J.,* 3, 569, 1969.
12. **Simard, D. and Paulson, O. B.,** Cerebral vasomotor paralysis during migraine attack, *Arch. Neurol.,* 29, 207, 1973.
13. **Edmeads, J.,** Cerebral blood flow in migraine, *Headache,* 17, 148, 1977.
14. **Olesen, J., Larsen, B., and Lauritzen, M.,** Focal hyperemia followed by spreading oligemia and impaired activation of rCBF in classic migraine, *Ann. Neurol.,* 9, 344, 1981.
15. **Olesen, J., Lauritzen, M., Tfelt-Hansen, P., Henriksen, L., and Larsen, B.,** Spreading cerebral oligemia in classical- and normal cerebral blood flow in common migraine, *Headache,* 22, 242, 1982.
16. **Andersen, A. R., Friberg, L., Skyhøj Olsen, T., and Olesen, J.,** Delayed hyperemia following hypoperfusion in classic migraine, *Arch. Neurol.,* 45, 154, 1988.
17. **Lauritzen, M. and Olesen, J.,** Regional cerebral blood flow during migraine attacks by Xenon-133 inhalation and emission tomography, *Brain,* 107, 447, 1984.

18. **Kobari, M., Meyer, J. S., Ichijo, M., Imai, A., and Oravez, W. T.,** Hyperperfusion of cerebral cortex, thalamus and basal ganglia during spontaneously occurring migraine headaches, *Headache,* 29, 282, 1989.
19. **Kobari, M., Meyer, J. S., Imai, A., Oravez, W., and Ichijo, M.,** Cross-sectional imaging of cerebral blood flow during migraine headaches, *Headache,* 28 (Abstr.), 295, 1988.
20. **Sakai, F. and Meyer, J. S.,** Regional cerebral hemodynamics during migraine and cluster headaches measured by the ^{133}Xe inhalation method, *Headache,* 18, 122, 1978.
21. **Levine, S. R., Welch, K. M. A., Ewing, J. R., Joseph, R., and D'Andrea, G.,** Cerebral blood flow asymmetries in headache-free migraineurs, *Stroke,* 18, 1164, 1987.
22. **Schlake, H.-P., Böttger, I. G., Grotemeyer, K.-H., and Husstedt, I. W.,** Brain imaging with ^{123}I-IMP-SPECT in migraine between attacks, *Headache,* 29, 344, 1989.
23. **Schlake, H.-P., Böttger, I. G., Grotemeyer, K.-H., Husstedt, I. W., Oberwittler, C., and Schober, O.,** The influence of acetazolamide on cerebral low-flow regions in migraine an interictal 99m-Tc-HMPAO SPECT study, *Cephalalgia,* 12, 284, 1992.
24. **Hachinski, V. C., Olesen, J., Norris, J. W., Larsen, B., Enevoldsen, E., and Lassen, N. A.,** Cerebral hemodynamics in migraine, *Can. J. Neurol. Sci.,* 4, 245, 1977.
25. **Lauritzen, M., Skyhøj Olsen, T., Lassen, N. A., and Paulson, O. B.,** Regulation of regional cerebral blood flow during and between migraine attacks, *Ann. Neurol.,* 14, 569, 1983.
26. **Lagrèze, H. L., Dettmers, C., and Hartmann, A.,** Abnormalities of interictal cerebral perfusion in classic but not common migraine, *Stroke,* 19, 1108, 1988.
27. **Donley, R. F., Sundt, T. M., Jr., Anderson, R. E., and Sharbrough, F. W.,** Blood flow measurements and the "look through" artifact in focal cerebral ischemia, *Stroke,* 6, 121, 1975.
28. **Skyhøj Olsen, T., Friberg, L., and Lassen, N. A.,** Ischemia may be the primary cause of the neurologic deficits in classic migraine, *Arch. Neurol.,* 44, 156, 1987.
29. **Skyhøj Olsen, T. and Lassen, N. A.,** Blood flow and vascular reactivity during attacks of classic migraine-limitations of the Xe-133 intraarterial technique, *Headache,* 29, 15, 1989.
30. **Skyhøj Olsen, T., Larsen, B., Skriver, E. G., Enevoldsen, E., and Lassen, N. A.,** Focal cerebral ischemia measured by the intra-arterial ^{133}Xenon method, *Stroke,* 12, 736, 1981.
31. **Bolmsjö, M.,** Hemispheric cross talk and signal overlapping in bilateral regional cerebral blood flow measurements using Xenon 133, *Eur. J. Nucl. Med.,* 9, 1, 1984.
32. **Leao, A. A. P.,** Spreading depression of activity in the cerebral cortex, *J. Neurophysiol.,* 7, 359, 1944.
33. **Leao, A. A. P.,** Pial circulation and spreading depression of activity in the cerebral cortex, *J. Neurophysiol.,* 7, 391, 1944.
34. **Leao, A. A. P. and Morison, R. S.,** Propagation of spreading cortical depression, *J. Neurophysiol.,* 8, 33, 1945.
35. **Lauritzen, M., Skyhøj Olsen, T., Lassen, N. A., and Paulson, O. B.,** Changes in regional cerebral blood flow during the course of classic migraine attacks, *Ann. Neurol.,* 13, 633, 1983.
36. **Gloor, P.,** Migraine and regional cerebral blood flow, *Trends Neurosci.,* 9, 21, 1986.
37. **Wilkinson, M., and Blau, J. N.,** Are classical and common migraine different entities?, *Headache,* 25, 211, 1985.
38. **Barkley, G. L., Tepley, N., Nagel-Leiby, S., Moran, J. E., Simkins, R. T., and Welch, K. M. A.,** Magnetoencephalographic studies of migraine, *Headache,* 30, 428, 1990.

V. Index

INDEX

A

A23187, 236–238, 345
Acetylcholine (ACh)
with aging, 346
basilar artery response to, 359–362
cerebral arteries and, 136
cerebral blood flow, metabolism, and, 134–136, 138
colocalization with neuropeptide Y, 151
in fetal cerebral arteries, 385–386
historical background, 130–131
metabolism, 139–140
perinatal response, 383
pial arteriole response, 355, 356, 360
relaxation effect, 237
release, 238
response to, 235, 236, 346
vasoconstrictive effect, 303–305
Acoustic Doppler technology, 15–16
Action potential, 35
Adenosine, 226
arterial dilation with, 229
in autoregulation, 286–287
in cerebral circulation, 283–293
cerebrovascular effects, 282
in cerebrovascular flow regulation, 282–293
hydrogen ions and, 276
in hypercapnia, 256, 288–290
in hypocapnia, 257, 291–292
in hypotension, 259–261, 286
in hypoxia, 251–252, 283–285
interstitial fluid levels, 49–50
in ischemia/reperfusion, 292
in neonate, 388
in seizures, 285–286
uptake, 254
Adenosine deaminase inhibitors, 252
ADP
aging and, 346–347
basilar artery response to, 358
pial arteriole response to, 355–357, 360
relaxation effect, 237
Adenosine triphosphate, see ATP
Adenylate cyclase
activation, 120–121
H_2 receptors and, 118–119
Adrenergic neuron blocking agents, 226
Aging
cardiovascular system in, 342
cerebral circulation during, 342–348
neuropeptide Y in, 150
Allopurinol, 251
α-noradrenergic receptors, 83, 87–88
Alzheimer's disease, 139
Angiotensin-converting enzyme (ACE), 317
Angiotensin-converting enzyme inhibitors, 316
Angiotensin I, 318
Angiotensins, 238–239, 318
Annihilation photons, 21
Antihypertensive treatment, 333
Antimigraine compounds, 108
Apoplexy, 5
Aprotinin, 322
Arachidonic acid
in arterial muscle, 39
kallikrein-kinin and, 321
metabolism, 300–301, 305
metabolites, 298–299
Arecoline, 134
Arginine vasopressin, 236
antidiuretic effects, 214
in cerebral arteries, 220
vasodilating action, 220–221
Arterial baroreceptors, 48
Arterial blood pressure, see also Hypertension; Hypotension
adenosine and, 259–261
autoregulation and, 46
cholinergic agonists and, 134–135
Arterial hypertension, chronic, 47
Arterial hypotension, 54
Arterial oxygen tension, 292–293
Arterioles
adenosine and diameter changes in, 282, 283
dilatation, 238–239
Arteriovenous malformations, 291–292
Asparagine amide, C terminal, 166
Asphyxia, neonatal, 390–392
ATP, 228
dilating effect, 253–254
inhibiting effect, 229
intracellular, 36, 40

relaxation effect, 237
release, 226
response, 236
Atropine, 137, 226, 238
Autacoids, 316
Autoradiographic tissue sampling technique, 9
Autoregulation, cerebral, see Cerebral autoregulation

B

Basal nucleus, 137
Basilar artery
CGRP in, 186
endothelium-dependent response during diabetes mellitus, 357–358, 360–362
impaired contractile response with aging, 344
VIP in, 170
Bernard, Claude, 80
β-noradrenergic receptors, 84, 87
Blood-brain barrier
catecholamines acting through, 71
disruption, 337
in neonate, 384–385
permeability of, 68, 85, 90
bradykinin and, 318–319
histamine and, 115, 119–121
neuropeptide Y and, 159–160
regulation, 122
serotonin and, see Endothelium-derived relaxing factor
Blood flow, see also Cerebral blood flow; Cerebrovascular blood flow
dynamic coupling of function metabolism to, 275–277
perfusion pressure and, 46–48
regional, 4
static coupling of function and metabolism to, 271–273
uncoupling of metabolism from, 277
Blood sampling, 4
Blood-tissue exchange equation, 8
Blood vessel wall, 114–115
Bolus fractionation principle, 21
Bradykinin, 300
basilar artery response to, 357–362
in blood-brain barrier permeability, 318–319
in brain edema mediation, 322
in cerebral microcirculation, 316–322
kininase II inhibitors and, 317–318
mechanisms mediating, 320–322
prostacyclin and, 345
receptors in cerebral arteries, 319–320
relaxation effect, 236–237
vasomotor response, 316–317
Brain
adenosine in blood flow regulation of, 282–293
autoregulation and injury, 53–54
blood flow in, 80
blood supply to, 250–261
capillary perfusion in, 273–275
central noradrenergic innervation, 84–90
cervical sympathetic innervation of macrovessels, 80–84
eicosanoids in injury of, 305
macrovessels, 89–90
metabolism and blood flow in, 270–277
microvessels, 84–90
in newborn, 382
traumatic injury of, 368–375
Brain edema
bradykinin mediation of, 322
radiation-induced, 121
stab wound-induced, 122
Burimamide, 172

C

C fibers, unmyelinated, 180
Caffeine, 256
Calcitonin gene-related peptide, 180
with aging, 343–344
in cerebral hyperperfusion syndromes, 190
immunoreactivity of, 202
in migraine, 188–189, 205
sensory fibers and, 185–187
structure-function relations in, 187–188
in subarachnoid hemorrhage, 189–190, 205
vascular sensory fibers and, 180–181
vasodilatory activity of, 182–185
Calcitonin gene-related peptide-immunoreactive fibers, 200
Calcium, extracellular, 156
Calcium ion
action potential and, 40
cystolic concentration of, 117
in EDRF release, 237
ionophore A23187 of, 236–238, 345

Calcium ion channel blockers, 35
Calcium ion channels, 37, 38
Capillaries
  cycling, 273
  perfusion, 273–275
  permeability, 66, 67
Capsaicin, 190
Carbachol, 134
Carbon dioxide
  extracellular levels, 288–290
  inhalation, 405
  levels, 250–261
  reactivity, 372–374
  vasodilatation and, 389
Carotid bubble-flow meters, internal, 5
Carotid vessels, innervation of, 81
Catalase, 346
Catecholamines
  adrenally derived, 71
  in cerebral blood vessel innervation, 80–90
  extravascular application of, 84
CBF, see Cerebral blood flow
Central nervous system, 4, 114–115
Central neural pathways
  in CBF regulation, 66–71
  cholinergic role in, 137
  fastigial nucleus in, 69–70
  locus ceruleus in, 66–68
  raphe nucleus in, 68–69
Central noradrenergic innervation
  anatomical evidence, 84–85
  biochemical and pharmacological evidence of, 87–88
  pathophysiological evidence, 86–87
  physiological evidence of, 85–86
Central noradrenergic nerve, degeneration of, 88
Centromedian-parafascicular complex, 71
Cerebral arterial muscle
  calcium ion channels in, 37
  electrophysiological mechanisms of activation, 34–42
  factors affecting membrane electrical events in, 37–42
  membrane potential and, 34–37
  P_{CO2} and pH effects on, 41–42
  P_{O2} effect on membrane properties of, 40–41
  potassium ion currents, 35–36
  pressure-induced activation of, 40
  regulation of tone, 34–37
  transmural pressure and electromechanical coupling in, 37–39
Cerebral arteries
  acetylcholine effects on, 136
  constriction of, 219
  contractile action in, 83, 117–118
  dilation of, 115–116
  in fetus and neonate, 382
  innervation of, 334–335
  kinin receptors in, 319–320
  occlusion of, 70
  purinergic transmission in, 226–230
  trauma to, 54
  vasopressin receptors in, 214–222
Cerebral arterioles
  atrophy of, 342
  during diabetes mellitus, 354–355
  smooth muscle cells of, 354
Cerebral autoregulation, 46–54
  adenosine in, 286–287
  factors affecting, 51–54
  hypertension and, 332–338
  impaired, 372
  limits, 82
  mechanisms, 48–51
  in neonate, 387–389
  perfusion pressure and, 46–48
Cerebral blood flow (CBF)
  adenosine in regulation of, 282–293
  aging and, 342–343, 347–348
  autoradiograms, 103
  in autoregulatory range, 46–47
  brain metabolism and, 270–277
  central nervous system stimulation and, 137
  central neural pathways in regulation of, 66–71
  cerebral blood volume and, 371–372
  cerebral glucose utilization and, 102–105, 108
  cholinergic agonists and, 134–136
  cholinergic control of, 130–140
  cholinergic nerve stimulation and, 136–137
  in common and classic migraine, 405–406
  Doppler flowmetry of, 15–17
  factors regulating, 332
  glucose utilization rate and, 137–140
  headache localization and, 404
  historical background on, 5
  hydrogen clearance polarography of, 14–15

hypertension and autoregulation of, 332–338
independence, 46
metabolism and, 102–106, 342–343
migraine and, 400–409
neural regulation, 166–174
O_2 and CO_2 levels in, 250–261
perfusion pressure and, 46–48
physiologic changes in migraine, 404–405
positron emission tomography of, 21–23
posttraumatic reduction in, 370–371
regional, 80, 401–402
changes in, 4
CT images of, 23–24
patterns in migraine, 405–406
sensory fibers and, 187
serotonin and, 101
single photon emission computed tomography of, 20–21
stable xenon enhanced computed tomography of, 19–20
studies of migraine pathogenesis, 407–408
systemic serotonin administration of, 100
tachykinins and, 196–205
tissue indicator uptake measurement of, 5–14
traumatic brain injury and, 368–375
ultrafast computed tomography of, 23–24
vascular and neuronal theories of migraine and, 408–409
vasopressin and, 216
very fast nuclear magnetic resonance imaging of, 24–26
^{133}xenon clearance of, 17–18
Cerebral blood vessels
bradykinin vasomotor action in, 316–317
catecholaminergic innervation of, 80–90
cervical sympathetic innervation of macrovessels, 80–84
choline-acetyltransferase expression, 131
cholinergic receptors in, 134
dilator pathways, 70
histamine effects on, 121
hypertrophy, 332
innervation, 68–69
response during diabetes mellitus, 354–363
tachykinins in, 204
tritium efflux from, 133
Cerebral blood volume, 371–372, 375
Cerebral circulation
aging and, 342–348
in neonate, 383–384
neural influence on, 343–344
neuropeptide Y and, 148–161
serotonin and, 98–108
Cerebral cortex, 137
Cerebral glucose utilization, 101, 102; see also Glucose utilization
blood flow and, 272–273
cerebral blood flow and, 108, 137–140
cholinergic agonists and, 135
local cerebral blood flow and, 102–105
Cerebral hemodynamics
eicosanoids in, 298–305
histaminergic effects, 114–122
Cerebral hyperperfusion syndromes, 190
Cerebral ischemia, 53, 305; see also Ischemia
Cerebral macrovasculature, 80–84, 89–90
Cerebral metabolic rate of oxygen utilization ($CMRO_2$), 250, 370, 374
Cerebral microvasculature, 84–90, 316–322
Cerebral perfusion
age-related changes in, 386–387
in neonate, 391–392
Cerebral vascular system
in apoplexy, 5
hypercapnia and, 255–257
hypocapnia and, 257–258
hypotension and, 258–261
hypoxia and, 250–255
serotonergic innervation of, 98–99
Cerebral vasospasm, 205
Cerebroarterial relaxation, 234–242
Cerebrospinal fluid (CSF)
hypotension and, 388
increased levels of, 50
pressures of, 46–48
Cerebrovascular blood flow
adenosine regulation, 282–293
methodology, 6
Cerebrovascular reactivity
disturbances, 372–375
in perinatal period, 382–383
Cerebrovascular responses
dilatory, 54
sympathetic nerves and, 52–53
Cerebrovascular serotonergic system, 107–108
Cerebrovascular smooth muscle, 157
Cerebrovascular spasm, 371
Cerebrovascular system

innervation in fetus and neonate, 385–386
regulation in fetus and neonate, 382–392
vasoactive intestinal peptide effect, 169–173
vasoactive intestinal peptide localization in, 166–169
Cerebrovascular tone, 67
Cervical sympathetic ganglia, 151
Cervical sympathetic nerves, 81–82
anatomical evidence of, 80–81
pathophysiological evidence of, 82–83
pharmacological evidence of, 83–84
physiological evidence of, 81–82
CGRP, see Calcitonin gene-related peptide
2-Chloroadenosine, 282
Chlorpheniramine, 122
Choline, synthesis of, 130
Choline acetyltransferase (ChAT), 238
activity, 131
in cranial arteries, 132
Cholinergic agonists, 134–136
Cholinergic cerebrovascular innervation
histochemical and biochemical functions, 131–133
sources, 130
Cholinergic receptors, 134
Cholinergic system
cerebral blood flow and, 136–137
in glucose and oxygen utilization rates, 138–140
vasodilator, 136
Cholinesterase, 131
Cholinesterase inhibition, 137
Cimetidine, 122
Clamp-on electromagnetic flow devices, 5
Collagen, 382
Compton scattering, 18, 22, 406
Computed tomography
stable xenon enhanced, 17, 19–20
techniques, 19–24
ultrafast, 23–24
Cranial arteries, 132
Cranial nerves, stimulation of, 131
Cranial parasympathetic fibers, 130–131
Cranial parasympathetic ganglion, 151–152
Cromakalim, 255
CSF, see Cerebrospinal fluid
Cyclic adenosine monophosphate-dependent receptors, 214
Cyclooxygenase constrictor substance (EDCF), 362–363
Cytochrome P_{450} products, 298–299

D

Deferoxamine, 346
Denervation, chronic, 67
Denervation supersensitivity, 88
Deoxycoformycin, 252
2-Deoxyglucose method, 270–271
Desmopressin (DDAVP), 220–222
Development, 150
Dexamethasone, 122
Diabetes mellitus
basilar artery response during, 357–358
cerebral blood vessel response during, 354–363
cerebrovascular pathogenesis in, 354
endothelium morphology during, 354–355
impaired endothelium-dependent response in, 358–363
pial arteriole response during, 355–357
1,2-Diacylglycerol (1,2-DAG), see Protein kinase C
Dibutyryl-cAMP, 121
Dipyridamole, 256, 257
Dopamine beta-hydroxylase immunoreactive nerve fibers, 84–85
Doppler flowmetry, 15–16
Doppler migraine studies, 408
Dorsal raphe nucleus
cortical circulation and, 106–107
electrical stimulation of, 101–102
dPVDAVP, 215, 217
dVDAVP, 220

E

Echo-Planar Imaging (EPI), 25–26
EDRF, see Endothelium-derived relaxing factor
Eicosanoids
in cerebral hemodynamics, 298–305
in cerebral injury, 305
functional significance, 300–305
synthesis, 299
vascular activity, 298–299
Electromagnetic flowmeters, 4
Electromechanical coupling, 37–39
Electrophysiology, cerebral arterial muscle, 34–42
End-organ capillary embolization, 12
Endothelial cells, autoregulating effects, 373
Endothelially released factors, 259
Endothelium

aging and, 345–347
histaminergic relaxation, 119
morphology during diabetes mellitus, 354–355
neonatal, 384–385, 391
in neuropeptide Y potentiation, 155–156
vasopressin-induced contraction of, 219
Endothelium-dependent responses, 354–363
Endothelium-derived factors, 50
Endothelium-derived relaxing factor (EDRF), 198
aging and, 346–347
arteriolar dilation mediated by, 238–239
in cerebral arteries, 234–237
discovery of, 234
inhibiting effect, 100
modification effect of, 237–238
nitric oxide release and, 241, 242
release of, 229, 253, 321–322
Energy metabolism, 100–102
Environmental factors, 37–42
EPI, see Magnetic resonance imaging, echoplanar
Epoxide derivatives, 298–299
Eptastigmine, 134–135
Equilibration techniques, 7–10
Erythrohydroxynonyladeine (EHNA), 252
Extracellular fluid, 49

F

Fastigial nucleus, 69–70
Fetus, cerebrovascular regulation in, 382–392
Fick principle, 7, 8, 10, 14
Flowmetry, Doppler, 15–16
Fluorescein isothiocyanate (FITC), 119–120, 318
Fluorescence microscopy, intravital, 119–120
Fluorocarbons, 284, 286
Forebrain ischemia, 292
FURA-2, 39

G

G protein, 156, 157
Gamma-aminobutyric acid (GABA), 196
Gamma photons, 22
Gamma radiation spectroscopy, differential, 13
Gastric inhibitory polypeptide (GIP), 166
Glasgow coma scale score, 369–370
Glibenclamide, 255
Global brain flow measurements, see Whole brain flow measurements
Glucagon, 166
Glucose metabolism, 100–101
Glucose utilization, 102–105, 135
blood flow and, 272–273
cerebral blood flow and, 108, 137–140
regional, 271
Glycolysis, 105
Gray matter, blood flow to, 342–343
Growth hormone-releasing factor (GHRF), 166
Guanethidine, 226
Guanylate cyclase, 118–119

H

Harvey, William, 5
Head injury
brain ischemia with, 368–370
hyperemia and, 371–372
Headache, see Migraine
Hemodynamics
eicosanoids in, 298–305
histaminergic effects on, 114–122
in hypertension, 332–334
Hemoglobin, 234, 238, 239, 284
Hemolysate, 305
15-HETE, 298, 299
20-HETE, 39
5-HIAA, 99
Hippocampus, 137
Histamine
blood-brain barrier permeability and, 119–121
cerebral hemodynamics and, 114–122
contractile action, 117–118
derivation, 114
mediator function, 121
pathophysiological importance, 121–122
relaxant action, 118–119, 236
response, 236
sources in central nervous system, 114–115
vasomotor effects, 115–119
Histamine receptors, 118
adenylate cyclase and, 118–119
antagonists, 118, 122
blockade, 116
in cerebral microvessels, 120

in smooth muscle and endothelium, 115–116
Histidine-decarboxylase, 114
Hydrogen clearance, 14–15
Hydrogen ion concentration, 276
6-Hydroxydopamine, 86–87
5-Hydroxytryptamine, see Serotonin
Hypercapnia, 140, 250, 300–301
adenosine in, 256, 288–290
arterial, 67
cerebral vascular response to, 71, 255–257
in neonate, 389–390
nitric oxide in, 256–257
prostanoids in, 257
vasodilation in, 301–302
Hyperemia, 190
adenosine and, 251–252, 284–285
cerebral, 288–289
cerebral blood flow and, 371–372
cortical, 408
seizure-induced, 285–286
slowly resolving, 402–403
Hyperoxia, 49, 250
Hypertension
in autoregulation of cerebral blood flow, 332–338
chronic, 47
neuropeptide Y and, 159
pathogenesis, 214
sympathetic nerves in, 82–83
vascular changes in, 332–334
Hypocapnia
adenosine in, 291–292
cerebral vascular response, 257–258
Hypotension, 54
adenosine in, 286
cerebral vascular response to, 258–261
in neonate, 388–389
Hypothalamus, 71
Hypoxia, 250–251
adenosine and, 251–252
adenosine in, 283–285
ATP-sensitive potassium ion channels and, 254–255
brain capillary density and, 274
cerebral vascular response to, 250–255
cerebrovascular responsiveness to, 71
effect on arterial muscle, 40
in neonate, 389–392
nitric oxide and, 253–254
prostanoids, 254

I

ICGU, see Cerebral glucose utilization
Indicator backflux, 11–13
Indicator equilibration techniques, 9–10
Indicator fractionation techniques
permeable radiolabeled markers in, 10–12
radiolabeled microspheres in, 12–14
Indomethacin, 301
bradykinin inhibition with, 346
dilation effects, 302–303
pial arteriolar effects, 304–305, 360
Intracarotid injection technique, 406
Intracranial hemorrhage, 305
Intracranial pressure
cerebral blood volume and, 371–372
high, 371
Intraventricular hemorrhage, 390
Iodoantipyrine fractionation, 12, 13
Ionositol 1,4,5-triphosphate (IP_3), see Protein kinase C
Ischemia
acetylcholine metabolism in, 139
adenosine in, 292
cerebral blood flow and, 368–371
eicosanoids and, 305
in migraine, 406
in neonate, 392
in perinatal period, 390–391

K

Kallikrein-kinin, 321–322
Ketanserin, 154
Kety equations, 11, 20
Kety equilibrium techniques, modified, 22
Kety indicator equilibration techniques, 7–10
Kety-Sokoloff method, 10
Kinin receptors, 316, 319–320
Kininase II, 316
Kininase II-angiotensin-converting enzyme, 318
Kininase II inhibitors, 317–318
Kininogen, 317, 322
Kinins, 322
Krypton-85, 17

L

L-arginine, 236, 346
availability with aging, 346, 347

nitric oxide synthesis from, 384
L-NA, 234, 236, 237, 239, 256–257
L-NA methylester (L-NAME), 234, 253, 257
L-NMMA, 234, 238–239, 253, 256–257
L-NOARG, 227–228
Laser-Doppler flowmetry (LDF), 4, 16
Leukotrienes, 298
release, 321
vasoconstrictive effect, 305
Lipid bilayer, permeability, 85
Lipoxins, 299
Lipoxygenase pathways, 299
5-Lipoxygenase products, 298
Locus ceruleus (LC), 66–68
lesion, 85–88
stimulation, 85–86

M

MABP, 256, 258–260
Magnetic resonance imaging (MRI)
echoplanar, 19
ultrafast, 5
very fast, 19
Magneto encephalographic studies, 408
Mast cells, 114
Medulla, 71
Membrane potential
change and arterial tension, 35
regulation of cerebral arterial muscle tone and, 34–37
Mepyramine, 121, 122
Metabolism
age-related changes in, 386–387
in aging, 342–343
blood flow and, 270–277
in cerebral autoregulation, 49–50
cerebral blood flow and, 102–106
cholinergic agonists and, 134–136
dynamic coupling of blood flow to, 275–277
rate and blood flow, 270–271
regulation with brain injury, 374, 375
uncoupling of blood flow from, 277
Metiamide, 121
Microcirculatory cerebral flow, 16
Microspheres
liquid, 20
materials technology, 12–14
radiolabeled, 12–14
Migraine
between attacks of, 402–404
CBF studies in pathogenesis of, 407–408
cerebral blood flow and, 400–409
CGRP in, 188–189
classic and common, 405–406
history, 400–401
lab results in, 406
localization, 404
neurovascular theory, 107–108
physiologic changes in, 404–405
prodrome, 401–402
tachykinins in, 204–205
vascular and neuronal theories, 408–409
MRI, see Magnetic resonance imaging
Myogenic autoregulating mechanisms, 50
Myogenic constriction, 51

N

NADPH diaphorase, 239
Neonate
brain in, 382
cerebral autoregulation in, 387–389
cerebral circulation in, 383–384
cerebral endothelium in, 384–385
cerebrovascular innervation in, 385–386
cerebrovascular regulation in, 382–392
contractility in, 391
hypercapnic and hypoxic cerebral vasodilatation in, 389–390
Nerves
autoregulation and, 51–53
of brain arteries, 80–81
Neurogenic purinergic response, 226–228
Neurokinin A, 182, 184
distribution of, 196–197
immunohistochemistry, 203
migraine and, 188–189
in nerve fibers, 202
pharmacology of, 204
in sensory fibers, 180
Neurokinin B, see also Gamma-aminobutyric acid
distribution of, 196–197
in migraine, 205
in nerve fibers, 202
pharmacology of, 204
Neurolipomastocytes, 114
Neuronal-behavioral function, 4
Neuropeptide gamma, 196
Neuropeptide K, 196, 202, 204

Neuropeptide Y (NPY)
aging and, 343
amino acid sequences for, 149
cerebral blood flow effects, 157–161
in cerebral circulation, 148–161
cerebral vessel effects, 152–157
endothelial dependence of, 155–156
localization in cerebral vessels, 148–152
in modification of neurotransmitter effects, 155
in neonate, 386
origin of nerve fibers, 151–152
physiological and pathological significance, 160–161
posttraumatic increase, 371
receptors, 154–155
signal transduction and, 156
with vasoactive intestinal peptide, 169
vasomotor actions, 152–154
Neurotransmitters
cerebrovascular, 173–174
decreased, 66
excitatory amino acid, 370
in migraine, 205
neuropeptide Y and, 155, 160
Neurovascular system, neonatal, 385–386
Neutral endopeptidase (NEP), 317
Nitric oxide
arteriolar dilation mediated by, 238–239
basilar artery response, 357
in cerebroarterial relaxation, 234–242
in hypercapnia, 256–257
in hypoxia, 253–254
modification relaxation effect of, 237–238
relaxation mediated by, 234–237, 239–242, 321
synthesis of, 119, 240, 384
Nitric oxide synthase, 239–241
L-arginine for, 346
in neonate, 384
Nitric oxide synthase inhibitors, 234, 236, 239, 241, 253
Nitroglycerin, 355
NMDA, 346, 347
NOergic response, 227–228
"Non-filling" phenomenon, 371
Noradrenaline
colocalization with neuropeptide Y, 150–151
neuropeptide Y and, 157
Noradrenergic nerve fibers, 80–82, 84–90
Noradrenergic receptors, 84, 87–89
Norepinephrine
aging and, 343
in cerebral arterial contraction, 83
cerebral blood flow and, 84, 216–217
cerebral macrovessel effects, 87
perinatal response, 383
release, 226–227
Norepinephrine-containing nerve fibers, 200
Noroxia, 283
NPY, see Neuropeptide Y
Nuclear magnetic resonance imaging, very fast, 24–26

O

Oligemia, 408
Ouabain, 35
Oxidative metabolism, suppressed, 372–373
Oxotremorine, 134–135
Oxygen
age-related change in supply, 387
cerebral blood flow and utilization, 137–140
consumption and blood flow, 272–273, 277
coupling hypothesis, 387
extracellular levels, 288
levels, 250–261
metabolism in aging, 342–343
Oxyhemoglobin dissociation curve, 387
Oxymetrazole-induced seizures, 285
Oxypurinol, 251
Oxytocin, 236

P

PACAP (pituitary adenylate cyclase activating polypeptide), 166
$PaCO_2$, 250–255
Pancreatic peptides, 148
PaO_2, 250
Parasympathetic ganglia, 151–152
P_{CO2}, 41–42
PCO_2, 135, 255–257
Peptide histamine isoleucine (PHI), 166, 172–173, 182
Peptide YY (PYY), 148
Peptidergic nerve fibers, 196
Peptides
amino acid sequences for, 149
perivascular, 150–161

Perfusion pressure, 46–48
Perinatal period
  cerebral pathophysiology during, 390–392
  cerebrovascular reactivity in, 382–383
Peripheral artery resistance, 332–333
Perivascular nerve fibers
  immunohistochemical studies of, 148–149
  neuropeptide Y distribution in, 148–150
  pattern with aging, 343–344
  radioimmunoassay studies of, 149–150
  substance P containing, 199
Perivascular nerves
  activation of, 66
  vasoactive intestinal peptide in, 169
Periventricular hemorrhage, 390–391
Permeable radiolabeled markers, 10–12
PET, see Positron emission tomography
Petrosal nerve, superficial, 136–137
pH, 41–42
Phospholipase C, 38–39
Photohematochometer, 5
Physostigmine
  in Alzheimer's disease, 139
  cerebral blood flow, metabolism, and, 134–135
  cholinesterase inhibition with, 137
Pial arteries
  constriction of, 116–117
  transmural electrical resistance, 119
  vasoactive intestinal peptide in, 168
  vasoconstriction of, 214
Pial arterioles
  adenosine and, 284, 287, 289, 290
  bradykinin response of, 346
  dilatation of, 298–299, 346–347
  endothelium-dependent response during diabetes mellitus, 355–357, 360
  hypercapnia and, 291
  impaired response with aging, 344
  indomethacin effects on, 304–305
Pilocarpine, 134
PKC, see Protein kinase C
Plasma membrane
  electrical events at, 34
  physical and environmental factors affecting electrical events of, 37–42
  P_{O_2} effect on, 40–41
  potential of and regulation of cerebral arterial muscle tone, 34–37
Platelet-endothelial interaction, 347–348
P_{O_2}, 40–41
Polarography, hydrogen clearance, 14–15
Positron annihilation, 22
Positron emission tomography (PET), 19, 21–23, 270, 271
Postganglionic fibers, 136
Postocclusive hyperemia, 190
Potassium ion, 275–277
Potassium ion channel inhibitors, 234–236
Potassium ion channels, 119
  activity of, 40–41
  ATP-sensitive, 254–255
Potassium ion currents, 35–36, 41–42
Prazosin, 226
Prepro-VIP, 166, 167, 170
Preprotachykinin gene, 198
Pressure-sensor, 38
Propranolol, 226
Prostacyclin, 299
  in neonate, 384
  responses with aging, 345
Prostaglandin E, 383
Prostaglandin E_2, 116
Prostaglandin $F_{2\alpha}$, 384, 386
Prostaglandin H synthase, 298, 299
  arachidonic acid metabolism and, 300–301
  cerebral reperfusion and, 305
  dilation and, 300
  inhibition of, 301–303
  vasodilation effect of, 303
Prostaglandin I_2, 234
Prostaglandins, 171
  extracellular fluid levels of, 49–50
  in hypercapnia, 257
  neonatal cerebral circulation and, 383–384
Prostanoids
  constrictor, 303
  dilating, 321–322
  functional significance, 300–305
  in hypercapnia, 257
  in hypoxia, 254
  kallikrein-kinin and, 321
  metabolism, 384
  vascular activity, 298
  vasoconstrictor, 386
Protein kinase C (PKC)
  activation, 320, 360
  inhibition, 38–39
Purinergic receptor subtypes, 228–230
Purinergic transmission, 226–230
P_{2x}-purinergic receptors, 228–229
P_{2Y}-purinergic receptors, 228–229
2-Pyridylethylamine, 117

R

Radiation-induced brain edema, 121
Ranitidine, 121
Raphe nucleus, 68–69, 106–107
rCBF, see Cerebral blood flow, regional
Reactive hyperemia, 190
Red-cell velocity, 4
Regional blood flow, 4, 23–24
Reperfusion, 292
Resting membrane potential, 34
Resting tone, 51

S

Sagittal sinus blood flow, 135
Sapirstein method equation, 10–11
Scopolamine, 137
Scotomata, 408
Second messenger systems, 130
Seizures, 285–286
Sensory nerve fibers
  cerebral blood flow and, 187
  CGRP in, 180–181, 185–186
Serotonergic central neurons, 98
Serotonergic dysfunction, 107–108
Serotonergic nerves, 68–69, 98–99
Serotonergic system
  anatomical and functional role in cerebral vasculature, 106–107
  cerebrovascular effects, 101
  features, 98
  neurovascular theory of migraine and, 107–108
Serotonin
  aging and, 343–344
  arteriolar response with aging, 346–347
  basilar artery response to, 358
  cerebral blood flow and, 216–217
  cerebral circulation and, 98–108
  cerebrovascular effects of, 99–102
  energy metabolism and, 100–101
  perinatal response to, 383
  pial arteriole response to, 357
  release of, 68–69
  in situ reactivity, 100
  synthesis of, 98
  in vitro reactivity, 99–100
Single capillary pass markers, 13
Single photon emission computed tomography (SPECT), 19, 20–21, 402, 404–406
Soman, 134
Somatosensory cerebral cortex, 138
Sphenopalatine ganglia, 136–137
  neuropeptide Y in, 151–152
  vasoactive intestinal peptide in, 169
Spinal cord trauma, 368–370
Spreading depression, 407–408
SQ 29548, 360
Stab wounds, 122
Stretch-activated ion channel, 38
Strokeprone, 336
Subarachnoid hemorrhage
  cerebral vasospasm after, 205
  CGRP in, 189–190
  neuropeptide Y and, 160–161
Substance K, see Neurokinin A
Substance P, 182
  aging and, 343–344
  distribution of, 196–197
  extracellular, 185
  extraction, 196
  immunohistochemistry, 201
  in migraine, 188–189, 205
  pharmacology, 204
  relaxation effect, 237
  response, 235, 236
  in subarachnoid hemorrhage, 205
  vasodilatory response, 182–183, 185
Substance P-containing nerve fibers, 180
  distribution and running pattern, 199–200
  origin, 200–202
Superoxide, 305
Superoxide dismutase, 346, 360
Sympathectomy, 153
Sympathetic adrenergic fibers, 226–227
Sympathetic denervation, 335–338
Sympathetic ganglia, 151–152
Sympathetic nerves
  autoregulation and, 52–53
  of cerebral blood vessels, 68–69, 333–335
  in chronic hypertension, 82–83
  contractions induced by, 227
  neuropeptide Y and, 160
  physiological studies, 81–82
  trophic influence, 333–338
Sympathetic noradrenergic nerves, 81

T

Tachykinin receptors, 198
Tachykinins

in amphibians, 197
cerebral blood flow and, 196–205
in cerebral vasospasm, 205
in mammals, 197
in migraine, 204–205
morphology, 199–203
pharmacology, 204
Technetium-99m-hexamethylpropyleneamine single photon emission computed tomography, 369–370
Theophylline, 257
adenosine receptor blockade by, 290
cerebral hyperemia and, 288–289
in hypocapnia, 291
lipid soluble, 285
Thoracic aorta, 360
Thrombin, 345
Thromboxane, 299, 305
aging and, 348
pial arteriole response, 357
Thromboxane A_2, 298, 386
Thromboxane A_2/prostaglandin H_2 receptor, 304–305, 359–360, 362
Thromboxane analogue U46619, 358
Tilt-table test, 403, 404
Tissue equilibration techniques, 7–10, 14
Tissue indicator uptake methods, 5–7
indicator fractionation techniques, 10–14
tissue equilibration techniques, 7–10
whole brain flow measurements, 7
Tissue radioactivity, 20
Tissue saturation method, 10
Transmural electrical resistance, 119
Transmural pressure, 37–39
Traumatic injury, cerebral blood flow and, 368–375
Trigeminal ganglionectomy, 187
Tryptophan-hydroxylase (TPOH), 98, 99
Tryptophan-hydroxylase (TPOH)-immunoreactive fibers, 106–107

U

U46619 analogue, 344
Ultrafast computed tomography, 19, 23–24
Ultrasonography, Doppler flowmetry, 15–16

V

Varicose fibers, 114
Vascular resistance, 332–333
Vascular responses, 344
Vascular sensory fibers, 180–181
Vascular system
anatomy, 5
failure, 47
hypertrophy, 53
morphology and mechanics, 342
Vascular wall
distensibility, 332, 333
remodeling, 333
trophic influences, 333–338
Vasoactive factors, 345–347
Vasoactive intestinal peptide (VIP)
aging and, 343–344
in cerebral blood flow regulation, 166–174
as cerebrovascular neurotransmitter, 173–174
cerebrovascular responsiveness to, 169–173
CGRP and, 182
colocalization with neuropeptide Y, 151
immunocytochemical localization, 166–169
isolation, 166
neuropeptide Y and, 157
proteolytic processing, 167
receptors for, 172
vasodilatory response, 182–183, 185
Vasoactive intestinal polypeptide, 201, 386
Vasoactive substances
in cerebral arterial wall, 334
perinatal response to, 383
Vasoconstriction, 303–305
in neonate, 388–389
neuropeptide Y in, 152–153
in perinatal period, 390–391
Vasodilation
aging and, 344
autoregulatory cerebral, 302–303
blood supply and, 276
endothelial-dependent, 373–374
in hypercapnia, 301–302
in neonate, 388–390
Vasodilator nerves, 239–242
Vasomotor system, 115–119
Vasopressin
cumulative application, 217
EC_{50} values and maximal response, 218
effects, 214–215
in vitro experiments with, 217–221
in vivo experiments with, 215–217
lysine, 384

relaxation effect, 237
response, 236
Vasopressin receptors, 215
in cerebral arteries, 214–222
V_1, 217–220, 222
V_2, 220–222
Venous occlusion, 287
Venous outflow, 5
Vertebrobasilar system, 199
VIP, see Vasoactive intestinal peptide

W

Wepfer's studies, 5
Whole brain flow measurements, 7
Willis circle
first description of, 5
neuropeptide Y distribution in, 149–150

X

X-ray computerized tomography
ultrafast, 5
xenon enhanced, 17, 19–20, 368–369
Xanthine oxidase, 305
Xanthine oxidase inhibitors, 251
^{133}Xenon clearance, 17–18
Xenon computed tomography-cerebral blood flow method, 402, 404
^{133}Xenon inhalation method, 402–406
^{133}Xenon intracarotid technique, 401

Y

Y_1-receptors, 154–155
Y_2-receptors, 154–155

Z

Zolantidine, 122